DIAGNOSTIC PATHOLOGY

Placenta

SECOND EDITION

HEEREMA-MCKENNEY | POPEK | DE PAEPE

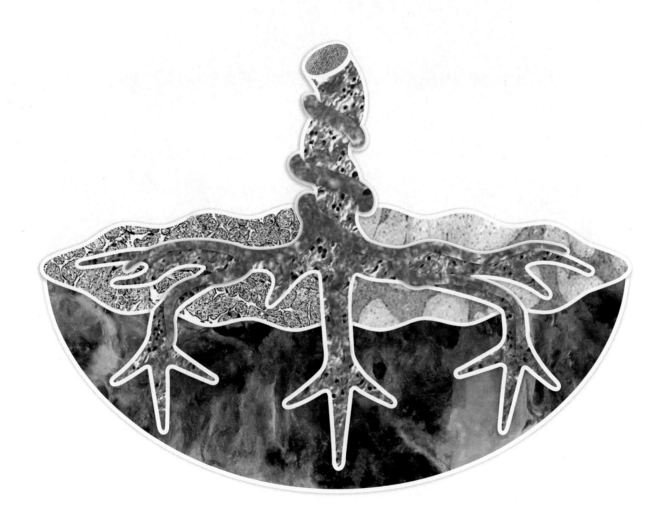

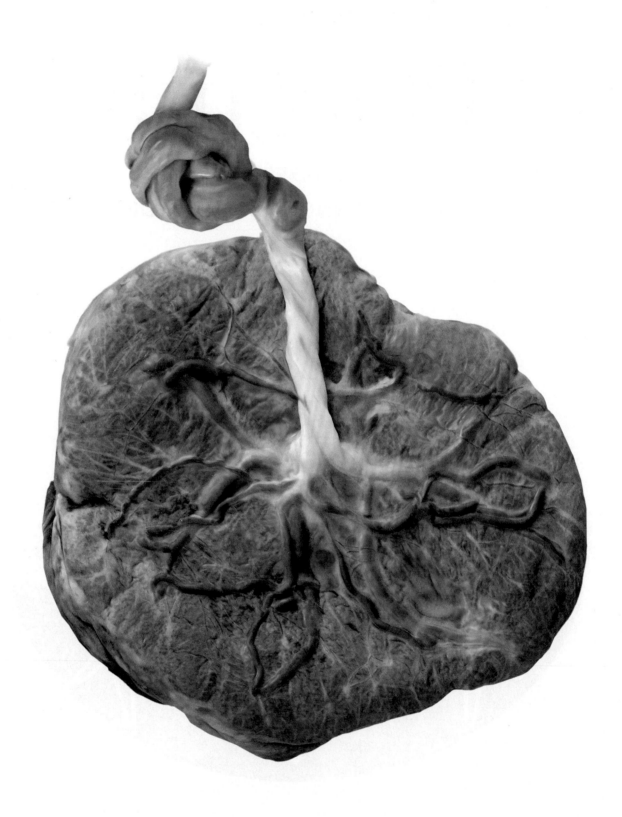

DIAGNOSTIC PATHOLOGY

Placenta

SECOND EDITION

Amy Heerema-McKenney, MD

Director of Perinatal Pathology
Robert J. Tomsich Pathology and Laboratory Medicine Institute
Division of Anatomic Pathology
Cleveland Clinic
Cleveland, Ohio

Edwina J. Popek, DO

Professor of Pathology and Pediatrics
Baylor College of Medicine
Texas Children's Hospital Pavilion for Women
Houston, Texas

Monique E. De Paepe, MD, MSc

Professor of Pathology and Laboratory Medicine
Women and Infants Hospital
Alpert Medical School of Brown University
Providence, Rhode Island

ELSEVIER

1600 John F. Kennedy Blvd.
Ste 1800
Philadelphia, PA 19103-2899

DIAGNOSTIC PATHOLOGY: PLACENTA, SECOND EDITION

ISBN: 978-0-323-60971-5

Library of Congress Control Number: 2018952970

Cover Designer: Tom M. Olson, BA
Printed in Canada by Friesens, Altona, Manitoba, Canada

Last digit is the print number: 9 8 7 6 5 4 3 2 1

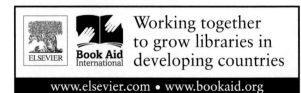

Dedications

For Jesse, with deepest gratitude for your support in all of my endeavors.

With warm gratitude and appreciation to my colleagues for their wisdom and patience in authoring this book together, and to Drs. Charles Zaloudek, Daniel Arber, and Milton Finegold for being my teachers and mentors in pathology.
AHM

In memory of my parents, Edward and Erma Popek, who saw that, despite multiple degrees and years of specialty training, I really was just like them: a teacher.
EJP

To the perinatal pathology assistants, unsung heroes whose diligent and tireless processing of the placentas forms the solid basis of our discipline—and this book. To Svetlana Shapiro and Lawrence E. Young, II, in particular.
MEDP

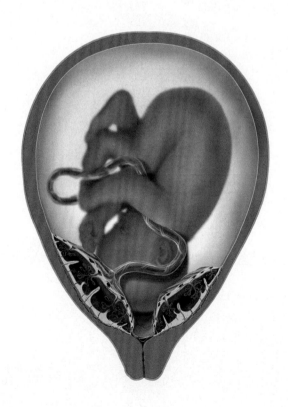

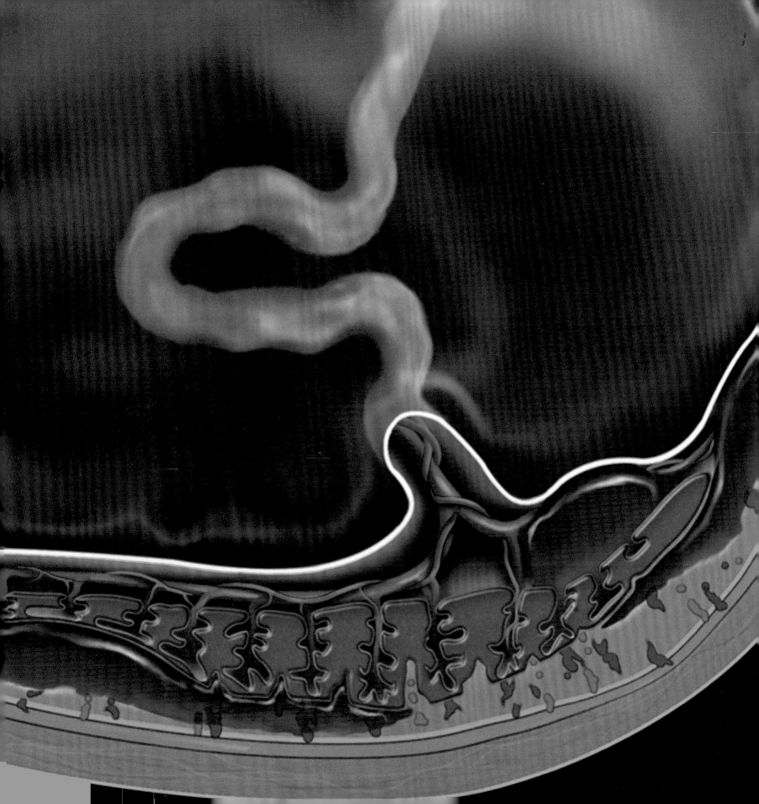

Contributing Authors

Linda M. Ernst, MD, MHS
Clinical Associate Professor
University of Chicago Pritzker School of Medicine
NorthShore University HealthSystem
Evanston, Illinois

Jason A. Jarzembowski, MD, PhD
Medical Director, Pathology and Laboratory Medicine
Children's Hospital of Wisconsin
Vice Chair (Pediatric Pathology) and Associate Professor, Department of Pathology
Medical College of Wisconsin
Milwaukee, Wisconsin

Philip J. Katzman, MD
Professor, Department of Pathology & Laboratory Medicine
University of Rochester Medical Center
Rochester, New York

Eileen Margaret McKay, MD
Associate Professor of Pathology & Immunology
Baylor College of Medicine/Texas Children's Hospital
Houston, Texas

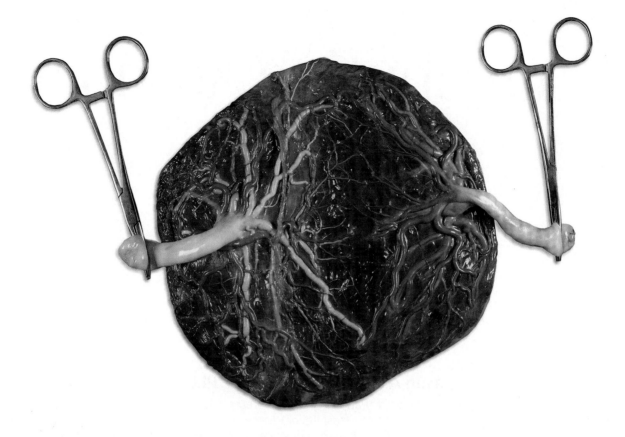

Preface

One of the more perplexing phenomena in the field of pathology is what could be termed the placenta paradox: The placenta is the most accessible human organ, yet, at the same time, it is also the most poorly understood. Attributable, in part, to the rather cursory attention devoted to the placenta in most training programs and to its ever-looming medicolegal ramifications, examination of the placenta often presents an intimidating task for the general surgical pathologist. The placenta probably does not deserve its enigmatic reputation. Many of the inflammatory, immune-mediated, or vascular processes seen in the placenta have analogies in other organ systems, such as the lung, liver, or kidney. And, as in these other organs, the placental pathologies have more or less constant—and increasingly better understood—clinical (fetal and/or maternal) correlates.

Even in this molecular era, placental pathology remains firmly entrenched in gross and microscopic morphology. As illustrated by the successful launch of the 1st edition of *Diagnostic Pathology: Placenta*, this practical, image-rich textbook has clearly filled a niche. The years since publication of the 1st edition have witnessed important advances in perinatal pathology, including the development and implementation of updated international consensus terminology for most prevalent placental conditions, based on meetings of placental experts in Amsterdam and most recently Dublin, and the more widespread application of molecular techniques (e.g., for work-up of stillbirth).

As with the 1st edition, *Diagnostic Pathology: Placenta*, the 2nd edition aims to be a practical and highly accessible complement to the existing excellent but somewhat more encyclopedic classic placental pathology literature. To this end, it uses the easy-to-access bullet format popularized by the Amirsys surgical pathology, histology, and radiology textbooks. The basic format of the book is continued. Throughout the text of the 2nd edition, we have updated terminology and diagnostic criteria to reflect the international consensus statements. The 1st section provides a systematic overview of the various placental compartments, each presented with their respective normal gross and microscopic appearance as well as their major pathological findings. The 2nd section addresses the most important placental pathology constellations and their typical clinical correlates. Infectious disease pathology of the placenta has been expanded and includes Zika virus infection; gestational trophoblastic disease continues to be a difficult diagnosis, especially in very early pregnancy, and we have expanded these chapters. The 3rd section continues focus on prevalent pregnancy complications and associated placental findings. We have added new chapters on complications of monochorionic pregnancy, maternal mortality, and the placental pathology of hypoxic-ischemic encephalopathy. The last section provides essential reference tables as well as proposed templates that may be useful for gross and microscopic placental description, utilizing the revised terminology of international consensus classification.

Finally, as with the 1st edition, we continue to hope that this text will enhance the readers' understanding of the placenta and, ultimately, their appreciation of the critical role it plays as the unique interface between mother and fetus. We hope we may have contributed to the demystification of the placenta. Enjoy the book.

Amy Heerema-McKenney, MD
Director of Perinatal Pathology
Robert J. Tomsich Pathology and Laboratory Medicine Institute, Division of Anatomic Pathology
Cleveland Clinic
Cleveland, Ohio

Edwina J. Popek, DO
Professor of Pathology and Pediatrics
Baylor College of Medicine
Texas Children's Hospital Pavilion for Women
Houston, Texas

Monique E. De Paepe, MD, MSc
Professor of Pathology and Laboratory Medicine
Women and Infants Hospital
Alpert Medical School of Brown University
Providence, Rhode Island

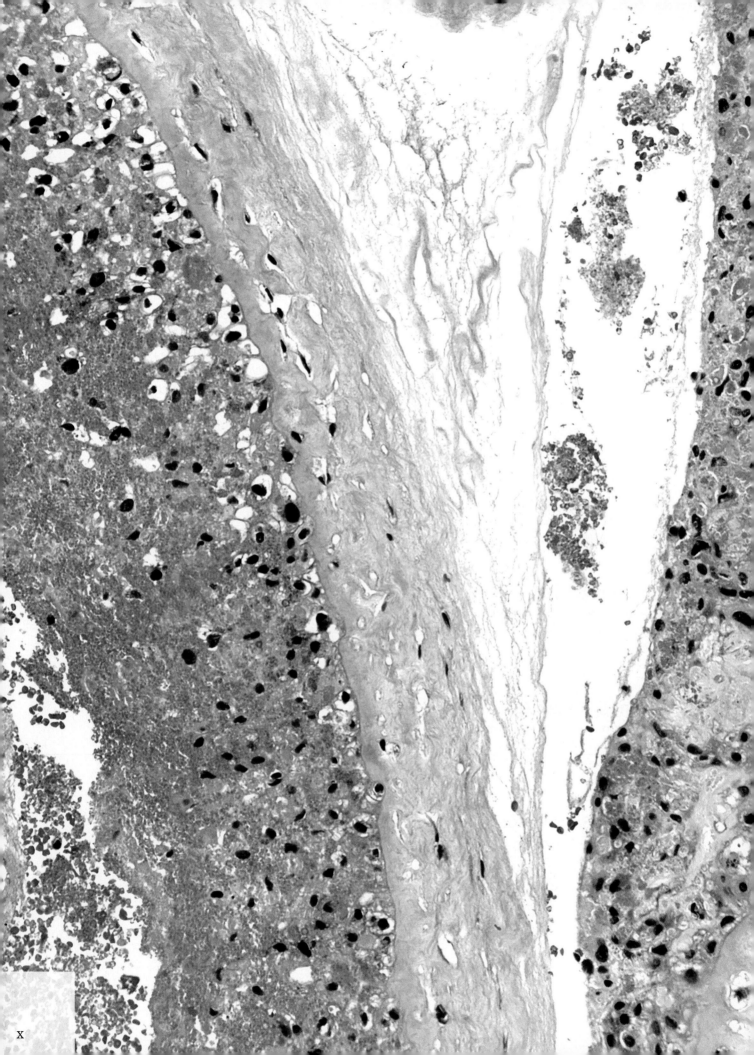

Acknowledgments

Lead Editor

Megg Morin, BA

Text Editors

Arthur G. Gelsinger, MA
Rebecca L. Bluth, BA
Nina I. Bennett, BA
Terry W. Ferrell, MS
Matt W. Hoecherl, BS
Joshua Reynolds, PhD

Image Editors

Jeffrey J. Marmorstone, BS
Lisa A. M. Steadman, BS

Illustrations

Richard Coombs, MS
Lane R. Bennion, MS
Laura C. Wissler, MA

Art Direction and Design

Tom M. Olson, BA
Laura C. Wissler, MA

Production Coordinators

Emily C. Fassett, BA
Angela M. G. Terry, BA

ELSEVIER

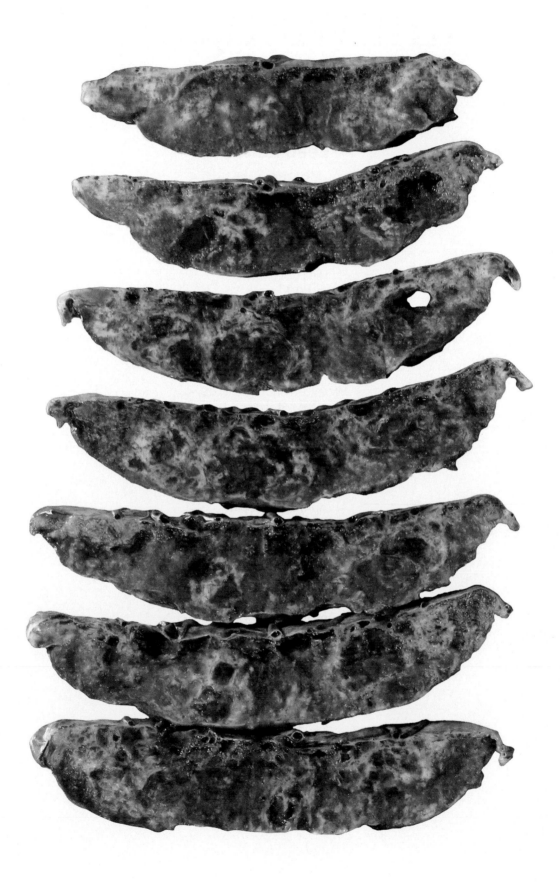

Sections

TABLE OF CONTENTS

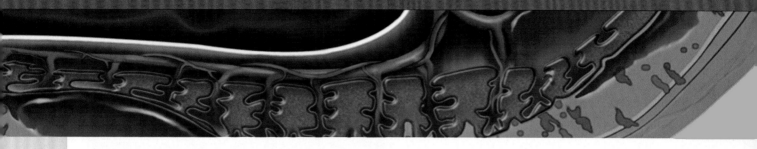

TABLE OF CONTENTS

DIAGNOSTIC PATHOLOGY

Placenta

SECOND EDITION

HEEREMA-MCKENNEY | POPEK | DE PAEPE

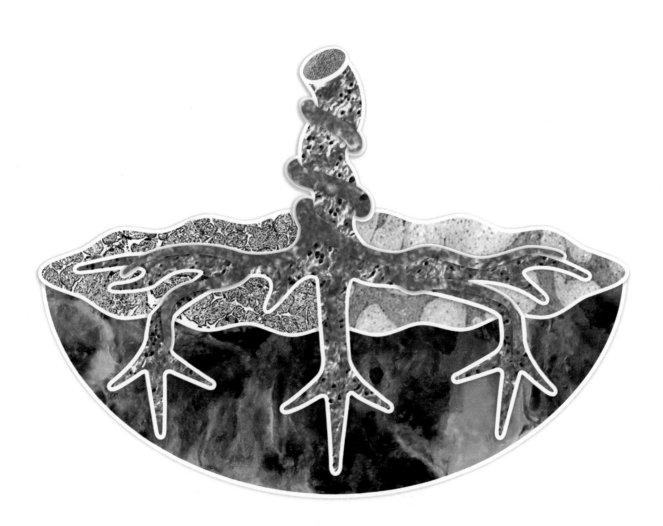

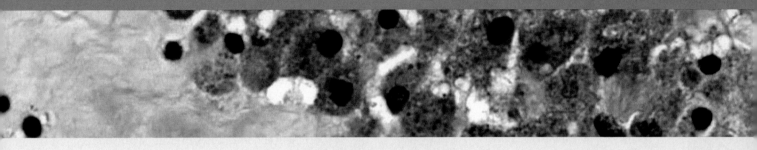

TERMINOLOGY

Synonyms

- Omphalomesenteric duct = vitelline duct
- Allantois = urachus = median umbilical ligament

GROSS EVALUATION

Gross Inspection of Cord

- Very important aspect of placental examination
- Abnormalities associated with fetal morbidity and mortality
  - Tight knots
  - Umbilical cord prolapse through or into cervix
  - Velamentous cord ± vasa previa
  - Abnormal cord length
  - Abnormal cord coiling, hypercoiling or hypocoiling
  - Hematoma/hemorrhage
  - Thrombosis
  - Hemangioma
  - Cord entanglement around neck or body
  - Cord entanglement between monoamniotic twins
- Every exam should document
  - Color, normally white
    - Green-brown discoloration with meconium staining
    - Yellow discoloration with meconium or inflammation
    - Red-brown discoloration after fetal demise
      - ☐ Discolored stripe may indicate thrombus
  - Total length
  - Diameter
  - Coiling
    - Count number of coils in total length to determine if undercoiled or overcoiled
  - Cord insertion site, distance from insertion to edge of placental disc
  - Presence of amniotic web
    - Extension of amnion from cord to chorionic plate tethers cord
      - ☐ May limit fetal mobility
      - ☐ Often mistaken for marginal or velamentous insertion on ultrasounds

- Presence of surface lesions
  - Small white plaques on surface of cord suggest peripheral funisitis due to *Candida* infection
  - Ulcerations may be secondary to meconium-associated smooth muscle necrosis
- True knots uncommon (< 2% of placentas) vs. pseudoknots very common
  - Tight knots have venous congestion on placental side
  - Pseudo or false knots are due to varicosities
- Number of vessels on cut section
- Lesions of vessels
  - Thrombi
  - Hematoma usually associated with disrupted vein during clamping of cord
  - Arc-like opacities of inflammatory debris oriented toward amnion surface
- Document abnormalities with gross photograph

Umbilical Cord Length

- Reference values for cord length are established for fresh cord at gross exam
  - > 70 cm at term considered excessively long
    - Fetal heart failure due to increased work of moving blood through long umbilical cord
    - Increased risk of cord wrapping around neck, body, or limbs, with potential effects on circulation through affected body part as well as through cord
    - Associated with increased fetal activity, male gender, increased maternal height, BMI and parity
  - < 35 cm at term considered short (clinical correlation necessary)
    - Associated with decreased fetal movement
    - Increased risk of premature placental separation or cord avulsion
    - Cord length shortens in fresh state approximately 3% in first 2 hours after delivery
    - Formalin fixation leads to further shortening of approximately 12% at 24-48 hours

---

Umbilical Cord False Knots

Wharton Substance

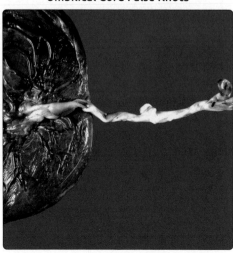
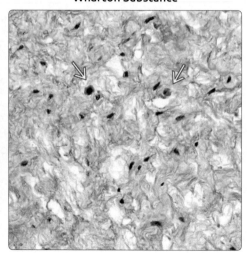

(Left) The umbilical vessels may have varicosities, commonly called "false knots," that usually arise from the vein. They are of little clinical significance. Rarely, they may contain thrombi. (Right) The umbilical cord is composed of myofibroblasts, found near the vessels and collagen fibers. Wharton substance is found between the cellular components. This includes fibroblasts, macrophages and mast cells ➡. Mast cells produce heparin-like substances to prevent thrombosis. The cord has no lymphatics or nerves.

– Length of cord received in pathology is usually < true total length, as segments may be sent from delivery room for blood gas analysis, cord blood banking, cytogenetics or cultures

Umbilical Cord Diameter

- Reference values for cord diameter on fresh cord
  o Cord diameter measured from slides will be approximately 0.1-0.2 cm smaller due to shrinkage with fixation and processing
- Thick cords (> 3 cm fresh) associated with large placenta, fetal macrosomia and hydrops
  o Usually due to increased volume of Wharton substance, may be secondary to increased umbilical vessel size
- Thin cords (< 8 mm measured off slides) associated with prematurity, postmaturity, fetal growth restriction, decreased uteroplacental blood flow, and oligohydramnios
  o Thinning usually due to decreased volume of Wharton substance or single umbilical artery
  o Usually has wrinkled cord surface
- Fetal end of cord is usually thicker than placental end

Umbilical Cord Coiling

- Helical coiling of umbilical arteries around vein
  o Coiling protects vessels from compression
  o 75% coil counterclockwise, leftward
- Average number of coils is reported as coiling index
  o Normal coiling ranges 1-3 twists per 10 cm of length
  o Calculate by counting total number of 360° twists, divide by length of cord
- Hypercoiled cords noted in 20%
  o May be associated with increased vascular resistance to blood flow through cord with increased afterload on fetal heart, torsions or strictures, further compromise flow
  o Chorionic plate and stem vessels may show thrombi
  o Hemodynamic effect of hypercoiling more severe in small-caliber arteries and excessively long cords
- Hypocoiled cords noted in 7.5%
  o May be more susceptible to kinking and acute obstruction of fetal blood flow
  o Associated with aneuploidy and single umbilical artery, meconium staining
  o Flat cords may be associated with nuchal or body wraps

Umbilical Cord Insertion

- Insertion is defined as point where cord vessels branch and are no longer covered with Wharton substance
- "Normal" cord insertion
  o Insertion within central 2/3 of disc (paracentral or eccentric insertion most common)
- Peripheral cord insertion, may be less efficient
  o Insertion within 3 cm of disc edge
- Marginal cord insertion, less efficient
  o Insertion within 1 cm of disc edge
- Velamentous cord insertion, less efficient
  o Insertion in membranes of placenta
  o Vessels coursing through membranes to disc are at risk for compression or disruption
    – No protection from compression by Wharton substance
    – Can tear if near site of membrane rupture

  o Measure length of longest intramembranous vessel and note thrombi or disruption
- Furcate (fork-like) cord insertion
  o Umbilical vessels branch before cord inserts onto placental surface
    – No protection by Wharton substance along branched segments
    – Increased risk of compression, thrombi, tearing

HISTOLOGIC COMPONENTS

Amniotic Epithelium

- Low cuboidal epithelium
- May become squamous, especially near term and near placental insertion site
- Skin covered component at fetal abdomen will have dermal appendages
- Tightly adherent to underlying connective tissue, unlike amnion of membranes

Umbilical Arteries

- 99% have 2 umbilical arteries
- Derived from allantoic vessels accompanying allantoic duct
- Continuation of internal iliac arteries in fetus
- Brings deoxygenated blood from fetus to placenta
- Thick, muscular vessels with 50-60 smooth muscle layers
  o No internal elastic lamina, but scant elastic fibers in wall
  o Smooth muscle arranged in helical bundles, allows for greater contractility
- Arteries frequently anastomose within 2-3 cm of cord insertion onto placental disc (Hyrtl anastomosis)
  o Equalizes pressure and ensures supply of blood throughout placenta if 1 umbilical artery is thrombosed
  o Various patterns of anastomosis, including varying length of fusion, or ≥ 1 communicating branch
- Single umbilical artery, 1% at term
  o Either left or right UA may be absent, more commonly left
  o More common in Caucasians
  o May see atrophic remnant of 2nd umbilical artery
  o More frequent in twins, usually in smaller twin when growth is discrepant
  o 20% have additional malformations with significant morbidity and mortality
    – Abnormal karyotype and multiple malformations are more common when left umbilical artery is missing
  o Associated with changes of fetal vascular malperfusion in small-for-gestational-age-growth fetus
- Discordant size, > 0.1-cm difference in arteries
  o Similar associations as single umbilical artery
- No vasa vasorum, thrombosis results in vessel necrosis

Umbilical Vein

- Paired in early gestation, singular with regression of right umbilical vein by 2nd month
  o Persistence of right umbilical vein is cause of true supernumerary vessels in < 1% of cords
    – Discern true supernumerary vessel from sectioning through varicosity with additional sections
- Returns oxygenated blood from placenta to fetus
- Derived from allantoic vessels accompanying allantoic duct

- Thin, muscular vessel with 30-40 layers, less well organized than arteries and less able to constrict
- Well-developed internal elastic lamina
- External diameter of vein is usually twice that of arteries
- No vasa vasorum, thrombosis results in vessel necrosis

Wharton Substance

- Mucoid extracellular ground substance protecting umbilical vessels from compression
- Rich in hyaluronic acid, chondroitin sulfate and collagen
- Scattered stellate myofibroblast-like cells, more concentrated toward vessels
- Scattered heparin producing mast cells and macrophages
- Derived from extraembryonic mesoderm
- Liquefies under pressure
  - Cystic degeneration seen in hydrops and with omphalocele
- No lymphatics or nerves are present in umbilical cord

Vestigial Remnants

- Present in 23% of cords
- Allantoic duct remnant, most common (63%)
  - Located between umbilical arteries
  - Lined by flattened, cuboidal or transitional-like urothelium, with occasional mucin-producing cells
  - Surrounded by concentric dense connective tissue, rarely smooth muscle
  - Frequently contains eosinophilic or calcified debris
  - May contain urine if urachus is patent
- Vitelline vessel remnants (30%)
  - May accompany omphalomesentic duct remnant
  - Lined by simple endothelium, with thin muscular wall
  - Variable number of channels
    - Commonly paired at fetal end of cord
    - May be singular at placental end of cord, continuing onto chorionic plate and yolk sac
  - May be associated with proliferation of small capillaries, so-called "hemangioma"
- Omphalomesenteric duct remnant, least common (7%)
  - Usually present at periphery of cord
  - Lined by various endodermal epithelia, typically small intestinal type (rarely gastric, hepatic, pancreatic)
  - Commonly has smooth muscle coat
  - May be cystic, contain eosinophilic or rarely meconium-like material
  - May be associated with other anomalies of persistent duct, such as Meckel diverticulum

ARTIFACTS, SPONTANEOUS AND IATROGENIC LESIONS

Gross Artifacts

- Hematomas
  - Usually due to clamping of cord during delivery of placenta
    - Usually disruption of thinner umbilical vein and extension of blood along perivascular spaces
    - Look for parallel clamp marks on cord surface
  - Small fresh hemorrhages may be due to cord blood sampling for gas analysis
  - Changes should not be confused with hemorrhages that occur before delivery
- Avulsion of cord usually occurs with delivery of placenta after birth
  - Communicate with obstetric team if timing of avulsion is uncertain

Microscopic Artifacts

- Inclusion "cyst" of amnion
  - Usually not true cyst but artifact due to tangential sectioning through spiral of cord
- Loss of 2nd umbilical artery due to incomplete sectioning
  - Section taken in area of Hyrtl anastamosis, close to placental end of cord
- > 3 vessels on section
  - Section taken in area of excessive coiling or varicosity of vessels, false knots

Umbilical Cord Rupture or Avulsion

- Rupture of cord prior to delivery of infant
  - Presents with bloody amniotic fluid and fetal distress
  - Associated with precipitous or uncontrolled delivery
  - Associated with short cords
- Avulsion of cord, partial or complete
  - True avulsion in utero is exceedingly rare
    - Increased risk with velamentous, marginal or furcate insertion
    - May be associated with vascular ectasia or focal segmental thinning of umbilical vessels
    - Rare complication of intrauterine pressure catheter
  - Presents with bloody amniotic fluid and fetal distress
    - Blood extravasates into Wharton substance and into subamniotic space on chorionic plate

Umbilical Cord Hematoma

- Small hemorrhages may be due to excessive coiling, entanglement of cord around fetal body, knots or thrombi
- Small hemorrhages may be complication of amniocentesis or cordocentesis
- Spontaneous hematomas are usually large, fusiform, and near fetal abdomen
- Rare complication of forceps delivery

SELECTED REFERENCES

1. Ayala NK et al: Is umbilical coiling genetically determined? J Perinatol. ePub, 2018
2. Linde LE et al: Extreme umbilical cord lengths, cord knot and entanglement: Risk factors and risk of adverse outcomes, a population-based study. PLoS One. 13(3):e0194814, 2018
3. Battarbee AN et al: Placental abnormalities associated with isolated single umbilical artery in small-for-gestational-age births. Placenta. 59:9-12, 2017
4. Downey A et al: Umbilical cord shortening: quantification postdelivery and postfixation. Pediatr Dev Pathol. 17(5):327-9, 2014
5. Jessop FA et al: Umbilical cord coiling: clinical outcomes in an unselected population and systematic review. Virchows Arch. 464(1):105-12, 2014
6. Ernst LM et al: Gross patterns of umbilical cord coiling: correlations with placental histology and stillbirth. Placenta. 34(7):583-8, 2013
7. Luo G et al: Peripheral insertion of umbilical cord. Pediatr Dev Pathol. 16(6):399-404, 2013
8. Proctor LK et al: Umbilical cord diameter percentile curves and their correlation to birth weight and placental pathology. Placenta. 34(1):62-6, 2013

Umbilical Cord Diameter (cm)

Gestational Age (Completed Weeks)	10th Percentile	50th Percentile	90th Percentile	N	Mean	Standard Deviation
18	0.36	0.46	0.61	4	0.53	0.08
19	0.43	0.54	0.68	10	0.51	0.12
20	0.50	0.60	0.73	8	0.72	0.30
21	0.56	0.67	0.79	9	0.61	0.14
22	0.62	0.72	0.84	17	0.69	0.09
23	0.67	0.78	0.88	14	0.75	0.20
24	0.72	0.83	0.93	18	0.84	0.13
25	0.77	0.87	0.97	9	0.86	0.12
26	0.80	0.91	1.01	9	0.93	0.13
27	0.83	0.94	1.05	7	0.93	0.09
28	0.85	0.97	1.09	4	1.04	0.06
29	0.87	1.00	1.12	9	0.92	0.16
30	0.88	1.02	1.15	16	1.04	0.18
31	0.88	1.03	1.18	13	1.06	0.16
32	0.88	1.05	1.20	10	1.04	0.14
33	0.88	1.05	1.22	16	1.06	0.20
34	0.87	1.06	1.23	23	1.03	0.24
35	0.86	1.06	1.24	17	0.97	0.13
36	0.85	1.05	1.25	33	1.03	0.17
37	0.84	1.05	1.24	40	1.02	0.14
38	0.83	1.03	1.23	54	1.04	0.18
39	0.82	1.02	1.22	58	1.01	0.15
40	0.81	1.00	1.19	59	1.04	0.14
41	0.80	0.98	1.16	40	1.05	0.17

Umbilical cord diameter (UCD) percentiles and mean and standard deviation of the cohort (N = 497) are shown. UCD was calculated using the formula: $UCD = 2 \times \sqrt{(weight/\pi \times length)}$. The substitution of weight in place of volume was used after showing that umbilical cord volume was similar to weight (p < 0.001; r = 0.997; y = 1.071x - 0.644).

Proctor LK et al: Umbilical cord diameter percentile curves and their correlation to birth weight and placental pathology. Placenta. 34(1):62-6, 2013.

Umbilical Cord Length at Various Gestational Ages

Gestational Age (Weeks)	N	Umbilical Cord Length (cm)
20-21	16	32.4 ± 8.6
22-23	27	36.4 ± 9.0
24-25	38	40.1 ± 10.1
26-27	59	42.5 ± 11.3
28-29	80	45.0 ± 9.7
30-31	113	47.6 ± 11.3
32-33	337	50.2 ± 12.1
34-35	857	52.5 ± 11.2
36-37	3,153	55.6 ± 12.6
38-39	10,083	57.4 ± 12.6
40-41	13,841	59.6 ± 12.6
42-43	4,797	60.3 ± 12.7

Data represent mean ± 1 standard deviation of cord length in fresh state after birth. Shortening occurs in fresh state and with formalin fixation.

Naeye RL: Umbilical cord length: clinical significance. J Pediatr. 107(2):278-81, 1985.

Candida Funisitis

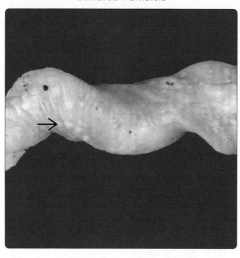

Vitelline Vessel Remnants in Cord

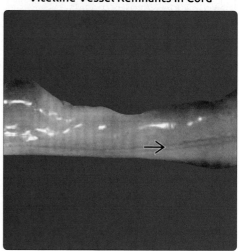

(Left) *Gross exam includes close inspection of the surface. The small, white plaques* ⇨ *on the cord surface are foci of peripheral funisitis. The lesion is nearly pathognomonic for candidal infection of the amniotic fluid.* (Right) *This segment of cord is hypocoiled. Vitelline vessels* ⇨ *may be visible on gross inspection. They are a remnant vasculature that accompanied the omphalomesenteric duct in early development. They are often paired on the fetal end of the cord.*

True Knot

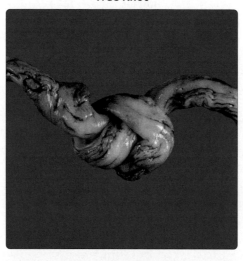

Umbilical Cord Coiling

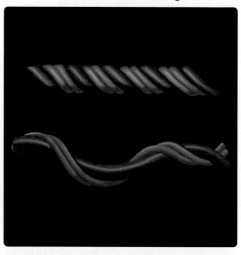

(Left) *True knots can be loose or tight. The lack of congestion on either side of this knot indicates that it is not a tight knot and may have had little clinical significance. The wrinkled cord surface indicates the loss of Wharton substance.* (Right) *Coiling index refers to the number of 360° coils made by the umbilical arteries (blue) around the umbilical vein (red). Normal coiling ranges from 1-3 per 10 cm length of cord. Both overcoiling (top) and undercoiling (bottom) have been associated with adverse outcome.*

Umbilical Cord Coiling

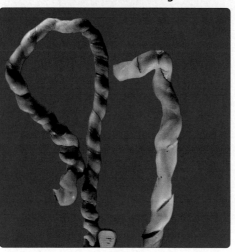

Umbilical Cord Torsion With IUFD

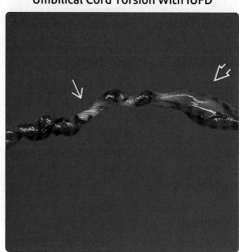

(Left) *The cause of overcoiling is unknown. The cords of these monochorionic twins are discrepant for coiling index and direction.* (Right) *The discoloration of the cord is an indication of prolonged fetal demise. The area of torsion* ⇨ *is toward the fetal end of the cord, and the* ⇨ *dilated area is toward the placental end.*

Hypercoiled Umbilical Cord

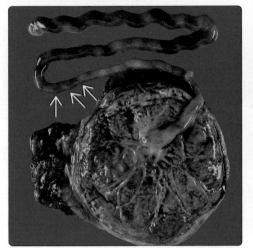

Undercoiled Umbilical Cord

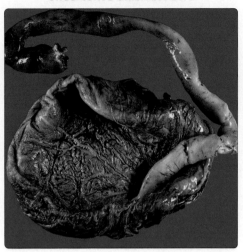

(Left) *This hypercoiled cord led to 2nd-trimester fetal demise. Mathematical modeling suggests that excessive coiling increases resistance to blood flow. Excessive length and hypercoiling increase the work required for placental perfusion. The hypercoiling ➡ is often difficult to appreciate.* (Right) *This undercoiled cord is from a case of severe, chronic meconium exposure and in-utero fetal demise. Undercoiled cords are more susceptible to acute occlusion from kinking.*

Umbilical Vein Thrombus

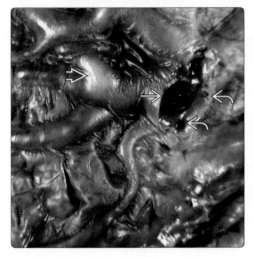

Umbilical Artery Thrombus

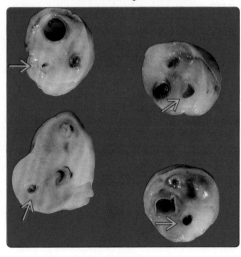

(Left) *Gross image shows a thrombus ➡ of the umbilical vein near the cord insertion. Note the smaller diameter of the 2 umbilical arteries ➡. The white discoloration ➡ of the proximal chorionic plate vein indicates extension of the thrombus.* (Right) *These cross sections of the cord show loss of the muscularis of one of the umbilical arteries ➡ due to longstanding thrombosis.*

Umbilical Cord Hematoma

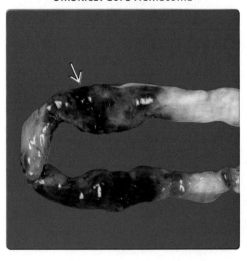

Umbilical Cord Hematoma

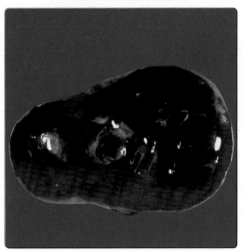

(Left) *Hemorrhage within the cord substance may be spontaneous, iatrogenic, or an artifact of delivery. The cord should be carefully inspected for clamp marks ➡ near the lesion.* (Right) *While the amount of blood that the fetus can lose in a cord hematoma is limited, the pressure may occlude flow through the remaining intact vessels.*

Umbilical Cord Insertion

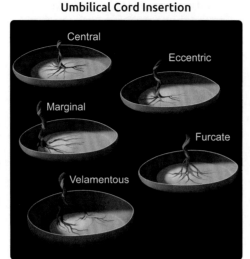

Marginal Umbilical Cord Insertion

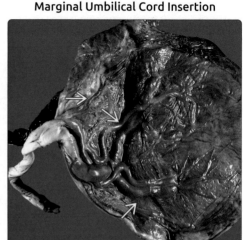

(Left) *Central and eccentric cord insertions are most common. Marginal, velamentous, and furcate are more often associated with pathology. Velamentous and furcate cords leave vessels vulnerable to injury. Marginal insertion may be less efficient for perfusion.* (Right) *Cords that insert at the margin, or within 1 cm of the margin, are deemed marginal. Marginal cord insertion is associated with magistral chorionic plate vasculature. There are few artery/vein pairs* ➡, *which show little decrease in diameter or branching.*

Velamentous Cord Insertion

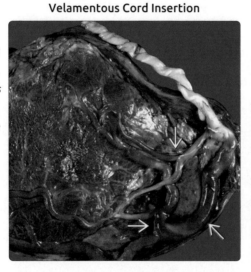

Marginal Cord Insertion

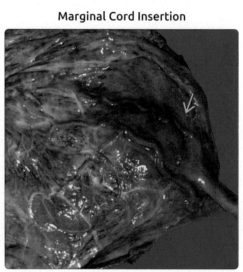

(Left) *Gross image shows vulnerable vessels* ➡ *in a velamentous insertion. Inspect closely for tears or thrombi and measure the length of the unprotected intramembranous vessels. All velamentous cord insertions are also furcate.* (Right) *Cords that insert at the disc margin* ➡ *frequently have vessels that may course through the membranes. These are also vulnerable to compression or tearing as in velamentous cord insertion.*

Furcate Cord Insertion

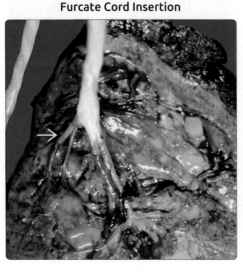

Amniotic Web of Tethered Cord

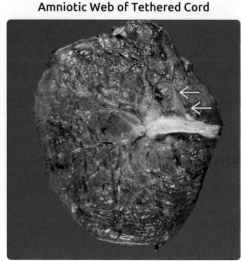

(Left) *In furcate cord insertion, the umbilical vessels branch* ➡ *like the tines of a fork before the cord inserts on the chorionic plate. Such vessels are vulnerable to compression or tearing. Tearing may be the source of subamniotic hemorrhage. Not all furcate cords are velamentous.* (Right) *In the amniotic web of the umbilical cord, an extension of amniotic membranes* ➡ *tethers the cord to the chorionic plate. This may limit cord mobility and cause the cord to be functionally short. Tearing of the web may result in subamniotic hemorrhage.*

10

Early 2nd-Trimester Cord

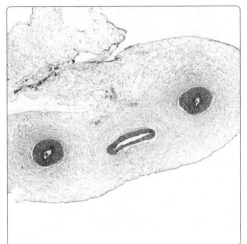

Single Umbilical Artery

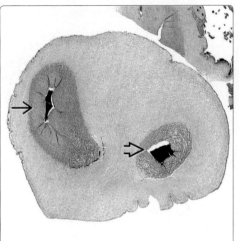

(Left) The thicker umbilical arteries are easily distinguished from the thinner-walled vein in this 15-week gestation cord. The loose stroma has an immature appearance. The umbilical vein is usually 2x the diameter of an artery but thinner walled. (Right) A single umbilical artery should be confirmed microscopically. There is 1 umbilical artery ➡ and 1 umbilical vein ⮕ present. This common anomaly has little clinical significance in the vast majority of newborns.

Umbilical Vein

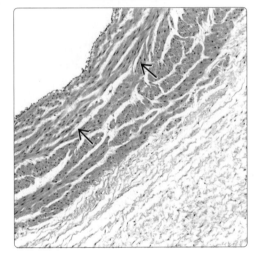

Umbilical Vein Elastin Stain

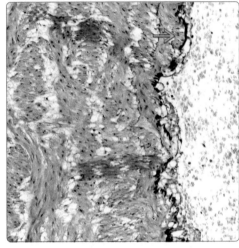

(Left) In contrast to the umbilical arteries, a vague resemblance to separate longitudinal and circular ➡ layers can be seen in the umbilical vein. The vein has limited ability to contract if damaged. (Right) The umbilical vein has an internal elastic lamina ➡.

Umbilical Artery

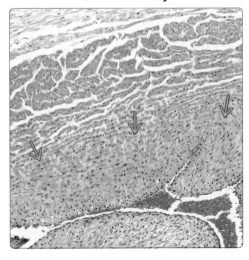

Umbilical Artery Elastin

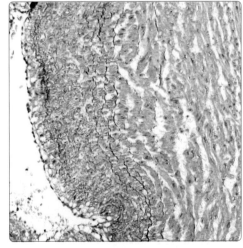

(Left) The muscle of the umbilical arteries consists of crossing spiral bundles of smooth muscle. The inner layers often appear less organized ➡, and may bulge into the lumen. The artery has more ability to contract, limiting bleeding. Desmin expression is often limited to the outer, more differentiated-appearing layers. (Right) The umbilical arteries lack a well-developed internal elastic lamina but have scattered circumferential elastic staining in the inner muscular layers.

2nd-Trimester Wharton Substance

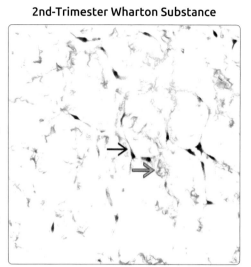

Wharton Substance

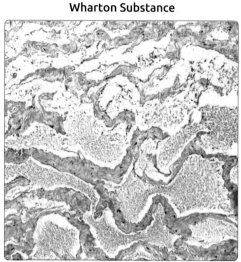

(Left) *The cord increases in diameter throughout gestation from growth of the vessels and increase in Wharton substance. This 2nd-trimester cord shows spindled fibroblasts ⊟ and few delicate collagen fibers ⊟. This connective tissue floats in a hyaluronic acid and proteoglycan-rich matrix termed "ground substance."* **(Right)** *The normal cord has variable amounts of fluid in the extracellular matrix. The blue staining of the hyaluronic acid component may be seen with certain hematoxylin and eosin stains.*

Umbilical Cord Squamous Metaplasia

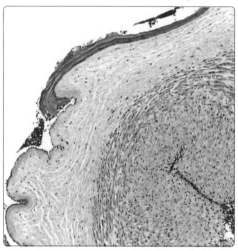

Hyrtl Anastomosis

(Left) *Squamous metaplasia is a feature of a mature cord and is most often seen at the placental end of the cord.* **(Right)** *This section came from the placental end of the cord. The 2 umbilical arteries on this section share a muscular wall. Sections from 1 side of this will have only 1 artery and the other side 2 arteries.*

Cystic Degeneration of Wharton Substance

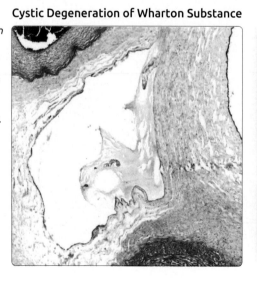

Body Stalk

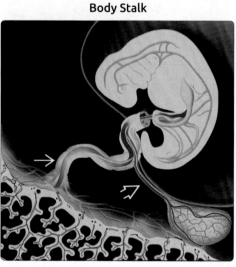

(Left) *Pseudocysts may form in areas of large accumulations of Wharton substance. There is no epithelial or endothelial lining, only condensed spindle cells. These are common near the fetal abdomen in association with omphalocele.* **(Right)** *The following are gathered by amnion into the body stalk: Paired allantoic arteries, initially paired allantoic veins (2nd vein regresses) ⊟ with allantoic duct (not shown), vitelline duct and vitelline vessels ⊟. The latter 3 structures can be seen as vestigial remnants in the mature cord.*

Omphalomesenteric Duct Remnant

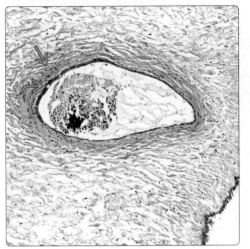

Omphalomesenteric Duct Remnant

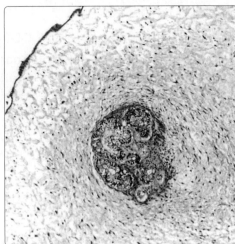

(Left) *Omphalomesenteric duct remnants are typically present at the periphery and may have a smooth muscle layer* ➡. *Various types of endodermal tissue may be seen, but typically they are lined by a cuboidal to low columnar epithelium, with occasional goblet cells* ➡. (Right) *This omphalomesenteric duct remnant has a smooth muscle coat and well-differentiated intestinal-type mucosa.*

Capillary Proliferation (Hemangioma) Associated With Vitelline Vessel Remnants

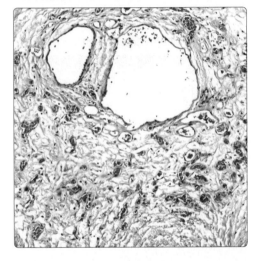

Extramedullary Hematopoiesis

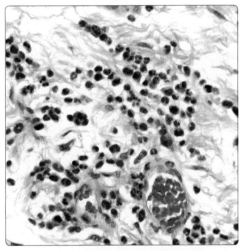

(Left) *Vitelline vessel remnants are usually found paired on the fetal end of the cord. They may have an associated capillary proliferation as seen in this image.* (Right) *Vitelline vessels once communicated with the embryonic yolk sac, the primary source of hematopoiesis in the early embryo. Remnants in the mature cord may also feature extramedullary hematopoiesis as seen here.*

Allantoic Remnant

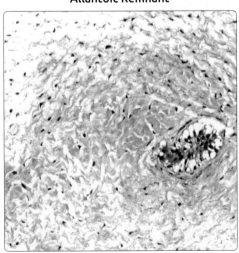

Allantoic Remnant

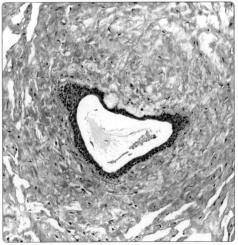

(Left) *Allantoic remnants are usually located between the 2 umbilical arteries. The epithelium is typically cuboidal or transitional. They are usually of no clinical significance.* (Right) *The allantoic remnant occasionally shows a patent lumen. Rarely, large patent allantoic remnants communicate with a persistent urachus in the fetus. Urination into the cord may occur.*

TERMINOLOGY

Definitions

- True knot
  - Intertwining looped segment of umbilical cord that can lead to cord compression
- False knot (a.k.a. pseudoknot)
  - Appear to be knots but are truly
    - Focal accentuations of vascular spirals
    - Local redundancies/looping of umbilical vessels, (nodus spurious vasculosis), most commonly of arteries, sometimes vein
    - Excessive amounts of Wharton substance present (nodus spurious gelatinous)

EPIDEMIOLOGY

Incidence

- 0.35-2.10% of umbilical cords contain true knot
- True knots represent ~ 4% of all cord complications

- Equal frequency of true knots in fetal demise and term live birth
- 0.1% of umbilical cords contain double true knots

ETIOLOGY/PATHOGENESIS

True Knot Formation

- Created by cord forming loop with diameter large enough to allow fetus to move through it
- Proposed to develop early in gestation when there is ample space for fetal movement and entanglement
  - Proposed to occur between 9- and 28-weeks gestation, after which cord length no longer increases significantly
  - Some narrow time period of knot formation to between 9- and 12-weeks gestation
- Depends on cord that is long enough to create loop and factors that create more room, allowing for exaggerated fetal movement
- Proposed that knots can also result from descent of fetus through loop of cord during labor

Tight Complex Knot

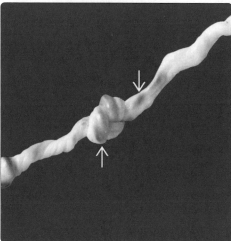

Tight Simple Knot

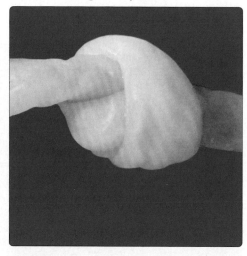

(Left) Gross photograph shows a tight, complex (2 loops) true knot of the umbilical cord with vascular congestion and dilation of the vessels, predominately on the placental side of the knot 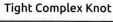. This fetus was small for gestational age and had meconium-stained amniotic fluid at birth. (Right) This photograph shows a tight, simple (1 loop) true knot of the umbilical cord. Note that there is no vascular congestion surrounding the knot. After untying the knot, there was underlying grooving of the cord.

Complex Multilooped Knot

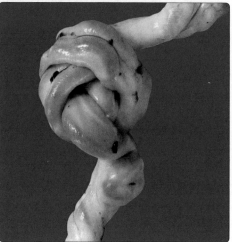

Loose Knot

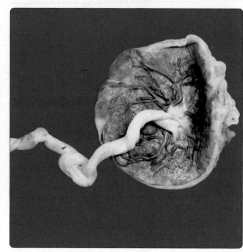

(Left) Gross photograph shows a complex, multilooped true knot with prominent vascular congestion. The fetus experienced distress during labor leading to cesarean delivery, suggesting transient tightening and vascular compression during labor. (Right) Gross photograph shows a loose true knot located 11.5 cm from the insertion site on the chorionic plate. Note that there is no vascular congestion or compression of the underlying umbilical cord. This fetus did not suffer any clinical sequelae.

- Further axial movements by fetus, such as changes in lie and presentation, could result in tightening of knot or formation of more complicated knot

Effects of True Knot Tightening

- Tightening of knot leads to compression of umbilical vessels with following effects
  - Umbilical venous stasis and congestion (dilation) on placental side of knot
  - Umbilical arterial stasis (less likely dilation) on fetal side of knot
  - Decreased delivery of oxygenated blood from placenta to fetus
  - Thrombosis in fetal vasculature of cord and placenta
    - Umbilical vein on placental side of knot and chorionic plate veins
    - Umbilical arteries on fetal side of knot, if severe enough
  - Avascular villi, secondary to stasis &/or decreased blood flow
- Tightening often occurs later in pregnancy secondary to increased traction on umbilical cord due to
  - Fetal descent into pelvis or through birth canal
  - Membrane rupture with loss of cushioning effect of amniotic fluid

Deleterious Fetal Effects

- Depend on increased venous perfusion pressure
  - In vitro studies show increase in venous pressure required to perfuse umbilical vein; occurs with
    - Tightening of knot
    - Increased number of knots in single cord
    - Even slack or loose knot
- Sublethal or lethal hypoxic fetal injury can result from true knots with
  - Complete umbilical blood flow obstruction
  - Critical reduction in umbilical blood flow associated with high venous pressure

Increased Risk of Fetal Vascular Compression Secondary to True Knot

- During uterine contractions
- After rupture of membranes
- With greater size or bulk of knot
- With increased complexity of knot

False Knot Formation

- Etiology currently unknown
- Suggested to signify temporal discrepancy of vascular growth with inadequate cord lengthening

CLINICAL IMPLICATIONS

Clinical Presentation

- True knots
  - Intrapartum death or intrauterine fetal demise represent most devastating presentation
  - Most fetuses with knots have completely normal pregnancy and delivery without complications or sequelae
  - Fetuses have increased risk during labor and delivery of
    - Nonreassuring fetal heart tracing, particularly variable decelerations

- Cord accidents at birth (cord prolapse and nuchal cord)
- Cesarean delivery
- Preterm delivery
- Low Apgar score at 1 and 5 minutes
- Meconium-stained amniotic fluid
- Need for neonatal intensive care
  - Fetal distress during labor may be temporary with quick recovery soon after birth attributed to transient tightening of knot during delivery
  - Poor fetal growth or varying degrees of neurologic injury may occur with chronic intermittent knot tightening without complete obstruction
  - Controversial association with abnormal artery cord pH with more normal venous cord pH
- False knots are typically of no clinical significance
  - Incidental findings during delivery
  - Often confused with true knots

Imaging Findings

- Prenatal diagnosis of true knot is rare and extremely difficult by ultrasound
- Larger &/or more complex knots are typically easier to visualize
- Color Doppler &/or 3D ultrasonography may be more helpful than typical 2D ultrasound technique for detection

Risk Factors for True Knot

- Long umbilical cord
- Hypercoiled umbilical cord
- Male gender (secondary to longer cords in male fetuses)
- Polyhydramnios
- Small-for-gestational-age fetus
- Monochorionic monoamniotic twin pregnancy (cord entanglement between twins)
- Prolonged gestation, often has decreased amniotic fluid
- Amniocentesis during pregnancy (secondary to increased rate of fetal movement and uterine contractions)
- Grand multiparous mother (secondary to lax abdominal &/or uterine wall muscles)
- Maternal chronic hypertension
- Gestational diabetes or diabetes mellitus (secondary to increased incidence of polyhydramnios)
- Advanced maternal age
- Maternal obesity
- Previous spontaneous abortion

Clinical Outcomes

- Most knots are not associated with adverse fetal outcomes
- Overall perinatal mortality rate of true knots: 8-11%
- 4x increased risk of stillbirth with true knot during pregnancy
  - In population study, 2% of fetuses with true knots were stillborn, which accounted for 5% of all stillbirths of infants weighing > 2,500 g
  - Stillbirth secondary to true knots seen at all gestational ages
- 25% morbidity and mortality in association with double true knots
- False knots have no clinical sequelae described

MACROSCOPIC

General Features of True Knots

- Gross pattern of knots
  - Single or simple (1 loop)
  - Complex (> 1 overhand loop)
    - Figure 8 pattern (2 loops)
    - Loop around fetal part with half-hitch knot
  - Multiple (≥ 2 separate knots of 1 umbilical cord)
  - Knot between 2 umbilical cords in monochorionic monoamniotic twin pregnancy secondary to entanglement of cords
- Indications of longstanding tight knot
  - Compression, grooving, and loss of Wharton substance at site of knot
  - Cannot easily move or untie loops of knot with gentle tugging
  - Even when untied, unknotted cord curls and grooving persists
- Indications of true obstruction of umbilical cord by knot
  - Umbilical venous congestion and dilation on placental side of knot
  - Venous distention may extend to chorionic plate vessels
  - Thrombus formation in umbilical or chorionic vessels ± thrombosis (depending on chronicity)
- Tightness of knot does not necessarily indicate clinical significance without other suspicious features, as knot may have tightened transiently during delivery
- Indications of newly formed or loose knot (typically not clinically significant)
  - No loss of Wharton substance
  - No marked groove at site of knot
  - No curling of cord after untying

General Features of False Knots

- Can be quite large and complex, often bulbous
- Appears as vascular protrusion or outpouching of Wharton substance
- Can have redundancy of 1 umbilical vessel
- Do not cause compression of umbilical vessels; therefore, distention, congestion, &/or edema are not typically seen

Specimen Handling

- Document whether knot is tight or loose
- Document if congestion is present on either side of knot
- Photograph knot, showing distance from chorionic plate
- Untie knot and document whether it stays curled, implying chronicity
- Sections should be taken through knot after untying or on either side of knot if left intact
  - Sections should be designated as knot, fetal or placental side of knot and placed in different cassettes

MICROSCOPIC

General Features of True Knots

- Commonly have completely normal histology of umbilical cord
  - Acute tightening may have early intraluminal thrombus in umbilical vein or chorionic vessels
  - Normal histology does not exclude acute tightening of cord knot

- Fetal vascular malperfusion changes are seen when more subacute to chronic tightening occurs
  - Intramural fibrin deposition or complete occlusion of umbilical vein by thrombus can be seen
    - At site of knot or within umbilical vein between placenta and knot
    - In fetal chorionic or stem vessels
  - Umbilical and chorionic veins become thickened and may exhibit subendothelial, dome-shaped, myxoid-appearing intimal protrusions (sometimes called cushions)
    - Associated with venous hypertension
    - Can have intramural fibrin deposition overlying these intimal cushions
  - Villous stromal-vascular karyorrhexis or avascular villi may also be present in distal villous tree
  - Differential congestion or dilation of vessels is easier to see on histology

General Features of False Knots

- Generally have focal increase of Wharton substance with normal histology of umbilical vessels
- May have focal dilation of umbilical vessels &/or ≥ 2 veins or ≥ 3 arteries in section
- Rarely can have thrombus present

REPORTING CRITERIA

Include in Gross Description

- Location of true knot in relation to umbilical cord insertion into chorionic plate
- Whether true knot is tight or loose
- Number of knots &/or complexity of true knot
- Note any vascular distention, congestion or thrombosis of umbilical or chorionic plate vessels
- After untying knot
  - Note whether it stays curled
  - Note if grooving or loss of Wharton substance are seen
- Presence and number of false knots

Include in Final Diagnosis

- Presence of true knot and whether it is tight or loose
- Presence of thrombus in umbilical, chorionic, or stem vessel
- Distal villous changes of fetal vascular malperfusion
- Note false knots only if thrombus is present

SELECTED REFERENCES

1. Linde LE et al: Extreme umbilical cord lengths, cord knot and entanglement: risk factors and risk of adverse outcomes, a population-based study. PLoS One. 13(3):e0194814, 2018
2. Baergen RN: Umbilical cord pathology. Surg Pathol Clin. 6(1):61-85, 2013
3. Räisänen S et al: True umbilical cord knot and obstetric outcome. Int J Gynaecol Obstet. 122(1):18-21, 2013
4. Rodriguez N et al: Three-dimensional high-definition flow imaging in prenatal diagnosis of a true umbilical cord knot. Ultrasound Obstet Gynecol. 39(2):245-6, 2012
5. Tantbirojn P et al: Gross abnormalities of the umbilical cord: related placental histology and clinical significance. Placenta. 30(12):1083-8, 2009
6. Tuxen AJ et al: Factors affecting umbilical venous perfusion during experimental cord knotting. Placenta. 26(10):753-7, 2005
7. Airas U et al: Clinical significance of true umbilical knots: a population-based analysis. Am J Perinatol. 19(3):127-32, 2002

Stillbirth With Tight True Knot

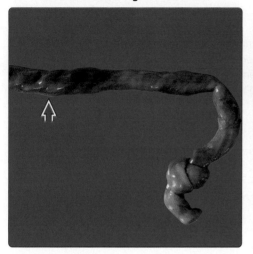

Recent Thrombosis of Umbilical Vein

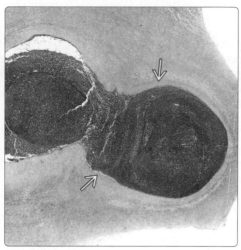

(Left) *Gross photograph shows a tight true knot in the cord of a stillborn infant. There is prominent congestion and vascular distention of the umbilical vessels suggestive of thrombosis ➡. Thrombosis of the umbilical vein at the site of the knot was seen along with multiple thrombi of the chorionic plate vessels.* (Right) *This low-power H&E shows the umbilical vein distended by a recent thrombus, associated with a nearby umbilical cord knot. Note the adherence to the wall, distension, and the lines of Zahn ➡.*

Multiple Knots

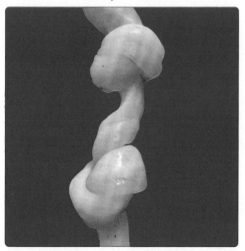

Monochorionic Monoamnionic Twin Placenta With Cord Entanglement

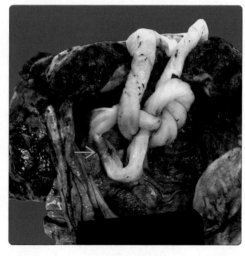

(Left) *Gross photograph shows 2 simple, tight true knots of a single umbilical cord. The pregnancy was complicated by oligohydramnios and 2-vessel umbilical cord. Histologically, a mural thrombus was identified in a stem vessel.* (Right) *This photograph of a monochorionic, monoamnionic twin placenta shows that the cord insertions are very close together ➡. The cords are knotted and entangled around each other, but they do not show any differential congestion.*

False Knot

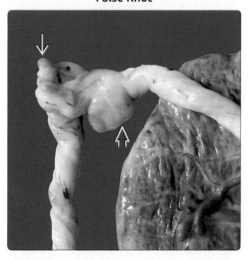

False Knot

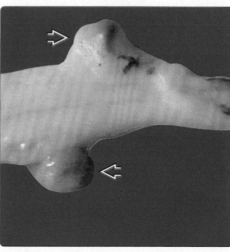

(Left) *Gross photograph shows a complex false knot with multiple protrusions of Wharton substance ➡ and redundant vessels ➡.* (Right) *Gross photograph shows pseudoknots composed of vascular protrusions ➡, most likely redundant umbilical veins. Note that there is no congestion of the umbilical vessels proximal or distal to these protrusions. These false knots were found adjacent to a true knot, which is not an uncommon finding in umbilical cords with true knots.*

TERMINOLOGY

Definitions

- Thick umbilical cord
  - Diameter is > 90th percentile for gestational age
    - Separate reference values are available for measurement by ultrasound in utero, gross evaluation, and on microscopic slides
    - In general, > 3 cm at term is considered thick
  - Thickening may be focal or diffuse and is usually equated with edema of cord
- Thin umbilical cord
  - Diameter is < 10th percentile for gestational age
    - At term, < 0.8 cm, measured off of slides, is considered thin
  - Thinning may be focal or diffuse
- Stricture
  - Sharply defined narrowed segment with decreased Wharton substance &/or vascular constriction

EPIDEMIOLOGY

Incidence

- Thick cord
  - By definition, 10% of infants have excessively thick cords
  - Localized edema is rare
    - Often near fetal end; common finding with omphalocele
    - May be focal or multifocal
- Thin cord
  - By definition, 10% of infants have excessively thin cords
    - Associated with growth restriction and postmaturity
- Strictures
  - 5/1,369 deliveries (0.4%)
  - 9/297 spontaneous abortions (3%)

ETIOLOGY/PATHOGENESIS

Thick Cord

- Amount of Wharton substance decreases near term
  - Cord reaches maximum diameter at 36 weeks

Thick Umbilical Cord

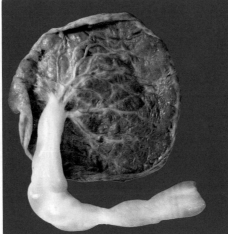

Thin Umbilical Cord

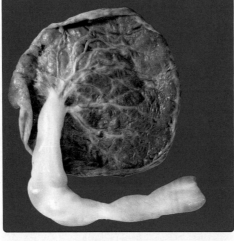

(Left) *This small placenta has a massively edematous, thick, swollen umbilical cord with a low coiling index. Severe edema was associated with hydrops of this fetus.* (Right) *A long segment of umbilical cord thinning ⇥ with a separate, unattached, normal-thickness segment of cord ⇥ is shown. Note the low coiling index of the thin cord and meconium staining.*

Thick Umbilical Cord, Localized

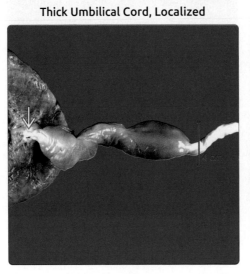

Localized Cord Edema With Vascular Malformation

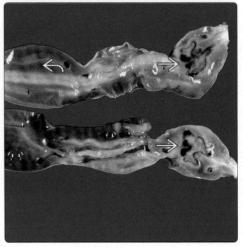

(Left) *Massive localized edema, measuring nearly 4 cm in diameter, is seen in this cord. Note the swollen and glistening surface of the cord with decreased Wharton substance near the cord insertion site ⇥.* (Right) *Localized edema may be associated with a vascular malformation ⇥ of the cord. Degeneration of Wharton substance ⇥ is also seen with brown discoloration of the gelatinous stroma.*

- Diffuse edema
  - Mechanism of edema similar to that of other tissues
    - Reduced oncotic pressure
    - Elevated hydrostatic pressure
    - Increased water content (water content of edematous cords is up to 93.5%)
    - Leaky endothelium secondary to inflammation
    - Umbilical cord does not have lymphatics
- Localized swelling/edema
  - Effect of local injury
    - Meconium
    - Cord compression from entanglement, nuchal cord, or limb/body wraps
    - Swelling between amniotic bands
    - Swelling on placental side of tight knot
  - Omphalocele at umbilicus
  - Cysts
    - Allantoic remnant cyst (1 in ~ 200,000) may communicate with bladder and contain urine near fetal end (patent urachus)
    - Omphalomesenteric duct cyst is more common at fetal end of cord
    - Amniotic epithelial inclusion cyst
    - Mucoid degeneration, pseudocyst filled with liquefied Wharton substance without amniotic lining
  - Vascular lesions
    - Cord hemangioma/chorangioma
    - Cord hematoma, accumulations of blood in Wharton substance are often attributed to traumatic or mechanical damage occurring during delivery of placenta
    - Idiopathic/aneurysmal dilation of umbilical vein

Thin Cord

- Diffuse thinning (sometimes referred to as "lean cord" or "thin cord syndrome")
  - Due to significant decrease/loss of Wharton substance volume; usually with decreased water content
    - Fetal volume depletion is secondary to longstanding uteroplacental underperfusion, leading to decreased extracellular fluid/Wharton substance
  - Due to overall decrease in cross-sectional area of umbilical cord vessels
    - Single umbilical artery
- Localized thinning
  - Focal reduction in diameter of fetal umbilical vessels
  - Thinned segment may be associated with increased coiling
- Stricture
  - Most commonly found at fetal end of cord near umbilical insertion
    - Unclear if etiology is secondary to excessive coiling or due to primary deficiency of Wharton substance
  - Multiple strictures can be seen between helices in some cases of extreme overcoiling

CLINICAL IMPLICATIONS

Thick Cord

- Diffuse edema
  - Typically have normal outcome

- More common in premature infants
- Associated with
  - Gestational diabetes
  - Funisitis in amniotic fluid infection syndrome
  - Fetal hydrops
  - Aneuploidy
    - Midtrimester ultrasound, aneuploidy associated with thicker cords than euploidy
  - Transient respiratory distress and respiratory distress syndrome, likely related to gestational diabetes
- Localized edema
  - Umbilical cord remnant cysts
    - At umbilicus, must clinically exclude patent urachus or herniated fetal intestine
    - Large omphalomesenteric or allantoic cysts have separate clinical associations
    - Venous obstruction due to these conditions is suggested to be one cause of mucoid degeneration elsewhere in cord
  - Localized cysts noted on 3rd-trimester ultrasound are associated with multiple congenital anomalies, especially in cases of trisomy 18
    - Omphalocele may also be present in some cases; others show only mucoid degeneration
  - Need to differentiate swelling of edema from hemorrhage
    - Umbilical cord hematomas are most commonly artifacts of cord clamping after birth
    - In true intrafunicular hemorrhage, perinatal mortality rate can be as high as 40-50% secondary to fetal blood loss or compression of umbilical vessels
  - May be due to mass-forming lesions of cord, such as hemangioma with its own clinical associations

Thin Cord

- Diffuse thinning
  - Complete absence of Wharton substance is associated with fetal death in utero
  - Meconium-stained amniotic fluid is often present
  - Associated with
    - Preeclampsia
    - Intrauterine growth restriction
    - Postterm pregnancy
    - Single umbilical artery
    - Oligohydramnios
    - Fetal intolerance to labor
- Localized thinning and stricture
  - Associated with
    - Intrauterine fetal demise/macerated fetuses
    - Fetal intolerance to labor
  - Stricture
    - Can recur in subsequent pregnancies
    - Proposed to be one cause of nonimmune hydrops
    - Rarely occur in hypocoiled or normally coiled cords

MACROSCOPIC

General Features of Thick Cord

- Diffuse thickening
  - Cord appears diffusely swollen and glistening
- Focal thickening

- o Segment of cord appears swollen and is often more translucent than adjacent segments
- o Transilluminate to identify cysts or other lesions
- True hematoma
  - o Red-purple, elongated, and fusiform throughout cord length, or focally, usually at fetal end
  - o Hemorrhage replaces Wharton substance on cut section
  - o No clamping or puncture marks on surface
- Artifactual cord hematoma
  - o Look for clamp marks or needle puncture sites
  - o Perivascular blood displaces Wharton substance

General Features of Thin Cord

- Diffuse thinning
  - o Single umbilical artery may be present
  - o Tends to have lower coiling index
  - o May have wrinkled appearance
  - o Associated with marginal insertion of umbilical cord
  - o Associated with gross placental features of uteroplacental malperfusion
- Focal thinning and strictures
  - o Associated with excessively long and hypercoiled cords
  - o Congestion and dilation of umbilical vessels may be seen between lesion and placenta
  - o Umbilical vein may be severely compressed
  - o Thrombi may be seen in vessels within or near stricture

Specimen Handling

- Note length and location of focal thickening or thinning of cord and presence of additional lesions identified on cut section
- If hemorrhage or hematoma is present, note extent and vessel involvement
  - o Note associated puncture or clamp marks
    - – If associated with clamp marks, unlikely to be significant
    - – If associated with punctures, need to assess whether there was cordocentesis in utero or after delivery
- Document significant associated findings, such as hematoma or other lesions with gross photograph

MICROSCOPIC

General Features of Thick Cord

- Diffuse edema
  - o Increased amount of Wharton substance ± increased mast cells and empty spaces without lining
  - o Fetal inflammatory response (umbilical phlebitis, umbilical vasculitis, &/or funisitis) in amniotic fluid infection sequence
- Localized edema, depending on etiology, may manifest as
  - o Bland degeneration of Wharton substance (pseudocyst)
  - o Degeneration of Wharton substance with inflammation and possible thrombi of umbilical vessels
  - o Effects of severe and prolonged meconium deposition with rare pigmented macrophages, vascular muscle necrosis, inflammation, and thrombi
  - o Vascular lesion of cord
  - o Cysts

- – Allantoic remnant cyst: Located between 2 umbilical arteries and flattened to cuboidal epithelium, surrounded by variable amount of smooth muscle or fibrous connective tissue
- – Omphalomesenteric duct cyst: Found near periphery of cord and lined by columnar cells similar to that seen in intestinal epithelium

General Features of Thin Cord

- Wharton substance appears condensed or fibrotic
  - o Vessels are close together and close to amnion surface
  - o Invaginations of surface amnion epithelium extend into cord substance
- Reduced cross-sectional area of umbilical vein
- Single umbilical artery may be present
- Stricture
  - o Overall decreased Wharton substance
  - o Associated thrombi in large vessels, cord, chorionic plate, or stem vessels
  - o Villous capillary congestion
  - o Compression &/or distension of umbilical vessels, especially vein
  - o May see degeneration of umbilical vessels, usually with prolonged in utero demise-to-delivery interval

Method to Assess Cord Diameter From Histologic Sections

- Submit sections of umbilical cord from fetal end and placental end
- Measure 2 cord diameters at right angles to each other from each histologic section
- Average 2 diameters
- In order to account for cord shrinkage caused by fixation and processing, correction coefficient should be used
  - o < 28 weeks = + 0.11 cm
  - o > 28 weeks = + 0.17 cm
  - o Proctor et al (2013) provide more specific ranges

SELECTED REFERENCES

1. Rippinger N et al: Lean umbilical cord: a case report. Geburtshilfe Frauenheilkd. 76(11):1186-1188, 2016
2. Baergen RN: Umbilical cord pathology. Surg Pathol Clin. 6(1):61-85, 2013
3. Proctor LK et al: Umbilical cord diameter percentile curves and their correlation to birth weight and placental pathology. Placenta. 34(1):62-6, 2013
4. Gupta N et al: Allantoic cyst: an unusual umbilical cord swelling. J Surg Case Rep. 2011(4):5, 2011
5. Schaefer IM et al: Giant umbilical cord edema caused by retrograde micturition through an open patent urachus. Pediatr Dev Pathol. 13(5):404-7, 2010
6. Goynumer G et al: Umbilical cord thickness in the first and early second trimesters and perinatal outcome. J Perinat Med. 36(6):523-6, 2008
7. Ghezzi F et al: Sonographic umbilical vessel morphometry and perinatal outcome of fetuses with a lean umbilical cord. J Clin Ultrasound. 33(1):18-23, 2005
8. Emura T et al: Omphalocele associated with a large multilobular umbilical cord pseudocyst. Pediatr Surg Int. 20(8):636-9, 2004
9. Predanic M et al: Fetal aneuploidy and umbilical cord thickness measured between 14 and 23 weeks' gestational age. J Ultrasound Med. 23(9):1177-83; quiz 1185, 2004
10. Sepulveda W et al: Pseudocyst of the umbilical cord: prenatal sonographic appearance and clinical significance. Obstet Gynecol. 93(3):377-81, 1999
11. Babay ZA et al: A case of varix dilatation of the umbilical vein and review of the literature. Fetal Diagn Ther. 11(3):221-3, 1996

Umbilical Cord Edema and Thinning

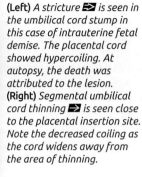

Umbilical Cord Stricture

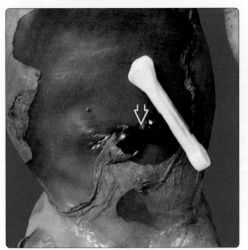

Segmental Umbilical Cord Thinning

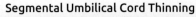
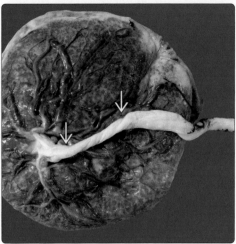

(Left) *A stricture* ⮕ *is seen in the umbilical cord stump in this case of intrauterine fetal demise. The placental cord showed hypercoiling. At autopsy, the death was attributed to the lesion.* **(Right)** *Segmental umbilical cord thinning* ⮕ *is seen close to the placental insertion site. Note the decreased coiling as the cord widens away from the area of thinning.*

Monochorionic Placenta With Discordant Umbilical Cord Thickness

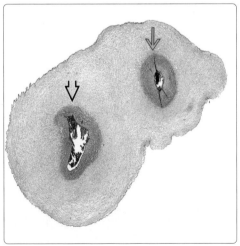

Dichorionic Placenta With Discordant Umbilical Cord Thickness

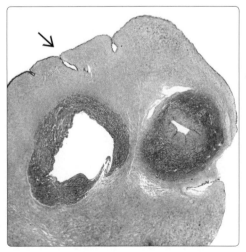

(Left) *This monochorionic twin placenta has a thick* ⮕ *and a thin* ⮕ *umbilical cord. The placental parenchyma shows unequal sharing with the smaller cord associated with a smaller allocation. This may be associated with twin-twin transfusion or selective fetal growth restriction.* **(Right)** *Discordant fetal growth may be reflected in thick and thin cords, as in this dichorionic placenta. The smaller twin was associated with the thinner umbilical cord* ⮕ *and the larger twin with the thicker cord* ⮕. *The placentas are also discordant in weight.*

Thin Umbilical Cord With Single Umbilical Artery

Thin Cord With Decreased Wharton Substance

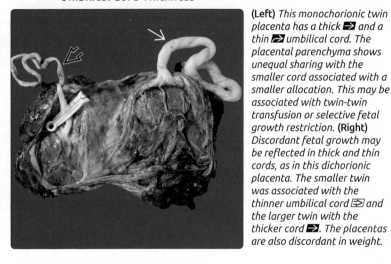

(Left) *This cross section of a thin umbilical cord at term (0.7 cm in diameter) shows only 2 vessels: A single umbilical artery* ⮕ *and vein* ⮕. **(Right)** *This cord has decreased Wharton substance. The cord substance is condensed, and there is very little white space. The vessels are close together and close to the amnion surface. There are deep invaginations of the amnion epithelium into the cord* ⮕, *suggesting a loss of volume. The 2nd artery is out of the field.*

21

TERMINOLOGY

Definitions

- Umbilical phlebitis: Fetal neutrophils in wall of umbilical vein
- Umbilical arteritis: Fetal neutrophils in wall of umbilical artery
- Panvasculitis: Fetal neutrophils in wall of vein and both arteries
- Funisitis: Neutrophils in Wharton substance
- Peripheral funisitis: Accumulation of neutrophils beneath amniotic surface
- Meconium-associated vascular necrosis: Necrosis of vascular smooth muscle in prolonged meconium exposure

Abbreviations

- Umbilical artery (UA)
- Umbilical cord (UC)
- Meconium-associated vascular necrosis (MAVN)

INFLAMMATION OF CORD

Acute Inflammation

- Fetal inflammatory response to stimulus
  - Amniotic fluid infection
    - Most common etiology
  - Chemical irritant, such as meconium
    - Must be localized to area of meconium changes, not associated with other changes of amniotic fluid infection sequence
    - Debate among experts as to whether or not meconium causes acute inflammatory response
  - Local injury
    - E.g., cordocentesis, UC prolapse
- Localization of inflammation correlates with acuity and severity of amniotic fluid infection
  - Early response
    - Phlebitis
  - Intermediate response
    - Arteritis
    - Panvasculitis
  - Late response
    - Funisitis
    - Necrosis
    - Perivascular calcifications
- Fetal inflammatory response in UC associated with
  - Acute chorioamnionitis (maternal inflammatory response)
  - Chorionic plate vasculitis (fetal inflammatory response)
  - Fetal thrombi (when fetal inflammation is severe or prolonged)

Peripheral Funisitis

- Frequent association with *Candida* species
  - May or may not be associated with congenital candidiasis in newborn
    - *Candida* may not be clinically suspected if newborn does not have rash
    - Finding of peripheral funisitis with fungi should prompt call to pediatrician/neonatologist regarding possibility of congenital candidiasis
- Microabscesses elsewhere on amniotic surface with fungal organisms
- Also seen with *Fusobacterium* species

Chronic Inflammation of Cord

- Very uncommon; suggests prolonged infection
- Plasma cell funisitis seen in congenital HSV infection and congenital syphilis
- Fetal eosinophilic/T-cell vasculitis uncommonly seen in umbilical vessels
- Lymphocytes may be seen with neutrophils in ascending pattern of HSV infection

Meconium-Laden Macrophages

- Inflammation in cord usually associated with prolonged meconium exposure
- Similar clinical associations as cases of MAVN

Peripheral Funisitis

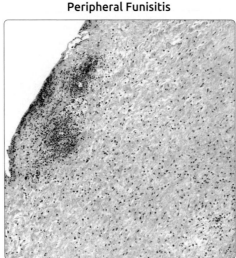

Candida Funisitis

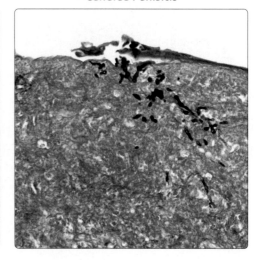

(Left) The term "funisitis" is very general; more specific terms have better clinical relevance. For example, peripheral funisitis (as depicted here) is strongly associated with congenital candidiasis. (Right) A PAS stain highlights the candidal organisms. The clinical team caring for the baby should be notified of such a result as a critical value in placental surgical pathology.

VASCULAR LESIONS OF CORD

Umbilical Cord Thrombi

- ~ 1 in 1,000 deliveries
- More frequent in high-risk pregnancies (1 in 250)
- Incidence of vessel involvement
  - 71% vein alone
    - Based on older studies with less stringent definitions of "thrombosis" than common today
    - Luminal fibrin more common in vein, but true occlusive thrombosis not compatible with life, rare
  - 11% artery alone
  - 18% artery and vein
- Etiology reflected in Virchow triad
  - Blood stasis
    - Cord compression, kinking of undercoiled cord, tight knots, strictures
    - Heart failure, excessively long cord, or increased resistance to flow in severely overcoiled cord
  - Vessel injury
    - Injury to endothelium from severe inflammation, MAVN, or vessel rupture
  - Hypercoagulable state
    - Increased red blood cells in gestational diabetes
    - 3rd spacing of intravascular volume
    - Genetic conditions that cause increased clotting
- Clinical significance
  - Lethal if vein or both arteries occluded
  - Liveborn infants often have neonatal distress or die in newborn period
  - Survivors may have long-term sequelae such as neurologic injury
- Occlusive thrombus
  - Thrombus filling lumen, commonly associated with ischemic necrosis of vessel wall
    - Endothelial cells, myocytes depend on fetal blood for oxygen
  - If older lesion, may see calcification
- Nonocclusive thrombus
  - Thrombus does not fill lumen; may see organization in vessel wall
  - Residual blood flow in part of vessel; vascular wall remains viable
  - Calcification in older lesion
- Associated histopathologic findings in UC
  - Fetal inflammatory response to amniotic fluid infection
  - Meconium-associated vascular necrosis
- Associated histopathologic findings in placenta (fetal vascular malperfusion)
  - Chorionic plate vessel thrombi and obliterative changes
  - Stem villous vessel thrombi and obliterative changes
  - Villous stromal/vascular karyorrhexis and avascular villi

Meconium-Associated Vascular Necrosis

- ~ 1% of meconium-stained placentas
- Meconium deposition leads to myocyte apoptosis in portion of vessel wall underlying meconium staining
- Meconium substance on vascular smooth muscle causes vasoconstriction

- May have linear ulceration overlying necrotic region of vessel
- Clinical implications
  - Frequent Cesarean section delivery due to fetal distress
  - Low Apgar scores
  - Acidemia on UC gases
  - Survivors may have long-term sequelae such as neurologic injury
- Microscopic changes of MAVN
  - Hypereosinophilia of myocytes with pyknotic nuclei
  - Reactive and necrotic changes to amnion associated with meconium
  - Meconium-laden macrophages in cord stroma and membranes
  - May see occlusive or nonocclusive thrombi
  - May see acute and chronic inflammatory cells reacting to meconium
    - Distinguish from amniotic fluid infection by extent of inflammation, with amniotropism elsewhere
    - Meconium deposition and amniotic fluid infection frequently coexist

Vascular Tumors

- Terminology varies in literature: Hemangioma, angioma, angiomyxoma
  - Small lesions composed of prominent capillary proliferations surrounding vitelline vessels
  - Larger lesions with abnormal stroma
    - Myxomatous with cystic degeneration of Wharton substance
    - Fibromuscular stroma, often in continuity with UA
- Very rare, true incidence unknown
- Clinical associations
  - Large lesions may be associated with hydrops due to high-output cardiac failure
  - Rare case reported as arteriovenous malformation at fetal end of cord
    - Associated with lesional thrombi and disseminated intravascular coagulation
    - Unclear if histology of this lesion differs from that most commonly described
  - ~ 1/3 with fetal or neonatal mortality, 1/3 with morbidity, and 1/3 with favorable outcome
  - Associated vascular malformation in neonate in subset of cases (port-wine stain)
- Gross features
  - Often associated with localized edema of UC
  - Reported greatest dimension ranges from 3-18 cm
  - Arise from 1 or both umbilical arteries
  - Most common at placental end of cord, but may be seen at either end
- Microscopic features
  - Irregular proliferation of capillaries separated by myxoid stroma, or sometimes bundles of vascular smooth muscle and fibrovascular connective tissue
- Differential diagnosis
  - Persistence of vitelline vessels
    - Capillary channels form wreath around remnants of vitelline vessels that accompanied omphalomesenteric duct
    - Lacks complexity of vascular angioma

Grading and Staging of Fetal Inflammatory Response in Acute Chorioamnionitis

Diagnostic Category	Suggested Terminology	Definition
Stage 1	Umbilical phlebitis	Involves umbilical vein (and/or chorionic plate vessels)
Stage 2	Umbilical vasculitis (1 umbilical artery and vein) or umbilical panvasculitis (all 3 umbilical vessels)	Involves 1 or both umbilical arteries ± scattered neutrophils in Wharton substance
Stage 3	Necrotizing funisitis, concentric umbilical perivasculitis	Concentric acute inflammation with karyorrhectic debris, eosinophilia of matrix ± mineralization
Grade 1 (mild-moderate)	No additional terminology	Scattered neutrophils beneath endothelium or in vascular smooth muscle, not confluent
Grade 2 (severe)	With a severe fetal inflammatory response	Confluent neutrophils beneath endothelium or in vascular smooth muscle with attenuation of vascular smooth muscle
Other patterns	Peripheral funisitis	Focal aggregates of neutrophils at the umbilical cord surface

Adapted from the Society for Pediatric Pathology Perinatal Section paper: Redline RW et al: Amniotic infection syndrome: nosology and reproducibility of placental reaction patterns. Pediatr Dev Pathol. 6(5):435-48, 2003.

- Abnormal vessels are in Wharton substance, not smooth muscle/fibrous tissue
    - Intrafunicular hematoma
        - Dissection of fetal blood into Wharton substance due to tearing of umbilical vessel (usually vein)
        - Fetal blood in spaces resembles vascular malformation
        - No endothelial lining around blood collections
        - No smooth muscle/fibrous tissue component
        - Up to 50% perinatal mortality
        - May represent delivery artifact with no clinical significance

Segmental Thinning of Umbilical Vessels

- Incidence 1.5%, associated with congenital malformations
- Usually affects < 1/3 of circumference, focal when multiple cord sections submitted
- Media reduced to only 1 or 2 cell layers
- Vein involved 76%, artery involved 24%
- Theoretically increased risk for injury to vessels
- Etiology unclear, dysplastic, or possibly meconium-associated in rare cases

ABNORMALITIES OF CORD STROMA

Decreased Wharton Substance

- Thin UC with reduced cross sectional surface area due to diminished ground substance
- Associated with intrauterine growth restriction
- Associated with reduced umbilical vein flow

Cord Stricture

- Localized absence of Wharton substance causing narrowing of cord and constriction of vascular lumens
- Associated with hypercoiling
- Cause of 2nd- and 3rd-trimester fetal demise
    - Debated whether cause or result of fetal demise
    - Association with hypercoiling and thrombi suggests stricture as cause of demise

SELECTED REFERENCES

1. Doty MS et al: Histologic funisitis and likelihood of intrauterine inflammation or infection: a case-control study. Am J Perinatol. 35(9):858-864, 2018
2. Cimic A et al: Meconium-associated umbilical vascular myonecrosis: correlations with adverse outcome and placental pathology. Pediatr Dev Pathol. 19(4):315-9, 2016
3. Park CW et al: Mild to moderate, but not minimal or severe, acute histologic chorioamnionitis or intra-amniotic inflammation is associated with a decrease in respiratory distress syndrome of preterm newborns without fetal growth restriction. Neonatology. 108(2):115-23, 2015
4. Baergen RN: Cord abnormalities, structural lesions, and cord "accidents". Semin Diagn Pathol. 24(1):23-32, 2007
5. Lee SE et al: The intensity of the fetal inflammatory response in intraamniotic inflammation with and without microbial invasion of the amniotic cavity. Am J Obstet Gynecol. 197(3):294, 2007
6. Redline RW: Inflammatory responses in the placenta and umbilical cord. Semin Fetal Neonatal Med. 11(5):296-301, 2006
7. Sato Y et al: Umbilical arterial thrombosis with vascular wall necrosis: clinicopathologic findings of 11 cases. Placenta. 27(6-7):715-8, 2006
8. Daniel-Spiegel E et al: The association of umbilical cord hemangioma with fetal vascular birthmarks. Prenat Diagn. 25(4):300-3, 2005
9. Korkmaz A et al: Placental apoptosis in pregnancies with intrauterine meconium passage. Am J Perinatol. 22(3):133-8, 2005
10. Redline RW: Severe fetal placental vascular lesions in term infants with neurologic impairment. Am J Obstet Gynecol. 192(2):452-7, 2005
11. Redline RW et al: Amniotic infection syndrome: nosology and reproducibility of placental reaction patterns. Pediatr Dev Pathol. 6(5):435-48, 2003
12. Di Naro E et al: Umbilical vein blood flow in fetuses with normal and lean umbilical cord. Ultrasound Obstet Gynecol. 17(3):224-8, 2001
13. Yoon BH et al: The relationship among inflammatory lesions of the umbilical cord (funisitis), umbilical cord plasma interleukin 6 concentration, amniotic fluid infection, and neonatal sepsis. Am J Obstet Gynecol. 183(5):1124-9, 2000
14. Qureshi F et al: Candida funisitis: a clinicopathologic study of 32 cases. Pediatr Dev Pathol. 1(2):118-24, 1998
15. Richards DS et al: Prenatal diagnosis of fetal disseminated intravascular coagulation associated with umbilical cord arteriovenous malformation. Obstet Gynecol. 85(5 Pt 2):860-2, 1995
16. Qureshi F et al: Marked segmental thinning of the umbilical cord vessels. Arch Pathol Lab Med. 118(8):826-30, 1994
17. Altshuler G et al: Meconium-induced umbilical cord vascular necrosis and ulceration: a potential link between the placenta and poor pregnancy outcome. Obstet Gynecol. 79(5 Pt 1):760-6, 1992
18. Altshuler G et al: Meconium-induced vasocontraction: a potential cause of cerebral and other fetal hypoperfusion and of poor pregnancy outcome. J Child Neurol. 4(2):137-42, 1989
19. Heifetz SA: Thrombosis of the umbilical cord: analysis of 52 cases and literature review. Pediatr Pathol. 8(1):37-54, 1988

Umbilical Arteritis

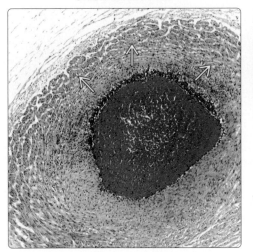

Moderate Umbilical Vein Vasculitis and Funisitis

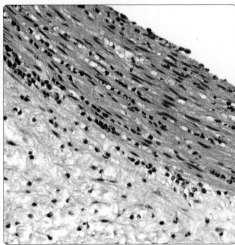

(Left) *In amniotic fluid infection, fetal inflammatory cells migrate toward ➡ the stimulus in the amniotic fluid.* (Right) *The fetal inflammatory response is graded and staged for better clinicopathologic correlation. This image shows a fetal inflammatory response at grade 1 (scattered neutrophils, not confluent). Staging is based upon involvement of the umbilical artery (UA) and necrosis.*

Severe Umbilical Arteritis

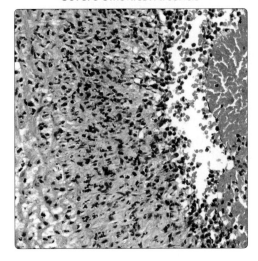

Necrotizing Severe Umbilical Arteritis

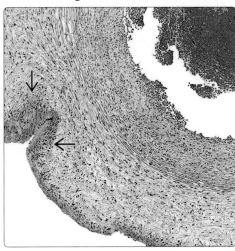

(Left) *The confluence of neutrophils with attenuation of the vascular smooth muscle makes this a grade 2 (severe) fetal inflammatory response. It is stage 2 because it involves the UA.* (Right) *The presence of concentric necrosis around the vessel makes this a grade 2 (severe), stage 3 (necrotizing funisitis) fetal inflammatory response. Also present is peripheral funisitis ➡. Branching hyphae of Candida were easily identified on GMS stain.*

Subacute Necrotizing Funisitis

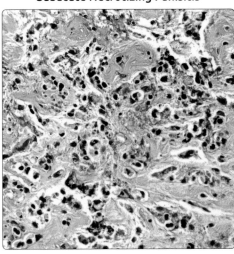

Meconium-Laden Macrophages

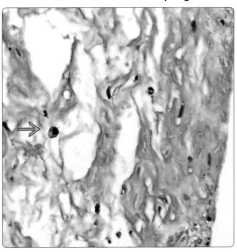

(Left) *This case of necrotizing funisitis contains karyorrhectic cells and mononuclear cells. Plasma cells are uncommon in the cord. Longstanding bacterial infection may have plasma cells, but it is always prudent to exclude herpes simplex virus infection or syphilis in such cases.* (Right) *Meconium-laden macrophages ➡ are not as common in the cord stroma as in the membranes. Identification requires careful searching. Similar to meconium-associated vascular necrosis (MAVN), they are associated with poor clinical outcomes.*

(Left) *This flattened area* 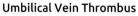 *of the cord shows an umbilical vein (UV) thrombus in a case of fetal demise. These findings suggest compression from limb/body entanglement, such as a nuchal cord.* **(Right)** *Laminations attest to in vivo clot formation in this UV thrombus.*

Umbilical Vein Thrombus

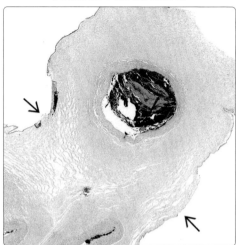

Umbilical Vein Thrombus

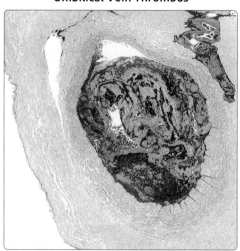

(Left) *This liveborn neonate had extensive changes of fetal vascular malperfusion in the placenta.* **(Right)** *The nonocclusive thrombus of the UV is not associated with necrosis of the media.*

Nonocclusive Umbilical Vein Thrombus

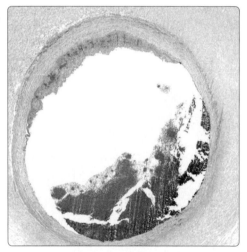

Nonocclusive Umbilical Vein Thrombus

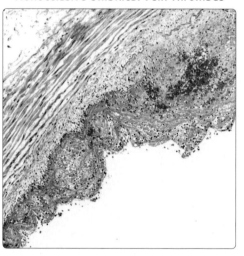

(Left) *Low-power clues to thrombosis include lines of Zahn (layering of fibrin)* 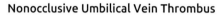 *in the lumen and pallor of the media* 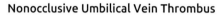*.* **(Right)** *The vascular smooth muscle is losing viability with loss of nuclear basophilia* 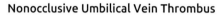*.*

Umbilical Artery Thrombus

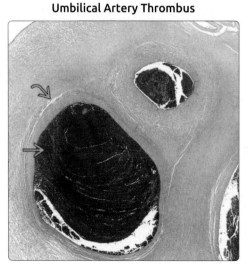

Umbilical Artery Thrombus

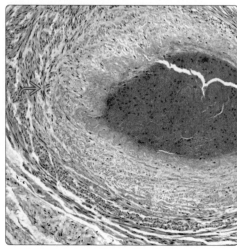

Meconium-Associated Vascular Necrosis

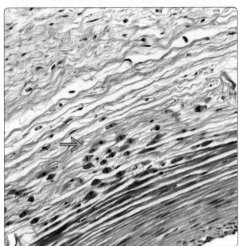

Umbilical Cord Torsion

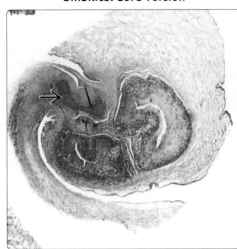

(Left) *MAVN is the result of toxic effects of meconium on the vascular smooth muscle. Apoptosis* ⇨ *of smooth muscle cells is seen in the outer layer.* (Right) *Spiraling is evident on this cross section through a stricture. The vessels are partially collapsed. The UV contains some degenerated blood product* ⇨*, while the arteries are empty.*

Segmental Thinning of Umbilical Vein

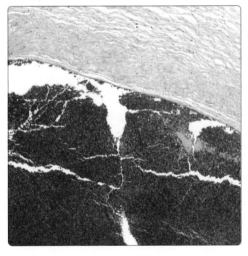

Segmental Thinning of Umbilical Vein

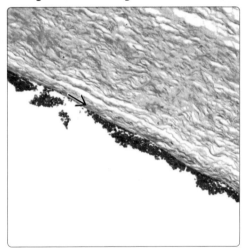

(Left) *Approximately 30% of the perimeter of the UV on this section shows marked thinning of the media with no visible smooth muscle layers.* (Right) *Trichrome staining shows only a minimal residual layer* ⇨ *of lavender-appearing smooth muscle in this UV.*

Angiomyxoma

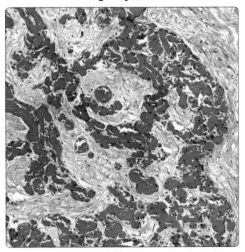

Angiomyxoma

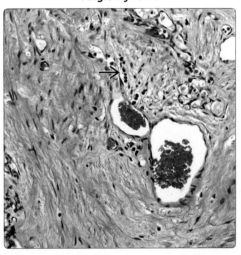

(Left) *An irregular proliferation of small capillaries is set in a loose myxomatous stroma.* (Right) *Extramedullary hematopoiesis* ⇨ *frequently accompanies the vascular proliferation.*

TERMINOLOGY

Definitions

- Extraplacental membranes: Amnion, chorion, and decidua extending from edge of placental disc
- Extrachorial placentation: Insertion of extraplacental membranes inside boundary of placental disc
- Chorion laeve: Membranous chorion
- Decidua capsularis: Layer of gestational endometrium overlying implanted conceptus
- Decidua parietalis: All decidua not overlying or underneath implanted conceptus

Synonyms

- Decidua parietalis and decidua vera

GROSS EVALUATION

Integrity

- Amnion normally loosely adherent to chorion
  - May slip entirely from chorion when edematous, but remains strongly attached to cord
- Amount of decidua present is variable
- Membranes excessively torn and shredded in hydropic placenta
- Torn membranes often discarded in delivery room

Color and Opacity

- Normal: Pink-white, variably translucent, glistening
- Chorioamnionitis: Usually yellow-white, opaque appearing
- Meconium: Variable with extent and chronicity
  - Recent: Blue-green, glistening, may have fresh meconium on surface
  - Subacute: Dark green-brown, slippery, and edematous
  - Chronic: Diffusely muddy brown (especially cord surface), dull appearing
- Retromembranous hemorrhage
  - Older hemorrhage is green-brown or yellow-tan on decidual side

Insertion

- Normal insertion of membranes is at disc margin
  - Fusion of chorionic plate and basal plate at margin create inner boundary of intervillous space
- Extrachorial placentation, 2 types
  - Circumvallate and circummarginate
    - Circumvallate placenta: Important diagnosis
      □ Membranes fold onto themselves, forming lip at junction of extraplacental membranes and chorionic disc
  - Circummarginate placenta
    - Membranes arise inside circumference of margin with flat junction
    - Thin fibrin ring may be present
    - Relatively common (6-20% of placentas)
    - No definite clinical significance

Measurements

- Distance from point of membrane rupture to disc margin
  - Only relevant in vaginal delivery with relatively intact membranes
  - Gives estimate of distance between placental implantation site and cervical os
  - Measurements < 2 cm suggest **placenta previa**
    - Placental implantation in lower uterine segment, with disc parenchyma overlying cervical os
    - ~ 1 in 2,500 gestations
    - Recognized clinically on US
    - Associated with marginal retroplacental hemorrhage, placenta accreta
    - May present with diffuse vaginal bleeding, premature labor
    - Risk of fetal exsanguination secondary to tearing of placental parenchyma
    - Partial placenta previa defined as disc edge within 2 cm of cervical os

---

Gross Appearance of Membranes

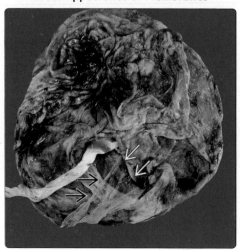

Normal Histology of Membranes

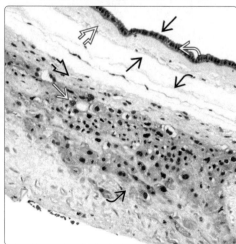

(Left) *This image shows membranes in anatomic position. Note the thin, translucent amnion ➡ partially separated from the thicker chorion and decidual layers ➡.* **(Right)** *Layers include amnion ➡ (amniotic epithelium with basement membrane ➡, connective tissue ➡) and chorion ➡ (chorionic mesoderm ➡ and cellular chorion ➡ with intermediate extravillous trophoblast).*

SECTIONS TO BE SUBMITTED

Membrane Rolls

- 2 membrane rolls ideal for identification of significant pathology
- Multiple methods described; following is useful for fresh or fixed tissue and involves tools present in most surgical pathology grossing stations
  - Instruments: Grooved forceps without teeth, 2 pins, cork board, scissors, and scalpel
  - Cut strip 2-4 cm in width perpendicular to site of rupture, leaving attachment to disc margin
  - Roll membranes around forceps grasping site of membrane rupture perpendicular to strip
  - Transfix roll to cork board at disc margin with 2 pins going through roll and center of forceps
  - Remove forceps, roll should remain intact
  - Take 2 sections of roll, ~ 5 mm in width sectioning on either side of pins
- If amnion stripped from chorion, submit representative sample separate from roll

MICROSCOPIC EVALUATION

Amnion

- Extension of fetal skin
- Normal histology
  - Single layer of cuboidal epithelial cells overlying basement membrane, adherent to connective tissue layer
  - Squamous metaplasia
    - May see full stratified squamous epithelium with keratinization
    - More common near term
    - More common near cord insertion
    - Excessive squamous metaplasia occurs with abrasion or trauma

Chorion

- Normal histology
  - Composed of trophoblast and connective tissue
    - Inner cellular layer of chorionic mesoderm
    - Reticular layer
    - Pseudobasement membrane layer
    - Outer trophoblastic layer

Decidua

- Gestational endometrium
- Normal histology
  - Decidual stromal cells
  - Spiral arteries
  - Veins
  - Endometrial glands: Uncommon in 3rd-trimester membranous decidua
  - Scattered lymphocytes and uterine NK cells

PLACENTAL DIAGNOSES FROM GROSS EXAM OF MEMBRANES

Placenta Membranacea

- Incidence
  - Rare (1 in 3,000-4,000 gestations)

- Etiology/pathogenesis
  - Extraplacental membranes fail to form
  - Chorionic villi covering early gestational sac do not regress
- Gross appearance
  - Cotyledons scattered throughout what should be membranes
  - Villous parenchyma diffusely thin (1-2 cm)
- Clinical associations
  - Vaginal bleeding
  - Placenta previa and accreta
  - Preterm delivery, fetal and neonatal morbidity
  - Should be suspected clinically, ensure membranes were not discarded at delivery

Circumvallate Placenta

- Incidence
  - Occurs in 1-2% of placentas
- Etiology/pathogenesis
  - Most likely marginal abruptions with fibrin accumulation
- Gross appearance
  - Membranes fold onto themselves, forming lip at junction of extraplacental membranes and chorionic disc
- Microscopic findings
  - Fibrin, infarcted villi of margin folded over surface with doubled membranes
- Clinical associations
  - Intrauterine growth retardation
  - Intrauterine fetal demise
  - Low Apgar scores
  - Oligohydramnios
  - Placental abruption
    - Clinically described entity: Chronic abruption-oligohydramnios sequence with severe circumvallation
    - May have diffuse chorioamniotic hemosiderosis of membranes on microscopic examination

SELECTED REFERENCES

1. Ravangard SF et al: Placenta membranacea. Arch Gynecol Obstet. 288(3):709-12, 2013
2. Suzuki S: Clinical significance of pregnancies with circumvallate placenta. J Obstet Gynaecol Res. 34(1):51-4, 2008
3. Winters R et al: What is adequate sampling of extraplacental membranes?: a randomized, prospective analysis. Arch Pathol Lab Med. 132(12):1920-3, 2008
4. Ohyama M et al: Maternal, neonatal, and placental features associated with diffuse chorioamniotic hemosiderosis, with special reference to neonatal morbidity and mortality. Pediatrics. 113(4):800-5, 2004
5. Elliott JP et al: Chronic abruption-oligohydramnios sequence. J Reprod Med. 43(5):418-22, 1998

Origin of Membrane Layers

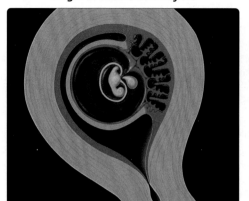

Membrane Color

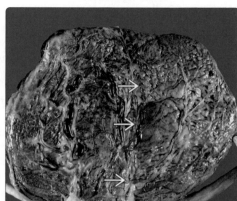

(Left) *The distinct membrane layers arise from separate structures. Amnion (green) surrounds the embryo. As the amniotic sac enlarges, amnion covers the cord and is apposed to the chorion (blue). The decidua capsularis (light pink) is the gestational endometrium overlying the conceptus. The decidua basalis is in purple. The rest of the decidua (fuchsia) eventually becomes apposed to the decidua capsularis.* (Right) *The membrane color is noted on gross exam. The membranes of one twin are green ➡, suggesting meconium.*

Membrane Opacity

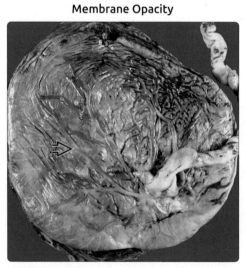

Gross Evaluation of Membranes

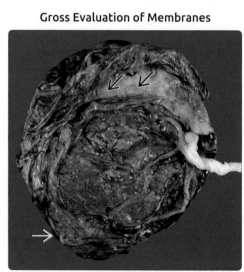

(Left) *Membrane opacity is best appreciated on the disc surface. The milky white opacity ⊃ here suggests acute inflammation (chorioamnionitis).* (Right) *The point of membrane rupture ➡ is assessed in vaginal deliveries. The shortest distance from the edge of the membranes to the disc insertion is measured. Values < 2 cm suggest a low-lying placenta. Note partial circumvallate insertion ⊃.*

Extrachorial Placentation

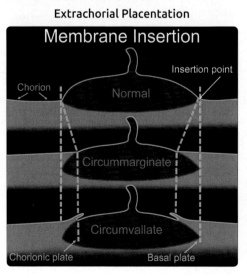

Circummarginate Membrane Insertion

(Left) *Membranes normally insert at the disc margin where the chorionic plate and basal plate meet. With circummarginate and circumvallate insertion, the membranes arise from within the circumference of the disc (lavender line). Circummarginate insertion is flat; circumvallate insertion is raised by a fold.* (Right) *In circummarginate membrane insertion, a fibrin ring ➡ delineates the site of membrane insertion inside the circumference of the disc margin. The insertion is flat.*

Circumvallate Membrane Insertion

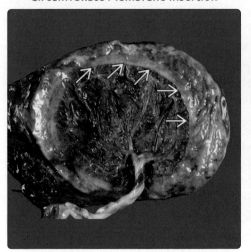

Circumvallate Membrane Insertion

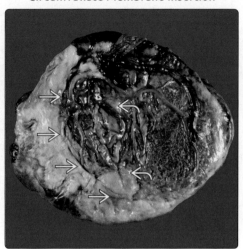

(Left) *Membrane insertion is circumvallate* ➡ *for 50% of the circumference and circummarginate for the remainder. The circumvallate insertion is raised from the surface, whereas the circummarginate portion is flat.* **(Right)** *Partial circumvallate membrane insertion* ➡ *is shown. The yellow discoloration suggests old hemorrhage and necrosis, consistent with chronic abruption. An older hematoma* ➡ *beneath the chorion is consistent with extension of a marginal hemorrhage.*

Circumvallate Membrane Histology

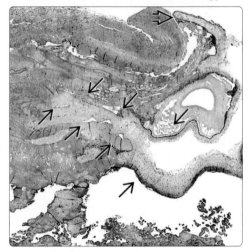

Amnion Nodosum

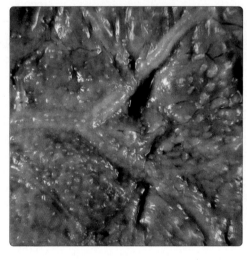

(Left) *The fold in circumvallate membrane insertion is easily recognized microscopically. The membranes fold over* ➡ *before the free edge* ➡ *arises. Abundant old hemorrhage is present behind the membrane.* **(Right)** *Amnion nodosum is noted on gross exam. The amnion is covered in small white plaques, strongly associated with oligohydramnios. In oligohydramnios, fetal squames become concentrated and deposited on the surface of the placenta.*

Histology of Membranes

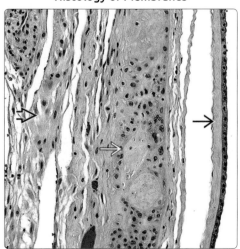

Maternal Spiral Arteries

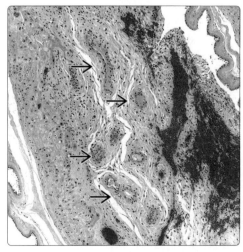

(Left) *Normal membrane histology is shown. The amnion epithelium* ➡ *is low cuboidal, separated from the chorion by a space. The cellular chorion* ➡ *contains extravillous trophoblast as well as occasional regressed villi from the chorion frondosum of the gestational sac. The adherent decidua* ➡ *is viable with scattered lymphocytes.* **(Right)** *The amount of decidua found in membrane rolls is variable. The membranous decidua is often the best place to observe maternal spiral arteries* ➡.

CONTENT

Scope of Discussion

- Changes of amnion and chorion of placental membranes
- Membranous decidua discussed separately

CHANGES OF AMNION

Reactive Changes

- Low cuboidal epithelium of amnion becomes columnar or pseudostratified columnar
  - Rarely becomes hyperplastic with polypoid projections
- Cytoplasm becomes vacuolated
  - Gastroschisis associated with diffuse, fine vacuolization

Amniocyte Necrosis

- Early: Loss of nuclear basophilia
- Later: Cell dropout
- Occurs in response to toxic substance (e.g., meconium, blood) or severe prolonged inflammation (necrotizing chorioamnionitis)

Edema

- Amnion slips from underlying chorion
- Basement membrane becomes thickened and eosinophilic
- Occurs with meconium, severe chorioamnionitis, fetal hydrops

Amnion Nodosum

- Deposition of fetal squames as nodules on surface of amnion
- Associated with severe prolonged oligohydramnios, anhydramnios

Amniotic Bands

- Amnion degenerates, separates from chorion during pregnancy, usually in 1st or early 2nd trimester
- Strips of amnion or connective tissue from extraembryonic celom may twist around limbs or face causing amputations or other disruptions

- Cause of separation unclear; possible associations include maternal hyperglycemia, high-altitude pregnancies, genetic abnormalities, collagen and connective tissue disorders, trauma, and prior uterine surgeries

Squamous Metaplasia

- Common change at term
- More often seen in amnion of cord and overlying chorionic plate

CHANGES OF CHORION

Changes in Chorionic Trophoblast Cell Number

- Usually decrease in number by term
- May proliferate as small cuboidal cells or cuboidal vacuolated cells

Microscopic Chorionic Cysts

- Chorionic trophoblast cells secrete extracellular matrix-forming microscopic cysts filled with homogeneous-appearing pink fluid
- Microscopic chorionic cysts are type of extravillous trophoblast cysts discussed separately

Chorionic Trophoblast Nuclear Pleomorphism

- Some degree of nuclear pleomorphism is common; may be related to tendency for extravillous trophoblast to become polyploid
  - Marked pleomorphism described in membranous chorionic trophoblast after cytotoxic chemotherapy
  - Some authors associate finding with hypoxia

Chorion Nodosum

- Nodules of fetal squames embedded in chorionic mesenchyme
- Uncommon finding, only seen when chorion is exposed to fetal squames in amniotic fluid for prolonged period of time
  - Early amnion rupture with amniotic bands, extraamniotic pregnancy, rarely in severe cases of amniotic fluid infection or meconium exposure when amnion has disintegrated

(Left) Acute chorioamnionitis is a maternal inflammatory response ➡ and the hallmark of amniotic fluid infection. Grading and staging the inflammatory response is helpful for clinical correlation. Mild acute chorioamnionitis may be clinically silent. (Right) Meconium deposition in the placenta causes characteristic reactive and necrotic ➡ changes in the amnion. This early change is characteristic but not entirely specific. Meconium pigment should be sought for diagnosis.

Mild Acute Chorioamnionitis

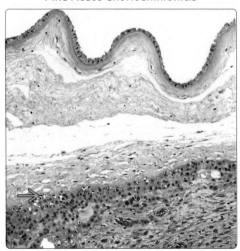

Reactive and Necrotic Changes of Amnion

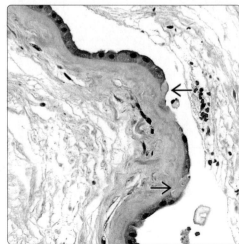

Grading and Staging of Maternal Inflammatory Response in Acute Chorioamnionitis

Category	Suggested Terminology	Definition
Stage 1: Early	Acute subchorionitis (chorionic plate) or chorionitis (membranes)	Acute inflammation limited to subchorionic space or membranous trophoblast, not extending into fibrous chorion
Stage 2: Intermediate	Acute chorioamnionitis	Diffuse or patchy acute inflammation of fibrous chorion &/or amnion
Stage 3: Advanced	Necrotizing chorioamnionitis	Necrotizing acute inflammation of chorion and amnion characterized by neutrophil karyorrhexis, amniocyte necrosis, ± amnion basement membrane thickening or hypereosinophilia
Grade 1: Mild-moderate	(No additional descriptor recommended)	Scattered neutrophils, insufficient in extent to meet criteria for "severe"
Grade 2: Severe	Severe acute chorioamnionitis **or** with subchorionic microabscesses	Confluent neutrophils (> 10 x 20 cells in extent); ≥ 3 isolated foci or in continuous band

Excerpted from Redline RW et al: Amniotic infection syndrome: nosology and reproducibility of placental reaction patterns. Pediatr Dev Pathol. 6(5):435-48, 2003.

- After fetal surgery

CHORIOAMNIONITIS

Acute Inflammation

- Hallmark of amniotic fluid infection
- Prominent cause of premature birth, especially in cases of premature rupture of membranes
- Frequently no association with clinical signs of chorioamnionitis
- Associated with ascending infection of membranes and amniotic fluid by genitourinary organisms
- Chorioamnionitis is maternal inflammatory response with migration of maternal neutrophils toward infected amniotic fluid
  - Maternal neutrophils migrate from intervillous blood space across chorionic plate and from decidual vessels across chorion and amnion
- Several grading systems exist, including one proposed by Society for Pediatric Pathology Perinatal Section, adopted by international consensus committees
  - Grading and staging system terminology aims to describe extent and severity of inflammation

Chronic Inflammation

- Usually lymphocytic, termed chronic chorioamnionitis
  - Also maternal inflammatory response but less commonly associated with infectious causes; usually associated with chronic villitis
  - Associated with late preterm birth
- Grading and staging of chronic chorioamnionitis
  - Grade 1: > 2 foci of inflammation or patchy inflammation
  - Grade 2: Continuous diffuse inflammation
  - Stage 1: Inflammation limited to chorionic trophoblast layer, sparing chorioamniotic connective tissue
  - Stage 2: Inflammation extends into chorioamniotic connective tissue
- Numerous histiocytes in chorion underlying necrotizing acute inflammation is termed subacute chorioamnionitis
  - Associated with chronic lung disease in infants

- Histologically and clinically distinct from chronic chorioamnionitis

PIGMENTED MACROPHAGES

Meconium

- Yellow-brown pigment found in amnion or chorion
- Characteristic reactive and necrotic changes in amnion

Diffuse Chorioamniotic Hemosiderosis

- Hemosiderin deposition in chorion and amnion of membranes and chorionic plate
  - Iron stain is positive
- Involves 1-2% of placentas submitted for pathologic examination
- Strongly associated with recurrent venous hemorrhage at margin of placenta (chronic abruption) as well as prematurity
  - Associated with circumvallate membranes, massive subchorial hematoma, chronic abruption-oligohydramnios sequence, persistent pulmonary hypertension, and rarely pulmonary hypoplasia in neonate
- May have amnion necrosis, acute chorioamnionitis, subacute chorioamnionitis

SELECTED REFERENCES

1. Khong TY et al: Sampling and definitions of placental lesions: Amsterdam Placental Workshop Group consensus statement. Arch Pathol Lab Med. 140(7):698-713, 2016
2. Kim CJ et al: Chronic inflammation of the placenta: definition, classification, pathogenesis, and clinical significance. Am J Obstet Gynecol. 213(4 Suppl):S53-69, 2015
3. Yamada S et al: Pulmonary hypoplasia on preterm infant associated with diffuse chorioamniotic hemosiderosis caused by intrauterine hemorrhage due to massive subchorial hematoma: report of a neonatal autopsy case. Pathol Int. 62(8):543-8, 2012
4. Abellar RG et al: Effects of chemotherapy during pregnancy on the placenta. Pediatr Dev Pathol. 12(1):35-41, 2009
5. Stanek J et al: Chorion nodosum: a placental feature of the severe early amnion rupture sequence. Pediatr Dev Pathol. 9(5):353-60, 2006
6. Redline RW et al: Amniotic infection syndrome: nosology and reproducibility of placental reaction patterns. Pediatr Dev Pathol. 6(5):435-48, 2003

Amnion in Gastroschisis

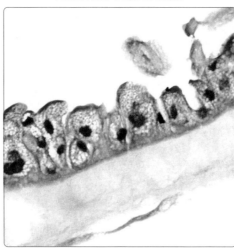

Coarse Vacuolation of Amnion

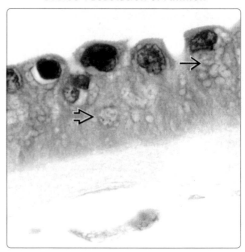

(Left) *The vacuolation in gastroschisis is fine and diffuse.* **(Right)** *With meconium exposure, the vacuolation ⇥ is more coarse with greater variability in size than in gastroschisis. Traces of meconium pigment ⇥ can be seen in some vacuoles.*

Reactive Changes of Amnion

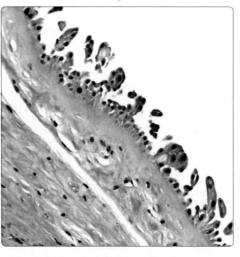

Reactive Amnion With Necrosis and Meconium Pigment

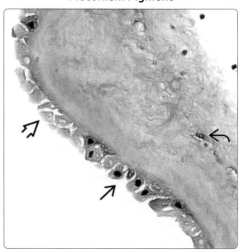

(Left) *In addition to vacuolation, the epithelium may become columnar or pseudostratified in reactive conditions.* **(Right)** *Meconium deposition is characteristically associated with reactive and necrotic changes in the amnion. The cells become columnar or pseudostratified ⇥ (reactive change) and lose nuclear basophilia ⇥ (necrotic change). Meconium pigment is present focally ⇥.*

Amnion Edema

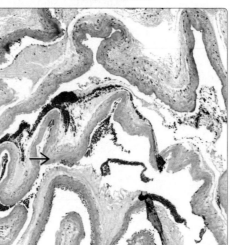

Amniotic Bands

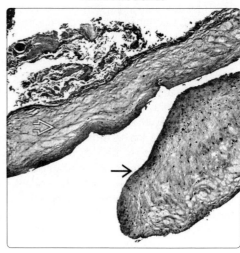

(Left) *Edematous amnion slips from the surface of the chorion and is difficult to sample in a membrane roll. It should be sampled separately. With edema, the amnion basement membrane is thickened and eosinophilic ⇥.* **(Right)** *Amniotic bands are strips of amnion that have separated from the chorion and float in the amniotic fluid. They may constrict fetal body parts and cause amputations or other disruptions. The epithelium is commonly eroded ⇥, and the mesenchyme appears edematous ⇥.*

Histopathologic Changes of Membranes

Amnion Nodosum

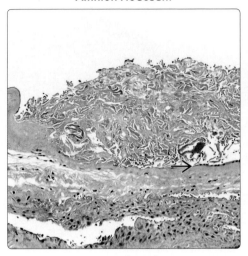

Squamous Metaplasia of the Amnion

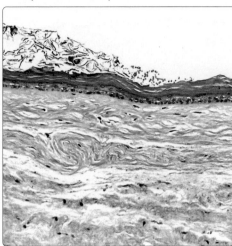

(Left) *Amnion nodosum is characterized by nodules of mostly anucleate squames deposited on the surface of the amnion. The amniotic epithelium is eroded or remains cuboidal ➡. Amnion nodosum is strongly associated with oligohydramnios.* (Right) *In contrast, squamous metaplasia is not necessarily a pathologic process. The cuboidal amniotic epithelium is replaced by squamous epithelium. Focal keratinization is seen mimicking amnion nodosum.*

Amnion Nodosum

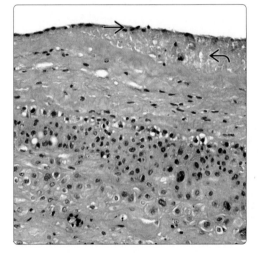

Chorion Nodosum

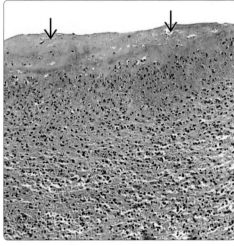

(Left) *Amnion nodosum can also form plaques on the amniotic surface ➡. Focal epithelial overgrowth ➡ suggests some chronicity.* (Right) *Chorion nodosum shows plaque-like deposits of fetal squames ➡ embedded in the chorion with no amnion. The amnion was disintegrated in this case of severe necrotizing acute chorioamnionitis. Chorion nodosum is also seen in cases of early amnion separation with amniotic bands.*

Microscopic Chorionic Cysts

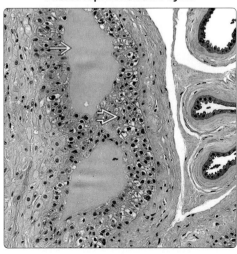

Chorionic Trophoblast Nuclear Pleomorphism

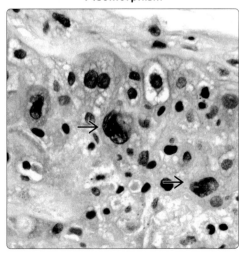

(Left) *The chorionic trophoblast ➡ may be abundant and form microscopic cysts ➡. When these trophoblast cells proliferate, they often have a smaller, cuboidal appearance with clear cytoplasm.* (Right) *Chorionic trophoblast cells normally show some degree of nuclear pleomorphism ➡. This pleomorphism may be exaggerated in some conditions, including postmaternal chemotherapy.*

Mild Acute Chorionitis

Moderate Acute Chorioamnionitis

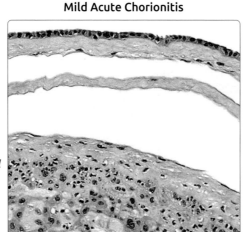
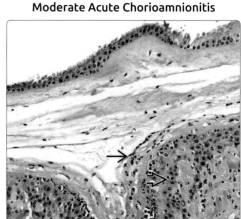

(Left) The earliest manifestation of amniotic fluid infection sequence is shown in this example of mild acute chorionitis, maternal inflammatory response grade 1, stage 1. Caution is warranted not to mistake karyorrhectic chorionic trophoblast for neutrophils. (Right) In this case of acute chorioamnionitis, the maternal inflammation is still limited in extent (grade 1, mild-moderate). Neutrophils ➡ extend above the cellular chorion ⇛ (stage 2, intermediate).

Severe Acute Chorioamnionitis

Necrotizing Severe Acute Chorioamnionitis

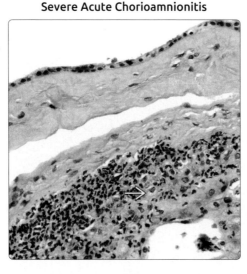

(Left) The intensity of the maternal neutrophilic response is greater in this case of acute chorioamnionitis (grade 2, severe). Neutrophils extend above the cellular chorion ⇛ (stage 2, intermediate). (Right) The large aggregates of neutrophils ⇛ define this as grade 2 (severe). Karyorrhexis of neutrophils ➡ with spotty amniocyte necrosis ➡ evince stage 3, necrotizing acute chorioamnionitis.

Necrotizing Severe Acute Chorioamnionitis

Subacute Necrotizing Chorioamnionitis

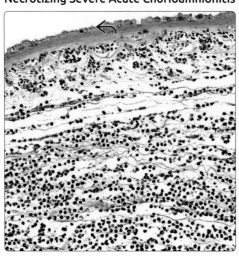
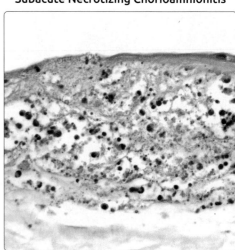

(Left) This amnion is severely inflamed and edematous. The epithelial cells are necrotic ➡. The maternal inflammatory response is grade 2 (severe), stage 3 (necrotizing). (Right) Subacute chorioamnionitis shows karyorrhexis of neutrophils. This inflammatory pattern is most often seen in early preterm births and suggests prolonged amniotic fluid infection.

Gram-Negative Rods in Membranes

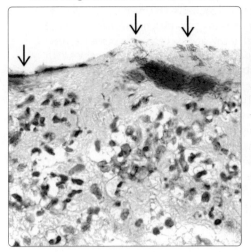

Necrotizing Acute Chorioamnionitis

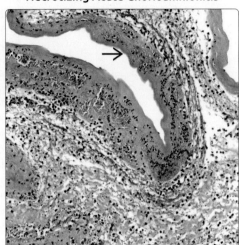

(Left) *Tissue Gram stains may identify organisms in acute chorioamnionitis. Numerous gram-negative rods ⊟ are present in this case.* (Right) *Severe prolonged amniotic fluid infection is manifest in this case of severe necrotizing acute and subacute chorioamnionitis (grade 2, stage 3). Note there is karyorrhexis of neutrophils and amniocyte necrosis with thickening and hypereosinophilia of the amnion basement membrane ⊟.*

Chronic Chorioamnionitis

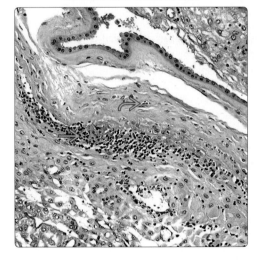

Granulomatous Chronic Chorioamnionitis

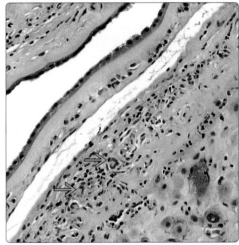

(Left) *Chronic chorioamnionitis shows a band-like infiltrate of lymphocytes ⊟ associated with degeneration or cell dropout of the chorionic trophoblast cells. Extension above the cellular chorion ⊟ is stage 2.* (Right) *Rarely, chronic chorioamnionitis has a granulomatous appearance with histiocytes admixed with the lymphocytes ⊟. Note the absence of chorionic trophoblastic cells.*

Hemosiderin Laden Macrophages

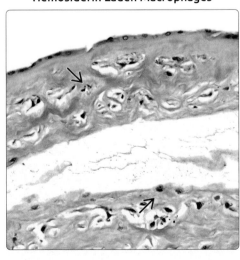

Chorioamniotic Hemosiderosis

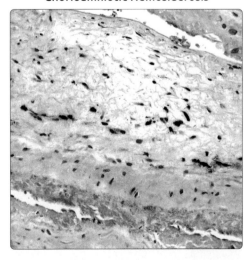

(Left) *Not all pigment in the membranes is meconium. Hemosiderin ⊟ is found with chronic abruption, cases of intraamniotic hemorrhage, or near a subchorionic hematoma.* (Right) *An iron stain shows extensive hemosiderin deposition in this case of diffuse chorioamniotic hemosiderosis (DCH). DCH has clinical correlations with prematurity, chronic abruption, and oligohydramnios as well as respiratory disease in the neonate.*

TERMINOLOGY

Abbreviations

- Chorionic plate (CP)

Synonyms

- Fetal surface of placenta

Definitions

- CP forms fetal surface of placental disc
  - Distinct from
    - Chorion frondosum, which is placenta villous tissue proper of disc
    - Chorion laeve, which is avascular membranous portion of chorionic sac
- CP vasculature
  - Represents branches of umbilical vessels that extend onto CP of placenta
  - Fetal in origin and carries only fetal blood

ETIOLOGY/PATHOGENESIS

Histogenesis

- CP development begins when 1st lacunae appear in syncytiotrophoblast layer (day 8 post conception)
- Hemangioblastic foci develop in CP from 4- to 9-weeks gestation
- Fetal allantoic blood vessels of umbilical cord connect with CP vessels in 2nd month of gestation
  - Full chorionic circulation between embryo and placenta established in early 2nd trimester

MACROSCOPIC

Shape of Chorionic Plate

- Reflects shape of entire placental disc
- Most are oval or elliptical, less commonly round
- ~ 10% of cases have variations of shape
  - Bilobed
    - 2-8% of placentas
    - ~ 2 equal-sized lobes are separated by membranes

- Umbilical cord most commonly inserts between 2 lobes (66%) or upon 1 of 2 lobes
- 2 lobes are connected by membranous vessels, vulnerable to compression, tear, and thrombosis
- Both bilobed and succenturiate placentas are associated with implantation over regions with variable uterine perfusion (leiomyomas, cornu, cervical os)
  - Succenturiate lobes/accessory lobes
    - 5-6% of placentas
    - Similar to bilobed but with unequal-sized lobes
    - Cord usually inserts in larger lobe
    - 2 lobes are connected by membranous vessels, vulnerable to compression, tear, and thrombosis
    - Infarction or atrophy of smaller lobe is common
  - Placenta membranacea
    - Very rare
    - Nearly all of fetal sac is covered by villous tissue; CP extends over all of what is usually extraplacental membranes
    - Typically, thin disc with limited villous growth
    - May have very large disc diameter with little to no attached free membranes
    - May appear as small disc with individual cotyledons scattered across free membranes
    - Can present clinically with 2nd-trimester vaginal bleeding and placenta previa
    - Often associated with abnormal implantation (placenta accreta, increta)
  - Placenta fenestra
    - Very rare
    - CP has defect within circumference
    - Underlying villous parenchyma is atrophied such that only tissue resembling free membranes is left covering defect
    - Atrophied region is likely due to implantation over focal region of poor perfusion, such as leiomyoma
    - Differentiate from missing cotyledon, which would have irregular, torn-appearing surface on basal surface, or iatrogenic villous sampling after delivery

CP Vasculature

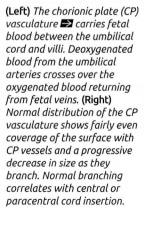

(Left) The chorionic plate (CP) vasculature ➡ carries fetal blood between the umbilical cord and villi. Deoxygenated blood from the umbilical arteries crosses over the oxygenated blood returning from fetal veins. (Right) Normal distribution of the CP vasculature shows fairly even coverage of the surface with CP vessels and a progressive decrease in size as they branch. Normal branching correlates with central or paracentral cord insertion.

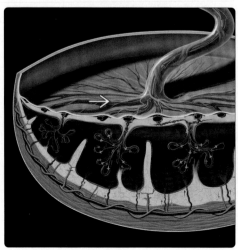

CP Vasculature

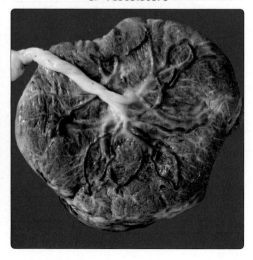

o Annular placenta (zonary)
  – Very rare
  – Disc is round or oval; villous parenchyma is distributed in ring underneath CP with central thinned area
  – Large central atrophic zone may represent implantation over cervical os with atrophy of central region not supported by decidua

Umbilical Cord Insertion

- CP is site of umbilical cord insertion in most placentas
- Eccentric insertions considered normal
- Other insertion types: Marginal, velamentous, furcate

Normal Gross Appearance and Physiology of Chorionic Plate Vessels

- CP vessels represent branches of umbilical vessels
- Artery-vein pairs generally travel together on CP
- Arteries traverse over veins
- Chorionic arteries carry deoxygenated blood toward placental cotyledon (villous parenchyma)
- Chorionic veins carry oxygenated blood away from placental cotyledon and toward umbilical vein to fetus
- Muscular chorionic vessels can experience rhythmic contraction and are responsive to vasodilatory and vasoconstrictive mediators

Vascular Distribution Pattern

- Mechanisms that determine this pattern are not fully understood
  o Study of placental vasculature casts reveals 2 patterns of chorionic vessel branching
    – Dichotomous pattern: Symmetrical branching into 2 fairly similar daughter vessels
    – Monopodial pattern: Main, long mother tube that courses for long distance with almost constant diameter and has only small-diameter daughter tubes that branch off to sides
  o Branching architecture is typically combination of dichotomous and monopodial patterns
  o First 2-3 generations are always dichotomous

Patterns of Chorionic Vessel Coverage of Plate

- Disperse
  o Fine network of vessels that course from cord insertion and extend fairly evenly over CP, diminishing in diameter as they extend distally
    – Most common type is present in ~ 2/3 of placentas
    – Associated with centrally and paracentrally inserted umbilical cord
- Magistral
  o Less evenly distributed vessels with arteries that course to edge of placenta without diminishing in diameter
    – Less common type is present in ~ 1/3 of placentas
    – Associated with marginal and velamentous umbilical cord insertion
- Morphometric evidence that, compared with eccentric/marginal cord insertion, central cord insertion is associated with denser vascular coverage of CP

Chorionic Plate Vasculature in Twin Placentas

- Features of CP in fused dichorionic, diamniotic placentas

o Percentage of shared placental disc that belongs to each twin is determined by position of dividing membrane on CP
o Dividing membrane is firmly attached to CP
o Thickened ridge (T-zone) at attachment of dividing membrane to CP usually visible
o Dividing membrane is thick and composed of 2 amnions and 2 fused chorions
o Chorionic vascular territory for each twin terminates at dividing membrane with no intertwin vascular connections

- Features of CP in monochorionic, diamniotic placentas
  o Percentage of shared placental disc that belongs to each twin is determined by outlines of CP vasculature
  o Dividing membrane is not firmly attached to CP and may tear away easily
  o No thickened ridge at attachment of dividing membrane to CP is present
  o Dividing membrane is thin and composed of only 2 amnions
  o Chorionic vascular territory for each twin does not terminate at dividing membrane
    – Vessels of either twin can traverse beneath dividing membrane
  o Intertwin vascular connections may be visible on CP (3 types)
    – Artery-to-artery connection
      □ Superficial connection/anastomosis, in which blood can be moved directly from artery of 1 twin into artery of other twin
    – Vein-to-vein connection
      □ Superficial connection/anastomosis, in which blood can be moved directly from vein of 1 twin into vein of other twin
    – Arteriovenous connection
      □ Unpaired artery from 1 twin enters cotyledon adjacent to unpaired draining vein from other twin
  o Unique features of acardiac twin/twin reversed arterial perfusion
    – Large intertwin artery-to-artery connection with accompanying large vein-to-vein connection
    – Acardiac twin shows loss of direct vascular connections with placenta; no arteries enter cotyledons on CP

Subchorionic Fibrin/Thrombi

- Yellow-white subchorionic plaques are not uncommon on CP
- Represent subchorionic intervillous thrombi related to stasis and turbulent blood flow beneath CP
- Are not considered abnormal unless extensive (> 40%) and/or excessively thick (> 1 cm in thickness)

Other Features/Variants of Normal on Chorionic Plate

- Chorionic cyst
  o Cyst on CP filled with gelatinous fluid
- Calcified remnant of yolk sac
  o Ovoid, chalky white disc located between amnion and chorion
- Iatrogenic defects in CP (usually due to sampling for cytogenetics by clinical team)

- Subamnionic hematoma
  - Usually associated with umbilical cord insertion site
  - Typically caused by excessive traction on cord during 3rd stage of labor with tearing of fetal vessels at insertion site

MICROSCOPIC

Chorionic Plate Layers

- Amnion
  - Loosely covers CP from ~ 17-weeks gestation
    - May detach when edematous
    - Can undergo similar changes as amnion of free membranes
  - Component layers (amnionic epithelium, basement membrane, mesoderm, and spongy layer) same as in free membranes
- Chorionic mesoderm
  - Cellularity consists of fibroblasts and myofibroblasts set in connective tissue
  - Chorionic vessels course through this mesoderm
- Extravillous trophoblast
  - Reserve of cytotrophoblast capable of proliferation and migration into extravillous fibrin
  - Origin of Langhans fibrinoid and extracellular matrix at base of CP
  - May form cysts
    - Microscopic to grossly visible chorionic cysts
- Syncytiotrophoblast
  - Continuous with syncytiotrophoblast of stem villi
  - Often eroded early in development, replaced by fibrin
- Subchorionic fibrin
  - Becomes more prominent over gestation
  - Blood type fibrin
  - Attributed to turbulent flow of maternal blood as it reaches intervillous space below CP

Chorionic Plate Vasculature

- Chorionic veins and arteries are indistinguishable histologically
- Layers of vessel wall
  - Intima
    - Intimal thickening with myxoid-appearing protrusions into lumen is commonly seen (intimal cushion)
    - Intimal asymmetry may represent response to turbulent flow or increased vascular resistance
    - Should be considered thrombi only if fibrin cap and/or calcifications are present
  - Media
    - Smooth muscle layer of variable thickness
    - Asymmetric thinning of fetal side of wall is not uncommon
- Mural fibrin or calcification is not normal
- Mural inflammatory cells are not normal

REPORTING CRITERIA

Gross Examination

- Note type of insertion of umbilical cord on CP
- Examination and description of appearance of CP vessels (before sectioning)
  - Distribution of chorionic vasculature

- Note any distended vessels or portions of vessels
- Note any firm segments of vessels
- Note any white discoloration or calcification of vessels
- Note any disruption of vessels
- Examination and description of cut surface of vessels after serial sectioning of placenta
  - Note any distended vessels or portions of vessels
  - Note any white discoloration or layered appearance of vascular contents
  - Note any chalky mural calcifications
- Note amount and distribution of subchorionic fibrin
- Full-thickness sections of placenta should include CP and representative chorionic vessels
- Gross features that should prompt additional sampling of chorionic vessels to attempt detection of abnormalities
  - Dilation of chorionic vessel with firm intraluminal contents, possible thrombosis
  - Firm segments of chorionic vessels with white discoloration
  - Cut surface of chorionic vessel with intraluminal mural or occlusive contents, possible thrombosis
  - Mural hemorrhage

SELECTED REFERENCES

1. Burton GJ et al: Development of the Human Placenta and Fetal Heart: Synergic or Independent? Front Physiol. 9:373, 2018
2. Khong TY et al: Sampling and definitions of placental lesions: Amsterdam Placental Workshop Group consensus statement. Arch Pathol Lab Med. 140(7):698-713, 2016
3. Aplin JD et al: Hemangioblastic foci in human first trimester placenta: Distribution and gestational profile. Placenta. 36(10):1069-77, 2015
4. De Paepe ME et al: What-and why-the pathologist should know about twin-to-twin transfusion syndrome. Pediatr Dev Pathol. 16(4):237-51, 2013
5. Ravangard SF et al: Placenta membranacea. Arch Gynecol Obstet. 288(3):709-12, 2013
6. De Paepe ME et al: Correlation between cord insertion type and superficial choriovasculature in diamniotic-monochorionic twin placentas. Placenta. 32(11):901-5, 2011
7. Schwartz N et al: Placental morphologic features and chorionic surface vasculature at term are highly correlated with 3-dimensional sonographic measurements at 11 to 14 weeks. J Ultrasound Med. 30(9):1171-8, 2011
8. De Paepe ME et al: Placental markers of twin-to-twin transfusion syndrome in diamniotic-monochorionic twins: a morphometric analysis of deep artery-to-vein anastomoses. Placenta. 31(4):269-76, 2010
9. Pathak S et al: Cord coiling, umbilical cord insertion and placental shape in an unselected cohort delivering at term: relationship with common obstetric outcomes. Placenta. 31(11):963-8, 2010
10. Suzuki S et al: Clinical significance of pregnancies with succenturiate lobes of placenta. Arch Gynecol Obstet. 277(4):299-301, 2008
11. Gordon Z et al: Anthropometry of fetal vasculature in the chorionic plate. J Anat. 211(6):698-706, 2007
12. De Paepe ME et al: Vascular distribution patterns in monochorionic twin placentas. Placenta. 26(6):471-5, 2005
13. Benirschke K: Remarkable placenta. Clin Anat. 11(3):194-205, 1998
14. Nordenvall M et al: Placental morphology in relation to umbilical artery blood velocity waveforms. Eur J Obstet Gynecol Reprod Biol. 40(3):179-90, 1991
15. Nordenvall M et al: Relationship between placental shape, cord insertion, lobes and gestational outcome. Acta Obstet Gynecol Scand. 67(7):611-6, 1988

Cut Surface of the CP

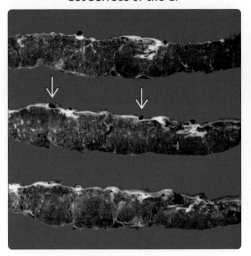

Bilobed Placenta

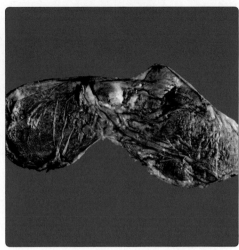

(Left) *Examination of the CP vasculature on a cut section shows the large fetal vessels on the upper edge of each slice* ➡. *This is an important opportunity to identify thrombi.* (Right) *Although it is usually round to oval, the CP, and therefore the placental disc itself, can have variant configurations, such as this bilobed placenta.*

Accessory Lobes

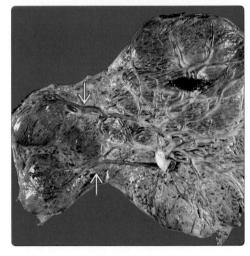

Placenta Membranacea

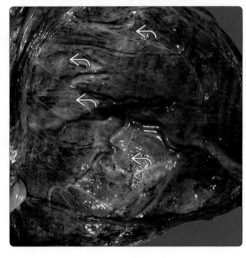

(Left) *This placenta has 2 accessory (succenturiate) lobes. Note that each are fed with branches of the CP vasculature* ➡. *These vessels can lie over the cervical os and present risk of fetal hemorrhage (vasa previa).* (Right) *Placenta membranacea is a rare abnormality. It may have a diffusely thinned disc with little to no membranes, or it may have cotyledons loosely scattered about the membranes* ➡, *as in this case.*

Normal Artery-Vein Pairs on CP

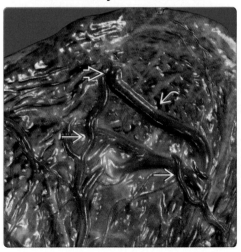

Disperse Pattern

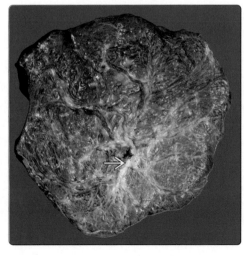

(Left) *The distal-most extent of the artery* ➡ *enters the underlying cotyledon, as a vein* ➡ *of similar caliber emerges from the same spot* ➡. *Similar pairings are present all over the surface of the placenta.* (Right) *The fetal blood vessels form a disperse (normal) branching pattern on the chorionic plate of this trimmed placenta. Note the paracentral umbilical cord insertion* ➡. *The cord insertion site can be traced back from the CP vasculature when avulsed.*

Magistral CP Vessel Distribution

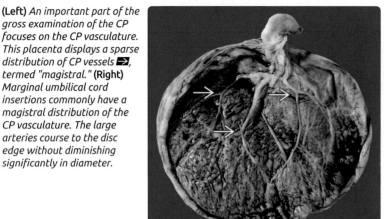

Magistral Distribution, Marginal Cord Insertion

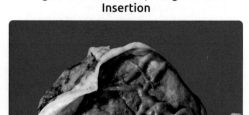

(Left) *An important part of the gross examination of the CP focuses on the CP vasculature. This placenta displays a sparse distribution of CP vessels* ➡, *termed "magistral."* **(Right)** *Marginal umbilical cord insertions commonly have a magistral distribution of the CP vasculature. The large arteries course to the disc edge without diminishing significantly in diameter.*

Magistral Distribution, Velamentous Cord Insertion

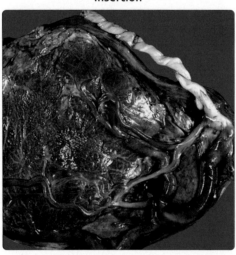
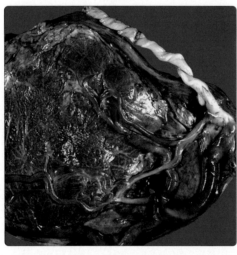

Magistral Distribution, Marginal Cord Insertion

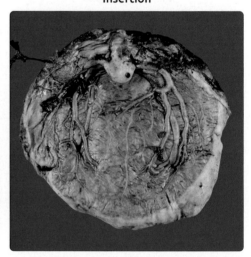

(Left) *Similarly, velamentous cord insertions often have magistral vasculature. There are no precise measurements that discern magistral from normal. The appearance of large sparse vessels leaving large areas of the disc without CP vessels is consistent with the magistral pattern.* **(Right)** *This placenta also illustrates a magistral CP vascular distribution associated with a marginal cord insertion.*

Chorionic Vessel Thrombosis

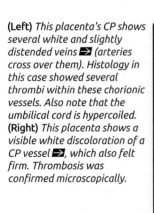
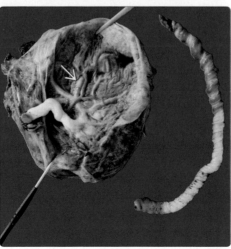

CP Vessel Thrombosis

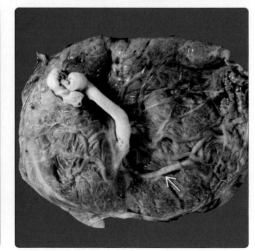

(Left) *This placenta's CP shows several white and slightly distended veins* ➡ *(arteries cross over them). Histology in this case showed several thrombi within these chorionic vessels. Also note that the umbilical cord is hypercoiled.* **(Right)** *This placenta shows a visible white discoloration of a CP vessel* ➡, *which also felt firm. Thrombosis was confirmed microscopically.*

Gestational Sac With Primary CP

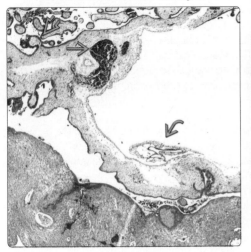

CP Histology

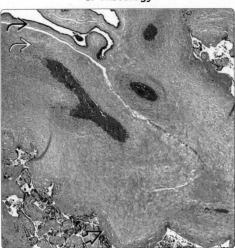

(Left) The primary chorionic plate forms the gestational sac. Primary and secondary villi ➥ bud from the outer surface. Hemangioblastic foci ➥ give rise to the future chorionic plate vasculature. The amnion is not seen in this image. The yolk sac ➥ is present, which may be seen as a yellow dot on the chorionic plate of the mature placenta. (Right) At term, shown here, layers of CP that are distinguishable include amnion ➥, chorionic mesoderm ➥, and subchorionic fibrin ➥.

CP Vessel Asymmetry

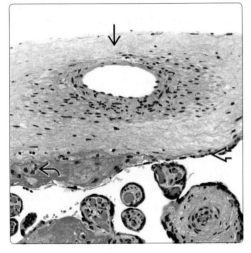

CP Vessel Intimal Cushion

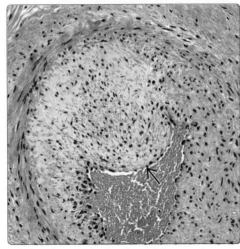

(Left) Amnion has slipped from the surface in this section of CP. The CP vessel shows asymmetry of the wall with thinning of the muscle on the side of the vessel closest to the amniotic sac ➥. Also seen are extravillous cytotrophoblast cells ➥ in Langhans fibrinoid and the syncytiotrophoblast layer ➥. (Right) CP vessel shows a myxoid intimal protrusion into the lumen ➥. There is no endothelial disruption. No fibrin cap is present. This finding does not merit a diagnosis of thrombosis or fetal vascular malperfusion.

CP Vessel Asymmetry

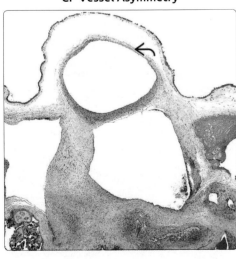

CP Vessel Wall Histology

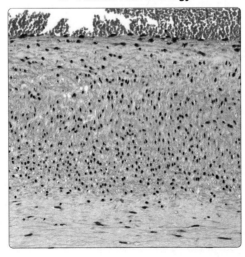

(Left) In this section of the CP, there is asymmetric thinning of the muscular wall on the top 1/2 of the superficial vessel ➥. The arrangement suggests that this is an artery overlying a vein, but such histologic designation is not reliable. (Right) The CP vessel wall typically has a thin endothelium overlying a thick media. There is no fibrointimal proliferation in this vessel.

TERMINOLOGY

Abbreviations

- Amniotic fluid infection (AFI), amniotic fluid infection sequence (AFIS)
- Maternal inflammatory response (MIR), fetal inflammatory response (FIR)

MICROSCOPIC

Pigmented Macrophages

- Meconium
  - Meconium-laden macrophages may accumulate in chorionic plate
    - Dull, tan-brown pigment
      - □ Can be solid appearing or more diffusely particulate in cytoplasm
    - Iron stains negative
  - May see reactive changes, necrosis &/or edema in overlying amnion
  - Green to brown discoloration on gross exam
  - Possible meconium-associated vascular necrosis in chorionic plate vasculature if meconium exposure is prolonged
- Diffuse chorioamniotic hemosiderosis
  - Hemosiderin-laden macrophages accumulate in chorionic plate
  - Brown, somewhat refractile pigment; iron stains positive
  - Usually premature birth with 2nd-trimester vaginal bleeding
    - May have chronic abruption-oligohydramnios sequence with respiratory failure in neonate
  - Also seen over large subchorionic hematoma
  - Associated gross features
    - Brown discoloration
    - Marginal hemorrhage (chronic abruption)
    - Circumvallate membrane insertion

Acute Inflammation

- Acute subchorionitis
  - Sensitive site for detecting MIR to AFI

- Aggregates of maternal neutrophils present beneath chorionic plate in subchorionic fibrin
  - Migrating from maternal intervillous blood space to chemoattractants in amniotic fluid
    - □ Usually microbes present in amniotic fluid
  - Confluent aggregates of ≥ 10 x 20 neutrophils are considered grade 2 (severe), fewer are grade 1
  - If MIR is limited to subchorionitis, stage is early (stage 1)
- Acute chorioamnionitis
  - Maternal neutrophils present in chorionic plate connective tissue
    - Usually accompanied by acute chorioamnionitis in free membranes
    - Confluent aggregates of ≥ 10 x 20 neutrophils are considered grade 2 (severe), fewer are grade 1
    - Indicates intermediate stage of AFIS, MIR stage 2
- Necrotizing acute chorioamnionitis
  - Chorionic plate and membranes are severely inflamed
  - Amnion necrosis, basement membrane hypereosinophilia, and/or karyorrhexis of neutrophils
    - Indicates late-stage MIR (stage 3)
  - Associated with prolonged, premature rupture of membranes
- Subacute chorioamnionitis
  - Infiltrate of histiocytes underlies superficial acute inflammation in chorionic plate
    - Neutrophils usually karyorrhectic
  - Usually seen with necrotizing acute chorioamnionitis
  - Associated with vaginal bleeding and chronic lung disease in infants with necrotizing and subacute chorioamnionitis
    - Diffuse chorioamniotic hemosiderosis also found with this histology; look for hemosiderin

Chorionic Vasculitis

- Fetal neutrophils migrate from chorionic plate vasculature toward stimuli in amniotic fluid (amniotropism)
- Sensitive site to detect fetal inflammatory response to AFI

Chorioamniotic Hemosiderosis

Hemosiderin Granules

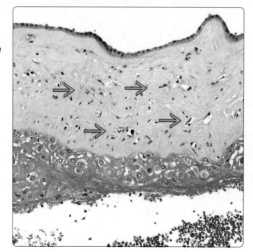 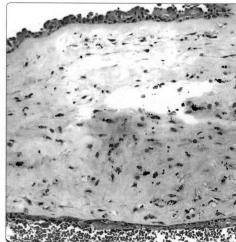

(Left) This 26-week gestation placenta had diffuse hemosiderin deposition ➡ in the chorionic plate. (Right) An iron stain demonstrates the presence of numerous hemosiderin granules in the chorionic plate.

o Grade 2 (severe) inflammation may be termed "intense" chorionic vasculitis

o If fetal inflammatory response is limited to chorionic plate vasculature, stage is early (FIR stage 1)

- May be complicated by thrombi
  o Strongly associated with neurologic impairment in affected neonate
- Mild chorionic plate vasculitis may be seen due to meconium effects alone, but difficult to exclude AFI
  o Look for features of AFIS elsewhere

Chronic Inflammation

- Chronic chorionitis
  o Infiltrate of maternal lymphocytes and histiocytes in chorionic plate, usually in lower 1/2
  o Associated with chronic villitis of unknown etiology
  o May see basal chronic villitis in parenchyma and chronic chorioamnionitis in membranes
  o Rarely associated with hematogenous infections such as herpes simplex virus
  o Infiltrate can involve chorionic plate vasculature

Eosinophilic/T-Cell Chorionic Vasculitis

- Fetal T cells and eosinophils migrating from chorionic plate vasculature preferentially, but not exclusively, toward underlying intervillous space
- Rare finding, in ~ 0.2% of placentas submitted for pathologic examination
- Associated with chronic villitis of unknown etiology (VUE)
  o Only small minority of placentas with VUE will have eosinophilic/T-cell vasculitis, but 30-40% of cases with eosinophilic/T-cell vasculitis will have associated chronic villitis
- May be associated with fetal thrombi in affected vessel or elsewhere
  o Most placentas with fetal thrombi will not have eosinophilic/T-cell vasculitis, but 40% of cases with eosinophilic/T-cell vasculitis will have thrombi
- Clinical significance of isolated eosinophilic/T-cell vasculitis without other associated findings is unclear

Chorionic Plate Vessel Thrombi

- May be occlusive or nonocclusive; and acute, subacute, or remote
  o Most commonly nonocclusive with fibrin adhering to wall
    – Most commonly in chorionic plate veins
  o With chronicity, develop mural calcification, become incorporated into vessel wall
    – Patent lumen with fibrin and calcification in fibrointimal protrusion indicates old, organized thrombus
- Look for associated villous changes of fetal vascular malperfusion
  o Thrombi, fibromuscular sclerosis, or septation of stem villous vessels
  o Villous stromal vascular karyorrhexis or avascular villi
- Associations include severe chorionic plate vasculitis, extension from umbilical cord thrombi, hypercoiled cord, meconium-associated vascular necrosis

Chorionic Plate Vasoocclusive Changes

- Endothelial breakdown, extravasation of red blood cells, fibrous septation of lumen with organization into small, residual, multiple vascular channels
- Occurs with cessation of fetal blood flow or markedly reduced perfusion
  o Due to fetal demise, heart failure, or obstructed proximal flow
  o Similar changes described as "hemorrhagic endovasculosis"
  o Part of spectrum of changes seen with fetal vascular malperfusion

Meconium-Associated Vascular Necrosis

- Severe, prolonged meconium deposition leads to apoptotic cell death of vascular smooth muscle
- Begins at site of meconium deposition on amniotic surface
- May be complicated by thrombi, likely impairs perfusion even without thrombi
- Associated with pronounced meconium changes: Amnion edema and necrosis, numerous pigmented macrophages

Massive Dilatation of Chorionic Plate Vessel

- Dilatation of chorionic plate vessel > 4x neighboring vessels
- Attributed to marked congestion from umbilical cord obstruction
  o Look for gross cord lesions or venous thrombi that support cord obstruction
  o Look for villous congestion or intravillous hemorrhage
  o Look for thrombi, changes of fetal thrombotic vasculopathy in villous parenchyma
- Exclude tangential sectioning as cause of enlargement along axis of chorionic plate

SELECTED REFERENCES

1. Katzman PJ et al: Eosinophilic/T-cell chorionic vasculitis and chronic villitis involve regulatory T cells and often occur together. Pediatr Dev Pathol. 16(4):278-91, 2013
2. Salas AA et al: Histological characteristics of the fetal inflammatory response associated with neurodevelopmental impairment and death in extremely preterm infants. J Pediatr. 163(3):652-7, 2013
3. Ryan WD et al: Placental histologic criteria for diagnosis of cord accident: sensitivity and specificity. Pediatr Dev Pathol. 15(4):275-80, 2012
4. Jacques SM et al: Eosinophilic/T-cell chorionic vasculitis: a clinicopathologic and immunohistochemical study of 51 cases. Pediatr Dev Pathol. 14(3):198-205, 2011
5. Wintermark P et al: Placental pathology in asphyxiated newborns meeting the criteria for therapeutic hypothermia. Am J Obstet Gynecol. 203(6):579, 2010
6. Ohyama M et al: Maternal, neonatal, and placental features associated with diffuse chorioamniotic hemosiderosis, with special reference to neonatal morbidity and mortality. Pediatrics. 113(4):800-5, 2004
7. Redline RW et al: Amniotic infection syndrome: nosology and reproducibility of placental reaction patterns. Pediatr Dev Pathol. 6(5):435-48, 2003

(Left) Acute subchorionitis is an early indication of amniotic fluid infection (AFI) ▱. Maternal neutrophils accumulate between the syncytiotrophoblast layer or subchorionic fibrin and chorionic plate connective tissue. **(Right)** The fetal and maternal inflammatory responses to AFI are evaluated in the chorionic plate. The maternal inflammatory response ▱ is seen in subchorionic fibrin and connective tissue. The fetal inflammatory response ▱ is seen on the side of the vessel near the amniotic fluid.

Early Indication of Amniotic Fluid Infection

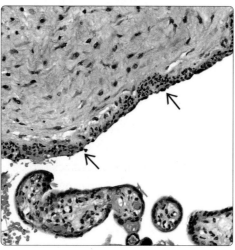

Signs of Amniotic Fluid Infection in the Chorionic Plate

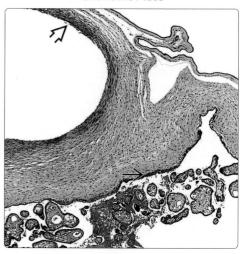

(Left) The fetal inflammatory response can be subtle. Only scattered neutrophils and eosinophils are seen in the intima of this chorionic plate vessel ▱ (AFIS FIR grade 1, stage 1). **(Right)** This image shows intense chorionic plate vasculitis complicated by thrombus formation ▱. This severe fetal inflammatory response is an ominous sign for neonatal morbidity and should not be missed.

Early Fetal Inflammatory Response

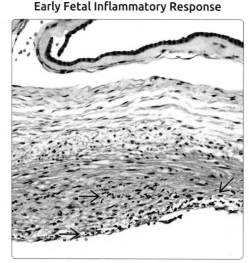

Intense Chorionic Plate Vasculitis With Thrombus

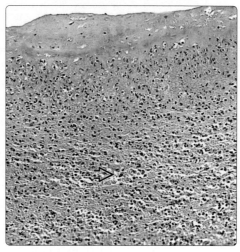

(Left) In prolonged necrotizing acute chorioamnionitis, a mononuclear cell infiltrate ▱ can also be seen in the chorionic plate, termed "subacute chorioamnionitis." **(Right)** This chorionic plate vessel has undergone partial necrosis due to severe necrotizing chorioamnionitis affecting the chorionic plate. A thrombus ▱ has formed.

Subacute Chorioamnionitis

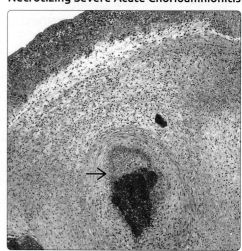

Necrosis of Chorionic Plate Vessel in Necrotizing Severe Acute Chorioamnionitis

Eosinophilic/T-Cell Vasculitis

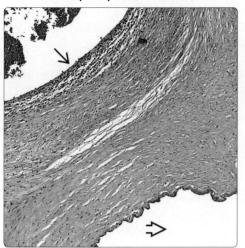

Fetal Inflammatory Response With Eosinophils

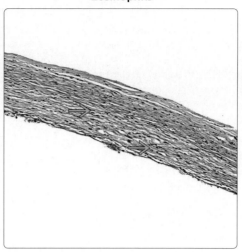

(Left) *This image shows true eosinophilic/T-cell vasculitis. The infiltrate ⊟ of eosinophils and lymphocytes from the fetal blood is directed predominantly toward the intervillous space ⊟.* **(Right)** *This image of the amniotic side of a chorionic plate vessel shows scattered eosinophils ⊟. Eosinophils are a frequent component of the very premature FIR to AFI.*

Chorionic Plate Thrombus

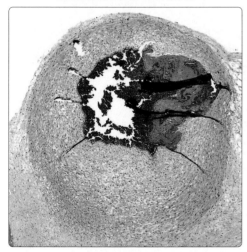

Thrombosis and Collapse of Chorionic Plate Vessel

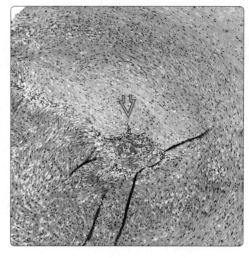

(Left) *This chorionic plate thrombus was associated with meconium deposition in the placenta.* **(Right)** *This chorionic plate vessel thrombus ⊟ from a twin placenta does not distend the vessel; instead, it appears collapsed, perhaps reflecting obstruction of arterial perfusion. With umbilical venous obstruction, the vessel may be markedly dilated.*

Meconium-Associated Vascular Necrosis

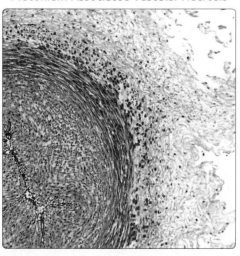

Meconium-Associated Vascular Necrosis

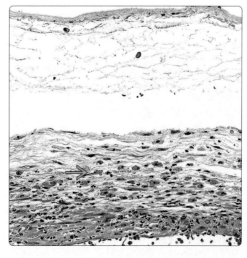

(Left) *The umbilical cord and chorionic plate vessels may show meconium-associated vascular necrosis. Individual vascular smooth muscle cells facing the amnion become separated, rounded, and pyknotic.* **(Right)** *This section shows the amniotic aspect of a chorionic plate vessel with heavy meconium and meconium-associated vascular necrosis. The vascular smooth muscle cells closest to the site of deposition become apoptotic ⊟. Chorionic plate vasculitis is present as well.*

TERMINOLOGY

Definitions

- Stem villi: Placental villi containing muscular vessels and dense fibrous stroma comprising > 1/2 of core connective tissue
  - Located in center of villous tree; can be likened to trunk
- Immature intermediate villi: Precursor chorionic villi that mature into stem villi and mature intermediate villi

MACROSCOPIC

Normal Gross Appearance of Stem Villi

- Villous fibrous tissue appears as tan-white vertical streaks extending down from chorionic plate; only largest stem villi are grossly visible
- When in cross section, artery and vein may be visible

Stem Villous Abnormalities on Gross Exam

- Marked vascular dilatation ± thrombi
  - Marked vascular dilatation defined as lumen diameter that is 4x neighboring vessels
  - Look for associated umbilical cord abnormalities and chorionic plate vessel thrombi or marked dilatation
  - Look for pale parenchymal foci of avascular villi resulting from fetal vascular malperfusion
- Cysts
  - Cysts of stem villi usually only grossly visible in placental mesenchymal dysplasia
- Chorangiomas
  - Commonly arise from stem villi under chorionic plate
    - Appear as oval, smooth, dark-red to tan-fibrous masses
    - Usually singular; may infarct over time, appearing tan
  - Multifocal chorangiomatosis
    - Rarely described gross appearance with multiple nodular lesions

MICROSCOPIC

Normal Histology of Stem Villi

- Classically described as trunci chorii, rami chorii, and ramuli chorii based on progressively smaller size and predominant location
- Range: 5,000 μm near chorionic plate to 80 μm in smaller branches
- Larger stem villi contain arteries and veins, smaller forms contain arterioles and venules, usually > 1 artery and vein
- Subset connects chorionic plate to basal plate and septa (anchoring villi)
- Syncytiotrophoblast layer is often replaced by perivillous fibrin at term

Stem Villous Heterogeneity

- 3 types of stem villi described based on size and location of myofibroblasts and smooth muscle cells
  - Type 1: 5,000-250 μm; myocontractile cells present in media of arteries and veins as well as surrounding central stroma
    - Supply peripheral number of > 100 terminal villi via subsequent type 2 and 3 branches
  - Type 2: 300-120 μm; myocontractile cells present only in media of arteries and veins
    - May branch into further type 2 villi up to 2x before branching into type 3 stem villi
    - Supply terminal villi via branching into 2-12 type 3 stem villi
  - Type 3: 150-80 μm; myocontractile cells present only in media of arteriole
    - Rarely branch into further type 3 villi
    - Branch into 2 or 3 mature intermediate villi, which further branch into 12-24 terminal villi

SELECTED REFERENCES

1. Benirschke K: Recent trends in chorangiomas, especially those of multiple and recurrent chorangiomas. Pediatr Dev Pathol. 2(3):264-9, 1999
2. Demir R et al: Classification of human placental stem villi: review of structural and functional aspects. Microsc Res Tech. 38(1-2):29-41, 1997

Placental Circulation

Prominent Stem Villus Vessels on Gross Exam

(Left) Stem villi ➡ take fetal blood to and from distal villi and chorionic plate vasculature, provide structural support, and likely play a role in fetal regulation of intervillous space volume by anchoring to the basal plate. (Right) The numerous white foci containing vessels in the parenchyma are larger stem villi ➡. A subset ➡ shows marked dilatation of 1 vessel with congestion, related to the chorionic plate thrombus ➡.

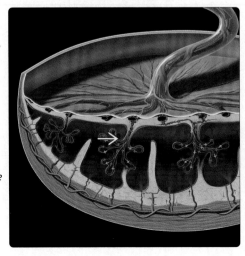

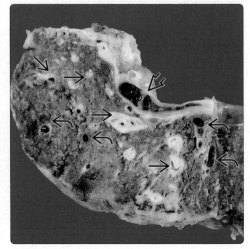

Mature Stem Villi

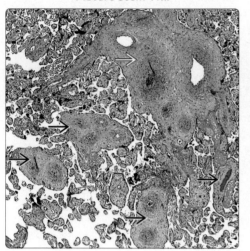

Loose Adventitia in Large Stem Villi

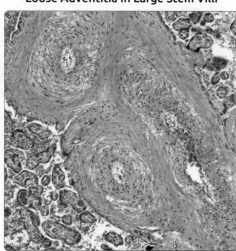

(Left) *The sizes of mature stem villi ⇨ vary greatly with the larger forms ⇨ emanating from the chorionic plate.* **(Right)** *The stem villous vasculature undergoes many nonspecific changes. The adventitia may seem loose and edematous and appear strikingly prominent at low power. In the absence of inflammation or infection, this change is of no defined significance.*

Stenotic-Appearing Stem Villous Vessels

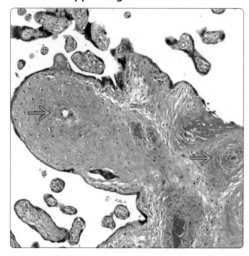

Stromal Clefts in Stem Villi

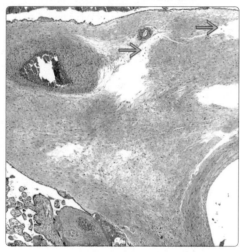

(Left) *In contrast, the vessels may also seem stenotic with prominent stromal collagen ⇨. While these changes may accompany changes of maternal vascular malperfusion, they are not diagnostic in isolation.* **(Right)** *The stroma may contain loose areas resembling empty clefts. These areas are likely in continuity with reticular spaces, as they sometimes contain Hofbauer cells ⇨.*

Syncytiotrophoblast Inclusions in Stem Villi

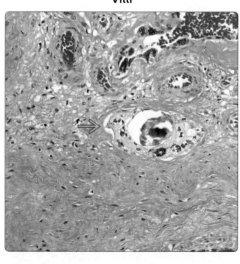

Myocontractile Cells in Stem Villi

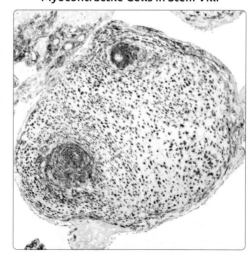

(Left) *Syncytiotrophoblast inclusions ⇨ may be seen in stem villi, reflecting the irregular villous contour likely related to branching of villi. They are more frequent in the preterm placenta.* **(Right)** *In addition to the vascular smooth muscle, the stem villous stroma also contains numerous myocontractile cells. As seen in this smooth muscle actin stain, these are postulated to regulate intervillous space volume through contraction in anchoring villi.*

MICROSCOPIC

Acute Inflammation

- Acute villitis
  - Accumulation of neutrophils underneath syncytiotrophoblast layer; may also have bacteria in fetal capillaries
  - Associated with fetal sepsis due to
    - *Escherichia coli*
    - Group B *Streptococcus*
    - Other streptococcal infections
  - May or may not be accompanied by intervillous abscess formation
    - When intervillous abscesses present, consider *Listeria monocytogenes*
  - Most commonly seen with acute chorioamnionitis
- Stem villus vasculitis
  - Fetal inflammatory response similar to that seen in chorionic plate and umbilical cord
  - May be seen with active intervillous inflammation when organisms spread to placenta from maternal bloodstream
    - Maternal bacterial sepsis, such as group A streptococcal sepsis or gram-negative septicemia
    - Herpes simplex virus (HSV) infection
    - Varicella-zoster virus (VZV) infection
    - Rickettsial infections

Chronic Inflammation

- Proximal chronic villitis (chronic villitis affecting larger 1st branches of stem villi)
  - Most cases are villitis of unknown etiology (VUE)
    - Less commonly caused by placental infection
  - Lymphohistiocytic infiltrate of proximal stem villi, usually affecting distal villi as well
  - Mostly composed of maternal T cells with fewer numbers of fetal histiocytes (Hofbauer cells)
  - Associated with obliterative changes in stem villus vasculature
    - Impaired perfusion of distal villous trees

- Avascular villi resulting from vascular obstruction
  - Can severely compromise placental function as proximal lesions cause loss of distal villous function
    - Single proximal stem villous supplies fetal blood to > 100 distal villi, sites of gas and nutrient exchange
- Eosinophilic/T-cell vasculitis
  - Fetal eosinophils and lymphocytes migrate from stem villous vessels toward intervillous space
  - More commonly seen in chorionic plate vasculature but occasionally seen in stem villi
  - Associated lesions include chronic villitis (VUE) and fetal vascular malperfusion
- Syphilis-associated proliferative vasculopathy
  - Originally described as part of histologic constellation for syphilis in placenta, along with large, hypercellular villi, acute or chronic (histiocyte-predominant) villitis, and necrotizing umbilical perivasculitis
  - Lesion affects all types of stem vessels (arteries, veins, arterioles, venules)
  - Vessel walls appear thickened with concentric perivascular stromal fibrosis
  - Some authors include changes of vascular occlusion with lesion
  - Unclear if there is increase in fibrosis, or if normal connective tissue stroma is accentuated by edema and inflammation

Thrombosis

- Part of spectrum of changes of fetal vascular malperfusion
- May extend from chorionic plate or umbilical cord thrombus, usually affecting vein
- Acute occlusive thrombi/emboli
  - Platelets and fibrin fully fill lumen of vessel with attachment to endothelium
    - Uncommon finding
- Recent thrombi
  - Dense luminal fibrin is adherent to endothelium, usually nonocclusive
  - May see extravasation of RBC into vessel wall
- Organizing

Chorangioma

Stem Vessel Obliteration in Chronic Villitis

(Left) Chorangioma is characterized by a stem villus proliferation of capillaries and pericytes in a variably fibrotic background. Chorangiomas are most commonly found beneath the chorionic plate or at the margin of the disc. (Right) Vasodestructive lesions ⊞ of proximal chronic villitis ⊞ are important to recognize, as they affect perfusion of potentially large areas of distal villi, thereby impairing placental function.

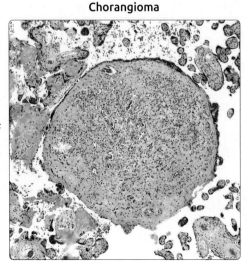
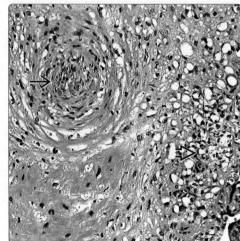

- o Fibrin becomes incorporated into vessel wall (intramural fibrin deposition)
  - – Small, delicate eosinophilic fibrin strands in endothelial cushion may be seen, unclear if these lesions relate to disturbance of fetal blood flow
    - □ Level sections can be helpful to look for more convincing fibrin deposition
- Remote
  - o Organized mural thrombus with calcification (intramural fibrin deposition)
- Causes of thrombi include Virchow triad
  - o Blood stasis
    - – Sluggish flow may be due to cord compromise, velamentous vessel occlusion, polycythemia, or fetal right heart failure
  - o Endothelial injury
    - – Severe fetal inflammatory response to amniotic fluid infection, or inflammation of marked chronic villitis
  - o Hypercoagulable state
    - – Fetal disseminated intravascular coagulation or rare inherited thrombophilias affecting fetal circulation

Other Occlusive Changes

- Large vessel fetal vascular occlusion
  - o Series of similar histopathologic changes occur downstream of vascular occlusion or with markedly diminished perfusion, especially after fetal demise
    - – Loss of endothelium with ingrowth of spindled cells, extravasation of red blood cells, eventual organization into multiple small channels
- Fetal arteriolar narrowing
  - o Stem villous arterioles appear to have thickened walls and luminal obliteration
  - o Strict morphometric assessments have shown associations with
    - – Small placentas
    - – Intrauterine growth restriction
    - – Increased resistance of umbilical artery wave flow
  - o Thickening of arteriolar wall of smaller stem villi (type 3) is normal feature of placental maturity
    - – Lumina remain patent

Marked Dilatation

- Enlargement of 1 stem villous vessel > 4x that of neighboring vessels of similar villous caliber
- Associated with umbilical cord compression or obstruction
  - o Dilated vessel probably stem villous vein
  - o May see intravillous hemorrhage in distal villi
  - o Look for thrombi, other lesions of fetal vascular occlusion, gross cord abnormalities

Chorangioma

- Expansile mass of capillaries and pericytes with variable degree of fibrosis
- Usually arises from stem villi, at peripheral areas of relatively poor perfusion
  - o Under chorionic plate, peripheral margin of disc
- Most are small, < 0.5 cm in size
- May also be massive

- o Larger sized lesions may be more clinically significant for shunting of significant amount of fetal blood, leading to high-output cardiac failure, risk of fetal-maternal hemorrhage
- Most commonly singular lesions, rarely multiple

Chorangiomatosis

- Peripheral stem villous proliferation of capillaries and pericytes that may extend into contiguous branches of smaller stem villi
- May be localized or diffuse
  - o Localized chorangiomatosis
    - – Restricted to single focus of multiple affected villi on slide
  - o Diffuse chorangiomatosis
    - – Present in multiple placental regions
    - – Most commonly seen in very preterm placentas (< 32 weeks), associated with intrauterine growth restriction

Edema

- Appearance of mesenchymal and immature intermediate villi may suggest edema because of their pallor at low magnification
  - o These are not necessarily edematous changes
  - o Stroma of these precursor villi is normally hypovascular with prominent spaces
  - o Normal in center of lobules, usually < 10 villi
- Residual reticular spaces in maturing stem villi may become markedly enlarged with numerous Hofbauer cells, resembling edema

Cysts

- Large proximal cysts found in placental mesenchymal dysplasia
  - o Often associated with thrombi in stem villous vasculature

Rests

- Small foci of hepatic tissue are rarely seen in stem villous stroma
  - o Rare
  - o Cleared cytoplasm of immature liver may resemble adrenal tissue
  - o Likely related to yolk sac progenitors

SELECTED REFERENCES

1. Khong TY et al: Sampling and definitions of placental lesions: Amsterdam Placental Workshop Group consensus statement. Arch Pathol Lab Med. 140(7):698-713, 2016
2. Bagby C et al: Multifocal chorangiomatosis. Pediatr Dev Pathol. 14(1):38-44, 2011
3. Redline RW: Severe fetal placental vascular lesions in term infants with neurologic impairment. Am J Obstet Gynecol. 192(2):452-7, 2005
4. Redline RW et al: Fetal vascular obstructive lesions: nosology and reproducibility of placental reaction patterns. Pediatr Dev Pathol. 7(5):443-52, 2004
5. Mitra SC et al: Placental vessel morphometry in growth retardation and increased resistance of the umbilical artery Doppler flow. J Matern Fetal Med. 9(5):282-6, 2000
6. Ogino S et al: Villous capillary lesions of the placenta: distinctions between choriangioma, choriangiomatosis, and choriangiosis. Hum Pathol. 31(8):945-54, 2000
7. Mitra SC et al: Morphometric study of the placental vessels and its correlation with umbilical artery Doppler flow. Obstet Gynecol. 89(2):238-41, 1997

Proximal Chronic Villitis

Late Vascular Obliterative Changes in Proximal Chronic Villitis

(Left) *This proximal stem villus is infiltrated by maternal lymphocytes [villitis of unknown etiology (VUE)]. The endothelium is breaking down* ⇨ *as the vessel begins the process of occlusion.* (Right) *Later in the affected stem villi of chronic villitis, the stem villus vessel lumina become progressively obliterated* ⇨. *Prolonged inflammation has also led to increased perivillous fibrin deposition.*

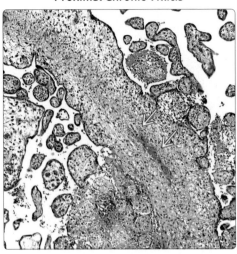
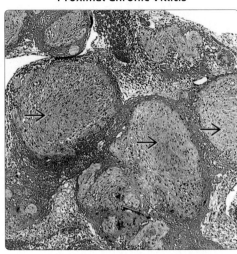

Stenotic Stem Vessel Arteriole

Stem Villus Vessel Thrombosis

(Left) *The lumen of this stem vessel arteriole is markedly narrowed with concentric thickening of the wall. These changes can be seen in small placentas associated with intrauterine growth retardation.* (Right) *This thrombosed stem villus vessel has lost endothelial integrity as the process of organization proceeds.*

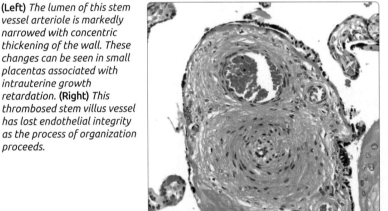
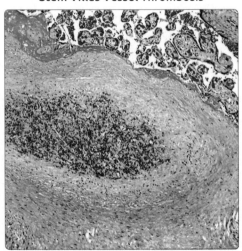

Intramural Fibrin Deposition

Organizing Thrombi of Stem Vessels

(Left) *This stem villus vessel shows focal intramural fibrin deposition, a form of a nonocclusive organizing mural thrombus.* (Right) *This large stem villus shows occlusive changes in the vessels. Residual fibrin thrombi* ⇨ *can be difficult to find as the organizational changes proceed.*

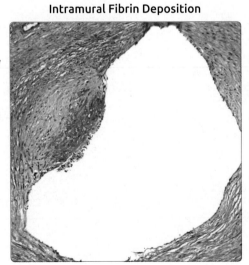
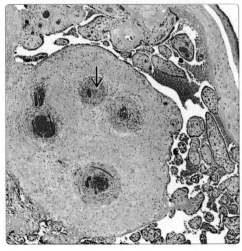

Early Stem Vessel Occlusion

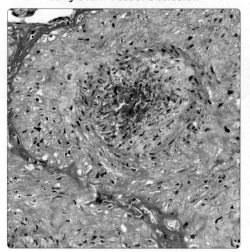

Late Stem Vessel Occlusive Changes

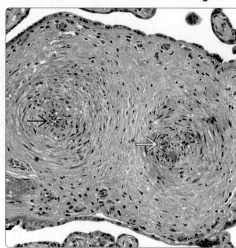

(Left) *Early occlusive changes in stem villi show loss of the endothelium with a proliferation of spindled intimal cells and extravasation of red blood cells.* (Right) *Later in the organizing process, only small residual channels* ➡ *remain. The neighboring vessel shows luminal narrowing* ⇨.

Localized Chorangiomatosis

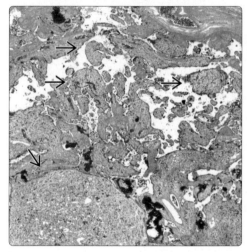

Hypervascular Stem Villi

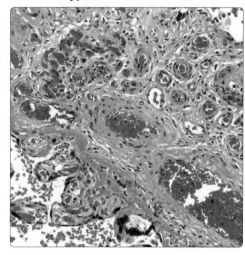

(Left) *In localized chorangiomatosis, vascular proliferations* ⇨ *resembling chorangioma extend into contiguous stem villous branches.* (Right) *Stem villi can appear hypervascular with numerous arterioles and capillaries. This lesion is distinct from chorangioma and is more similar to chorangiosis.*

Concentric Perivascular Fibrosis

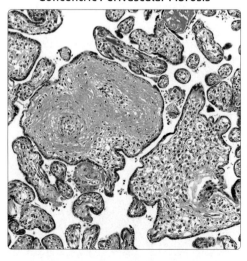

Hepatic Rest in Stem Villus

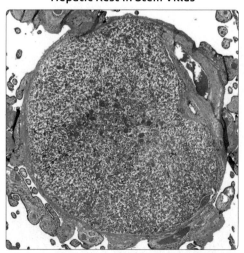

(Left) *Concentric perivascular fibrosis has been described as a feature of placental syphilis. However, distinguishing this change from the normal maturation of immature intermediate villi into stem villi, or from effects of edema on stem villi, has proven difficult.* (Right) *Rarely, isolated nodules of fetal liver tissue can be seen in stem villi. These rests may be related to remnants of the yolk sac. In contrast, metastatic hepatoblastoma diffusely involves chorionic villus vessels.*

TERMINOLOGY

Synonyms

- Distal villi and terminal villi
- Rounded intraplacental hematoma and infarction hematoma

MACROSCOPIC

Gross Appearance of Normal Villous Parenchyma

- Thickness
  - Measured as part of 3 dimensions of disc
  - Increases with gestational age; increases with placental edema
    - Thickness generally correlates with infant birthweight
  - Large discs may be thin, conserving overall volume
- Color
  - Degree of redness or pallor reflects fetal blood content of villi
    - 1st- and 2nd-trimester placentas contain less fetal blood; they are normally tan white
    - Mature placentas have higher fetal blood content and appear dark red
    - Pathology that removes fetal capillaries from villi leads to focal pallor with retention of villous granularity
  - Fibrin and remotely infarcted villi appear tan
    - Distinction between intervillous hematoma and remote infarct can be difficult grossly
- Consistency
  - Normal villous parenchyma is finely granular because of 3D texture of villi
  - Loss of villus architecture leads to homogeneous smooth texture
    - Chorangiomas, infarcts, and intervillous lesions with fibrin deposition all may have smoother consistency
  - Marked edema exaggerates texture; parenchyma appears stringy
  - Flow voids, spaces filled with jets of maternal blood in utero, appear as Swiss cheese-like holes on cut section
    - No known pathologic associations

Gross Appearance of Pathologic Lesions

- Tan, homogeneous-appearing lesions (infarcts, intervillous thrombi, and intervillous fibrin plaques)
  - Infarcts that are singular, up to 1 cm in size, within 1 cm of disc margin are normal at term
    - Preterm, multiple, central, and larger-sized infarcts are significant
  - Intervillous thrombi vary in size and location within parenchyma
    - Angular intraparenchymal lesions more likely to contain fetal blood
    - Plaque-like basal and paraseptal intervillous thrombi more likely related to stasis of maternal blood
    - Rounded intraplacental thrombohematoma, distinct lesion
      - □ Microabruptions near basal surface containing maternal blood
      - □ When surrounded by infarcted villi, they are also termed infarction hematoma
- Dark red lesions
  - Acute infarcts may appear hemorrhagic or dark red
  - Acute infarction hematoma resembles rounded recent thrombi
  - Areas of intravillous hemorrhage
- Tan, granular lesions
  - Lack or reduction of fetal villous capillaries in mature placenta leads to pale foci on gross exam; only grossly visible when large areas affected
    - Avascular villi of fetal vascular malperfusion
    - Large foci of chronic villitis
    - Large foci of relatively immature villi
    - Subacute infarct
- Increased fibrin
  - Fibrin in mature placenta is usually restricted to margins, subchorionic region, and minimally along basal plate
  - Fibrin in parenchyma and basal surface is markedly increased in massive perivillous fibrin deposition/maternal floor infarction

Pale Parenchyma

Dark Red Mature Parenchyma

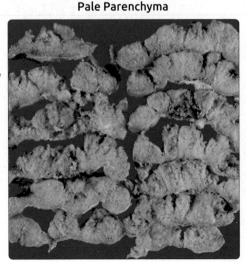
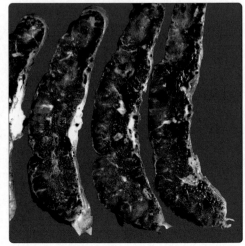

(Left) Color is an important gross observation of the villous parenchyma. Color depends on the fetal blood content. Diffuse pallor, as seen here, indicates either an immature placenta or marked edema/fetal anemia. (Right) The normal color of the mature placenta is dark red; fixation turns it dark brown. The placenta should be sliced at 1 cm intervals to look for parenchymal lesions.

– Increased perivillous fibrin noted as tan streaks extending from chorionic plate to basal plate; parenchyma may appear partitioned into rounded nodules
– Increased fibrin present on basal surface appears as rind, usually > 3 mm in thickness
- Abscesses
  o Rarely encountered in placental examination, have liquefactive necrotic contents
  o Cultures and touch preparation for Gram stain are strongly recommended

Checklist for Gross Parenchymal Lesions
- Note number of foci for focal lesions, size, color, texture, distance to margin or cord insertion, and percentage of parenchyma affected by lesion(s)
- Include representative section of lesion in addition to routine sections of normal-appearing parenchyma

MICROSCOPIC

General Features
- Nomenclature of villous development can be confusing; different words often describe same structures

Early Villous Development
- Primary, secondary, and tertiary villi describe 1st villous structures arising from days 13-28 post conception
  o Develop from cytotrophoblast and mesenchyme of primary chorionic plate and grow into trabeculae formed from early mass of syncytiotrophoblast and lacunar spaces
  o Primary villi: Outer syncytiotrophoblast layer and inner cytotrophoblast core
  o Secondary villi: Mesenchymal cells from chorionic plate extend into primary villi
  o Tertiary villi: Capillaries develop in mesenchyme of secondary villi; fetus is not required
- Villogenesis proceeds from these 1st villi in similar fashion: Budding of trophoblast, investment by mesenchyme, formation of vessels

Normal Appearance of 1st-Trimester Villi
- Mesenchymal villi develop from tertiary villi around 5 weeks post menstruation
  o Thick cytotrophoblast layer, loose mesenchyme with polygonal cells and few small vessels derived from mesenchyme, lined only by simple endothelium (vasculogenesis)
  o Give rise to immature intermediate villi, more mesenchymal villi
    – Source of early maternofetal nutrient exchange
- Immature intermediate villi develop from mesenchymal villi ~ 8 weeks post menstruation
  o Thick cytotrophoblast layer, reticular stroma with numerous round spaces filled with fluid, numerous Hofbauer cells (fetal macrophages)
  o Anchoring villi connect with basal plate and septa, have proliferations of immature extravillous trophoblast (cell columns) that become intermediate trophoblast of basal plate, implantation site decidua and invasive trophoblast that will remodel vasculature

  o Give rise to new mesenchymal villi and mature into stem villi
- Stem villi mature from immature intermediate villi with progressive stromal development
  o Minor population in 1st trimester, reticular stroma still present underneath cytotrophoblast layer in early stages

Normal Appearance of 2nd-Trimester Villi
- Continue to see numerous mesenchymal villi
- Angiogenesis 26 weeks to term, vessels formed by proliferation of endothelium
- Major population consists of immature intermediate villi with variable degrees of stromal maturation
- Stem villi include mostly 1st and 2nd ramifications

Normal Appearance of 3rd-Trimester Villi
- Tertiary branches of stem villi become numerous (also called mature intermediate villi), branch into distal villi
  o Long and slender, contain arteriole and venule with no media, as well as numerous capillaries
  o Multiple mature intermediate villi connect outpouchings of distal villi in series
  o Site of further elongation of fetal vessels, as well as branching angiogenesis
- Distal villi defined as having > 50% of volume consisting of vascular lumen
  o Form as coils of capillary loops that elongate and bulge out from surface of mature intermediate villi
  o Lined by thin trophoblast layer (mostly only syncytiotrophoblast), overlying capillary-rich stroma with minimal connective tissue and few Hofbauer cells
  o Vasculosyncytial membranes form where capillary abuts syncytiotrophoblast without intervening nucleus or visible connective tissue
    – Normally number 1 to several per mature distal villus; essential for optimal gas and nutrient exchange
  o Syncytiotrophoblast nuclei pile up in aggregates or knots
    – Increases free surface of vasculosyncytial membranes to promote efficient gas and nutrient exchange
- Immature intermediate villi become progressively less frequent as they mature into stem villi; < 5% of villi at term, usually in center of lobules
- Mesenchymal villi similarly comprise progressively smaller percentage of population; only 1% of villi at term
- Changes with maturation
  o Fibrin replaces syncytiotrophoblast around larger stem villi
  o More vasculosyncytial membranes: 1-6 per distal villus at term
  o More syncytial knots: Bridging knots contact 2 villi, nonbridging knots (aggregates of ≥ 5 nuclei) seen in < 1 in 5 villi before 34 weeks and up to 1 in 3 villi at term

SELECTED REFERENCES

1. Loukeris K et al: Syncytial knots as a reflection of placental maturity: reference values for 20 to 40 weeks' gestational age. Pediatr Dev Pathol. 13(4):305-9, 2010
2. Salafia CM et al: Placental growth patterns affect birth weight for given placental weight. Birth Defects Res A Clin Mol Teratol. 79(4):281-8, 2007
3. Kingdom J et al: Development of the placental villous tree and its consequences for fetal growth. Eur J Obstet Gynecol Reprod Biol. 92(1):35-43, 2000

Gross Appearance of Parenchyma

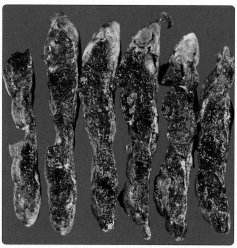

Marginal Parenchymal Lesions

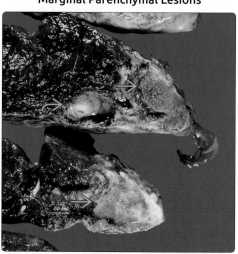

(Left) *The mature placenta shows a variegated texture reflecting the microscopic architecture. The granular texture appears softer and less well defined in the fresh cut section.* (Right) *Tan lesions are common at the margin of the mature placenta. The margin is a site of numerous changes, as it is relatively poorly perfused. This image shows an infarct ⊡ and an adjacent intervillous thrombus ⊿. These lesions are often found in the same region and can be difficult to distinguish on gross exam.*

Intervillous Thrombus

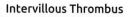
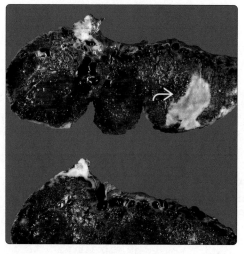

Multiple Infarcts

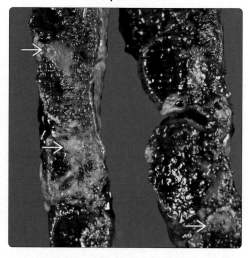

(Left) *The irregular contour of this tan lesion ⊿ suggests a remote intervillous thrombus. These lesions are often located near the septa and basal plate.* (Right) *Cross sections of this thin placenta show multiple tan, firm infarcts ⊡. Each lesion should be described and sampled. It is also important to estimate the volume of parenchyma that is involved.*

Infarction Hematoma

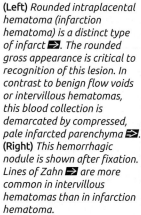
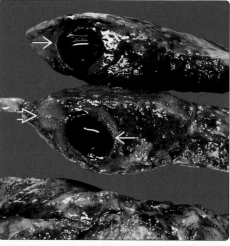

Laminated Intervillous Hematoma

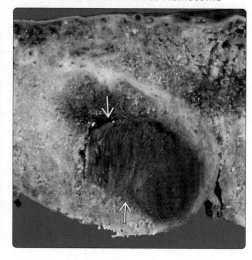

(Left) *Rounded intraplacental hematoma (infarction hematoma) is a distinct type of infarct ⊡. The rounded gross appearance is critical to recognition of this lesion. In contrast to benign flow voids or intervillous hematomas, this blood collection is demarcated by compressed, pale infarcted parenchyma ⊡.* (Right) *This hemorrhagic nodule is shown after fixation. Lines of Zahn ⊡ are more common in intervillous hematomas than in infarction hematoma.*

Gross Evaluation and Normal Histology of Chorionic Villi

Intervillous Hemorrhage

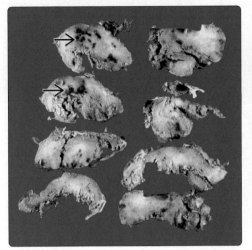

Intervillous Thrombus

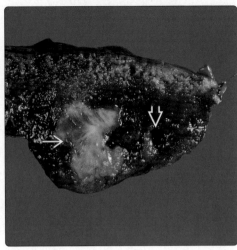

(Left) *Blood in the intervillous space is normally maternal. In cases of fetal-maternal hemorrhage ➡ the blood may be fetal. The edematous, pale parenchyma is consistent with fetal anemia. Microscopic examination shows fetal blood in the intervillous space. These breaks in the maternal fetal barrier are termed "Kline hemorrhages."* (Right) *This tan lesion shows fine striations, consistent with laminations of an intervillous thrombus ➡. Also present is a benign (physiologic) flow void ➡.*

Massive Perivillous Fibrin Deposition

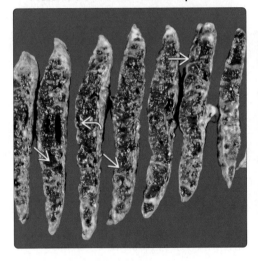

Massive Perivillous Fibrin Deposition

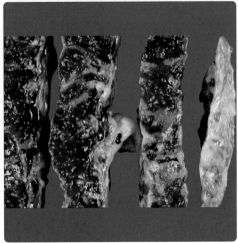

(Left) *These sections show a diffuse increase in fibrin, both crossing from the chorionic plate to basal plate ➡ and localized at the decidua basalis ➡, consistent with massive perivillous fibrin deposition. The terms "fibrin" and "fibrinoid" are often used interchangeably in this disorder.* (Right) *Tan-white strands cross the parenchyma. The fibrin is homogeneous and shiny on the cut section. The percentage involvement must be assessed on gross exam; 50% of the parenchyma should be affected for a diagnosis of MPVFD.*

Gross Exam in Chronic Villitis

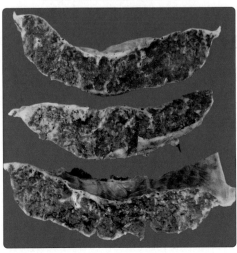

Large Focus of Avascular Villi

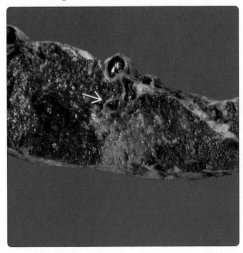

(Left) *Chronic villitis is a microscopic diagnosis; on gross examination, the disc may be small for age. Careful inspection may show coarsened granularity of the parenchyma, increased fibrin deposition, and vague areas of pallor.* (Right) *Large foci of fetal vascular malperfusion can be seen on gross exam. The lesion is tan, but finely granular villous texture is preserved. The associated stem vessel is dilated and contains some fibrin ➡.*

1st-Trimester Gestational Sac

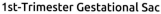

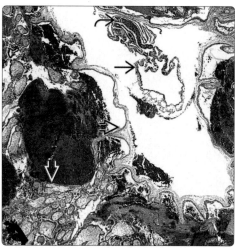

Early Villogenesis

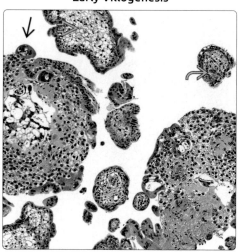

(Left) *The earliest villi form from the chorionic disc as projections into lakes of maternal blood. This image from an ectopic pregnancy shows an embryo ➡, yolk sac ➡, and chorionic plate ➡ with primary, secondary, and tertiary villi ➡.* (Right) *Villous sprouts begin as projections of syncytiotrophoblast ➡ invested with cytotrophoblast. The developing mesenchymal stroma contains mostly polygonal stromal cells ➡. Capillaries form in situ from the stroma ➡.*

Mesenchymal Villi

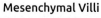

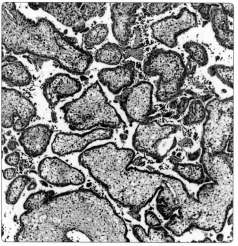

Immature Intermediate Villi

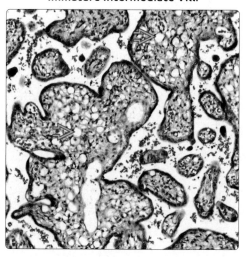

(Left) *These 1st-trimester villi have polygonal stromal cells in a loose mesenchyme. Similar-appearing mesenchymal villi may be seen throughout gestation in limited numbers. They are a source for further villogenesis.* (Right) *The 2nd-trimester placenta has numerous immature intermediate villi. These villi have a loose reticular stroma full of rounded spaces ➡, many of which contain fetal macrophages (Hofbauer cells).*

Immature Intermediate Villi

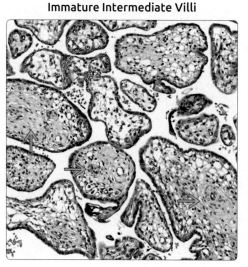

Late 2nd-Trimester Villi

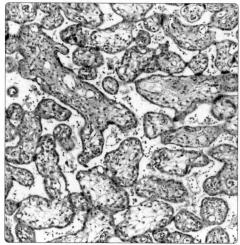

(Left) *These 2nd-trimester villi show maturation of the immature intermediate villi with development of vascular smooth muscle and collagenization of the stromal core ➡.* (Right) *These 28-weeks-gestation villi retain the loose reticular stroma of immature intermediate villi. This immature morphology can be difficult to distinguish from villous edema.*

Intermediate Villi

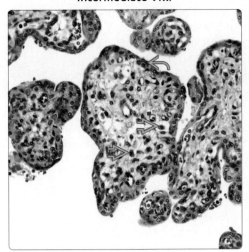

Intermediate Villi and Distal Villi

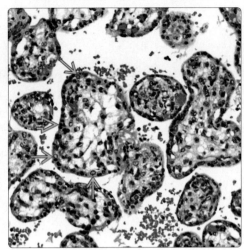

(Left) This 27-weeks-gestation villus shows classic features of 2nd-trimester villi. Syncytiotrophoblast and cytotrophoblast nuclei ⇨ are easily identified, as are Hofbauer cells ⇨. There are few stromal capillaries. These intermediate villi will bring blood to and from terminal villi, which are yet to fully form. (Right) Late in the 2nd trimester, villi of smaller diameter are more abundant. Syncytiotrophoblast nuclei remain evenly spaced ⇨. The more vesicular cytotrophoblast nuclei ⇨ are still present but discontinuous.

Distal Villi

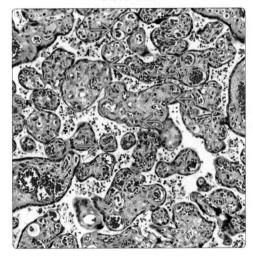

Mature Terminal Villi

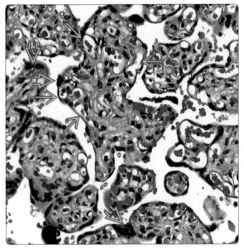

(Left) Early in the 3rd trimester, distal villi are formed ⇨. The larger intermediate villi in the center ⇨ have few vasculosyncytial membranes compared to mature distal villi. (Right) Mature villi are optimized for gas and nutrient exchange. Syncytiotrophoblast nuclei are gathered into knots, and cytotrophoblast nuclei are rare, leaving a thin vasculosyncytial membrane ⇨. Approximately 1/3 of villi show syncytial knots ⇨.

Bridging Syncytial Knots

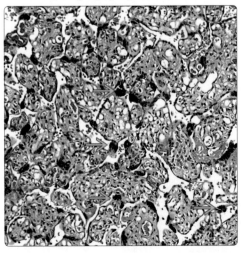

Normal Perivillous Fibrin

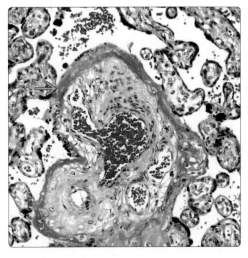

(Left) These mature villi show bridging knots ⇨ joining adjacent villi. Standards for quantification of knots exclude bridging knots and include only aggregates of > 5 syncytiotrophoblast nuclei that protrude above the villus contour. (Right) The presence of fibrin around proximal stem villi and at the subchorionic plate (Langhans stria) is seen with maturity. Over time, the syncytiotrophoblast is no longer replenished by cytotrophoblast and is replaced by fibrin ⇨.

OVERVIEW

Spectrum of Changes

- Chorionic villi vary in appearance
  - Variation over time with different morphology at different stages of development
  - Variation also in different regions of placenta
  - Variation between patients at similar gestational ages
- Histopathologic changes due to
  - Abnormal maturation
  - Inflammation/infection
  - Ischemia (from inadequate maternal or fetal perfusion)
  - Trauma
- These changes are part of broader constellation of clinically significant findings explored in greater detail elsewhere in text

DISORDERS OF VILLOUS MATURATION

General Features

- Villi become smaller as they mature
  - Accelerated villous maturation: Smaller terminal villi in greater proportion than expected for age
  - Delayed villous maturation: Larger villi than expected for age
- Gradient of maturity in normal placenta
  - More mature histology beneath chorionic plate, at periphery of lobule
  - Least mature histology near base, in center of lobule
  - Gradient exaggerated in states of abnormal villous maturation
- Vasculosyncytial membranes (VSM) signify full maturity in terminal villus
  - VSM: Area of broad contact between capillary and syncytiotrophoblast layer without intervening nucleus or connective tissue
    - Defined in mature placenta (after 34 weeks)
    - < 1 VSM per 4 small distal villi, on average, in count of 10 HPF (400x)

- VSM form as villous capillaries bulge against syncytiotrophoblast
  - May be absent if increased stromal volume from edema or immaturity
  - May be absent if collapse of fetal blood content or decreased perfusion pressure

Delayed Villous Maturation

- Failure to form appropriate proportion of terminal villi in mature placenta
  - Definition: Groups of at least 10 larger, immature-appearing villi, comprising at least 30% of parenchyma on full-thickness section
  - Villi appear larger with centrally located vessels
  - May have reticular stroma (rounded clear spaces ± Hofbauer cells)
  - More common histology in basal 1/3 of villi
    - Single foci not meeting criteria above may be physiologic growth centers, usually at center of villous tree, near base
  - Difficult to diagnose before 34-weeks gestation
  - Histologic overlap with changes of villous edema
    - Both processes feature larger villous size, loose stroma, fewer VSM
- Failure to form sufficient VSM
  - Seen in 6% of placentas after 34 weeks
    - Associated with fetal demise ~ 38 weeks
    - Associated with hypercoiled umbilical cords
- Increased numbers of villous cytotrophoblast
  - Villous cytotrophoblasts normally inconspicuous in term distal villi, ~ 1 cell per villus
  - Rarely may persist as continuous layer under syncytiotrophoblast, similar to early gestation
  - Increase more often seen as 2 or more villous cytotrophoblast per mature distal villous
- Clinical associations with delayed maturation include gestational diabetes and prediabetes
- Difficult diagnosis to make, even among experts
  - Look for enlarged villi with poor VSM formation

Distal Villous Immaturity

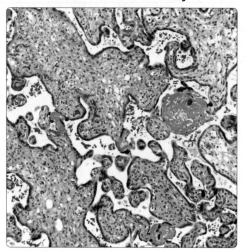

Accelerated Villous Maturation

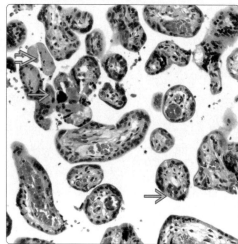

(Left) These villi from a 39-week pregnancy are large with poor vascular development. At this gestational age, the majority of villi should be small vascular distal villi. (Right) These villi are too small for normal development at 25-weeks gestation. They are not as widely spaced or very small, as seen in distal villous hypoplasia. Syncytial knots ➡, a feature of maturity, are seen. There is also fibrinoid necrosis of individual villi ➡, an uncommon feature in the 2nd trimester.

- o Don't over call congested villi as delayed villous maturation or chorangiosis

Chorangiosis

- Excess of capillary profiles per villus due to increased length of capillary causing excessive coiling
  - o Defined as > 10 capillaries per villus in > 10 villi in multiple (10) HPF
- Commonly seen together with delayed villous maturation

Hypovascular Villi

- Common histology that lacks consensus definition and has not been well studied
  - o Similar lesion termed "reparative villitis" or stromal fibrosis, assumed to be reparative stage after chronic villitis
    - − Unclear if this predominant etiology
  - o Can be seen in continuity with uninjured mesenchymal-appearing villi of growth centers
  - o Precursor shows immature villi with some but not all vessels showing karyorrhexis
- Villi often large like immature villi, but stroma appears mature and collagen rich

Accelerated Villous Maturation

- Villi appear more mature than expected histology for gestational age
  - o Difficult to diagnose after 36 weeks
  - o Increased numbers of smaller villi with VSM
  - o Increased syncytial knotting for age
  - o Usually accompanied by increased perivillous fibrin along stem villi and beneath chorionic plate
- Associated conditions include changes of maternal vascular malperfusion, prematurity, and twin gestations

Distal Villous Hypoplasia

- Sparse, small, elongated distal villi
  - o Some villi appear to be single capillary loop with syncytiotrophoblast knot
  - o Few distal villi present between stem villi
- Associated with other changes of maternal vascular malperfusion
- Diagnostic criteria: Involves > 30% of parenchyma
  - o Normal change at extreme periphery of lobule
  - o Focal: > 30% on 1 slide
  - o Diffuse: > 30% on > 1 slide

Increased Syncytial Knots

- Feature of maternal vascular malperfusion and accelerated maturation
- Defined as knots in > 20% of villi preterm (before 34 weeks) or 30% of villi at term (after 38 weeks)
- Tenney-Parker change: Increased syncytial knots that stand out from villous surface as polypoid projections, often seen with distal villous hypoplasia

INFLAMMATION

Acute Villitis

- Accumulation of neutrophils in villus, usually between syncytiotrophoblast layer and stroma, usually focal, associated with fetal sepsis in amniotic fluid infection

Chronic Villitis

- Infiltrate of lymphocytes with histiocytes, rarely plasma cells
- May be subchorionic, mid-parenchymal, paraseptal, or basal in distribution
- Grading (Amsterdam consensus)
  - o Low grade: < 10 villi affected per focus, can be focal (1 slide) or multifocal (> 1 slide)
  - o High grade: > 10 villi affected in any focus, can be patchy or diffuse if > 30% of parenchyma affected
- May have associated chronic chorioamnionitis, fetal vasculopathy, or increased perivillous fibrin

CHANGES OF FETAL VASCULAR MALPERFUSION

Villous Stromal-Vascular Karyorrhexis

- Reflects early change of interrupted or insufficient fetal perfusion of villi
- Definition: Karyorrhexis of fetal blood cells, endothelial cells, and stromal cells in villus
  - o Affects groups of villi
  - o Usually affects all 3 components (blood cells, endothelial cells, stromal cells) in segmental lesions or after fetal demise
  - o May affect only subset of villous vessels in edematous/immature-appearing villi

Avascular Villi

- Later distal villous lesion of interrupted or insufficient fetal perfusion
- Definition: Groups of homogeneously pink villi, may contain stromal cells but lack capillaries; syncytiotrophoblast layer viable
  - o Affects groups of villi
    - − Small: 2-4 villi affected in ≥ 3 foci
    - − Intermediate: 5-10 villi per focus
    - − Large: > 10 villi per focus

EDEMA

Multifocal Edema

- Markedly enlarged reticular spaces, often with frequent reactive Hofbauer cells, present in multiple foci

Villous Edema/Dysmaturity

- Enlarged villi, loose mesenchymal-appearing stroma, central thin-walled vessels
  - o Pallor suggests edema; poor vascular development suggests immaturity

Villous Hydrops

- Increased placental weight and bulk; villi diffusely edematous
- Usually in setting of hydropic infant
- Often with separation of syncytiotrophoblast from villous stroma

ISCHEMIC CHANGES AND VILLOUS INJURY

Villous Agglutination

- Microscopic lesion showing adherent clusters of villi not separated by maternal blood space

- Often with damage to syncytiotrophoblast and thin rim of perivillous fibrin deposition

Infarct

- Grossly visible lesion showing degeneration with progressive loss of nuclear basophilia of all components of distal villi
  - Usual infarct shows loss of intervillous space with agglutination of dead villi
  - Subset shows separation of dead villi by intervillous fibrin

Intravillous Hemorrhage

- Fetal blood hemorrhage into villous stroma
  - Associations include venous obstruction, ischemia, and bruising of villi from abdominal trauma or placental abruption

Fibrinoid Necrosis

- Perivillous fibrin incorporated into villous stroma; stroma adjacent to fibrin becomes avascular
- Typically affects only single or small groups of villi in mature placenta
- Considered normal in term placenta when confined to < 3% of distal villi
- Abnormal preterm, may accompany accelerated maturation
- Attributed to syncytiotrophoblast injury with exhaustion of cytotrophoblast population for regeneration

DISORDERS OF FETAL BLOOD COMPONENTS

Increased Nucleated Red Blood Cells

- > 10 NRBCs in 10 HPF (400x) of distal villi in mature placenta; associated with fetal stress
  - No standards for preterm placenta

Erythroblastosis Fetalis

- Numerous circulating fetal precursor NRBCs, often with immature forms
  - Associated with immune- and nonimmune-mediated hemolysis, severe fetal-maternal hemorrhage, Parvovirus B19, and CMV infection

Myeloid Proliferation of Down Syndrome

- Leukemia-like condition of Down syndrome fetus with numerous circulating immature myeloid cells, including megakaryoblasts and NRBCs
- Regresses in most patients by 3 months (transient abnormal myelopoiesis); some develop myelodysplastic syndrome and acute myeloid leukemia
  - Can cause fetal demise with fibrosis of liver, heart, and other organs

CHANGES OF PERIVILLOUS SPACE

Increased Perivillous Fibrin

- Injury, degenerative changes of syncytiotrophoblast leads to deposition of fibrin
  - Can be focal or diffuse
  - Diffuse cases evident grossly as massive perivillous fibrin deposition/maternal floor infarction
- Often seen with fibrinoid necrosis of villi

Perivillous Trophoblast Proliferations

- Reactive proliferations of intermediate-type extravillous trophoblast adjacent to villi
  - Many so-called "cell islands" have focal perivillous connection
- May be associated with local ischemia, but not well studied
- May show marked enlargement and atypia of trophoblast
  - Distinguish from true neoplastic trophoblast in intraplacental choriocarcinoma
    - Reactive proliferations often show larger cells than intraplacental choriocarcinoma
    - Reactive proliferations usually involve only 1 villus; incidental microscopic finding
    - Intraplacental choriocarcinoma usually identified as lesion on gross exam, often mistaken as infarct

OTHER CHANGES

Vacuolation of Syncytiotrophoblast

- Prominent cytoplasmic clearing in syncytiotrophoblast
  - Associated with fetal metabolic storage diseases
    - Mucopolysaccharidoses, sphingolipidoses, mucolipidoses, and other lipidoses, oligosaccharidoses, and glycogen storage disease
    - Some entities show storage material in other cells, such as Hofbauer cells

Dysplastic Changes Associated With Abnormal Chromosomes

- Abnormal villus contour: Irregular shape; sectioning may show trophoblast inclusions
- Stromal cell cytomegaly: Marked cytomegaly (3x variation in size) with hyperchromasia
- Abnormal vasculature: Maze-like, irregular vascular proliferations

SELECTED REFERENCES

1. Khong TY et al: Sampling and definitions of placental lesions: Amsterdam placental workshop group consensus statement. Arch Pathol Lab Med. 140(7):698-713, 2016
2. Al-Adnani M et al: "Delayed Villous Maturation" in Placental Reporting: Concordance among Consultant Pediatric Pathologists at a Single Specialist Center. Pediatr Dev Pathol. 18(5):375-9, 2015
3. Redline RW: Elevated circulating fetal nucleated red blood cells and placental pathology in term infants who develop cerebral palsy. Hum Pathol. 39(9):1378-84, 2008
4. Redline RW et al: Maternal vascular underperfusion: nosology and reproducibility of placental reaction patterns. Pediatr Dev Pathol. 7(3):237-49, 2004
5. Stallmach T et al: Rescue by birth: defective placental maturation and late fetal mortality. Obstet Gynecol. 97(4):505-9, 2001
6. Salafia CM et al: Intrauterine growth restriction in infants of less than thirty-two weeks' gestation: associated placental pathologic features. Am J Obstet Gynecol. 173(4):1049-57, 1995
7. Roberts DJ et al: Diagnosis of unsuspected fetal metabolic storage disease by routine placental examination. Pediatr Pathol. 11(4):647-56, 1991

Delayed Villous Maturation

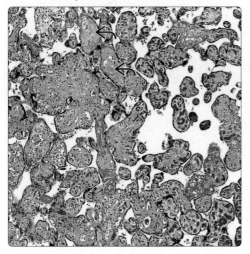

Poor Vasculosyncytial Membrane Formation

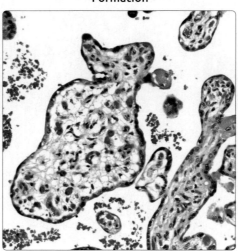

(Left) *These villi are too large and hypervascular for term. Note the fibrinoid necrosis ⟶. There are too few vasculosyncytial membranes, indicating a villous maturation defect. Distal villous immaturity represents a villous maturation defect, but not all cases with villous maturation defect have distal villous immaturity.* (Right) *The hypervascular villus of this term placenta fails to show gestational age-appropriate apposition of capillaries to thinned syncytiotrophoblast in regions without knots.*

Chorangiosis

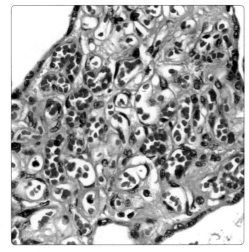

Hypovascular Villus

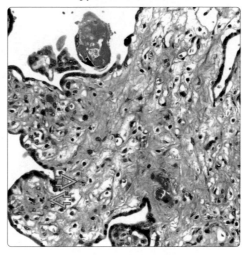

(Left) *This villus is enlarged by multiple coils of the capillary loops.* (Right) *In contrast, this term villus is enlarged and hypovascular. Note the karyorrhexis ⟶ limited to a subset of the villous vessels. There are overlapping features of dysmaturity, edema, and fetal vascular malperfusion.*

Increased Numbers of Villous Cytotrophoblast

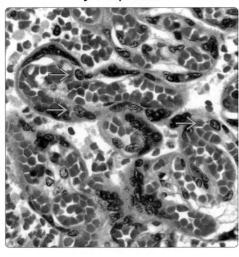

Persistence of Continuous Cytotrophoblast Layer

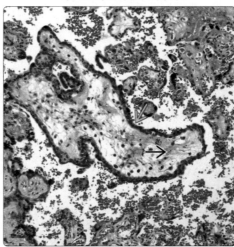

(Left) *Two or more cytotrophoblast/villus ⟶ in multiple villi (10) in multiple HPF is recognized as a pattern of increased villous cytotrophoblast numbers by international placental consensus groups; this is difficult to recognize in daily practice.* (Right) *Persistence of a continuous cytotrophoblast layer ⟶ in the mature placenta is almost always a focal finding, usually in a growth center. This immature villus in a 41-week placenta also shows vascular karyorrhexis ⟶.*

Accelerated Maturation

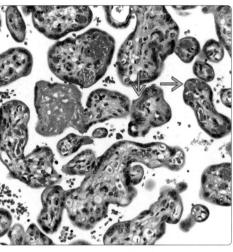

Distal Villous Hypoplasia

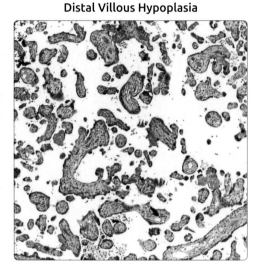

(Left) These 2nd-trimester villi are smaller than expected and have multiple vasculosyncytial membranes ➡. These changes should be a major pattern, not a focal finding, to make the diagnosis of accelerated maturation. (Right) These villi from a 30-week placenta are sparse and very small for age. Some consist of only a single capillary loop and syncytium. The villi are smaller and more sparse than in accelerated maturation.

Distal Villous Hypoplasia With Tenney-Parker Changes

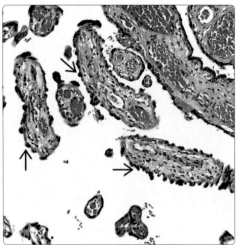

Distal Villous Hypoplasia

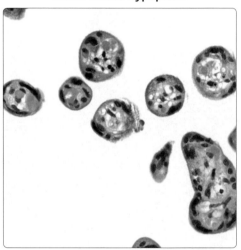

(Left) These villi of distal villous hypoplasia (DVH) in a 27-week placenta complicated by severe preterm preeclampsia also show Tenney-Parker changes with numerous small, polypoid syncytial knots ➡. This may reflect attempts at villogenesis, as trophoblast sprouting is the initial stage in new growth. (Right) Villi begin as trophoblast sprouts from the surface of stem or intermediate villi. In DVH, very little development of mesenchyme or capillary elongation occurs to increase the villous volume.

Increased Syncytial Knots

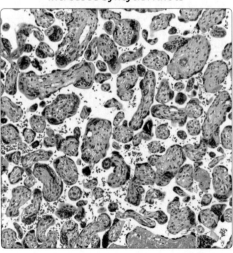

Fibrinoid Necrosis of Individual Villi

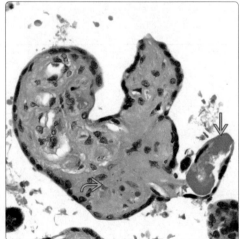

(Left) Increased syncytial knotting is another feature of accelerated maturation. It may be a feature of maternal vascular malperfusion in the appropriately mature placenta as well. (Right) Damage to the syncytiotrophoblast leads to fibrin deposition ➡. Nodules of fibrin may be surrounded by syncytiotrophoblast. The underlying villus becomes progressively avascular ➡. This change is normally present in up to 3% of villi at term. In contrast to avascular villi, single villi are affected.

Acute Villitis

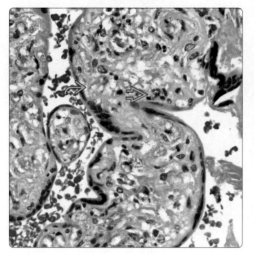

Acute Villitis

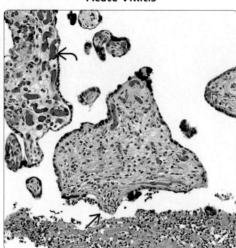

(Left) *This fetal demise due to E. coli maternal sepsis was associated with subtle neutrophil infiltrates ⊟. The fetal blood appears blue-tinged from bacterial overgrowth ⊟.* **(Right)** *Acute villitis ⊟ is a rare but important finding, associated with fetal sepsis due to ascending infection (amniotic fluid infection sequence). These villi are also hypervascular (chorangiosis) ⊟.*

Chronic Villitis

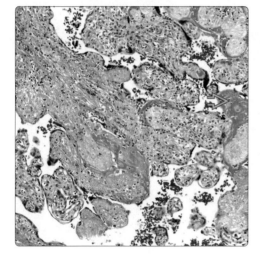

Chronic Villitis

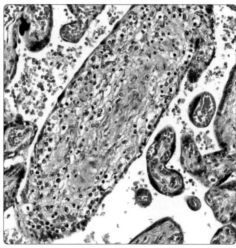

(Left) *Chronic villitis is characterized by an infiltrate of maternal T cells into the villous stroma. It may feature trophoblast injury with perivillous fibrin deposition ⊟ and inflammation &/or involution of the fetal vessels.* **(Right)** *In this image, the inflammation is low grade (< 10 villi per focus). The syncytiotrophoblast is intact, but fetal vessels are indistinct.*

Chronic Villitis With Plasma Cells

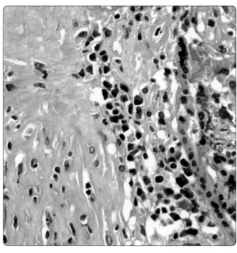

Hofbauer Cell Hyperplasia

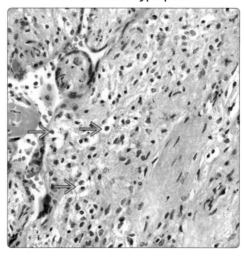

(Left) *The presence of plasma cells in chronic villitis should prompt exclusion of infections, especially CMV.* **(Right)** *Increased numbers of stromal Hofbauer cells ⊟ (macropahges) is also termed "histiocytic villitis." This villus with Hofbauer cell hyperplasia is from an intrauterine fetal demise due to undiagnosed syphilis.*

(Left) *At low power, the fetal vessels are indistinct. A stem villus shows early vascular obliterative changes* ⮕. **(Right)** *The dusty debris of karyorrhexis is admixed with calcifications in this focus of villous stromal-vascular karyorrhexis. In general, karyorrhexis eventually affects fetal blood cells, endothelial cells, and stromal cells.*

Villous Stromal-Vascular Karyorrhexis

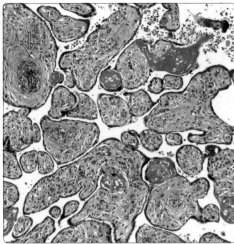

Villous Stromal-Vascular Karyorrhexis

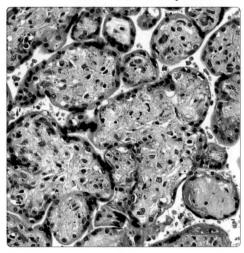

(Left) *Avascular villi appear at a later stage of fetal vascular malperfusion. In contrast to fibrinoid necrosis, whole groups of villi are affected. At low power, the homogeneous pink appearance of the villi* ⮕ *stands out in contrast to the variegated appearance of normal villi at the lower left.* **(Right)** *This pattern suggestive of edema shows marked enlargement of reticular spaces* ⮕ *in what appear to be mature villi. These spaces are not vessels. They may contain Hofbauer cells* ⮕.

Avascular Villi

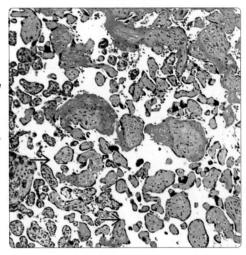

Villous Edema With Prominent Reticular Spaces

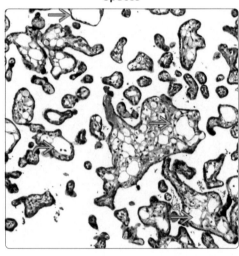

(Left) *In some cases, it may be impossible to distinguish edema from immaturity. These 36-week villi differ from immature villi in that the syncytiotrophoblast* ⮕ *layer appears thin without cytotrophoblast.* **(Right)** *In placental hydrops, edema may cause separation of the syncytiotrophoblast layer from the stroma* ⮕. *Note the numerous nucleated red blood cells* ⮕ *in the fetal circulation in this case of severe fetal anemia.*

Villous Edema/Dysmaturity

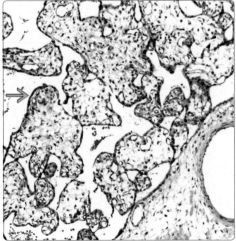

Villous Edema in Hydrops

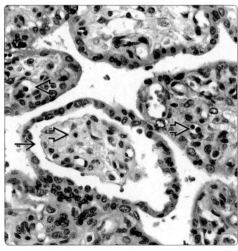

Villous Agglutination

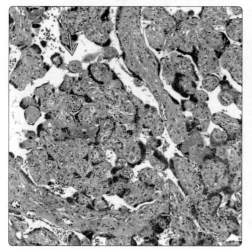

Infarct

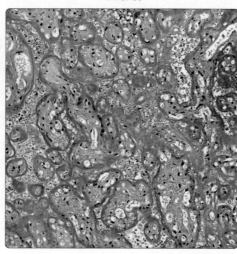

(Left) *These villi are coalesced* ⬆ *with smudging of the syncytiotrophoblast. Villous agglutination is a microscopic change on the progression to villous infarction.* (Right) *Infarcts become progressively pink over time as villi lose nuclear basophilia.*

Intravillous Hemorrhage

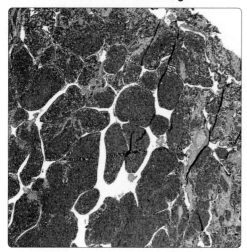

Myeloid Proliferation of Down Syndrome

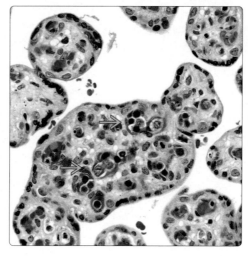

(Left) *These villi were injured from an acute placental abruption.* (Right) *Myeloid proliferation of Down syndrome [a.k.a. transient abnormal myelopoiesis (TAM)] is the most common cause of blasts and hematopoietic precursors* ➡ *in the fetal blood. It is usually a mixed population of immature erythroid cells, myeloblasts, and abnormal megakaryocytes.*

Syncytiotrophoblast Vacuoles

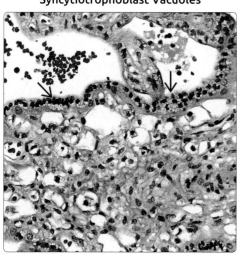

Cytotrophoblast Pleomorphism

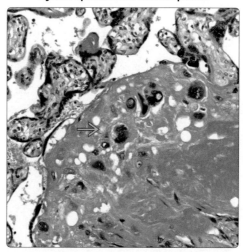

(Left) *The syncytiotrophoblast in this case shows cytoplasmic vacuolization* ➡. *This uncommon change suggests a metabolic storage disease in the fetus, and clinical correlation is imperative. Some liposomal drug formulations can cause similar changes.* (Right) *Extravillous cytotrophoblasts are often abundant in foci of perivillous fibrin deposition. The cells may become enlarged and bizarre appearing* ➡ *as a reactive change.*

TERMINOLOGY

Abbreviations

- Extravillous trophoblast (EVT) cells

Definitions

- Septum: EVT-derived connections from lateral anchoring villi to basal plate
  - Defines lateral margins of cotyledons
- Intervillous space: Maternal blood space between chorionic villi
  - Bound by chorionic plate, septa, basal plate, and marginal sinus
- Basal plate: EVT-derived interface between villous parenchyma and decidua basalis

MACROSCOPIC

Septa

- Thin, white lines extending into parenchyma perpendicularly from basal plate
- Gross lesions
  - Smooth-walled, fluid-filled cysts lined by EVT
  - Hemorrhage/thrombohematoma within septum

Intervillous Space

- Usually not visible unless replaced by fibrin
- Gross lesions
  - Perivillous/intervillous fibrin: Serpiginous-appearing, tan-white strands, firm to touch
  - Intervillous fibrin plaque: Tan, firm lesion, thinner than thrombus or infarct, no lamination or lines of Zahn
  - Intervillous thrombus: Laminated lesion may appear red-tan in recent lesions or tan-white in older lesions

Basal Plate

- Thin rim of tan-white or translucent tissue on maternal surface of placenta
  - Gives rounded, intact appearance to cotyledons
- Torn-appearing cotyledons lack basal plate, may signify incomplete removal

- Gross lesions
  - Maternal floor infarct
  - Basal intervillous thrombus/intervillous fibrin plaque

NORMAL HISTOLOGY

Septa

- Wedge-shaped projections from basal plate into intervillous space
- Connect with anchoring villi on lateral aspects
- Lined by syncytiotrophoblast, becomes replaced by fibrin over time
- Cellularity: Mostly EVT embedded in matrix-type fibrinoid
  - In lower 1/2, may contain core of decidual cells
- Often see openings of maternal vessels at base where septum connects with basal plate

Intervillous Space

- Normally contains mostly maternal red blood cells; frequent nucleated cells pathologic

Basal Plate

- Contains matrix-type fibrinoid, blood fibrin, and EVT
  - May see "foot" of anchoring villus embedded and surrounded by fibrinoid
  - Profiles of maternal vessels show large lumens surrounded by fibrinoid and EVT with no residual muscle
- Aspect-facing intervillous space lined by syncytiotrophoblast in some regions, and elsewhere, maternal endothelial cells
  - Fibrin deposited on this side called "Rohr's fibrinoid"
- On decidual side, EVT and fibrinoid appose decidual cells
  - Fibrin termed "Nitabuch's fibrinoid"

SELECTED REFERENCES

1. Ockleford CD: The allo-epi-endothelial lining of the intervillous space. Placenta. 31(12):1035-42, 2010
2. Salafia CM et al: Morphometry of the basal plate superficial uteroplacental vasculature in normal midtrimester and at term. Pediatr Dev Pathol. 8(6):639-46, 2005

Normal Basal Plate With Prominent Septum

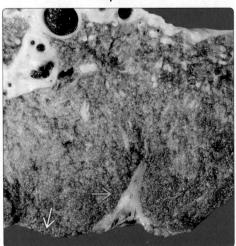

Septum

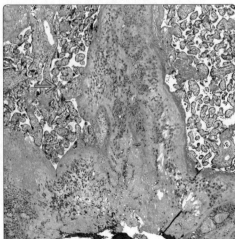

(Left) A normal basal plate ➡ appears as a thin, tan-white layer adherent to the villous parenchyma. Folds of the basal plate and decidua into the parenchyma form septa ➡. (Right) Septa ➡ are not seen connecting to the basal plate on every full-thickness section. Villi attach to the sides of septa, providing extravillous trophoblast (EVT) from cell columns. The amount of EVT present generally correlates with the thickness of the septa.

Gross Evaluation and Normal Histology
of Septa, Intervillous Space, and Basal Plate

Expanded Septum

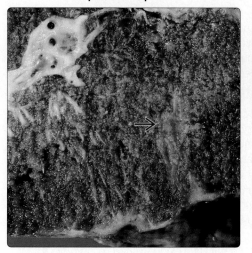

Villous Lakes

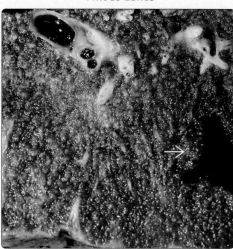

(Left) *Expanded septa ➡ appear gray and mucoid on gross exam. Rounded EVT-lined cysts may be seen. These are generally considered insignificant changes unless multiple (> 3) cysts are seen.* (Right) *The intervillous space is inconspicuous in normal circumstances. Expansions without thrombosis ➡ can be seen and are termed "villous lakes" or "flow voids." They have no known significance.*

Increased Perivillous Fibrin Deposition

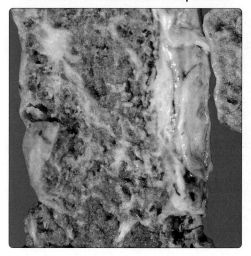

Maternal Floor Infarction

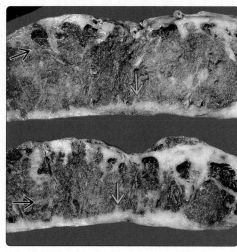

(Left) *Increased perivillous fibrin appears as serpiginous, tan-white, firm stranding of the parenchyma. When > 50% of the total parenchyma is affected, the term "massive perivillous fibrin deposition" is used.* (Right) *Maternal floor infarction (MFI) is part of the same spectrum as massive perivillous fibrin deposition; however, in MFI, the fibrin is localized to the basal plate. In this case, the basal plate appears flattened and thickened from excessive fibrinoid ➡. The speckled gray areas correspond to numerous EVT-associated microcysts ➡.*

Maternal Blood Returning via Septum

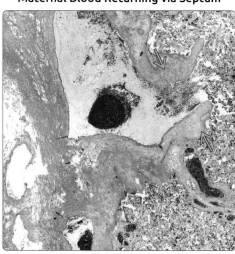

Basal Plate

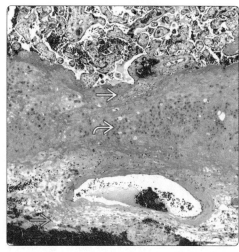

(Left) *Intervillous blood returns to the maternal venous circulation through openings ➡ in the septa and marginal sinus.* (Right) *The basal plate forms the maternal surface boundary of the intervillous space. It contains a variable amount of decidua basalis ➡, maternal vessels, embedded anchoring villi ➡ with EVT ➡, and fibrinoid. The inner lining is maternal endothelium in some areas, syncytiotrophoblast elsewhere, and fibrin deposition where both are absent.*

TERMINOLOGY

Abbreviations

- Extravillous trophoblast (EVT) cells

Synonyms

- Intervillous fibrin and intervillous fibrinoid, often used interchangeably in literature

Definitions

- Fibrin/fibrinoid: Dense, pink extracellular material deposited in placenta may be maternal blood fibrin or fibrinoid, product of EVT cells
  - Blood fibrin is usually red on trichrome, EVT-associated fibrinoid is usually blue, with EVT embedded in material
  - For simplification and consistency, both products are referred to as fibrin

MICROSCOPIC

Histopathologic Changes of Septa

- Septal cysts
  - EVT-lined cysts, similar to those seen in membranes, chorionic plate, and basal plate
- Septal hematoma
  - Can see hemorrhage into septa, usually at base, likely from decidual vessels

Histopathologic Changes of Intervillous Space

- Acute intervillositis
- Chronic histiocytic intervillositis
  - Important not to miss diagnosis; associated with recurrent pregnancy complications (intrauterine growth rate, fetal demise)
  - Often associated with increased perivillous fibrin deposition
- Placental malaria
- Maternal leukemia
- Fetal nucleated red blood cells in intervillous space
- Maternal sickle cell disorders
- Increased intervillous fibrin

- Excessive perivillous fibrin deposition
  - Localized
  - Massive perivillous fibrin deposition/maternal floor infarction
- Intervillous thrombus/thrombohematoma, intervillous fibrin plaque
- Frequent cell islands (> 3 foci in mature placenta)

Histopathologic Changes of Basal Plate

- EVT proliferation
  - EVT may accumulate in basal plate, as under chorionic plate, membranous chorion, cell islands, and septa
  - Often associated with EVT cysts
- Maternal floor infarction
  - Fibrin and matrix type fibrinoid continuous with basal plate surround basal villi
  - Often with EVT embedded in fibrin
- Basal plate plaque
  - Localized basal plate plaque, similar to intervillous thrombus, localized to intervillous surface of basal plate
- Myometrium adherent to basal plate without intervening decidua
- Thrombosis of maternal vessels
  - Pathologic preterm
  - Significance at term unclear, may be preparation for parturition
- Uteroplacental chronic vasculitis
  - Lymphocytes embedded within fibrin surrounding transformed spiral arteries, often associated with dropout of trophoblast
  - May be physiologic preparation for end of pregnancy at term, not normal preterm

SELECTED REFERENCES

1. Chen A et al: Placental pathologic lesions with a significant recurrence risk - what not to miss! APMIS. ePub, 2017
2. Mekinian A et al: Chronic histiocytic intervillositis: outcome, associated diseases and treatment in a multicenter prospective study. Autoimmunity. 48(1):40-5, 2015
3. Stark MW et al: Histologic differences in placentas of preeclamptic/eclamptic gestations by birthweight, placental weight, and time of onset. Pediatr Dev Pathol. 17(3):181-9, 2014

Maternal Sickle Cell Trait

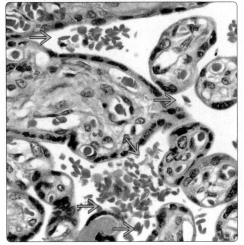

Frequent Cell Islands

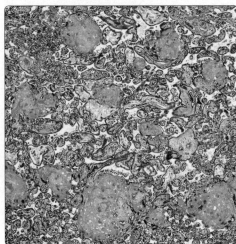

(Left) The intervillous space normally contains mostly red blood cells, reflecting the distribution of the maternal complete blood count. As in a blood smear, ↑ numbers of nucleated cells are abnormal. Sickled red blood cells ⇨ are easily seen in this placenta from a mother with sickle cell trait. (Right) Rounded formations of fibrinoid and extravillous trophoblast (EVT) are called cell islands. Continuity with a villus may be seen. They are similar to areas of contact of anchoring villi with septa or basal plate but are free floating.

Chronic Histiocytic Intervillositis

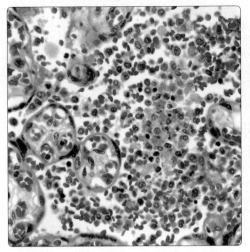

Fetal Nucleated Red Blood Cells in Intervillous Space

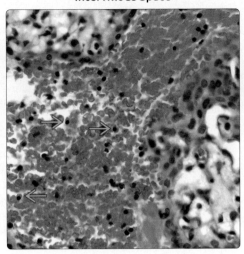

(Left) *Large numbers of nucleated cells in the intervillous space are abnormal. This placenta showed numerous histiocytes in the intervillous space. Chronic histiocytic intervillositis is an important diagnosis to recognize, associated with recurrent pregnancy loss, intrauterine growth restriction (IUGR), and maternal autoimmune conditions.* (Right) *These nucleated cells ⇾ are fetal erythroid cells in a case of chronic fetal-maternal hemorrhage with fetal hydrops.*

Increased Perivillous Fibrin

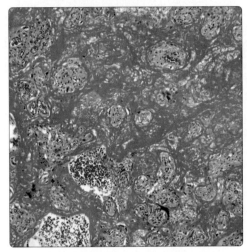

Blood-Fibrin Type Fibrin

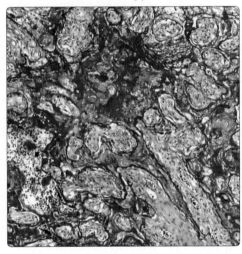

(Left) *The intervillous space is obliterated by fibrin. The villous stroma remains mostly viable. When > 50% of the parenchyma is involved on gross or microscopic exam of generalized lesions, the diagnosis of massive perivillous fibrin deposition is used. It is associated with IUGR, neurologic impairment, fetal demise, and recurrence risk.* (Right) *Trichrome staining shows that the fibrin filling the intervillous space is mostly dark red, similar to blood fibrin associated with clotting. No EVT proliferations are seen within the fibrin.*

Maternal Floor Infarction

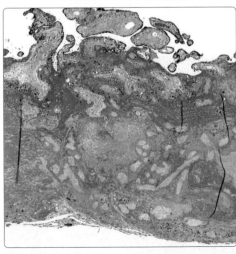

Extravillous Trophoblast Cysts

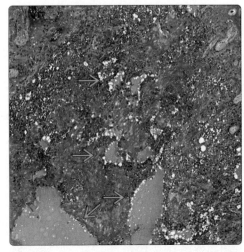

(Left) *Maternal floor infarction is an uncommon presentation of massive perivillous fibrin deposition where the excessive intervillous fibrin is deposited as a thick rind along the basal plate. The entrapped villi are infarcted. More than 25% of the basal plate should be involved to make the diagnosis. It is associated with IUGR and fetal demise.* (Right) *EVT in the septa, basal plate, or cell islands can form cysts ⇾, which may be visible grossly.*

TERMINOLOGY

Definitions

- Decidua: Endometrium in pregnancy
  - Decidua capsularis: Decidua overlying implanted blastocyst; progressively atrophies as gestational sac enlarges; not distinguished after 22 weeks
  - Decidua vera, decidua parietalis: All decidual lining of uterine cavity except that of implantation site
  - Decidua basalis: Decidua underlying placenta at implantation site
- Marginal sinus: Region where decidua vera meets decidua capsularis at edge of placental disc and where intervillous space connects with uteroplacental veins

Synonyms

- Decidua vera, decidua parietalis, and membranous decidua are synonyms

NORMAL FUNCTION OF DECIDUA

Facilitates Implantation

- Cytokines and cell surface molecules facilitate apposition, attachment, and penetration of blastocyst into gestational endometrium

Endocrine Function

- Decidual cells produce growth factors and cytokines that sustain embryo development

Immune Function

- Dendritic cells and uterine NK cells migrate to decidua from 6th-11th week post conception
  - Influence stromal cell differentiation and interact with extravillous trophoblast (EVT) in vascular remodeling

Facilitates Parturition

- Mechanical function
  - Latin root "deciduus" means "with tendency to fall off or shed"; decidua facilitates separation of placenta and membranes from uterus
  - Degenerative changes in upper decidua begin prior to labor and delivery in preparation for shedding
  - Absence of decidua leads to placenta accreta, increta, percreta wherein placenta remains firmly attached to maternal tissues
- Endocrine function
  - Decidual prostaglandin production markedly increases during labor and plays role in cervical ripening and myometrial contraction

MACROSCOPIC

Gross Appearance of Decidua

- Tan-yellow to gray tissue firmly adherent to membranes and basal surface of delivered placenta
  - Present in variable amounts, generally less in spontaneous term deliveries
- Decidua basalis vessels
  - Spiral arteries run perpendicular to surface in central placenta and more parallel at margins
    - Appear as punctate erosions
    - Estimated to number 0.5-1.0 per square centimeter of basal surface
  - Uteroplacental veins generally lay parallel to basal surface
    - Difficult to see; may appear as small white serpentine line segments

Pathologic Changes on Gross Examination

- Adherent blood clot
  - May be on basal surface, behind membranes, or at margin
    - Retroplacental hematoma may indent basal surface
  - Measure and weigh any well-formed hematomas
- Shaggy red-brown myometrial fibers on basal surface
  - Indicate occult placenta accreta
  - Take sections of suspicious areas
- Incomplete basal cotyledons
  - Suggest possible incomplete removal of placenta
- Spiral artery thrombi in decidua basalis (rare)

Types of Decidua

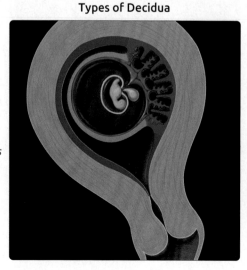

Decidua With Placental Circulation

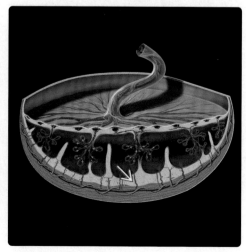

(Left) This diagram demonstrates the 3 types of decidua from early gestation. The decidua capsularis is in light pink, the decidua vera is in dark pink, and the decidua basalis is in purple. (Right) The decidua provides the only opportunity to evaluate maternal blood vessels ➡ in the delivered placenta. Vessels from all other sites are fetal. Maternal vessels are remodeled in pregnancy to optimize placental perfusion.

Decidual Vascular Remodeling in Pregnancy

Vasculature	1st Trimester	2nd Trimester	3rd Trimester	Postpartum
Spiral arteries of membranous decidua	Media thins out	Media remains thin	Media remains thin	Normal thickness resumes
Spiral arteries of decidua basalis	Extravillous cytotrophoblast cells invade wall and form luminal plugs; smooth muscle is replaced by fibrin	Lumen is enlarged and becomes patent; trophoblast cells embed in mural fibrin; 2nd wave of invasion goes deeper into arteries; ~ 1/3 of arteries invaded	All spiral arteries in central 2/3 are remodeled (90% of spiral arteries)	Placental bed vessels thrombose; trophoblasts in and near walls regress or die; smooth muscle regrows
Myometrial arteries	Media thins and lumen dilates	Arteries proximal to placental bed get remodeled with 2nd wave; all lumina remain dilated	Remodeling continues; vessel lumina remain dilated	Remodeled vessels thrombose; trophoblasts in and near walls regress or die; smooth muscle and elastica regrows; other lumina return to normal size; media thickens to prepregnant state
Veins	Lumen dilates	Veins underlying placental bed and at margins may have ingrowth of villi	Veins underlying placental bed may have ingrowth of villi; villous growth at margins facilitates lateral placental growth	Lumina return to normal size

MICROSCOPIC

Components of Decidua

- Endometrial stromal cells become decidual stromal cells under influence of progesterone
  - Polygonal stromal cells rich in glycogen and lipid
  - Proliferate and differentiate in pregnancy, become polyploid
  - Comprise 30% of cellularity in 1st trimester, 30-55% at term
- Immune cells
  - Uterine NK cells: 40% of cellularity in 1st trimester; 4-9% at term; secrete cytokines that aid in stromal cell differentiation and vascular remodeling
  - Macrophages and dendritic cells: 20% of cellularity in 1st trimester; 20-40% at term; aid in support of decidual function
  - T cells: 8-10% of cellularity in 1st trimester; 8-17% at term; play role in tolerance of fetal antigens
    - Subset appears primed to react to fetal antigens
    - Subdued during pregnancy but can be activated to respond to infection
  - B cells and plasma cells: Very rare in normal pregnancy, comprise < 1% of decidual cells
- Vasculature
  - Spiral arteries
    - In membranous decidua: Have thinned walls and do not undergo trophoblast-mediated vascular remodeling
    - In decidua basalis: Undergo trophoblast-mediated remodeling for optimal uteroplacental perfusion
  - Veins do not undergo trophoblast-mediated remodeling and have dilated lumina with inconspicuous to absent smooth muscle
    - May see ingrowth of villi
- EVT cells

  - Present at interface of membranous chorion or basal plate and decidua; stationary EVT cells secrete extracellular matrix; invasive EVT cells migrate to underlying tissues
  - Subset of invasive EVT cells remodels spiral arteries of decidua basalis (endovascular trophoblast); others remain outside of vessels (intermediate trophoblast)
- Multinucleated trophoblastic giant cells
  - Uncommon in normal decidual basalis; not seen in membranous decidua; thought to be derived from fusion of invasive EVT cells at end of their journey
- Glandular epithelium
  - Prominent in 1st-trimester specimens and uncommonly seen in delivered placental tissues
    - May show Arias-Stella reaction with nuclear enlargement and polymorphism as result of polyploidy

SELECTED REFERENCES

1. Crespo ÂC et al: Cytotoxic potential of decidual NK cells and CD8+ T cells awakened by infections. J Reprod Immunol. 119:85-90, 2017
2. Powell RM et al: Decidual T cells exhibit a highly differentiated phenotype and demonstrate potential fetal specificity and a strong transcriptional response to IFN. J Immunol. 199(10):3406-3417, 2017
3. Blois SM et al: Decidualization and angiogenesis in early pregnancy: unravelling the functions of DC and NK cells. J Reprod Immunol. 88(2):86-92, 2011
4. Whitley GS et al: Cellular and molecular regulation of spiral artery remodelling: lessons from the cardiovascular field. Placenta. 31(6):465-74, 2010
5. King A et al: Human uterine lymphocytes. Hum Reprod Update. 4(5):480-5, 1998
6. Dietl J et al: The decidua of early human pregnancy: immunohistochemistry and function of immunocompetent cells. Gynecol Obstet Invest. 33(4):197-204, 1992
7. Robertson WB et al: Uteroplacental vascular pathology. Eur J Obstet Gynecol Reprod Biol. 5(1-2):47-65, 1975

Decidua Basalis

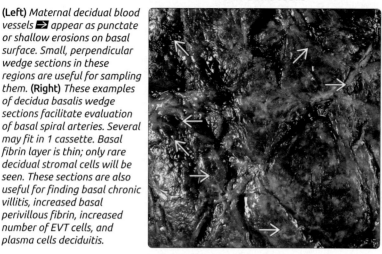

Wedge Sections to Visualize Decidua Basalis

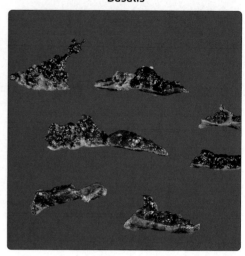

(Left) *Maternal decidual blood vessels* ⇒ *appear as punctate or shallow erosions on basal surface. Small, perpendicular wedge sections in these regions are useful for sampling them.* (Right) *These examples of decidua basalis wedge sections facilitate evaluation of basal spiral arteries. Several may fit in 1 cassette. Basal fibrin layer is thin; only rare decidual stromal cells will be seen. These sections are also useful for finding basal chronic villitis, increased basal perivillous fibrin, increased number of EVT cells, and plasma cells deciduitis.*

Decidua

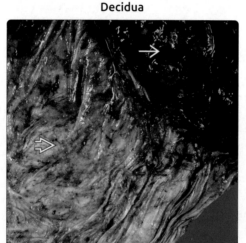

Membranous Decidua

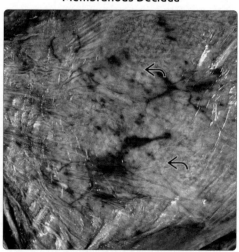

(Left) *Examination of the basal* ⇒ *and membranous* ⇒ *decidua provides an opportunity to evaluate the maternal vasculature. Viewed from the maternal side, the decidua is velvety tan-pink.* (Right) *Only a scant amount of residual decidua* ⇒ *is seen behind the placental membranes in this image. As the amount of membranous decidua is variable, submission of 2 membrane rolls is ideal.*

Membranous Decidua

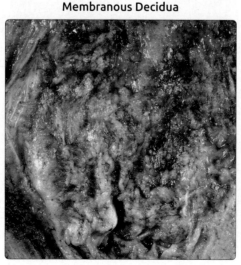

Retroplacental Hemorrhage

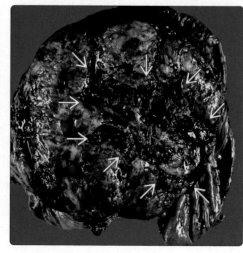

(Left) *In some specimens, membranous decidua is abundant, as seen in this image of the maternal surface of membranes. This is generally more common in nonspontaneous births.* (Right) *Retroplacental hemorrhage can be difficult to distinguish from nonspecific adherent blood. This case had a large marginal and retroplacental hemorrhage, which effaced and indented* ⇒ *the parenchyma.*

Vasculature of Membranous Decidua

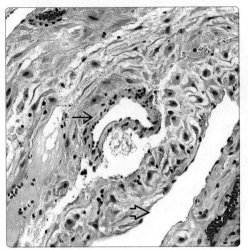

Decidual Glands

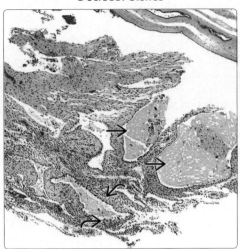

(Left) *This image shows a normal spiral artery ➡ and vein ⊟ of the membranous decidua. Arteries of the membranes do not get remodeled by trophoblast, but the musculature should appear appropriately thin (< 1/3 the diameter of the vessel). The vein has minimal to no smooth muscle.* **(Right)** *Membranous decidua may be abundant in the preterm placenta. This image shows glands ➡ with focal Arias-Stella change ⊟ characterized by hyperchromatic, enlarged nuclei.*

Minimal Decidua in Normal Membranes

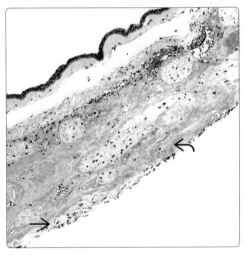

Minimal Decidua Basalis

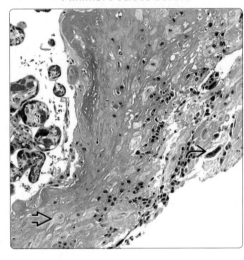

(Left) *Prior to labor and delivery, degenerative changes in the decidua ready the placenta and membranes for parturition. The membranes may only show fibrin ➡ with rare viable or necrotic residual decidual cells ➡.* **(Right)** *The basal plate may have minimal to no adherent decidua basalis. A multinucleated trophoblast cell ➡ is present. Rare decidual stromal cells ⊟ with pale nuclei and abundant cytoplasm are seen.*

Remodeled Spiral Artery of Decidua Basalis

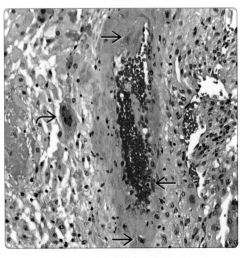

Decidua Basalis Veins

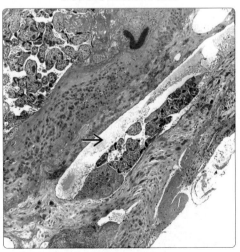

(Left) *This maternal spiral artery of the decidua basalis is adapted for pregnancy by trophoblast-mediated remodeling. The smooth muscle is replaced by fibrin ➡ encasing occasional trophoblast cells. Also present is a multinucleate trophoblast cell ➡.* **(Right)** *Decidua basalis veins are not remodeled by trophoblast but may show extension of villi ➡ into lumina. This is a normal mechanism of lateral placental growth and not evidence of placenta accreta.*

ACUTE INFLAMMATION

Acute Deciduitis

- Maternal neutrophils in decidua
  - May be earliest maternal inflammatory response to amniotic fluid infection (AFI)
    - Neutrophils migrate from decidual vessels toward membranes and amniotic fluid
  - If limited to decidua without chorioamnionitis
    - Look for fetal inflammatory response to further substantiate AFI sequence (AFIS)
    - Some cases of AFIS have more robust fetal response than maternal response, e.g., group B *Streptococcus*
    - Diffuse decidual leukocytoclastic necrosis also has neutrophils

CHRONIC INFLAMMATION

Plasma Cell Deciduitis

- Presence of plasma cells and lymphocytes in decidua
  - Also termed chronic deciduitis
  - Lymphocytes are normal constituent of decidua, but plasma cells are not
- Reflects abnormal immune environment; associations include
  - Chronic villitis of unknown etiology (VUE), especially basal VUE
  - AFIS
  - Hematogenous infections; look for additional changes
    - Cytomegalovirus
    - Herpes simplex virus
    - Syphilis
  - Preeclampsia, decidual arteriopathy
  - Severe immune Rh isoimmunization
  - Unclear association with chronic endometritis
- May be seen in decidua basalis or membranous decidua
- Plasma cell deciduitis present in ~ 10% of preterm placentas

Perivascular Chronic Inflammation

- Prominent cuff of lymphocytes around maternal decidual vessels
  - Seen in some cases of preeclampsia
- Perivascular lymphocytes are normal in 1st trimester
  - Uterine NK cells coordinate vascular remodeling

NECROSIS

Laminar Decidual Necrosis

- Bland, band-like necrosis of upper decidua
  - Loss of decidual stromal cell and vascular cell nuclear basophilia
- May be physiologic change in preparation for parturition
  - May be normal at term, pathologic preterm
- Associated with intrauterine hypoxia in some studies but not in others
  - Discrepancy in significance may reflect gestational age
- Leads to separation of placenta from decidua, often associated with vaginal bleeding

Decidual Leukocytoclastic Necrosis

- Similar necrosis of decidua associated with karyorrhectic debris
  - ± neutrophils
- Associated with early preterm birth and preeclampsia when diffuse
- Less commonly associated with positive amniotic fluid cultures or neonatal sepsis
- Can be difficult to distinguish from acute inflammation preceding AFIS
  - Karyorrhexis of neutrophils
  - Immediately surrounding decidua becomes necrotic as in laminar decidual necrosis

DECIDUAL ARTERIOPATHY

Incomplete Adaptation for Pregnancy

- Failure of maternal spiral arteries to undergo trophoblast-mediated vascular remodeling in decidua basalis

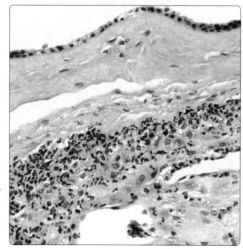

Acute Deciduitis and Chorionitis

(Left) *Acute deciduitis may be an early manifestation of the maternal inflammatory response to amniotic fluid infection (AFI). In AFI, maternal neutrophils migrate from decidual vessels toward the membranes.* (Right) *Although scattered lymphocytes are normal in the decidua, plasma cells ⇨ are not. The presence of plasma cells suggests an abnormal immune environment and has numerous clinical associations.*

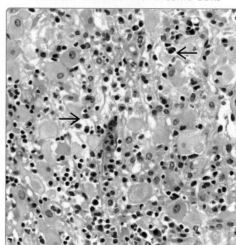

Chronic Deciduitis With Plasma Cells

- o Presence of vascular smooth muscle in decidua basalis spiral arteries of central 2/3 placenta is diagnostic
- o Persistence of luminal trophoblast in 3rd-trimester decidua basalis spiral arteries suggests incomplete remodeling

Hypertrophic Vasculopathy

- Thickened vascular media in decidual spiral arteries, most often seen in membranes
  - o Wall thickness > 1/3 of vessel diameter is diagnostic
  - o Associations
    - – Hypertension, pregnancy-associated hypertensive disorders
    - – Diabetes
- Intermediate stage to fibrinoid necrosis shows breakdown of muscle wall integrity before fibrin deposition

Fibrinoid Necrosis

- Eosinophilic necrosis of vessel wall in membranous decidua or decidua basalis
  - o Only unremodeled vessels are susceptible
  - o Associated with preterm preeclampsia, preeclampsia with fetal growth restriction
  - o May be complicated by thrombosis

Acute Atherosis

- Subintimal foamy macrophages in decidual vessel with fibrinoid necrosis
  - o Only unremodeled vessels are susceptible
  - o Associated with preterm preeclampsia
  - o May be complicated by thrombosis

HEMORRHAGE

Retroplacental Hematoma

- Pathologic correlate of placental abruption
  - o Hemorrhage in upper decidua basalis
  - o Significance depends on amount of placental bed separated from maternal blood supply
  - o Gross exam may show adherent clot with indentation of basal plate
  - o Microscopic findings
    - – Acute villous injury with intravillous hemorrhage
    - – Wedge-shaped dissecting hemorrhage from basal surface into villous parenchyma in acute lesions
    - – Recent or remote infarcts
    - – Hemosiderin-laden macrophages
- Marginal abruption
  - o May be chronic and repetitive throughout gestation
    - – Attributed to venous bleeding at marginal sinus
  - o Remote hemorrhage seen at margin, may extend behind placenta and membranes, circumvallate membranes
    - – May be associated with diffuse chorioamniotic hemosiderosis
  - o Clinical associations
    - – Vaginal bleeding
    - – Oligohydramnios
    - – Preterm birth
    - – Fetal growth restriction

Retromembranous Hemorrhage

- Adherent blood behind membranes is common and usually not significant
- Hemosiderin deposition in membranous decidua suggests chronicity
  - o More common in preterm births
  - o Associated with decidual necrosis
- Focal retromembranous hematomas may reflect amniocentesis sites

ABSENCE OF DECIDUA

Placenta Accreta, Increta, and Percreta

- Disorders of abnormal placental implantation in which placenta fails to separate from uterus
  - o Characterized by absence or deficiency of decidua
  - o Placenta implants in myometrium or scar
  - o Only fibrin and extravillous trophoblast cells separate villi from
    - – Myometrium in placenta accreta, placenta increta
    - – Serosa or adjacent organs in placenta percreta
- Associations all share deficiency of decidua
  - o Implantation in lower uterine segment or cornua
  - o Uterine scarring

Adherent Basal Plate Myofibrils

- Myofibrils adherent to basal plate of delivered placenta without intervening decidua
  - o May see shaggy red myometrial fibers attached focally to basal surface
  - o Microscopically, myometrial fibers are adjacent to basal fibrin with no intervening decidua
- Has been termed "occult placenta accreta," associated with morbidly adherent placenta
- Similar change can be seen in membranes with adherent myofibrils and little to no decidua

SELECTED REFERENCES

1. Ernst LM et al: Placental pathologic associations with morbidly adherent placenta: potential insights into pathogenesis. Pediatr Dev Pathol. 20(5):387-393, 2017
2. Hecht JL et al: Revisiting decidual vasculopathy. Placenta. 42:37-43, 2016
3. Elsasser DA et al: Diagnosis of placental abruption: relationship between clinical and histopathological findings. Eur J Obstet Gynecol Reprod Biol. 148(2):125-30, 2010
4. Tantbirojn P et al: Pathophysiology of placenta creta: the role of decidua and extravillous trophoblast. Placenta. 29(7):639-45, 2008
5. Goldenberg RL et al: The Alabama Preterm Birth Study: diffuse decidual leukocytoclastic necrosis of the decidua basalis, a placental lesion associated with preeclampsia, indicated preterm birth and decreased fetal growth. J Matern Fetal Neonatal Med. 20(5):391-5, 2007
6. Stanek J et al: Occult placenta accreta: the missing link in the diagnosis of abnormal placentation. Pediatr Dev Pathol. 10(4):266-73, 2007
7. Goldenberg RL et al: The Alabama Preterm Birth Project: placental histology in recurrent spontaneous and indicated preterm birth. Am J Obstet Gynecol. 195(3):792-6, 2006
8. Stanek J et al: Laminar necrosis of placental membranes: a histologic sign of uteroplacental hypoxia. Pediatr Dev Pathol. 8(1):34-42, 2005
9. Redline RW et al: Maternal vascular underperfusion: nosology and reproducibility of placental reaction patterns. Pediatr Dev Pathol. 7(3):237-49, 2004
10. Salafia CM et al: Histologic evidence of old intrauterine bleeding is more frequent in prematurity. Am J Obstet Gynecol. 173(4):1065-70, 1995

(Left) *Image of decidua basalis shows a spiral artery appropriately adapted for pregnancy and numerous surrounding plasma cells. The mother had recurrent preterm birth without further evidence of infection.* (Right) *This decidua basalis vessel has a prominent perivascular lymphoid infiltrate ⮕, a finding sometimes seen in preeclampsia with other features of maternal vascular malperfusion. As it resembles 1st-trimester changes, it may reflect a late attempt to remodel the vessel.*

Plasma Cell Deciduitis

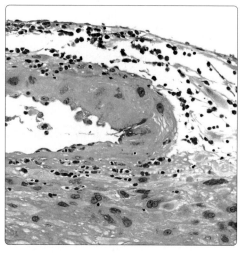

Perivascular Lymphoid Infiltrates

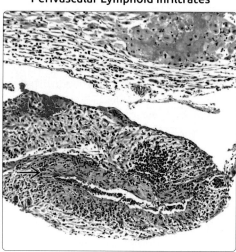

(Left) *Laminar decidual necrosis is bland necrosis of the upper decidua ⮕. It may be normal at term but is a pathologic finding preterm. Some experts attribute the finding to intrauterine hypoxia.* (Right) *Decidual leukocytoclastic necrosis is similar to laminar decidual necrosis with the addition of karyorrhectic debris ± neutrophils. It is associated with preterm birth and preeclampsia.*

Laminar Decidual Necrosis

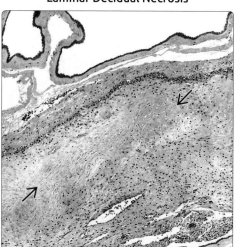

Decidual Leukocytoclastic Necrosis

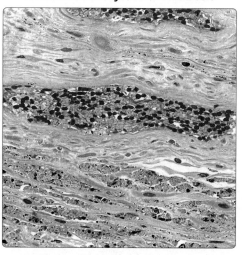

(Left) *Retromembranous hemorrhage is associated with decidual necrosis and extension of hemorrhage from a marginal abruption.* (Right) *Hemosiderin-laden macrophages impart chronicity to the hemorrhage. They are uncommonly found with retroplacental hematomas. Their presence has been associated with lesions that are 5-7 days old.*

Retromembranous Hemorrhage

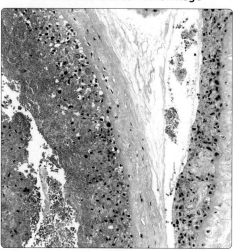

Hemosiderin-Laden Macrophages in Decidua

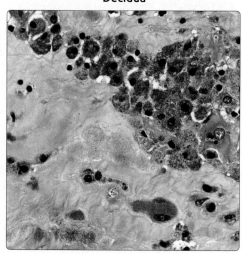

Persistence of Smooth Muscle in Spiral Arteries of Decidua Basalis

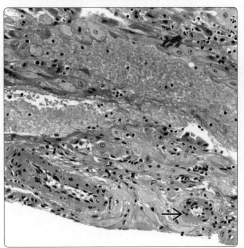

Hypertrophic Decidual Arteriopathy

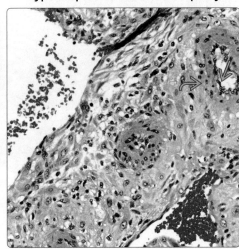

(Left) *Persistence of smooth muscle in central decidua basalis spiral arteries* ➡️ *is pathologic. It represents a failure of trophoblast-mediated vascular remodeling.* (Right) *Hypertrophic decidual arteriopathy is defined as a decidual vessel wall thickness > 1/3 of the total diameter. This image shows early progression to fibrinoid necrosis with separation of the endothelium* ➡️ *and fragmentation of the vascular smooth muscle* ➡️.

Fibrinoid Necrosis of Spiral Arteries

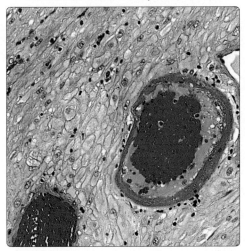

Thrombosis of Decidual Spiral Artery

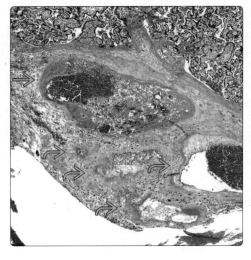

(Left) *Fibrinoid necrosis and acute atheromatous lesions are part of a spectrum of vascular injury seen in severe preterm preeclampsia. The necrotic vessel wall becomes intensely eosinophilic. In acute atheromatous lesions, foamy histiocytes accumulate beneath the endothelium.* (Right) *The multiple coils of this spiral artery show thrombosis* ➡️ *and necrosis of the vessel wall* ➡️. *An infarction hematoma was present elsewhere.*

Multinucleated Trophoblast Cells in Decidua Basalis

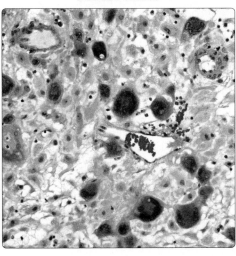

Placenta Increta

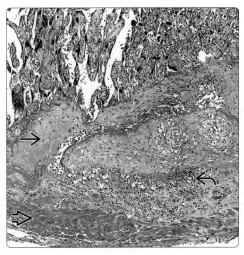

(Left) *Extravillous trophoblast cells are rarely multinucleate in the superficial decidua basalis. They typically become multinucleate at the end of migration. Their presence suggests superficial implantation.* (Right) *In placenta increta, the placenta basal plate, with Nitabuch fibrin layer* ➡️, *abuts the myometrium* ➡️ *without intervening decidua. Abnormal placentation, such as placenta increta, is often associated with excessive chronic inflammation* ➡️.

SECTION 2
Placental Diagnoses

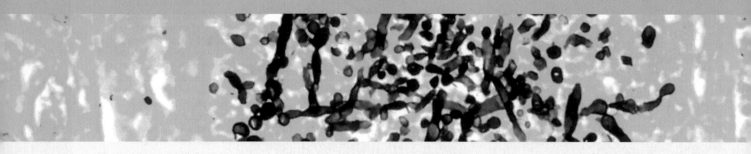

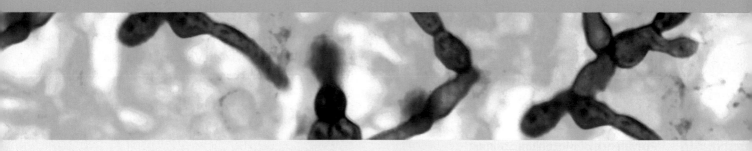

TERMINOLOGY

Definitions

- Meconium: Early, dark green feces composed of intestinal secretions, mucus, lanugo, bile, and intestinal epithelial cells
- Meconium aspiration syndrome (MAS): Early-onset respiratory distress and persistent pulmonary hypertension in meconium-stained term or near-term infant
- Meconium-associated vascular necrosis (MAVN): Apoptosis of vascular smooth muscle underlying meconium deposition in chorionic plate or umbilical cord

EPIDEMIOLOGY

Prevalence of Meconium Staining

- 19% of term placentas, 31% of postterm placentas
- Very rare to see placental staining before 30-weeks gestation
- 9-16% of pregnancies have meconium-stained amniotic fluid noted at delivery

Incidence of Meconium-Associated Vascular Necrosis

- ~ 1% of meconium-stained placentas demonstrate MAVN

ETIOLOGY/PATHOGENESIS

Meconium Passage In Utero

- Stimulated by hormone motilin
- Usually occurs in last month of pregnancy, more frequently in postterm, and rarely in midgestation
  - Some studies suggest fetal defecation is normal process from 2nd trimester throughout gestation
- Controversial association with fetal stress
  - Proposed association with preceding fetal distress and hypoxia
    - Other studies show no association with tocograms or fetal pH
    - May reflect complications of postterm infant
  - Meconium staining is not usually only pathologic change in cases with poor outcomes

- Likely contribution from other processes such as chorioamnionitis, vascular malperfusion vasculopathy, or extensive chronic villitis
- Timing of meconium exposure often medicolegal concern
  - In vitro studies suggest 24-48 hours of exposure required to see pigmented macrophages in membranes
  - In vivo study difficult to perform or interpret

Meconium-Associated Vascular Necrosis

- Prolonged meconium exposure is toxic to vascular smooth muscle cells of chorionic plate and umbilical cord
  - Not all fetal vessels exposed to meconium will show MAVN
- Meconium associated with vasoconstriction in vitro, even in absence of MAVN

CLINICAL IMPLICATIONS

Meconium Aspiration Syndrome

- Affects 2% of infants born with meconium-stained amniotic fluid

Meconium-Associated Vascular Necrosis

- Associated with CNS injury and significant neonatal morbidity and mortality
- Presence of meconium-laden macrophages in umbilical cord stroma has similar clinical and placental pathologic associations as MAVN, although acute inflammation is more common in MAVN

MACROSCOPIC

General Features

- Note color, consistency, and extent of staining on cord and membranes
  - Color ranges from bright green to muddy brown
  - Amnion may be edematous and slippery
- Follow routine protocol with particular attention to possibility of ulcerations &/or thrombi of umbilical cord and chorionic plate vasculature

Reactive and Necrotic Amnion With Pigment

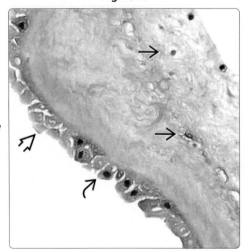

Bright Green Staining of Meconium

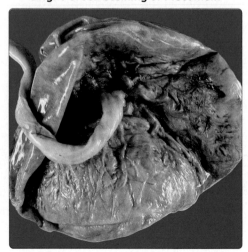

(Left) *Meconium is toxic to amnion cells, inducing characteristic columnar change associated with vacuolation ➡ and loss of nuclear basophilia ➡. Yellow-brown meconium particles ➡ are present.* (Right) *Gross photo shows diffuse bright green staining and a glistening appearance in recent meconium exposure.*

Chronicity of Meconium Staining, Gross Appearance and Associations

Chronicity	Gross Features	Clinical Outcomes	Placental Pathology
Acute	Blue-green discoloration, glistening surface, particulate slimy meconium present	Usually normal	Few associated placental lesions except low level of acute chorioamnionitis
Subacute	Slippery edematous membranes, dark discoloration	Outcomes of combined subacute and chronic: Lower 5-minute Apgar scores, umbilical artery acidosis	Pathologies of combined subacute and chronic: Associated with fetal thrombi, infarcts, acute chorioamnionitis, chronic villitis, meconium-associated vascular necrosis
Chronic	Dull appearance, diffuse muddy staining, cord stained		

Adapted from Benirschke et al: Anatomy and Pathology of the Placental Membranes. In Benirschke et al: Pathology of the Human Placenta. 6th ed. New York: Springer-Verlag. 275, 2012; Kaspar HG et al: The placenta in meconium staining: lesions and early neonatal outcome. Clin. Exp. Obst. & Gyn. 27(1): 63-6, 2000.

MICROSCOPIC

Meconium Staining

- Characteristic changes in amnion
  - Alternating areas of columnar reactive change with vacuolation and necrosis with loss of nuclear basophilia
  - Occasionally associated with marked epithelial hyperplasia
  - May see globular pigment in amniotic epithelium
  - May see free meconium particles above amnion in recent exposure
- May see mild "chemical chorioamnionitis"
  - Occasional neutrophils only, some experts dispute that meconium can cause inflammation
    - Note that meconium may promote bacterial growth; amniotic fluid infection is frequently present
  - Acute fetal inflammatory response without maternal inflammatory response may reflect fetal inflammatory response syndrome associated with chemical pneumonitis due to meconium aspiration
- Meconium-laden macrophages found in membranous amnion, chorion, decidua, chorionic plate, and umbilical cord stroma
  - Depth of their presence implies chronicity, cord affected rarely
  - Distinguish from hemosiderin-laden macrophages with Prussian blue stain
  - Luna-Ishak stain will positively stain bile with greenish hue to confirm meconium if needed
  - Immunohistochemical stain recently described for meconium: Zinc coproporphyrin I

DIFFERENTIAL DIAGNOSIS

Diffuse Chorioamniotic Hemosiderosis

- Most important distinction from meconium because it has its own clinical significance
- See hemosiderin deposition, from phagocytosis of lysed red cells
  - Dark yellow to brown pigment
- Does not have typical reactive and necrotic changes of amnion
- Usually associated with chronic abruption, circumvallation

- Prussian blue stain will identify iron in hemosiderin-laden macrophages

Other Pigments

- Other pigments that may be seen in placenta
  - Hematoidin
    - Brown pigment similar to bilirubin
    - Found at sites of prolonged blood accumulation, like old hemorrhages
    - Does not react with iron stain
  - Lipofuscin
    - Yellow to light brown pigment
    - Noted after 32-weeks gestation
    - Will not have characteristic amniotic changes associated with meconium
  - Melanin
    - Described with prolonged rupture of membranes
    - Associated with dermatopathic conditions in fetus
    - Similar distribution as meconium pigment, positive Masson-Fontana stain
  - Formalin pigment
    - Fixation artifact, often with acid or alkaline formalin solution and prolonged fixation
    - Black dots formed from degradation of hemoglobin
    - Found in areas of blood, e.g., around vessels of villi
    - No characteristic amnion changes as in meconium; distribution not similar to meconium

SELECTED REFERENCES

1. Cimic A et al: Meconium-associated umbilical vascular myonecrosis: correlations with adverse outcome and placental pathology. Pediatr Dev Pathol. 19(4):315-9, 2016
2. Furuta N et al: Immunohistochemical detection of meconium in the fetal membrane, placenta and umbilical cord. Placenta. 33(1):24-30, 2012
3. Funai EF et al: Timing of fetal meconium absorption by amnionic macrophages. Am J Perinatol. 26(1):93-7, 2009
4. Poggi SH et al: Variability in pathologists' detection of placental meconium uptake. Am J Perinatol. 26(3):207-10, 2009
5. Kaspar HG et al: The placenta in meconium staining: lesions and early neonatal outcome. Clin Exp Obstet Gynecol. 27(1):63-6, 2000
6. Burgess AM et al: Inflammation of the lungs, umbilical cord and placenta associated with meconium passage in utero. Review of 123 autopsied cases. Pathol Res Pract. 192(11):1121-8, 1996
7. Altshuler G et al: Meconium-induced umbilical cord vascular necrosis and ulceration: a potential link between the placenta and poor pregnancy outcome. Obstet Gynecol. 79(5 (Pt 1)):760-6, 1992

Recent Meconium Deposition

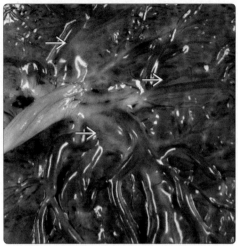

Discordant Meconium Staining in Twin Placenta

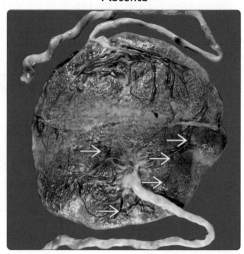

(Left) *Acute meconium deposition appears as a focal green-yellow discoloration* ➡. *Note the overall glistening appearance. The amnion remains attached to the surface.* **(Right)** *Comparison of the chorionic plate in a monochorionic diamniotic twin placenta shows that the recent meconium soilage* ➡ *is limited to the amniotic sac of the lower twin.*

Green Meconium Staining

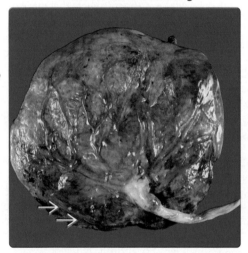

Meconium Staining After Formalin Fixation

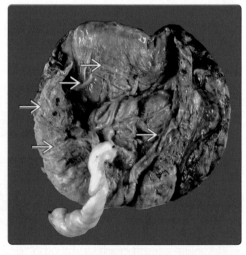

(Left) *Subacute meconium exposure is shown. The green-yellow discoloration is more diffusely distributed. Folds in the amnion* ➡ *on the surface of the chorionic plate attest to edema and slippage of the amnion.* **(Right)** *Subacute/chronic meconium exposure after formalin fixation is shown. The placenta and cord are diffusely yellow-brown stained. The crinkles and folds on the surface* ➡ *indicate that the edematous amnion has slipped from the dull-appearing chorionic plate surface.*

Prolonged Meconium Staining

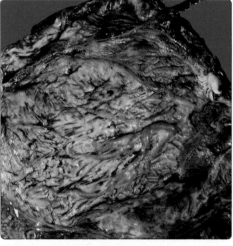

Linear Ulceration of Meconium-Associated Vascular Necrosis

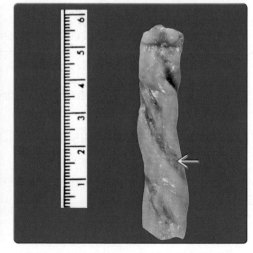

(Left) *Subacute/chronic meconium exposure with chorioamnionitis shows diffuse tan-brown staining and opacity surrounding the chorionic plate vasculature. Amniotic fluid infection sequence often complicates meconium spillage in the amniotic fluid.* **(Right)** *Meconium-associated vascular necrosis (MAVN) is rarely seen grossly with linear ulceration* ➡ *along the umbilical vessels. The umbilical arteries are more commonly affected than the umbilical veins. More often, MAVN is a focal finding in a stained umbilical cord.*

Vacuolization in Amnion With Meconium

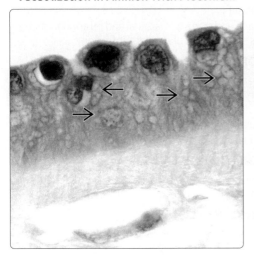

Meconium-Laden Macrophages in Membranes

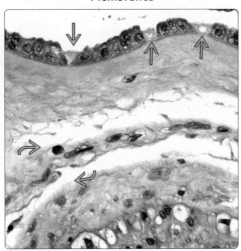

(Left) *Reactive changes in the amnion are shown. The normally cuboidal epithelium becomes columnar or pseudostratified with coarse cytoplasmic vacuolation ➡. The basement membrane remains mostly invisible at this early stage. Rare vacuoles contain pigment.* (Right) *This section of meconium-stained placental membranes shows the characteristic changes of a reactive amnion with spotty necrosis ➡ and pigmented macrophages in the amnion and chorion ➡.*

Meconium-Laden Macrophages in Decidua

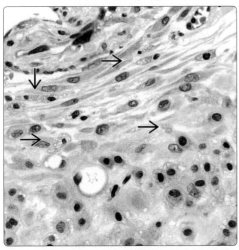

Meconium-Laden Macrophage in Umbilical Cord Stroma

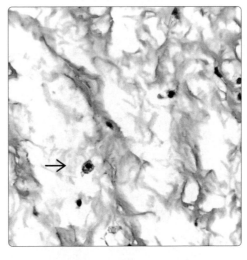

(Left) *In some cases, meconium-laden macrophages reach the membranous decidua. The faint pigment of meconium ➡ can be easy to miss without a careful search.* (Right) *Umbilical cords with dull, green-tan staining may show pigmented macrophages ➡ in the stroma. One study suggests this finding is also significant with similar associations as MAVN.*

Meconium-Associated Vascular Necrosis in Umbilical Artery

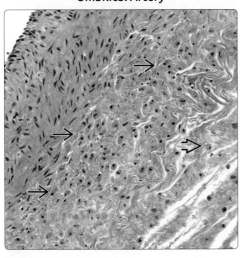

Meconium-Associated Vascular Necrosis in Chorionic Plate Vasculature

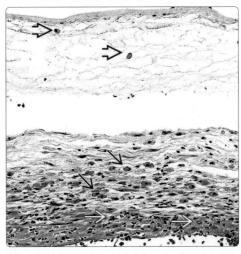

(Left) *MAVN occurs on the side of the vessel nearest to the amnion. Vascular smooth muscle cells lose connectivity, round up, and become pyknotic ➡. Note pigmented macrophages ➡.* (Right) *MAVN in chronic meconium staining is shown. Individual vascular smooth muscle cells ➡ become polygonal and apoptotic. Meconium particles ➡ are seen in media and above edematous amnion. The fetal inflammatory response is evidenced by neutrophils ➡.*

Amniotic Fluid Infection Sequence
(Maternal and Fetal Inflammatory Response)

TERMINOLOGY

- Amniotic fluid infection sequence (AFIS)
  - Maternal and fetal inflammatory responses to ascending infection of amniotic cavity by cervicovaginal flora
  - Maternal response seen in membranes, chorionic plate
  - Fetal response in umbilical and chorionic plate vasculitis
- Intraamniotic inflammation, infection, or both (triple I)
  - Term proposed to replace clinical (not histologic) diagnosis of chorioamnionitis

ETIOLOGY/PATHOGENESIS

- Preterm chorioamnionitis: Higher rate of positive cultures
- Term chorioamnionitis: Frequently has negative cultures and negative bacterial PCR, (sterile intraamniotic inflammation)

CLINICAL ISSUES

- 66-75% of women with significant inflammation within membranes are asymptomatic

- Nearly 40% of premature births associated with histologic chorioamnionitis
- Higher grade and stage of maternal and fetal inflammatory responses → higher risk of neonatal infection

MICROSCOPIC

- Maternal and fetal acute inflammatory responses graded for severity and staged for extent and implied duration of response
- Bacteria are rarely identified within membranes; their presence indicates heavy colonization

TOP DIFFERENTIAL DIAGNOSES

- Decidual leukocytoclastic necrosis: More similar to laminar decidual necrosis than AFIS

DIAGNOSTIC CHECKLIST

- Placental pathology showing maternal and fetal inflammatory responses confirms suspected diagnosis of triple I.

Infection In Utero

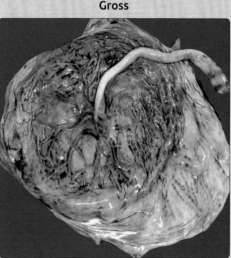

(Left) In utero infection is acquired in 2 ways: Ascending from the maternal genitourinary tract and hematogenous from the maternal bloodstream. Amniotic fluid infection is typically an ascending infection. (Right) Acute chorioamnionitis is rarely a gross diagnosis. This placenta has only slightly cloudy membranes, but significant histologic inflammation was present. A foul odor may accompany the infected membranes, depending upon the infectious organism.

Acute Chorioamnionitis Gross

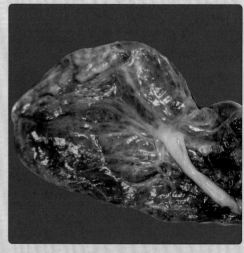

Severe Acute Necrotizing Chorioamnionitis Gross

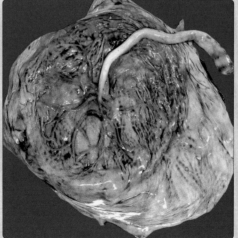

(Left) This placenta has advanced, severe chorioamnionitis, stage 3, grade 2, with nearly opaque free and attached membranes. (Right) This cord shows a severe advanced fetal inflammatory response, stage 3, grade 2. Degenerated inflammatory debris ➡ is present in Wharton substance (subacute necrotizing funisitis). Note the degeneration ➡ of the umbilical vein muscular wall.

Funisitis Fetal Inflammatory Response

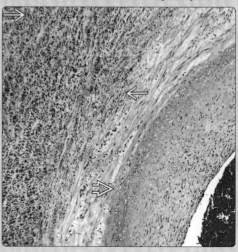

TERMINOLOGY

Abbreviations

- Amniotic fluid infection sequence (AFIS)
- Intraamniotic infection, inflammation, or both (triple I)

Definitions

- AFIS: Progression of maternal and fetal inflammatory responses (FIR) to ascending infection of amniotic cavity by cervicovaginal flora
  o Grade: Severity of inflammation
  o Stage: Chronicity, implied from progression of inflammation through tissue layers
- Maternal inflammatory response (MIR): Maternal neutrophils reacting to stimuli in amniotic fluid
  o Grade 1 (mild, moderate): Defined as not severe
  o Grade 2 (severe): Severe acute chorioamnionitis, ± subchorionic microabscesses, > 10 x 20 confluent neutrophils in at least 3 foci or in continuous band of membrane roll
  o Stage 1 (early): Acute subchorionitis or chorionitis
  o Stage 2 (intermediate): Acute chorioamnionitis, neutrophils in fibrous chorion &/or amnion
  o Stage 3 (advanced): Necrosis of amnion, amnion basement membrane thickening/hypereosinophilia, karyorrhexis of neutrophils
- FIR: Fetal neutrophils reacting to stimuli
  o Grade 1 (mild, moderate): Defined as not severe
  o Grade 2 (severe): Near confluent neutrophils in fetal vessels with attenuation of vascular smooth muscle
  o Stage 1 (early): Chorionic plate vasculitis or umbilical vein phlebitis
  o Stage 2 (intermediate): Inflammation of 1 or both arteries ± inflammation of vein
  o Stage 3 (advanced): Necrotizing funisitis (subacute) with neutrophils and debris (sometimes calcified) forming arcs oriented towards amnion surface around 1 or more vessels
- FIR syndrome
  o Clinical diagnosis, elevated fetal IL-6, IL-8, TNF-α, G-CSF with increased neutrophils and enhanced erythropoiesis

ETIOLOGY/PATHOGENESIS

Infectious Agents

- Histologic acute chorioamnionitis conventionally considered reaction to infectious microbe ascending from cervicovaginal region
  o Genital mycoplasmas (e.g., *Ureaplasma urealyticum),* *Escherichia coli, Fusobacterium* spp. most commonly involved
  o Higher rate of positive cultures in preterm chorioamnionitis, especially when fastidious organisms are specifically cultured
  o Chorioamnionitis at term, especially low grade, may have negative cultures
    – Possible maternal response to something other than bacteria (sterile intraamniotic inflammation)

Chronology of Histologic Changes

- Timing of infection dependent on many factors
  o Type (virulent or nonvirulent) and amount of bacteria

- o Immunocompetence of mother and fetus (primarily related to gestational age)
- o Maternal inflammation is generally present within 6-12 hours of infection; initially at subchorionic plate and decidua of free membranes over cervix
- o Involvement of amnion connective tissues probably develops over 12- to 36-hour period
- o Neutrophils begin to undergo karyorrhexis 36-48 hours after extension into tissues
  – Subacute chorioamnionitis possibly present for 2 weeks
- o The FIR may be delayed by hours to possibly days from onset of MIR
  – Necrotizing funisitis possibly present for weeks

CLINICAL ISSUES

Presentation

- Triple I
  o Proposed terminology to replace **clinical** diagnosis of "chorioamnionitis"
  o Categorized as "suspected" or "confirmed"
    – Confirmed triple I when amniocentesis yields positive Gram stain, low glucose or positive culture, or placental pathology diagnostic of infection
  o Documented fever = maternal temperature of > 39°C (102.2°F) or > 38°C (100.4°F) on repeated measurement (taken orally)
  o Suspected triple I: Maternal fever + 1 or more of following
    – Fetal tachycardia (> 160 bpm for 10 minutes or longer)
    – Maternal white blood cell count > 15,000 $10^3/\mu L$ in absence of corticosteroids
    – Purulent fluid from cervical os
  o Using criteria of triple I, fewer cases of histologic chorioamnionitis with funisitis are identified (low sensitivity), but specificity is very high
- 66-75% of women with histologic chorioamnionitis are asymptomatic
- Histologic chorioamnionitis is more frequent in preterm placentas
  o 40-50% < 27 weeks, 15% at 28-36 weeks, 2-10% at term
  o Preterm placentas often have chorionic plate vasculitis as initial fetal response
  o Term placentas often have inflammation of umbilical vein as initial fetal response

Treatment

- Once inflammatory cascade is activated, it is not stopped or reversed by antibiotics or tocolytics
- Antibiotics reduce risk of maternal sepsis and early-onset fetal sepsis and may delay delivery by a few days

Prognosis

- Chorioamnionitis may result in dysfunctional uterine contractions, ↑ incidence of cesarean section, ↑ risk for postpartum hemorrhage due to uterine atony
- FIR is associated with FIR syndrome with neonatal morbidity and risk of neurologic injury
  o Mechanisms of brain injury include cytokines, ischemia, and toxic injury by bacterial products or actual infection
- Meconium passage often accompanies chorioamnionitis

MACROSCOPIC

General Features

- Chorioamnionitis is often not recognized grossly
- Subacute chorioamnionitis has opaque yellow-white membranes
- Necrotizing funisitis may have barber pole appearance due to necrotic/calcified debris
- *Candida* funisitis has subamniotic yellow-white microabscesses on umbilical cord

MICROSCOPIC

Histologic Features

- Description of severity (grade) and location (stage) of inflammation of MIR and FIR provides clinically useful information
  - Higher grades and stages of both MIR and FIR have higher incidence of neonatal infection
  - Bacteria are rarely identified within membranes; their presence indicates heavy colonization
- MIR to intraamniotic infection
  - Acute deciduitis: Neutrophils in decidua parietalis
    - Severe inflammation and necrosis of decidua is frequently associated with midgestation marginal placental abruption (diffuse decidual leukocytoclastic necrosis) ± AFIS
  - MIR stage 1: Acute chorionitis or subchorionitis
    - Extraplacental membranes: Patchy to diffuse neutrophils in cellular or fibrous chorion, frequently lined up at junction between cellular and fibrous chorion
    - Chorionic plate: Neutrophils marginate in subchorionic fibrinoid and extend into chorion
  - MIR stage 2: Acute chorioamnionitis
    - Acute inflammation above cellular chorion, may or may not extend into amnion
  - MIR stage 3: Necrotizing acute chorioamnionitis
    - Amniocyte necrosis and neutrophil karyorrhexis, thickening and hypereosinophilia of amnion basement membrane
  - Subacute necrotizing chorioamnionitis
    - Amniocyte necrosis with heavy mixed inflammatory infiltrate, extensive karyorrhexis, histiocytic infiltrate in underlying chorion
- FIR to intraamniotic infection
  - Inflammation oriented toward amniotic fluid, in incomplete arcs, not circumferential around vessel
  - Neutrophils initially marginated on endothelium, then extend into muscle and out into Wharton substance or chorionic plate connective tissue
    - Inflammation in chorionic plate may be of either maternal or fetal origin
    - Eosinophils are generally FIR
  - Severe fetal vasculitis may be complicated by thrombi, ominous finding for neonatal morbidity

ANCILLARY TESTS

Placental Cultures

- Rarely positive and frequently contaminated with vaginal flora; organisms may be difficult to culture

Gram or Other More Specific Stains

- May be helpful when organisms visible on routine H&E

DIFFERENTIAL DIAGNOSIS

Chronic Chorioamnionitis

- Rarely due to amniotic fluid infection
  - Associated with chronic villitis of unknown etiology

T-Cell Lymphocytic and Eosinophilic Vasculitis

- Fetal chorionic plate vasculitis often oriented toward intervillous space, not amniotropic, not associated with infection

DIAGNOSTIC CHECKLIST

Clinically Relevant Pathologic Features

- Pathologic diagnosis should include MIR and FIR findings with full histologic terminology, that clearly describes the stage and grade

Pathologic Interpretation Pearls

- Most term babies with MIR and FIR have negative blood cultures
- Higher stage and more severe grade of MIR and FIR, more likely there will be neonatal infection
- Highest yield of positive placental cultures in preterm premature ruptured membranes
  - Positive placental cultures are associated with increased incidence of respiratory distress and positive neonatal cultures

SELECTED REFERENCES

1. Doty MS et al: Histologic funisitis and likelihood of intrauterine inflammation or infection: a case-control study. Am J Perinatol. ePub, 2018
2. Peng CC et al: Intrauterine inflammation, infection, or both (Triple I): A new concept for chorioamnionitis. Pediatr Neonatol. 59(3):231-237, 2018
3. Kim CJ et al: Acute chorioamnionitis and funisitis: definition, pathologic features, and clinical significance. Am J Obstet Gynecol. 213(4 Suppl):S29-52, 2015
4. Park CW et al: Timing of histologic progression from chorio-deciduitis to chorio-deciduo-amnionitis in the setting of preterm labor and preterm premature rupture of membranes with sterile amniotic fluid. PLoS One. 10(11):e0143023, 2015
5. Roberts DJ et al: Acute histologic chorioamnionitis at term: nearly always noninfectious. PLoS One. 7(3):e31819, 2012
6. Park CW et al: The involvement of human amnion in histologic chorioamnionitis is an indicator that a fetal and an intra-amniotic inflammatory response is more likely and severe: clinical implications. Placenta. 30(1):56-61, 2009
7. Redline RW: Inflammatory responses in the placenta and umbilical cord. Semin Fetal Neonatal Med. 11(5):296-301, 2006
8. Redline RW et al: Amniotic infection syndrome: nosology and reproducibility of placental reaction patterns. Pediatr Dev Pathol. 6(5):435-48, 2003
9. Ohyama M et al: Re-evaluation of chorioamnionitis and funisitis with a special reference to subacute chorioamnionitis. Hum Pathol. 33(2):183-90, 2002
10. Kim CJ et al: Umbilical arteritis and phlebitis mark different stages of the fetal inflammatory response. Am J Obstet Gynecol. 185(2):496-500, 2001

Initiation of Maternal Inflammatory Response

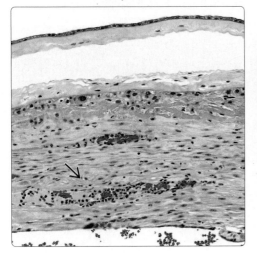

Decidual Leukocytoclastic Necrosis

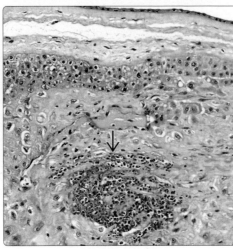

(Left) *The earliest stage of the maternal inflammatory response is margination of neutrophils within small vessels* ⮕ *in the decidua parietalis (mild, acute deciduitis).* (Right) *Small areas of acute inflammation with karyorrhexis and decidual necrosis* ⮕ *are frequently found in the decidua and may not indicate infection. They are often continuous with areas of laminar necrosis.*

Acute Chorioamnionitis

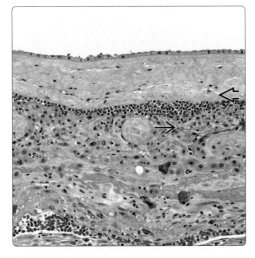

Acute Chorioamnionitis

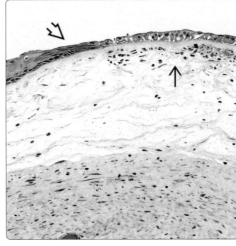

(Left) *Maternal neutrophils respond to chemotactic factors in the amniotic fluid and frequently marginate between cellular* ⮕ *and fibroblastic* ⮕ *chorion. The density of the connective tissue may impede further migration. This image shows moderate acute chorioamnionitis (maternal inflammatory response grade 1, stage 2).* (Right) *Neutrophil chemotaxis* ⮕ *toward substances within the amniotic fluid (amniotropic) is blocked by squamous metaplasia* ⮕*. The amnion is edematous.*

Acute Chorioamnionitis and 2nd-Trimester Abruption

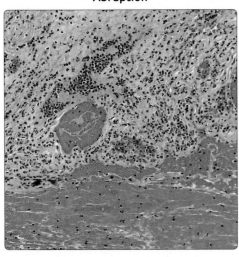

Villous Edema

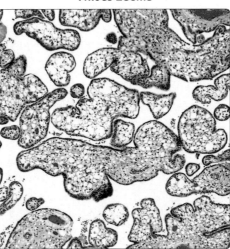

(Left) *Acute placental abruption occurring between 16- and 24-weeks gestation is commonly associated with chorioamnionitis and decidual necrosis. Abruption due to decidual arteriopathy associated with preeclampsia generally occurs after 24-weeks gestation.* (Right) *Villous edema is a common finding with both chorioamnionitis and abruption. It is sometimes difficult to distinguish villous immaturity from edema.*

Acute Subchorionitis of Chorionic Plate

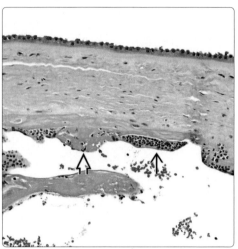

Acute Chorioamnionitis in Chorionic Plate

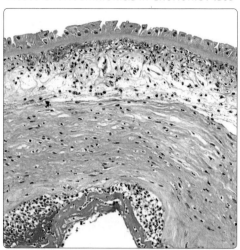

(Left) *Maternal neutrophils ⇥ are marginated in the subchorionic fibrin ⇥ (acute subchorionitis). This is a sensitive site for detecting amniotic fluid infection sequence (AFIS).* (Right) *The chorionic plate shows full thickness inflammation with thickening and eosinophilia of the amnion basement membrane. The diagnosis is acute necrotizing chorioamnionitis (maternal inflammatory response stage 3, grade 2) due to the karyorrhexis of the neutrophils.*

Subacute Necrotizing Chorioamnionitis

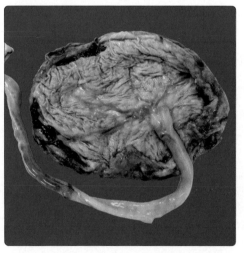

Subacute Necrotizing Chorioamnionitis

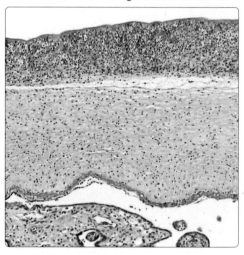

(Left) *A premature placenta with opaque membranes is characteristic of subacute necrotizing chorioamnionitis. The umbilical cord is also discolored, suggestive of funisitis.* (Right) *Subacute necrotizing chorioamnionitis is characterized by necrosis of the amnion epithelium, a heavy layer of necrotic neutrophils in the amnion and mononuclear cells in the chorion with very few remaining neutrophils. This type of inflammation is seen in extreme prematurity and may be present for up to 2 weeks prior to delivery.*

Fetal Lung With Congenital Pneumonia

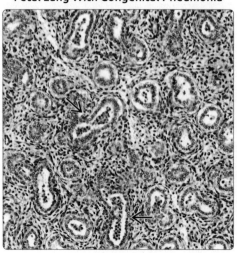

Fetal Stomach in Amniotic Fluid Infection

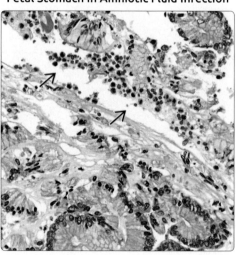

(Left) *This premature lung shows abundant neutrophils in the airways ⇥. Breathing movements bring debris from the amniotic cavity into the airways. The neutrophils are mostly fetal in origin. This is termed congenital pneumonia.* (Right) *The fetal swallowing mechanism is more robust than breathing in very immature fetuses and the inflammation ⇥ may be more apparent in the stomach than in the lungs. These findings support AFIS as a cause of fetal demise vs. postmortem change.*

Fetal Inflammatory Response

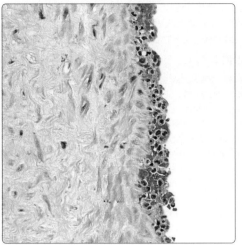

Fetal Inflammatory Response

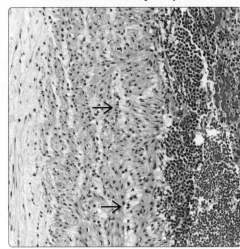

(Left) *Fetal neutrophils beneath the endothelium are the earliest feature of a fetal inflammatory response. Usually, this first occurs within the umbilical vein or chorionic plate vessels. Inflammation of the umbilical arteries is usually a later feature.* **(Right)** *Extremely heavy neutrophil response in the umbilical vein seen here is associated with extension of the neutrophils ➡ into the muscular wall of the vein (phlebitis).*

Necrotizing Funisitis

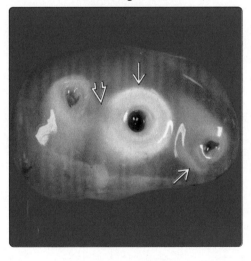

Mimic of Inflammation, Pseudofunisitis

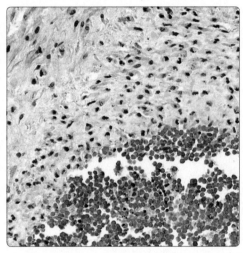

(Left) *This section of umbilical cord from a premature delivery has marked edema of Wharton substance and white exudate partially around the vessels ➡, which represents amniotropic inflammatory infiltrates. Note the lack of inflammation ➡ between the vessels.* **(Right)** *This section of umbilical cord is from a moderately macerated fetus and shows autolysis. The degenerative changes of the vascular smooth muscle nuclei resemble neutrophils. Immunohistochemistry for myeloperoxidase could be useful if in doubt.*

Chorionic Plate Vasculitis

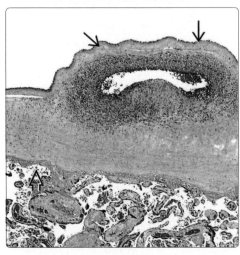

Chorionic Plate Vasculitis With Thrombosis

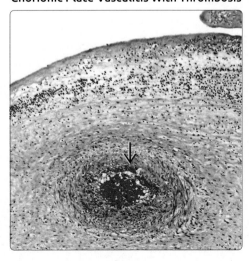

(Left) *Chorionic plate vasculitis ➡ exemplifies the fetal response. Note that there is very little maternal inflammation in contrast ➡. Discordance between fetal and maternal responses may be seen in group B Streptococcus infection, meconium aspiration syndrome, and maternal immunoincompetence.* **(Right)** *This case of acute necrotizing chorioamnionitis with severe chorionic plate vasculitis is complicated by a nonocclusive fibrin thrombus ➡ in the fetal vessel. This is associated with increased neonatal morbidity.*

Group B *Streptococcus*

ETIOLOGY/PATHOGENESIS

- *Streptococcus agalactiae* [group B *Streptococcus* (GBS)]
- Small Gram-positive cocci, in pairs or short chains
- Colonization of genitourinary tract occurs in 15-40% of women, majority of whom are asymptomatic
  - 40-50% recurrence of colonization in subsequent pregnancies
  - Invasive disease in one baby carries high risk for invasive disease in subsequent pregnancies

CLINICAL ISSUES

- GBS is a leading cause of neonatal sepsis
- 50% of infants born to colonized mothers are colonized at birth, and 1% develop GBS disease
- Early-onset disease is invasive and occurs < 7 days of life
  - Usually result of ascending infection
- Late-onset disease is diagnosed between 7 days and 3 months
  - Usually result of acquisition during birth

- Intrapartum antibiotics are effective in preventing early-onset disease but have not decreased late-onset disease
- Early-onset disease: 4-15% mortality
- Late-onset disease: 0-6% mortality

MICROSCOPIC

- GBS is frequently associated with minimal or no maternal inflammatory reaction
- GBS is associated with heavy colonization and large numbers of bacteria in 40% of cases
- Fetal inflammatory response may be more robust than maternal inflammatory response and include eosinophils
- Among infants dying of early-onset GBS sepsis, histologic chorioamnionitis and funisitis are more often seen in premature than term
- Heavy colonization and large numbers of bacteria in 40% of cases

Bacterial Overgrowth of GBS in Membranes

Subtle Presence of GBS Without Inflammation

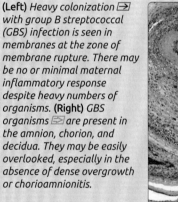

(Left) Heavy colonization ⇨ with group B streptococcal (GBS) infection is seen in membranes at the zone of membrane rupture. There may be no or minimal maternal inflammatory response despite heavy numbers of organisms. (Right) GBS organisms ⇨ are present in the amnion, chorion, and decidua. They may be easily overlooked, especially in the absence of dense overgrowth or chorioamnionitis.

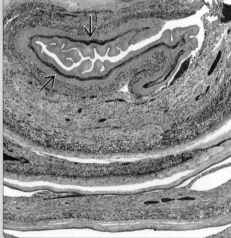

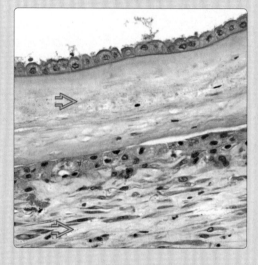

Fetal Inflammatory Response to GBS

Chorionic Plate Vasculitis in GBS

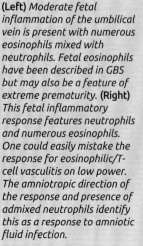

(Left) Moderate fetal inflammation of the umbilical vein is present with numerous eosinophils mixed with neutrophils. Fetal eosinophils have been described in GBS but may also be a feature of extreme prematurity. (Right) This fetal inflammatory response features neutrophils and numerous eosinophils. One could easily mistake the response for eosinophilic/T-cell vasculitis on low power. The amniotropic direction of the response and presence of admixed neutrophils identify this as a response to amniotic fluid infection.

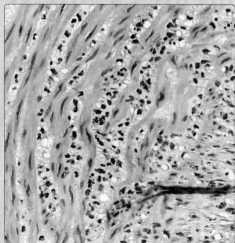

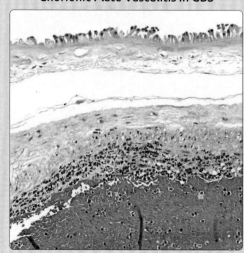

TERMINOLOGY

Abbreviations

- Group B *Streptococcus* (GBS)

ETIOLOGY/PATHOGENESIS

Infectious Agents

- *Streptococcus agalactiae* (GBS)
  - 9 serotypes, Ia, Ib, II, III, and V cause majority of neonatal disease
    - Type-specific antibodies provide immunity
- Small Gram-positive cocci, in pairs or short chains, mucoid white colonies with β-hemolysis
- Normally found in lower gastrointestinal tract
- Colonization of genitourinary tract occurs in 15-40% of women, majority of whom are asymptomatic
  - 40-50% recurrence of colonization in subsequent pregnancies
- Transmission of GBS from mother to fetus
  - Most often from ascending infection
  - Less commonly from colonization at time of delivery
  - Rarely acquired postnatally, from breast milk, nosocomially
- Capsular polysaccharides shield organism from complement-mediated destruction
  - Allows GBS to multiply in bloodstream

CLINICAL ISSUES

Presentation

- A leading cause of neonatal sepsis
- 50% of infants born to colonized mothers are colonized, and 1% develop GBS disease
- Heavy colonization, prematurity, prolonged rupture of membranes, and clinical chorioamnionitis are all associated with increased risk for neonatal disease
- Early-onset disease is invasive and occurs < 7 days of life
  - Usually result of ascending infection
  - Most present within 1st hours of life; also results in fetal demise
  - Sepsis (without source), neutropenia, respiratory distress, pneumonia, and, rarely, meningitis
  - Incidence of invasive early-onset neonatal sepsis 0.22/1,000 live births
- Late-onset disease is diagnosed between 7 days and 3 months
  - Usually result of acquisition during birth
  - Bacteremia, meningitis, or focal infections, such as osteomyelitis, septic arthritis, or cellulitis
  - Incidence: 0.3/1,000 live births

Laboratory Tests

- Screening of all pregnant women between 35- and 37-weeks gestation
  - Rectal and vaginal swabs submitted for cultures or PCR

Treatment

- Guidelines for screening and intrapartum treatment of GBS colonization during pregnancy have been established by consensus of American Academy of Pediatrics (AAP), American College of Obstetricians and Gynecologists (ACOG), and Centers for Disease Control and Prevention
- Screening and intrapartum antibiotics are effective in preventing early-onset disease but have not decreased late-onset disease

Prognosis

- Early-onset neonatal sepsis: 4-15% mortality
- Late-onset neonatal sepsis: 0-6% mortality
- Survivors of meningitis have substantial long-term deficits

MACROSCOPIC

General Features

- Chorioamnionitis may be associated with thickened, cloudy, white to yellow-green membranes

MICROSCOPIC

Histologic Features

- Frequently associated with minimal or no maternal inflammatory response
  - 38-75% have histologic chorioamnionitis, more common preterm than term
- Heavy colonization and large numbers of bacteria in 40% of cases
- Fetal inflammatory response may be more robust than maternal inflammatory response
  - Funisitis is present in 27-58% of cases, more common preterm than term
  - Fetal inflammatory response may include large numbers of eosinophils
- Villous edema may be seen, nonspecific feature
- Acute villitis may be associated with fetal sepsis

ANCILLARY TESTS

Immunohistochemistry

- Specific antibody to GBS available, useful when cultures are not available

DIFFERENTIAL DIAGNOSIS

Other Streptococcal Organisms

- Other *Streptococcus* species usually associated with severe chorioamnionitis

Staphylococcus aureus

- Methicillin-sensitive and methicillin-resistant *Staphylococcus aureus* are rare causes of chorioamnionitis

DIAGNOSTIC CHECKLIST

Pathologic Interpretation Pearls

- Heavy bacterial colonization of membranes with minimal maternal inflammation

SELECTED REFERENCES

1. Schrag SJ et al: Epidemiology of invasive early-onset neonatal sepsis, 2005 to 2014. Pediatrics. 138(6), 2016

GBS Without Chorioamnionitis

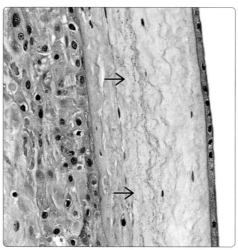

Gram Stain of GBS Without Chorioamnionitis

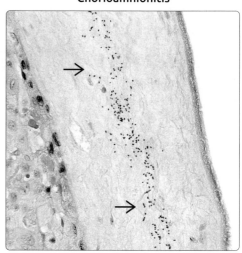

(Left) *Only a light sprinkling of bacteria* ➡️ *in the membranes is present in this case without a maternal inflammatory response. This is consistent with heavy GBS colonization but could be easily overlooked.* (Right) *Gram stain of the same section of membranes shows numerous gram-positive cocci* ➡️. *Gram stains rarely show organisms that are not visible on routine H&E stains.*

GBS Immunohistochemistry

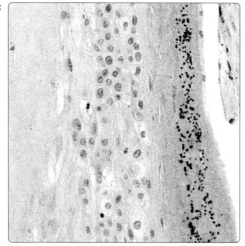

GBS Chorioamnionitis

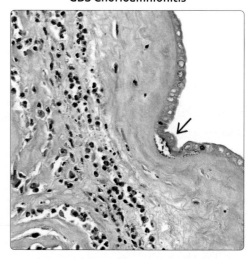

(Left) *Immunohistochemistry is very useful in confirming that these organisms are GBS. This may be useful for monitoring in subsequent pregnancies.* (Right) *In this case of chorioamnionitis, a single GBS colony* ➡️ *is found beneath the amnion epithelium.*

Acute Villitis With Fetal GBS Sepsis

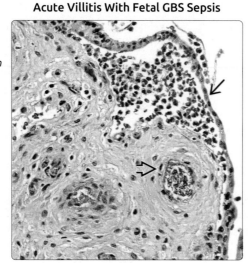

Gram Stain in GBS With Lethal Fetal Sepsis

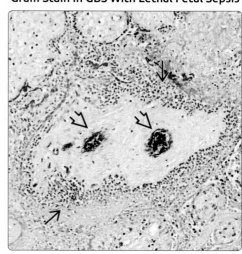

(Left) *The presence of acute villitis* ➡️ *heralds fetal sepsis. Large numbers of GBS bacteria* ➡️ *are present within fetal vessels. This kind of severe infection is only seen with fetal demise.* (Right) *Gram stain shows numerous gram-positive bacteria* ➡️ *within the fetal stem vessels. This stem villus also shows acute villitis* ➡️.

Autopsy Findings in Early-Onset Neonatal Sepsis

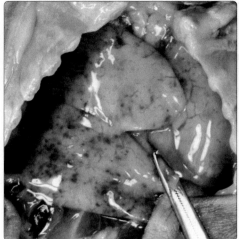

Lung Pathology in Early-Onset Neonatal GBS Sepsis

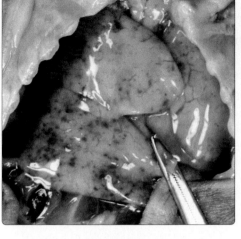

(Left) *Petechial hemorrhages are seen on the pleura in this extremely premature infant who died from early-onset GBS sepsis.* **(Right)** *Microscopic exam shows hyaline membranes ⇒. Focally, there is heavy colonization by GBS ⇒. This feature is referred to as dirty hyaline membranes.*

Yellow Hyaline Membranes With Hyperbilirubinemia

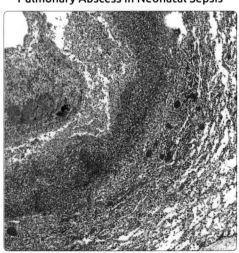

Pulmonary Abscess in Neonatal Sepsis

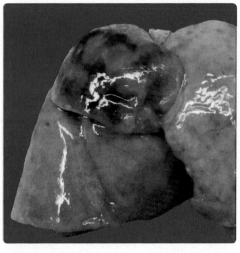

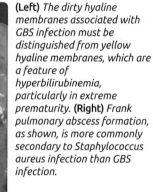

(Left) *The dirty hyaline membranes associated with GBS infection must be distinguished from yellow hyaline membranes, which are a feature of hyperbilirubinemia, particularly in extreme prematurity.* **(Right)** *Frank pulmonary abscess formation, as shown, is more commonly secondary to Staphylococcus aureus infection than GBS infection.*

Pulmonary Abscess in Neonatal Sepsis

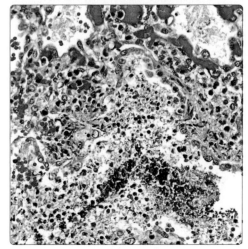

Staphylococcus aureus in Lung

(Left) *Lung abscess formation is more common with neonatal Staphylococcus infection in contrast to GBS. Subpleural abscesses may rupture and can result in a pneumothorax.* **(Right)** *The cocci of GBS should be distinguished from those of S. aureus. The heavy burden of large cocci in this newborn lung abscess is consistent with S. aureus.*

ETIOLOGY/PATHOGENESIS

- Gram-negative bacilli account for 1/3 of neonatal sepsis; *Escherichia coli* predominates
- *Staphylococcus aureus* is rare cause of chorioamnionitis but is particularly lethal
- Group B (*Streptococcus agalactiae*) is a leading cause of chorioamnionitis, fetal and neonatal infection
- Group A (*Streptococcus pyogenes*) is a leading cause of maternal septic shock, causes pharyngitis, tonsillitis, impetigo, necrotizing fascitis, chorioamnionitis
- *L. monocytogenes* is significant cause of 2nd- and 3rd-trimester fetal demise
  - Amniotic fluid appears meconium stained, even in extreme prematurity
- *Fusobacterium nucleatum* and *Fusobacterium necrophorum* are most often associated with extreme prematurity

CLINICAL ISSUES

- Maternal bacteremia, sepsis, and shock in pregnancy
- Bacteremia occurs in 8-10%
- Severe maternal sepsis in ~ 5 in 10,000 pregnant women
- 0-3% incidence of death in sepsis during pregnancy
- Group A streptococcal infections frequently involved

MACROSCOPIC

- *Listeria* is associated with multiple parenchymal micro- or macroabscesses

MICROSCOPIC

- Most of these bacteria have been implicated in acute chorioamnionitis but have no specific histologic features
- *Listeria monocytogenes*: Acute villitis with abscesses
- *Fusobacterium* spp.: Necrotizing chorioamnionitis, long, thin, filamentous rods, vertically oriented in amnion
- Acute villitis is frequently seen with fetal sepsis
- Placenta in maternal sepsis may show intervillous neutrophils, fibrin, maternal floor infarction

Subacute Necrotizing Chorioamnionitis

Polymicrobial Infection

(Left) *This 26-weeks-gestation placenta has nearly opaque membranes. This feature is characteristic of subacute necrotizing chorioamnionitis, a prolonged infection that usually occurs in extreme prematurity.* (Right) *Polymicrobial chorioamnionitis is common. Gram staining shows the gram-negative bacilli of Proteus ⮕ and gram-positive cocci of group B Streptococcus ⮕.*

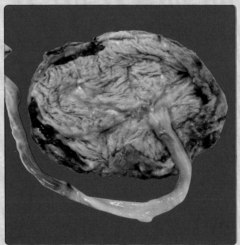

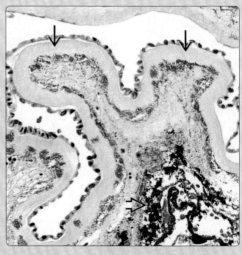

Maternal Sepsis

Fetal Sepsis

(Left) *In this case of maternal sepsis due to group A Streptococcus, Gram staining shows fibrin, neutrophils, and bacteria in the intervillous space.* (Right) *This pregnancy loss was associated with fetal sepsis. Note the numerous coccoid organisms in the fetal capillaries and villous stroma. The organism was not cultured.*

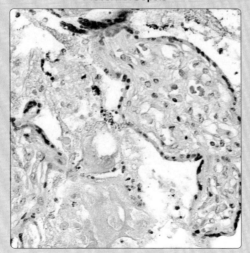

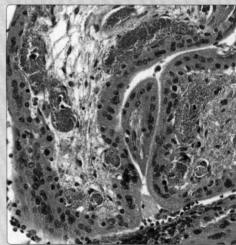

ETIOLOGY/PATHOGENESIS

Infectious Agents

- *Escherichia coli*
  - Gram-negative bacillus, normal flora of bowel and genital tract
- *Staphylococcus* spp.
  - Gram-positive coccus, occurring in pairs, chains, or grape-like clusters
  - Coagulase-negative *Staphylococcus* spp. currently consists of 29 different spp.
    - Normal skin flora
    - Most neonatal infections are nosocomial
  - *Staphylococcus aureus*, methicillin sensitive or methicillin resistant (MRSA)
- *Enterococcus faecalis* and *Enterococcus faecium*
  - Gram-positive, ovoid bacterium, occurring singly, in pairs, or in short chains
  - Normal flora of gastrointestinal tract; less common in genital tract
- *Streptococcus* spp.
  - Small, gram-positive cocci in pairs and chains
- *Listeria monocytogenes*
  - Facultative anaerobic, motile, gram-positive, β-hemolytic, small coccobacillus
  - Found in soil and livestock feeds
  - Food-borne illness; unpasteurized milk products, deli meats, and raw vegetables
    - Infections usually occur in small epidemics due to contaminated food
  - 17% of cases occur in pregnant women; also at risk are elderly and immunocompromised individuals
  - Incubation period of ~ 24 hours for gastrointestinal symptoms, 28 days for pregnancy complications
- *Fusobacterium nucleatum* and *Fusobacterium necrophorum*
  - Anaerobic, gram-negative, very long, thin, filamentous bacilli
  - Oral bacterium associated with gingivitis
- *Bacteroides fragilis* or *Bacteroides bivius*
  - Anaerobic, gram-negative bacillus
  - Normal flora of colon and genital tract; may be found in bacterial vaginosis
- *Prevotella* spp. (previously in *Bacteroides* spp.)
  - Gram-negative, anaerobic bacilli
  - Normal flora of oral cavity, intestinal and genitourinary tract
    - *Prevotella bivia* and *Prevotella disiens* associated with genital tract infections in women
- *Clostridium perfringens*
  - Anaerobic, large, gram-positive, spore-forming bacilli
  - Normal flora of colon
- *Gardnerella vaginalis*
  - Small, gram-negative coccobacillus
  - High potential for adhesion and cytotoxicity of epithelial cells and biofilm formation
  - Normal flora in 33-50% of women
- *Mycoplasma hominis/Ureaplasma* spp. (*Ureaplasma urealyticum* and *Ureaplasma parvum*)
  - Eubacteria are small, cell-associated organisms
  - Morphology: 0.2-0.3 μm cocci or 1-2 μm long, tapered rods
  - Organisms lack cell wall and will not stain with Gram stain
  - Fastidious growth requirements, special transport, and culture media are needed
  - 10% colonization rate in children, 20-50% in adults
- *Neisseria gonorrhoeae*
  - Gram-negative intracellular diplococci with adjacent flattened sides
  - Most common sexually transmitted infection; up to 1 million cases per year
- *Chlamydia trachomatis*
  - Obligate intracellular 200- to 400-μm organisms in membrane-lined phagosomes
  - High infection rate, up to 2-26%, highest in adolescents
- *Borrelia burgdorferi* (Lyme disease)
  - Spirochete transmitted to humans through deer tick bite
  - 1% incidence of seroconversion during pregnancy
  - Rare cases of maternal to fetal transmission
- *Mycobacterium tuberculosis*
  - *Mycobacterium* spp. are acid-fast bacilli (AFB)
  - Women at risk include those with HIV/AIDS and immigrants from regions with endemic tuberculosis

CLINICAL ISSUES

Maternal Bacteremia, Sepsis, and Shock in Pregnancy

- Bacteremia occurs in 8-10%
- Severe maternal sepsis in ~ 5 in 10,000 pregnant women
  - 0-3% incidence of death in sepsis during pregnancy
  - Group A streptococcal infections frequently involved

E. coli

- Maternal infection
  - Urinary tract infection, premature rupture of membranes, premature delivery, chorioamnionitis (ascending amniotic fluid infection)
- Fetal/neonatal infection
  - Gram-negative bacilli account for 1/3 of neonatal sepsis; *E. coli* predominates
    - Other gram-negative organisms include *Klebsiella*, *Enterobacter*, *Pseudomonas*, or *Proteus*
  - Early-onset neonatal infection has 40% mortality rate and high morbidity in survivors

Staphylococcus spp.

- Maternal infection
  - Rare cause of chorioamnionitis
  - *S. aureus* (including MRSA) common cause of postpartum infections
    - Perineal abscess, mastitis, episiotomy site infections, C-section wound infection
- Fetal/neonatal infection
  - High mortality rate in congenital infection with *S. aureus*

Enterococcus spp. (*E. faecalis* and *E. faecium*)

- Maternal infection
  - Urinary tract infection, premature rupture of membranes, premature delivery, chorioamnionitis
- Fetal/neonatal infection
  - Usually low-virulence organism, 0.1% of neonatal sepsis

– Early onset in 32% and late onset in 46%
- o Most infections iatrogenic, associated with central venous catheters or necrotizing enterocolitis
  – Up to 28% mortality when associated with necrotizing enterocolitis
- o Resistant to many antibiotics, including vancomycin-resistant *Enterococcus*

Other *Streptococcus* spp.

- Maternal infection
  - o Group B (*Streptococcus agalactiae*) leading cause of chorioamnionitis
  - o Group A (*Streptococcus pyogenes*) causes pharyngitis, tonsillitis, impetigo, necrotizing fasciitis, chorioamnionitis, and septic shock
  - o α- and nonhemolytic *Streptococcus* spp. uncommon causes of chorioamnionitis
- Fetal/neonatal infection
  - o Neonatal sepsis, congenital pneumonia

L. monocytogenes

- Maternal infection
  - o Asymptomatic or flu-like symptoms, fever, diarrhea, premature labor
    – Cause of up to 3% of 2nd-trimester abortions
    – Infection more common later in gestation, associated with preterm delivery
- Fetal/neonatal infection
  - o 9-17/100,000 births, 20-22% are stillborn
  - o Early onset: Erythematous papular rash, petechiae, sepsis, 20-70% mortality
  - o Late onset: Typically term, 1-8 weeks of age, 80% present with meningitis, < 10% mortality

F. nucleatum and *F. necrophorum*

- Maternal infection
  - o Most often associated with chorioamnionitis and prematurity (8-18%)
    – Ascending infection or hematogenous spread from mouth to decidua
    – May be found as single organism or with other organisms, such as group B *Streptococcus*
- Fetal/neonatal infection
  - o Associated with preterm and term stillbirths and congenital pneumonia
  - o Neonatal sepsis due to either organism; mortality 4-66%

Bacteroides spp.

- Maternal infection
  - o Preterm premature rupture of membranes, sepsis, bacterial vaginosis, intraabdominal abscesses, postpartum endometritis, salpingitis, tuboovarian abscesses, mastitis
- Early member of neonatal gut microbiome, rare cause of neonatal morbidity

Prevotella spp.

- Maternal infection
  - o Bacterial vaginosis, chorioamnionitis
- Frequently isolated in newborn meconium, rare cause of neonatal morbidity

C. perfringens

- Maternal infection
  - o Septic abortion with massive intravascular hemolysis, mahogany-colored urine, anemia, renal failure
- Fetal/neonatal infection
  - o Omphalitis, cellulitis, necrotizing fasciitis, sepsis, hemolysis, jaundice

G. vaginalis

- Maternal infection
  - o Bacterial vaginosis, endometritis, chorioamnionitis
    – Clue cells, vaginal squamous epithelium covered by bacteria on wet prep
- Fetal/neonatal infection
  - o Rarely associated with neonatal infection and meningitis

Mycoplasma, Ureaplasma spp.

- Maternal infection
  - o Both associated with bacterial vaginosis, postpartum endometritis, and pelvic inflammatory disease
    – *Ureaplasma* has stronger association with chorioamnionitis, preterm delivery, and fetal loss
    – Both associated with intraamniotic infection but rarely as single agent
- Fetal/neonatal infection
  - o Congenital pneumonia, meningitis, stillbirth
    – 50% of neonates are colonized with either or both agents; increased incidence in premature infants
  - o *Ureaplasma* associated with increased incidence of chronic lung disease in low-birth-weight infants

N. gonorrhoeae

- Maternal infection
  - o Most women asymptomatic, some have dysuria or erythematous friable cervix with purulent discharge
    – Up to 10% incidence in certain at-risk populations
    – Infection in 1st trimester may result in septic abortion
    – May play role in preterm premature rupture of membranes, chorioamnionitis, and preterm delivery
- Fetal/neonatal infection
  - o Gonococcal ophthalmia develops in 30-50% of exposed infants or 1/2,000 births
  - o 1% of exposed neonates will have disseminated disease, usually polyarticular septic arthritis

C. trachomatis

- Maternal infection
  - o Most women are asymptomatic (5-37% carrier rate) and some will have mucopurulent cervicitis, pelvic inflammatory disease, or endometritis
    – Lymphogranuloma venereum due to specific serotypes
    – Exposure to cervicitis results in higher incidence of neonatal infection
    – Definitive role in chorioamnionitis or preterm delivery has not been established
- Fetal/neonatal infection
  - o 35-50% of affected pregnancies will result in neonatal inclusion conjunctivitis
  - o 11-20% of affected pregnancies will result in congenital pneumonia

o Molecular studies demonstrate widespread presence of organisms in some cases of unexplained fetal demise

Borrelia burgdorferi (Lyme disease)

- Maternal infection
  o Flu-like symptoms, erythema chronicum migrans (expanding bull's-eye skin lesion at bite site), cardiac, musculoskeletal, and arthritic symptoms
- Fetal/neonatal infection
  o Most infants born to mothers with Lyme disease are normal
  o Associated with prematurity, cortical blindness, developmental delay, and rash
  o 26% of affected pregnancies result in stillbirth or neonatal mortality due to widely disseminated infection

Mycobacterium tuberculosis

- Maternal infection
  o Pulmonary and extrapulmonary diseases occur in pregnancy
    – Risk factors include HIV coinfection and residence in endemic region
- Fetal/neonatal infection
  o Infection via maternal bacteremia during primary infection, from direct extension into uterus/placenta from genitourinary tract involvement or through inhalation or ingestion of infected amniotic fluid
  o Congenital infection rare but particularly aggressive in infants with extrapulmonary and disseminated disease
  o Hepatosplenomegaly, fever, lymphadenopathy, or respiratory distress with progressive pulmonary infiltrates
  o Diagnosis difficult, frequently delayed, and usually fatal untreated

MACROSCOPIC

General Features

- *Listeria* associated with multiple parenchymal micro- or macroabscesses
  o Amniotic fluid generally appears meconium stained (even in extremely premature deliveries unlikely to pass meconium)
- Other organisms have nonspecific features of chorioamnionitis
- Some organisms, such as *E. coli*, result in foul or feculent odor

MICROSCOPIC

Histologic Features

- Most of these bacteria have been implicated in acute chorioamnionitis but have no specific histologic features
  o Regardless of organism, extreme prematurity has high incidence of subacute necrotizing chorioamnionitis
- Maternal sepsis and shock
  o May be associated with severe chorioamnionitis
  o May have large number of neutrophils and fibrin present in maternal intervillous space
    – Maternal floor infarction with increased perivillous fibrin and infarction of basal villi reported
  o May have large number of bacteria in intervillous space without maternal or fetal inflammatory response

- *Staphylococcus*
  o Fetus may show skin pustules, lung abscesses with increased incidence of pneumothorax and empyema, rarely osteomyelitis
- *Listeria monocytogenes*
  o Acute villitis with micro- or macroabscesses
    – Heavy colonization, possibly due to enhanced replication or impaired clearance
  o Chorioamnionitis with large number of organisms, extracellular and intracellular in amnion epithelium; funisitis
    – Tissue Gram stains may be misinterpreted as small gram-negative rods or gram-positive cocci
- *Fusobacterium* spp.
  o Very thin, long, filamentous rods, usually vertically oriented within amnion epithelium and connective tissue; difficult to see on H&E
  o Associated with severe acute necrotizing or subacute necrotizing chorioamnionitis
- *Mycobacterium* TB
  o Organisms rarely found in placenta
  o May have granulomatous villitis with multinucleated giant cells
  o AFB stains should be performed on all sections

ANCILLARY TESTS

Histochemistry

- Gram stain
  o May be helpful in cases wherein bacteria are seen on routine stains
- Warthin-Starry stain
  o Will stain all bacteria; shows morphology; useful with filamentous anaerobes, spirochetes

Immunohistochemistry

- Specific antibodies available for few of organisms

DIAGNOSTIC CHECKLIST

Clinically Relevant Pathologic Features

- 8-21% of still births may be due to fetal bacterial infection

Pathologic Interpretation Pearls

- Bacteria are rarely seen and, when present, usually indicate heavy infection or lack of antibiotic therapy

SELECTED REFERENCES

1. Acosta CD et al: Severe maternal sepsis in the UK, 2011-2012: a national case-control study. PLoS Med. 11(7):e1001672, 2014
2. Capoccia R et al: Ureaplasma urealyticum, Mycoplasma hominis and adverse pregnancy outcomes. Curr Opin Infect Dis. 26(3):231-40, 2013
3. Centers for Disease Control and Prevention (CDC): vital signs: Listeria illnesses, deaths, and outbreaks–United States, 2009-2011. MMWR Morb Mortal Wkly Rep. 62(22):448-52, 2013
4. Monari F et al: Fetal bacterial infections in antepartum stillbirth: a case series. Early Hum Dev. 89(12):1049-54, 2013
5. Han YW et al: Term stillbirth caused by oral Fusobacterium nucleatum. Obstet Gynecol. 115(2 Pt 2):442-5, 2010
6. Negishi H et al: Staphylococcus aureus causing chorioamnionitis and fetal death with intact membranes at term. A case report. J Reprod Med. 43(4):397-400, 1998

Umbilical Cord Vesicles

(Left) *This umbilical cord from a midgestation loss shows clear, fluid-filled vesicles due to Escherichia coli infection.* (Right) *Histology of the umbilical cord vesicle shows numerous rod-shaped bacteria* ⟹*, consistent with E. coli. Note that there is no inflammatory response, a feature not uncommon in extreme prematurity.*

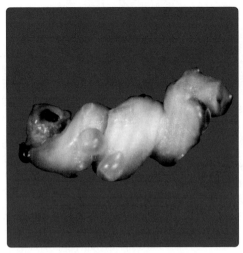

Escherichia coli Infection

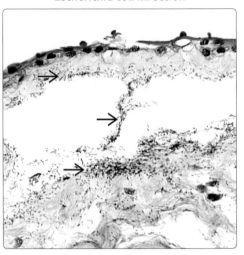

Escherichia coli in Amnion

(Left) *The amnion epithelium hosts a large number of gram-negative rods, consistent with E. coli.* (Right) *Acute villitis may occur with E. coli, often in maternal sepsis with pyelonephritis. The placenta is directly infected through the maternal bloodstream.*

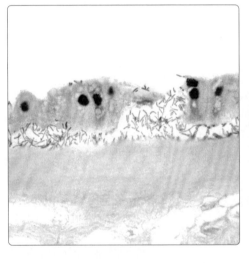

Escherichia coli Acute Villitis

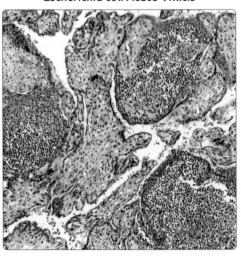

Fetal Sepsis With Acute Villitis

(Left) *Fetal sepsis is associated with acute villitis* ⟹*. In this case, a large number of organisms are present in the fetal capillaries* ⟹*. This type of fetal sepsis usually occurs in extreme prematurity.* (Right) *The H&E section of a lung from a case of E. coli chorioamnionitis shows a large number of rod-shaped organisms. Immunohistochemical staining for E. coli allows specific identification of the organism. This may be useful in cases wherein autopsy cultures were not obtained.*

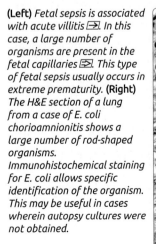

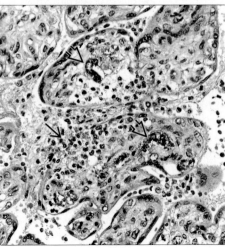

Congenital Pneumonia With *Escherichia coli*

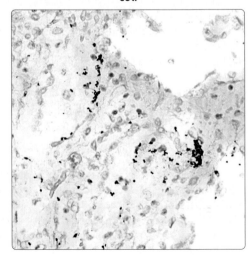

Listeria Microabscess in Placenta

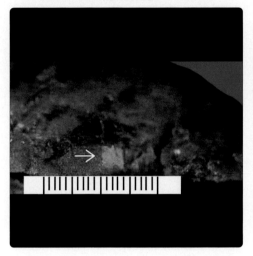

Listeria Abscess

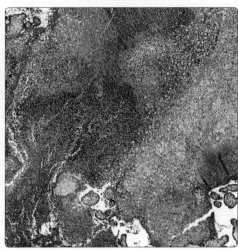

(Left) *This gross photograph of the maternal surface of the placenta shows a light yellow microabscess* ➡ *due to Listeria.* (Right) *Histologic section of a placental Listeria abscess shows necrotizing acute inflammation in the perivillous and intervillous space.*

Listeria in Amnion Epithelium

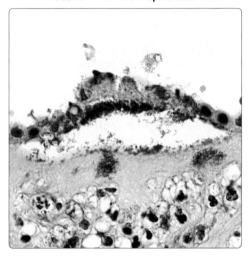

Listeria, Gram-Positive Organisms

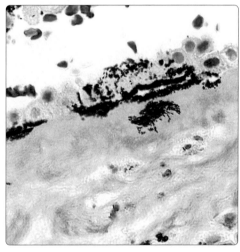

(Left) *This case of Listeria shows a large number of bacteria within the amnion. Heavy colonization is commonly seen with Listeria but can be seen with other microorganisms as well.* (Right) *Gram stain of the Listeria organisms shows gram-positive coccobacilli. Listeria may be mistakenly called gram-positive cocci or overgrowth of diphtheroids.*

Listeria Lung Abscesses

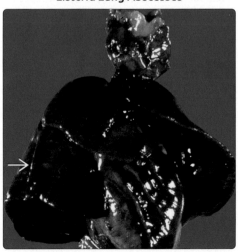

Listeria Congenital Pneumonia

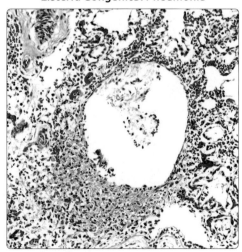

(Left) *This fetal lung at autopsy shows subtle microabscesses* ➡ *of Listeria in lung parenchyma.* (Right) *Microscopic exam shows congenital necrotizing pneumonia secondary to Listeria. Similar lesions are found in the liver and skin.*

Fusobacterium in Amnion

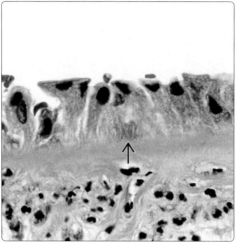

Fusobacterium Gram-Negative Filamentous Bacterium

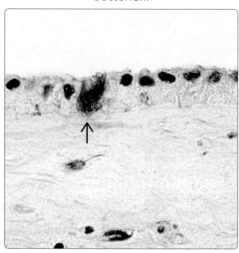

(Left) *Fusobacterium is a very long, thin filamentous bacterium ➡ usually found vertically oriented in the amnion. It is associated with severe chorioamnionitis.* **(Right)** *Fusobacterium is gram negative but generally poorly staining. The bacteria are visible in this section because of the large number of bacteria that are localized in the amnion epithelium ➡.*

Fusobacterium Necrotizing Chorioamnionitis

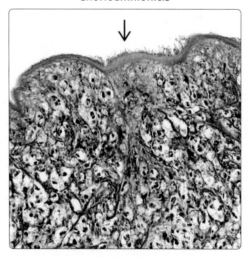

Fusobacterium Silver Stain

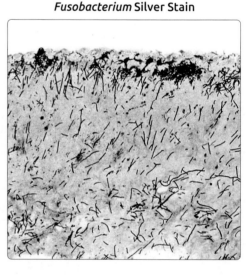

(Left) *Subacute necrotizing chorioamnionitis is associated with extreme prematurity. Fusobacterium spp. are a frequent causative organism. In this image, they impart a hairy appearance to the amnion ➡.* **(Right)** *Warthin-Starry stain is very useful in highlighting the organisms within the amnion and subamniotic connective tissue.*

Fusobacterium Involving 1 Twin

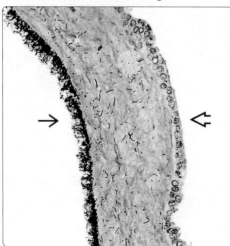

Fusobacterium and Group B *Streptococcus*

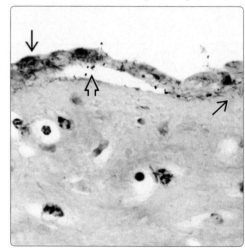

(Left) *This section shows monochorionic, diamniotic twin-dividing membranes with Fusobacterium infection in twin A ➡ but not in twin B ➡. Because twin A is usually located closer to the cervix, its amniotic sac is more susceptible to ascending infection than that of twin B.* **(Right)** *Gram stain shows mixed infection with gram-negative filamentous Fusobacterium spp. ➡ and gram-positive cocci ➡. Fusobacterium is a frequent component of polymicrobial infections.*

Neisseria gonorrhoeae

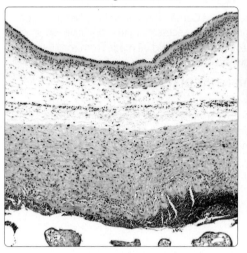

Group A *Streptococcus* Endometritis

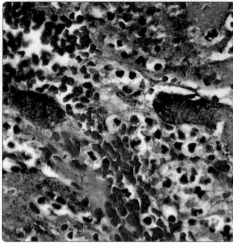

(Left) *This case of severe chorioamnionitis at 23-weeks gestation was attributed to Neisseria gonorrhoeae that had been incompletely treated earlier in gestation.* **(Right)** *This postpartum curettage shows severe postpartum endometritis with abundant cocci. The placenta was not submitted for examination. The organism was found to be group A Streptococcus, which may cause severe necrosis of the myometrium and fascia.*

Staphylococcus aureus Congenital Pneumonia

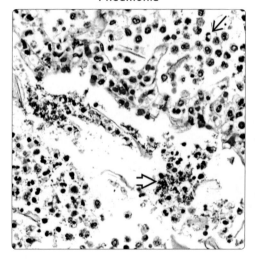

Staphylococcus aureus Meningitis

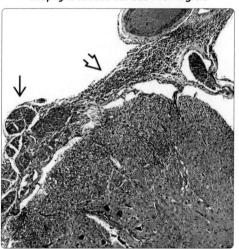

(Left) *This section of neonatal congenital pneumonia shows numerous intraalveolar neutrophils ⇨ and cocci ⇨. Cultures identified methicillin-resistant Staphylococcus aureus (MRSA).* **(Right)** *H&E section of the spinal cord shows the dorsal nerve roots ⇨ and meningitis ⇨ due to MRSA.*

Enterococcus Acute Chorioamnioitis

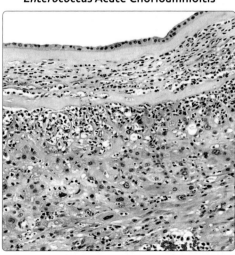

Mycobacterium tuberculosis

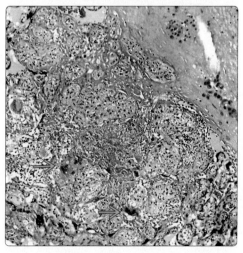

(Left) *This case of acute chorioamnionitis is attributed to Enterococcus spp. No organisms were identified on special stains of the membranes, but cultures from the baby were positive.* **(Right)** *This section of placental basal villi shows granulomatous villitis with Langhans-type multinucleated giant cells ⇨ due to Mycobacterium tuberculosis. Rare acid-fast organisms were noted in some but not all sections. (Courtesy P. O'Shea, MD.)*

KEY FACTS

CLINICAL ISSUES

- 20-50% of pregnant women have candidal colonization
- Identification of *Candida* funisitis in premature placenta is of critical lab value and neonatology should be notified
- Prematurity < 28 weeks is associated with increased incidence of disseminated disease with high mortality
- Higher mortality with *Candida albicans* infection compared with other *Candida* species

MACROSCOPIC

- Umbilical cord has superficial yellow-white plaques

MICROSCOPIC

- Subamniotic microabscesses, organisms are difficult to see with H&E
- Membranes rarely have chorioamnionitis and rarely have yeast

ANCILLARY TESTS

- Silver stain, such as Gömöri methenamine silver (GMS) or PAS, is almost always necessary to identify organisms
- Scrape or touch preps should be made from cord lesions for rapid diagnosis

TOP DIFFERENTIAL DIAGNOSES

- *Candida glabrata* is less likely to have umbilical cord microabscesses; usually has large number of microorganisms in membranes associated with chorioamnionitis and does not form pseudohyphae
- True fungi, *Aspergillus* spp., *Mucor*, or *Rhizopus* are generally acquired in postnatal period

Gross Appearance of Umbilical Cord in *Candida* Infection

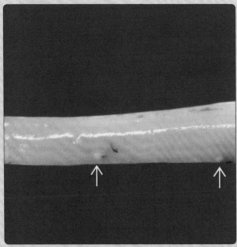

Pseudohyphae of *Candida*

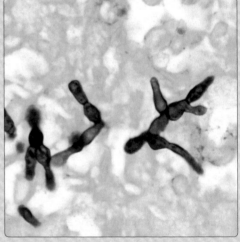

(Left) *This segment of umbilical cord has numerous subamniotic yellow-white plaques* ➡️, *which are microabscesses. This gross finding is characteristic of Candida infection.* (Right) *Formation of pseudohyphae with constrictions between elongated elements is characteristic of some, but not all, of the Candida spp. True hyphae have straight sides.*

Prominent Subamniotic Abscesses

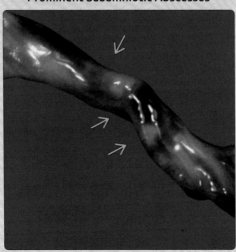

Rapid Evaluation for *Candida*

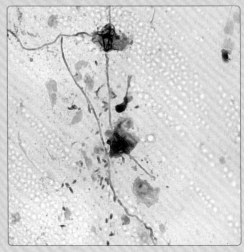

(Left) *These large subamniotic abscesses of Candida* ➡️ *are somewhat obscured by congested umbilical vessels. The gross appearance of these abscesses should prompt expedient evaluation for Candida.* (Right) *This scrape preparation was made from an umbilical cord plaque recognized on gross exam. Scrape preparations facilitate rapid communication of Candida funisitis to those caring for the neonate.*

TERMINOLOGY

Synonyms
- Candidiasis

Definitions
- Infection with *Candida albicans* or other *Candida* spp.

ETIOLOGY/PATHOGENESIS

Infectious Agents
- 80% due to *C. albicans*
  - Other less common species include
    - *Candida parapsilosis, Candida glabrata, Candida tropicalis, Candida kefyr*
- Vaginal candidiasis is common, ascending infection is uncommon
- Congenital candidiasis may occur with intact membranes

CLINICAL ISSUES

Epidemiology
- 20-50% of pregnant women have candidal colonization
  - 50% of infants are colonized, may have skin lesions
  - 10% develop systemic disease, usually in prematurity
- Higher incidence in pregnant women with intrauterine device or cerclage
- More commonly associated with late-onset neonatal sepsis

Presentation
- Most infants are asymptomatic; some will have pink macules or white skin pustules (cutaneous candidiasis)
- 50% of neonates with disseminated disease will have positive blood cultures, often persistent

Prognosis
- Prematurity < 28 weeks is associated with increased incidence of disseminated disease with high mortality
- Higher mortality with *C. albicans* infection compared with other *Candida* spp.

MACROSCOPIC

General Features
- Umbilical cord has superficial yellow-white plaques
  - Consider touch or scrape preparation or frozen section when identified at gross exam for rapid diagnosis
- Squamous metaplasia may produce white plaques only found near cord insertion and is normal finding

MICROSCOPIC

Histologic Features
- Umbilical cord
  - Subamniotic microabscesses, also termed peripheral funisitis
  - Rarely associated with necrotizing funisitis
  - Yeast forms, sometimes budding with pseudohyphae, difficult to see on H&E
- Membranes may or may not have chorioamnionitis and rarely have yeast
  - Severe chorioamnionitis may occur in some cases
- Villi
  - Granulomatous villitis is rarely reported
  - Rarely, organisms may be seen in intervillous space
  - Villous edema may be present, mostly as reaction to chorioamnionitis

ANCILLARY TESTS

Histochemistry
- Silver stain, such as Gomori methenamine silver (GMS) or PAS, almost always necessary to identify organisms in tissue section
- Yeast are gram positive
- Candida in tissue may appear more like true fungus, rarely even producing true hyphae

DIFFERENTIAL DIAGNOSIS

Other Fungal Organisms
- *C. glabrata*
  - Less likely to have umbilical cord microabscesses
  - Usually has large number of yeast in membranes associated with chorioamnionitis
  - Does not form pseudohyphae
- True fungi are generally acquired in postnatal period
  - *Aspergillus* spp.
  - Zygomycetes (*Mucor* or *Rhizopus*)

Bacterial Organisms
- Rare infections with certain species have been reported with similar pattern of peripheral funisitis
  - *Corynebacterium kutscheri, Haemophilus influenzae, Listeria monocytogenes*

DIAGNOSTIC CHECKLIST

Pathologic Interpretation Pearls
- Small white plaques on umbilical cord surface is nearly pathognomonic for *Candida*
- Identification of *Candida* in placenta/umbilical cord should be considered critical laboratory value, neonatology should be notified
- Scrape or touch preps from cord lesions facilitate rapid diagnosis
- Silver stains or PAS almost always necessary to identify organisms in tissue section

SELECTED REFERENCES

1. Kaufman DA et al: Congenital cutaneous candidiasis: prompt systemic treatment is associated with improved outcomes in neonates. Clin Infect Dis. 64(10):1387-1395, 2017
2. Pammi M et al: Candida parapsilosis is a significant neonatal pathogen: a systematic review and meta-analysis. Pediatr Infect Dis J. 32(5):e206-16, 2013
3. Pineda C et al: Maternal sepsis, chorioamnionitis, and congenital Candida kefyr infection in premature twins. Pediatr Infect Dis J. 31(3):320-2, 2012
4. Matsuzawa S et al: Congenital Candida glabrata infection without specific nodules on the placenta and umbilical cord. Pediatr Infect Dis J. 24(8):744-5, 2005
5. Diana A et al: "White dots on the placenta and red dots on the baby": congenital cutaneous candidiasis--a rare disease of the neonate. Acta Paediatr. 93(7):996-9, 2004
6. Qureshi F et al: Candida funisitis: a clinicopathologic study of 32 cases. Pediatr Dev Pathol. 1(2):118-24, 1998

Peripheral Funisitis

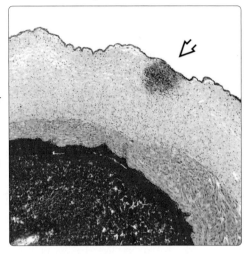

Necrotizing Funisitis

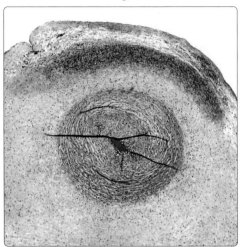

(Left) The classic presentation of Candida funisitis is peripheral funisitis, with triangular ⊟ subamniotic microabscesses. (Right) Necrotizing funisitis is usually evidence of a longstanding infection. While this may occur with Candida, it is much less common than the microabscesses. Necrotizing funisitis may also be seen in syphilis, toxoplasmosis, herpes simplex virus, group B Streptococcus, and Neisseria gonorrhoeae.

Peripheral Funisitis

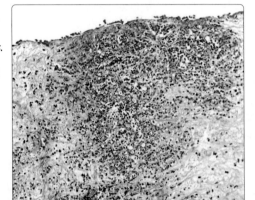

Surface Colonization of Cord

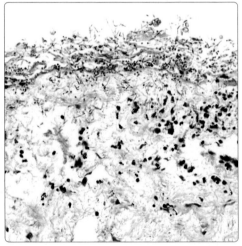

(Left) This high-power image of a subamniotic abscess shows degenerating neurophils and necrotic debris. (Right) This image shows the unusual finding of large yeast colony on the cord surface with many pseudohyphae.

Candida albicans

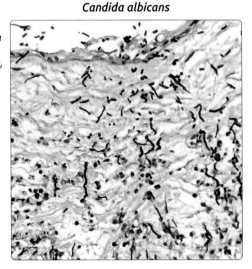

Candida albicans

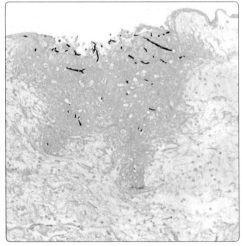

(Left) Microabscesses of peripheral funisitis may have a significant number of yeast when seen with a special stain, PAS in this case. (Right) GMS stain is also useful for visualizing the organism.

Severe Acute Chorioamnionitis

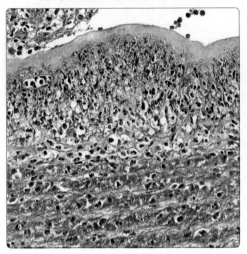

Candida albicans in Membranes

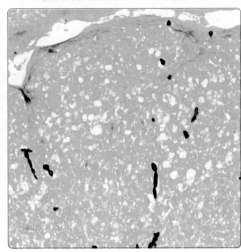

(**Left**) *Candida albicans may be associated with chorioamnionitis, which can be severe. It may be mixed with other microbes in ascending amniotic fluid infection. The multifocal subamniotic abscesses may also be seen overlying the chorionic plate* (**Right**) *Candida albicans-associated chorioamnionitis rarely has significant numbers of yeast and pseudohyphae in the membranes, even in the presence of severe chorioamnionitis.*

Candida glabrata

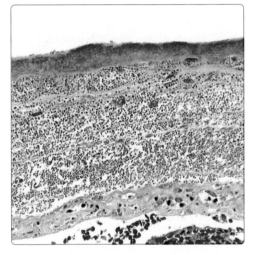

Candida glabrata

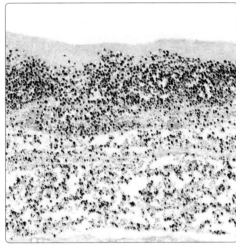

(**Left**) *Candida glabrata does not form pseudohyphae and is often found in large numbers in the membranes, but it is rarely associated with funisitis.* (**Right**) *Candida glabrata is gram positive, as are all fungi. The absence of pseudohyphae may be misdiagnosed as a coccoid bacterium.*

Candida glabrata

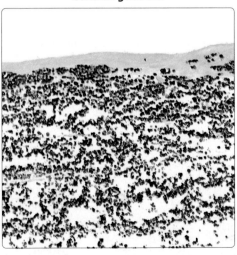

Disseminated Neonatal Candidiasis

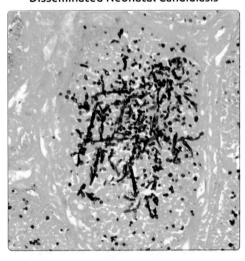

(**Left**) *Candida glabrata is positive with GMS stain, as are all fungi. Bacteria may also be weakly positive with GMS, but the yeast are significantly larger.* (**Right**) *This is a section of kidney from a case of disseminated candidiasis. With dissemination, the organisms may form colonies that can be misdiagnosed as true fungus. Rare true hyphae may be seen, but pseudohyphae and yeast will always be present as well.*

KEY FACTS

ETIOLOGY/PATHOGENESIS

- Cytomegalovirus (CMV): Most common congenital viral infection, occurring in 1% of newborns
- Congenital CMV may be transmitted vertically in utero, at time of delivery by cervical secretions, or through breast milk

CLINICAL ISSUES

- CMV is leading cause of nongenetic sensorineural hearing loss and a leading cause of neurodevelopmental abnormalities in children
  - Hearing loss is progressive over 1st year; infants may pass hearing screen at birth
- 85-90% of infected infants asymptomatic
- Central nervous system involvement includes meningoencephalitis, chorioretinitis, microcephaly, hydrocephalus, polymicrogyria, and periventricular calcifications

- Infected infants may have pancytopenia with hepatosplenomegaly, petechiae, and purpura
- Prematurity, hydrops, symmetric intrauterine growth restriction and intrauterine fetal demise with early in utero infection

MICROSCOPIC

- Lymphoplasmacytic villitis
- Avascular villi with hemosiderin
- Rare viral inclusions in Hofbauer cells and endothelium
- Eosinophilic necrotic debris in villi with suspicious viral inclusions

ANCILLARY TESTS

- Immunohistochemistry for CMV very useful in confirming diagnosis
- Unknown whether placental infection always means fetal infection

---

Lymphoplasmacytic Villitis

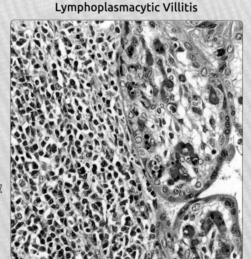

Chronic Villitis and Intervillositis

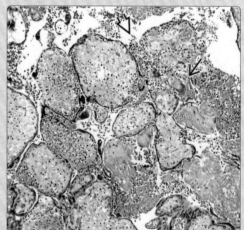

(Left) Cytomegalovirus (CMV) villitis is classically lymphoplasmacytic, but there is significant variability in the number of plasma cells. Confluent plasma cells are present within a villus adjacent to one without any inflammation. Note the increase in nucleated red blood cells. (Right) Lymphohistiocytic villitis with multinucleated giant cells ⊟ and maternal intervillositis ⊟. This has more of the appearance of villitis of undetermined etiology, but was due to CMV with HIV coinfection.

CMV Inclusion in Renal Tubules

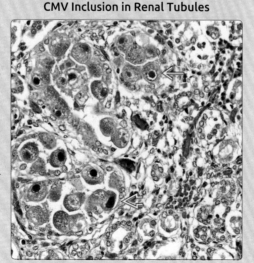

CMV Inclusion in Chorionic Villus

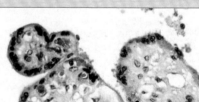
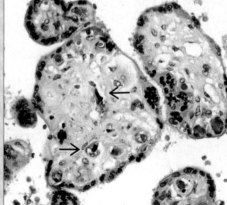

(Left) Renal tubule epithelium is shown in an 18-week fetal demise with large numbers of infected cells. Cowdry type A ⊟ (owl-eye) and Cowdry type B ⊟ (smudged nucleus) inclusions are present in addition to the basophilic cytoplasmic inclusions. (Right) Rare CMV inclusions ⊟ may be found in Hofbauer cells or endothelial cells of the villi. Hemosiderin is also noted, but little to no inflammation is present.

TERMINOLOGY

Abbreviations

- Cytomegalovirus (CMV)

ETIOLOGY/PATHOGENESIS

Infectious Agents

- Most common congenital viral infection, occurring in 1% of live births
- Congenital CMV may be transmitted from mother to child in 3 ways
  - In utero vertical transmission across placenta (hematogenous spread)
    - 30-50% of pregnant women during primary CMV infection
    - 1-3% of women with reactivation of CMV
  - Intrapartum transmission by cervical secretions
    - Women with primary or reactivated CMV infection may shed virus from cervix
    - 50% of women shedding virus from cervix will infect baby during vaginal delivery
  - Postpartum transmission through breast milk
    - 30-70% of women with primary or reactivated CMV infection shed virus in breast milk
- CMV antibody-negative women have 1-2% risk of primary CMV infection during pregnancy

CLINICAL ISSUES

Presentation

- CMV is leading nongenetic cause of sensorineural hearing loss and a leading cause of neurodevelopmental disabilities in children
- 85-90% of infected infants are asymptomatic
- Central nervous system manifestations
  - Meningoencephalitis, chorioretinitis, hydrocephalus, microcephaly, polymicrogyria, and periventricular calcifications
- Systemic manifestations
  - Intrauterine growth restriction, hepatosplenomegaly, anemia, neutropenia, thrombocytopenia with petechiae or purpura

Treatment

- Drugs
  - Treatment with intravenous ganciclovir or oral valganciclovir for symptomatic infants
  - Treatment of less severely affected or asymptomatic infants not yet routine
  - Treatment with hyperimmune globulin during pregnancy has not shown efficacy

Prognosis

- Mortality for symptomatic congenital CMV is ~ 30%
- Associated with prematurity, hydrops, intrauterine growth restriction and intrauterine fetal demise
- 70% of 1st-trimester infections have severe CNS injury
- 10-17% of asymptomatic infants at birth will develop unilateral or bilateral deafness

MACROSCOPIC

General Features

- Placenta may be hydropic

MICROSCOPIC

Histologic Features

- Lymphoplasmacytic villitis
- Avascular villi with hemosiderin
- Viral inclusions in Hofbauer cells and endothelium
  - May be rare
- Eosinophilic necrotic debris in villi with suspicious viral inclusions
  - Eosinophilic debris usually immunoreactive for CMV

ANCILLARY TESTS

Immunohistochemistry

- Anti-CMV antibodies against immediate-early, early, or late viral antigens available
- Can be useful in confirming diagnosis
  - Sensitivity not 100%
  - If lymphoplasmacytic villitis present, urine culture or other studies of neonate for CMV may be warranted

PCR

- PCR for CMV on formalin-fixed paraffin-embedded tissue may be more sensitive than immunohistochemistry
  - Has been negative in placenta of confirmed congenital CMV

DIFFERENTIAL DIAGNOSIS

Other Viral Infections

- Other viruses of herpes family will have similar intranuclear inclusions, but only CMV has intracytoplasmic inclusions

Fetal Vascular Malperfusion

- May occur in conjunction with CMV infection, especially when villitis affects proximal stem villi

Neonatal Alloimmune Thrombocytopenia

- May have lymphoplasmacytic villitis
- Congenital CMV should be clinically excluded with cultures

DIAGNOSTIC CHECKLIST

Pathologic Interpretation Pearls

- CMV should always be considered when there is lymphoplasmacytic villitis or hemosiderin deposition

SELECTED REFERENCES

1. Oosterom N et al: Neuro-imaging findings in infants with congenital cytomegalovirus infection: relation to trimester of infection. Neonatology. 107(4):289-96, 2015
2. Folkins AK et al: Diagnosis of congenital CMV using PCR performed on formalin-fixed, paraffin-embedded placental tissue. Am J Surg Pathol. 37(9):1413-20, 2013
3. Iwasenko JM et al: Human cytomegalovirus infection is detected frequently in stillbirths and is associated with fetal thrombotic vasculopathy. J Infect Dis. 203(11):1526-33, 2011
4. McDonagh S et al: Patterns of human cytomegalovirus infection in term placentas: a preliminary analysis. J Clin Virol. 35(2):210-5, 2006

(Left) *Lymphoplasmacytic villitis is prominent in this case associated with abundant hemosiderin.* **(Right)** *CMV inclusions are rare within the placenta. It is more common to see this eosinophilic granular material, which is strongly positive with CMV immunohistochemistry (IHC). The inflammation in this villus is minimal, possibly representing "burned-out" villitis.*

Lymphoplasmacytic Villitis

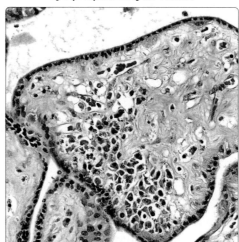

Eosinophilic Bodies Suspicious for CMV

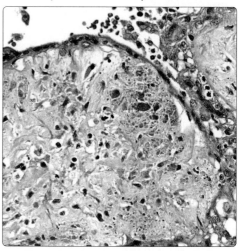

(Left) *An avascular villus is shown with rare plasma cells ⟶ but abundant granular hemosiderin ⟹, the result of endothelial injury by CMV.* **(Right)** *Iron stain is positive within Hofbauer cells in avascular villi without residual inflammation.*

Hemosiderin in Villus

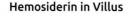

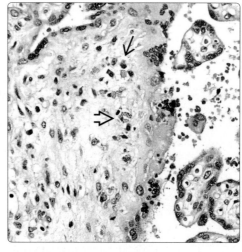

Villus Hemosiderin With Iron Stain

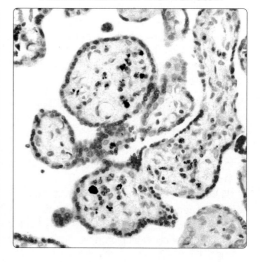

(Left) *Multiple CMV inclusions are present in what may be capillary endothelium. There is minimal lymphocytic villitis.* **(Right)** *IHC may identify numerous CMV(+) cells that are not suspected on routine H&E stains.*

Chronic Villitis With CMV Inclusions

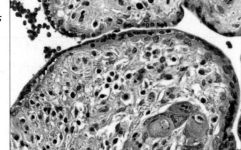

Villus With CMV Inclusions, IHC

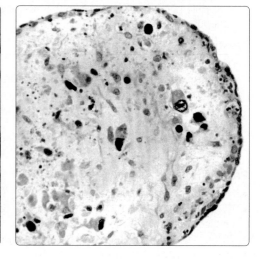

Eosinophilic Debris With Suspicious Viral Inclusions

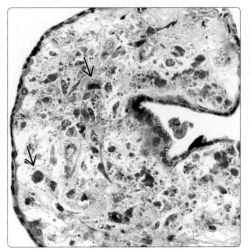

Eosinophilic Debris Positive for CMV, IHC

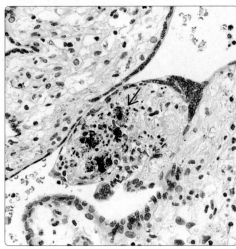

(Left) Villi may show stromal necrosis with abundant eosinophilic debris that may be calcified. Some nuclei ⊡ appear suspicious for viral inclusions. (Right) IHC for CMV will confirm the presence of the virus ⊡ in suspicious cells.

Fetal Vasculopathy Due to CMV

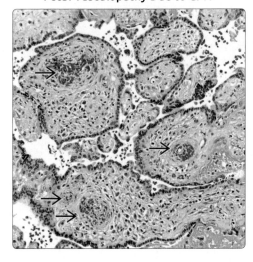

Fetal Erythroblastosis Due to CMV

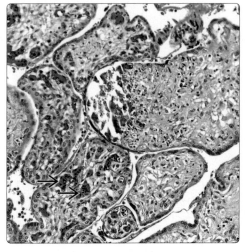

(Left) CMV infection may be associated with extensive fetal vascular occlusion ⊡ characterized by loss of endothelial integrity, red blood cell extravasation, and septation. This could result from proximal chronic villitis of stem villi, as in villitis of unknown etiology, or possibly from viral infection of the endothelium. (Right) A calcified, avascular, inflamed villus is found adjacent to normal-appearing villi with marked fetal erythroblastosis ⊡.

Basal Plate With Lymphoplasmacytic Inflammation

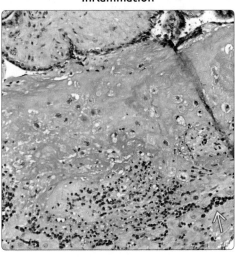

Basal Plate With Lymphoplasmacytic Inflammation

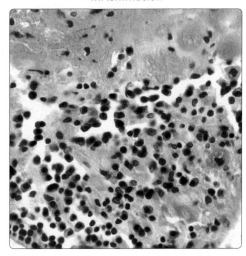

(Left) The placental basal plate in this case of CMV contains moderate chronic inflammation including plasma cells ⊡. (Right) Lymphoplasmacytic deciduitis is less specific for CMV infection than lymphoplasmacytic villitis.

Hepatomegaly Due to Congenital CMV

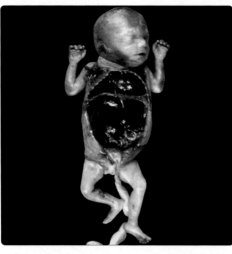

Hepatic Necrosis Due to CMV

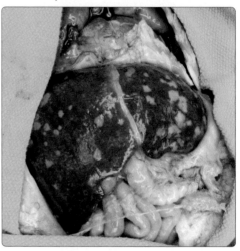

(Left) *There is massive hepatomegaly in this mildly hydropic previable fetus with congenital CMV infection.* (Right) *This neonate had symptomatic congenital CMV and survived for 4 months with persistent viremia despite antiviral therapy. The liver is markedly enlarged and shows numerous white areas of remote hepatic necrosis.*

Hepatic Necrosis Due to CMV

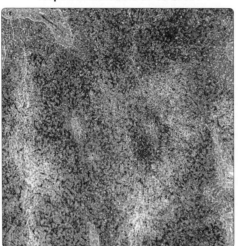

CMV in Biliary Epithelium

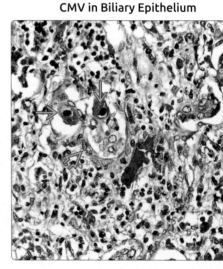

(Left) *Congenital CMV may cause massive hepatic necrosis. CMV inclusions are usually visible in biliary epithelium.* (Right) *Numerous CMV inclusions ➡ are noted within the liver bile duct epithelium ➡.*

Macerated Fetus Due to CMV

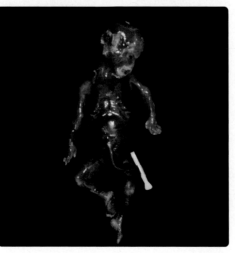

Multiple CMV Inclusions in Autolyzed Lung

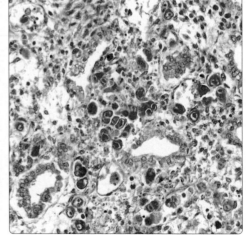

(Left) *Severely macerated fetus was found to have CMV infection on microscopic examination.* (Right) *Microscopic examination of tissues from macerated fetuses can be very useful. This section of lung shows numerous CMV inclusions, despite moderate autolysis of the tissue.*

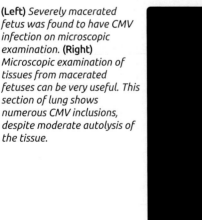

Brain CT With Periventricular Calcifications Due to CMV

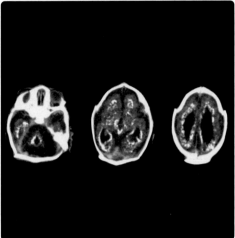

Microencephaly and Polymicrogyria Due to CMV

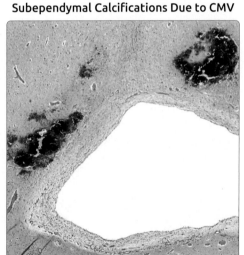

(Left) CT scan shows hydrocephalus with periventricular calcifications in a case of congenital CMV. (Right) CNS involvement with congenital CMV may show microencephaly with polymicrogyria, as in this case of demise at 36-weeks gestation.

Ventriculomegaly With Subependymal Calcifications Due to CMV

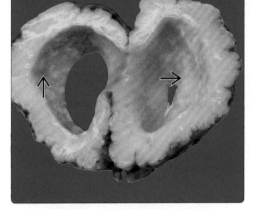

Subependymal Calcifications Due to CMV

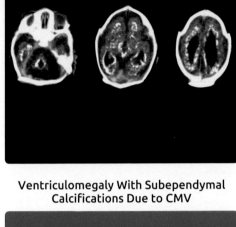

(Left) Hydrocephalus may be seen with congenital CMV, as in this case with multiple yellow subependymal calcifications ➡. (Right) Microscopic examination of the 4th ventricle shows periventricular block-like calcification.

Microcephaly Due to Congenital CMV

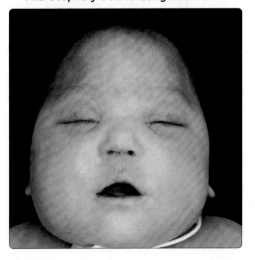

Brain Section With CMV Inclusion

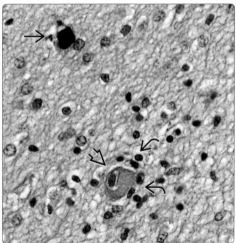

(Left) This baby, who survived 4 months with congenital CMV, shows severe microcephaly. (Right) This section of brain from the periventricular area shows microcalcification ➡ and a CMV inclusion cell ➡ that is partially surrounded by microglial cells ➡, forming a type of microglial nodule.

Parvovirus B19

ETIOLOGY/PATHOGENESIS

- Parvovirus B19 is single-stranded DNA member of Parvoviridae family
- Infection of fetal erythroid precursors results in severe anemia, high-output cardiac failure, and hydrops fetalis
- Infection of myocardium may contribute to cardiac dysfunction

CLINICAL ISSUES

- Parvovirus during pregnancy may result in nonimmune hydrops fetalis 4-6 weeks post exposure
- Vertical transmission occurs in 33% of women during primary infection
- Severe fetal anemia results in high-output cardiac failure
- 15% of nonimmune hydrops are due to parvovirus
- 5-10% of in utero infections result in lethal hydrops
- Survivors of in utero infection are generally normal with rare cases of neurodevelopmental disability reported

MICROSCOPIC

- Placenta
  - Mild to marked villous edema
  - Increased fetal nucleated red blood cells (NRBCs), many with intranuclear basophilic or eosinophilic inclusions
  - Usually without significant chronic villitis
- Fetal findings
  - Liver is most severely affected often with hemosiderosis
  - Bone marrow is hypocellular

DIAGNOSTIC CHECKLIST

- Marked increase in NRBCs (erythroblastosis fetalis) associated with hydropic pale placenta should prompt search for parvovirus inclusions
- Hydropic pale fetus, often with hepatic hemosiderosis is suggestive of parvovirus
- Immunohistochemistry is very useful, even in severely macerated tissues

Villous Edema and Fetal Anemia

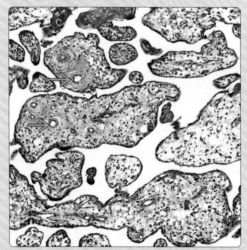

Villous Edema and Erythroblastosis

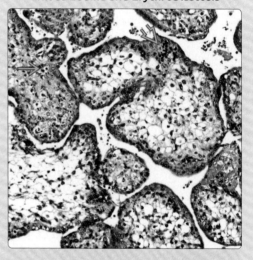

(Left) *Diffuse villous edema is seen in this case of parvovirus infection. Fetal blood spaces are mostly empty ➡, as is often seen in fetal anemia.* (Right) *These edematous villi contain numerous Hofbauer cells and rare probable lymphocytes ➡. Fetal capillaries contain numerous nucleated red blood cells ➡.*

Parvovirus Nuclear Inclusions

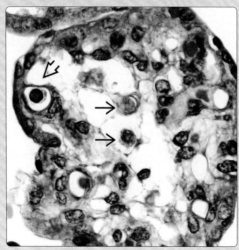

Fetal Liver in Parvovirus B19

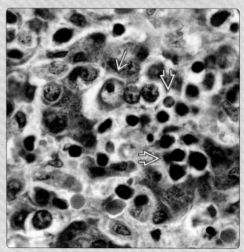

(Left) *An erythroid precursor in this villous capillary displays a characteristic intranuclear parvovirus inclusion ➡. A nonspecific feature of villous edema is prominent Hofbauer cells ➡.* (Right) *This section of fetal liver in a case of erythroblastosis fetalis due to parvovirus shows atypical pronormoblasts ➡, along with numerous normoblasts with intranuclear parvovirus inclusions ➡.*

TERMINOLOGY

Abbreviations

- Nucleated red blood cell (NRBC)

Synonyms

- Erythema infectiosum and 5th disease

ETIOLOGY/PATHOGENESIS

Infectious Agents

- Parvovirus B19-single-stranded DNA member of Parvoviridae family, species specific
  - Globoside or erythrocyte P antigen required for infection of host cell
    - Present on surface of syncytiotrophoblast and cytotrophoblast, erythroid precursors, red cells, some megakaryocytes, endothelial cells, and fetal myocardium

Nonimmune Hydrops Fetalis Due to Parvovirus B19

- Virus infects erythroid precursors
  - Shortened RBC survival with hemolysis and erythroid hypoplasia
  - Severe fetal anemia results in high-output cardiac failure
    - Characteristic elevated peak systolic velocity of middle cerebral artery on fetal Doppler imaging
- Parvovirus may also infect myocardium, contributing to cardiac dysfunction

CLINICAL ISSUES

Epidemiology

- Winter/spring epidemics
- Maternal parvovirus infection during pregnancy
  - ~ 50% of women are at risk for infection (nonimmune)
    - 1-5% incidence of seroconversion during pregnancy
    - Once woman has seroconverted, antibodies are protective for life
  - Vertical transmission occurs in 33% of women with primary infection during pregnancy
    - Fetus may develop nonimmune hydrops ~ 4 weeks after exposure
    - Estimated that 5-15% of nonimmune hydrops are due to parvovirus
    - 70-95% survival rate, higher rates after intrauterine transfusion

Presentation

- Nonimmune hydrops fetalis
  - Now accounts for 90% of cases of fetal hydrops
    - Fewer cases of Rh(D) alloimmunization with widespread use of Rh(D) immune globulin
    - Many causes, including cardiac dysfunction, hematologic abnormalities, twin-to-twin transfusion, placental dysfunction, and infection
  - Ultrasonographic findings
    - Presence of 2 or more abnormal fluid collections in fetus on ultrasound
      □ Ascites, pleural effusions, pericardial effusion, skin edema
    - Often accompanied by increased placental thickness and hydramnios

- - Maternal indirect Coombs test negative
- Erythema infectiosum (5th disease) described as 5th viral exanthem in childhood
  - In children
    - Petechial eruption in glove or stocking pattern with truncal reticular erythema and slapped cheek appearance
    - Rarely associated with hepatitis and acute renal failure
  - In adults
    - Commonly asymptomatic
    - Violaceous plaques or nodules; firm, flesh-colored papules; papular and eczematous eruptions
    - Polyarthritis
    - Rarely associated with hepatitis and acute liver failure
    - Transient aplastic crisis in sickle cell disease, chronic pure red cell aplasia in immunocompromised patients

Laboratory Tests

- Maternal serologies to parvovirus (IgM and IgG) for evidence of exposure
- Maternal serum α-fetoprotein may be elevated due to fetal hydrops
- Parvovirus PCR from amniocentesis or fetal blood sampling

Treatment

- No specific antiviral drug for parvovirus
- Immune globulin is used in immunoincompetent individuals
- Intrauterine transfusion treatment of choice for fetal anemia
  - There can be spontaneous recovery in utero

Prognosis

- 5-10% of in utero infections result in lethal hydrops
  - Infection during 2nd trimester is associated with greatest risk for hydrops
  - 1st trimester is associated with lower risk
  - 3rd trimester is associated with very low risk
- Resolution of hydrops may occur ± intrauterine transfusion
- Some survivors have hepatic fibrosis, possibly due to toxicity of hemosiderosis or inflammatory mediators
- Survivors may have neurodevelopmental disability, possibly related to anemia

MACROSCOPIC

General Features

- Placenta is large, pale, and friable

MICROSCOPIC

Histologic Features

- Placenta
  - NRBCs, many with intranuclear ground-glass inclusions
  - Diffuse villous edema, generally with delayed maturation
    - Delayed maturation persists in placenta even after intrauterine transfusions
  - Increased number of T lymphocytes within villi, but usual findings of chronic villitis are not present
- Fetal organs
  - Liver is most severely affected
    - Erythroid hyperplasia
    - Atypical giant pronormoblasts

- Moderate to marked hemosiderosis
- Rarely giant cell transformation of hepatocytes, cholestasis, and rare fibrosis
- Immunohistochemistry for parvovirus may be positive in liver but negative in placenta
- Bone marrow is hypocellular
- Myocarditis may be difficult to distinguish from circulating NRBCs with viral inclusions
- Parvovirus inclusions will be found in circulating NRBCs in all organs
- Stress reaction in fetal adrenal cortex with marked accumulation of lipid

ANCILLARY TESTS

Immunohistochemistry

- Immunostain for parvovirus is very useful for confirming viral inclusions in NRBCs
- Immunostains should be used on both placenta and liver if available

DIFFERENTIAL DIAGNOSIS

Erythroblastosis Fetalis Due to Immune-Mediated Hemolysis

- May appear similar in placenta and fetus
- Maternal antibody to fetal blood group antigen detected
- Lacks viral inclusions in NRBCs
  - Severe autolysis may result in pseudoinclusions in any condition

Fetal Hydrops Due to Chronic Fetal Maternal Transfusion

- May see numerous erythroblasts in villous capillaries
- No viral inclusions in NRBC
- Find evidence of fetal blood in maternal intervillous blood space
  - Confirm fetal-maternal transfusion by Kleihauer-Betke stain on maternal blood or flow cytometry

Increased Fetal Nucleated Red Blood Cells

- Severe hypoxic stress can cause increased NRBCs in fetal circulation
  - More often seen in 3rd-trimester placenta
    - e.g., after placental abruption
  - Mild elevations in NRBC seen with gestational diabetes
    - Usually < 10 NRBC in 10 high-power fields of terminal villi
- May be increased in response to anemia after severe acute fetal hemorrhage

Myeloid Proliferations of Down Syndrome

- May present in utero with hydrops, numerous nucleated precursor hematopoietic cells in peripheral blood
- Greater variety of precursor cell types (e.g., myeloid precursors, megakaryoblasts) than in parvovirus

Other Infections

- Congenital syphilis may have profound fetal anemia with hydropic placenta
  - Leukemoid reaction can mimic acute leukemia
  - Villous enlargement with numerous Hofbauer cells may appear similar

- May see chronic or acute villitis with proliferative vasculitis of fetal stem villous vasculature
- May see significant changes associated with ascending infection in syphilis, i.e., chorioamnionitis, necrotizing funisitis
- Maternal serologies indicate exposure to *Treponema pallidum*
- Warthin-Starry or immunohistochemistry demonstrates treponemes
- Cytomegalovirus may be associated with hydropic fetus and placenta with anemia
  - May see immature hematopoietic cells in fetal circulation
  - Viral cytopathic effects, plasma cell villitis, avascular villi with hemosiderin present

DIAGNOSTIC CHECKLIST

Pathologic Interpretation Pearls

- Marked increase in NRBCs (erythroblastosis fetalis) associated with hydropic placenta should prompt search for parvovirus inclusions
- Hydropic, pale fetus
- Placenta may only have rare inclusions, while liver contains numerous inclusions

SELECTED REFERENCES

1. McCarthy WA et al: Persistence of villous immaturity in term deliveries following intrauterine transfusion for parvovirus B19 infection and RhD-associated hemolytic disease of the fetus and newborn. Pediatr Dev Pathol. 20(6):469-474, 2017
2. Oliveira GM et al: Detection of cytomegalovirus, herpes virus simplex, and parvovirus b19 in spontaneous abortion placentas. J Matern Fetal Neonatal Med. 1-8, 2017
3. Ornoy A et al: Parvovirus B19 infection during pregnancy and risks to the fetus. Birth Defects Res. 109(5):311-323, 2017
4. Li JJ et al: Parvovirus infection: an immunohistochemical study using fetal and placental tissue. Pediatr Dev Pathol. 18(1):30-9, 2015
5. Society for Maternal-Fetal Medicine (SMFM) et al: Society for maternal-fetal medicine (SMFM) clinical guideline #7: nonimmune hydrops fetalis. Am J Obstet Gynecol. 212(2):127-39, 2015
6. Al-Buhtori M et al: Viral detection in hydrops fetalis, spontaneous abortion, and unexplained fetal death in utero. J Med Virol. 83(4):679-84, 2011
7. Young NS et al: Parvovirus B19. N Engl J Med. 350(6):586-97, 2004
8. Jordan JA et al: Placental cellular immune response in women infected with human parvovirus B19 during pregnancy. Clin Diagn Lab Immunol. 8(2):288-92, 2001
9. Jordan JA et al: Globoside expression within the human placenta. Placenta. 20(1):103-8, 1999
10. Essary LR et al: Frequency of parvovirus B19 infection in nonimmune hydrops fetalis and utility of three diagnostic methods. Hum Pathol. 29(7):696-701, 1998

Erythroblastosis in Fetal Capillaries

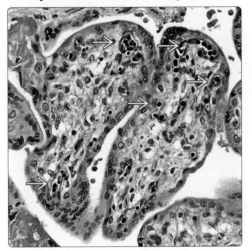

Immunohistochemistry for Parvovirus B19

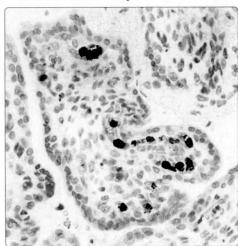

(Left) These villi show a marked increase in fetal nucleated red blood cells ➡ (erythroblastosis fetalis). (Right) Immunohistochemistry confirms the presence of parvovirus within many cells in the fetal capillaries. This stain is very useful in the differential diagnosis of erythroblastosis fetalis.

Resolving Villus Edema

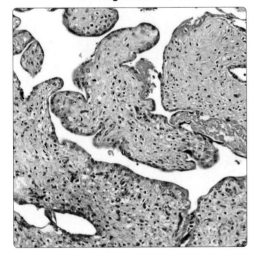

Resolving Villous Edema

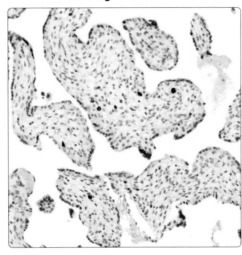

(Left) The villous stroma appears more condensed, and less edematous, while there is little vascular development. A subtle increase in mononuclear cells in the villous stroma suggests mild chronic lymphocytic villitis. (Right) Immunohistochemistry for CD3 is useful for recognition of T cells. The same cluster of villi shows only rare T lymphocytes stained with CD3. High-power examination is required to discern whether or not they are in the stroma (villitis) or circulating in the fetal blood in capillaries.

Parvovirus B19-Infected Erythroblasts

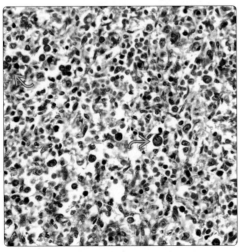

Immunohistochemistry for Parvovirus

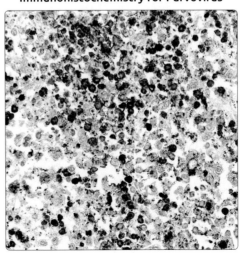

(Left) The fetal spleen shows increased extramedullary hematopoiesis. Nuclear clearing ➾ in some of the precursors suggests parvovirus infection. (Right) On this immunohistochemical stain for parvovirus in the spleen, the majority of erythroid precursor cells are clearly positive.

Nonimmune Fetal Hydrops

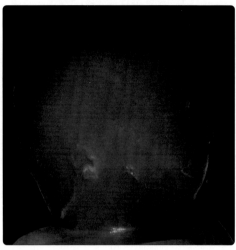

Nonimmune Fetal Hydrops

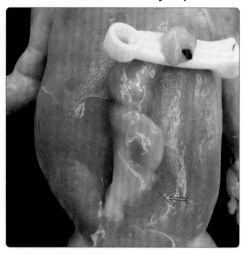

(Left) *Previable fetus with hydrops secondary to parvovirus infection is shown.* (Right) *Pale hydropic stillborn with subcutaneous edema and a thick, edematous umbilical cord with focal cystic* 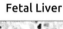 *degeneration of umbilical cord Wharton substanceis shown.*

Fetal Liver

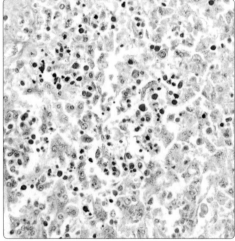

Hemosiderin in Fetal Liver

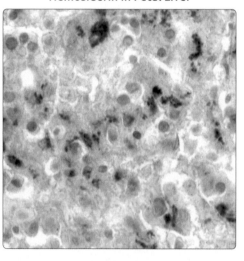

(Left) *Despite the moderate maceration of this fetal liver, parvovirus can be suspected due to the numerous intranuclear inclusions in erythroid precursors and abundant iron deposition.* (Right) *Iron staining confirms the abundant hemosiderin deposition associated with the increased red blood cell turnover with parvovirus.*

Neonatal Giant Cell Hepatitis in Parvovirus

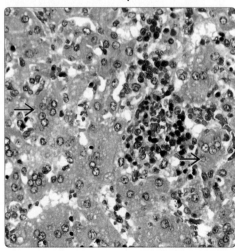

Late Effects of Congenital Parvovirus Infection

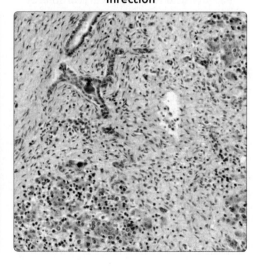

(Left) *A rare finding with congenital parvovirus is giant cell transformation of hepatocytes* 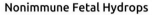. (Right) *This stain of the liver shows the unusual finding of cholestasis and fibrosis in a parvovirus-infected baby who survived for a short time after delivery. Hepatic fibrosis is also associated with myeloid proliferations of Down syndrome, an important differential diagnosis.*

Severely Macerated Liver

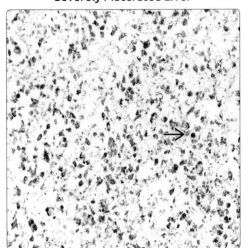

Iron Staining in Severely Macerated Liver

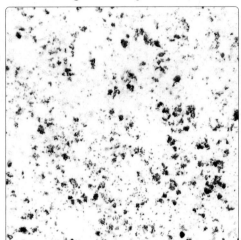

(Left) In this severely macerated fetal liver, cytologic detail is very poorly preserved. Pigment is present, which could represent either iron or formalin pigment. A rare intact cell shows a possible viral inclusion ➡️. (Right) The same fetal liver shows diffuse positive iron staining.

Severely Macerated Liver

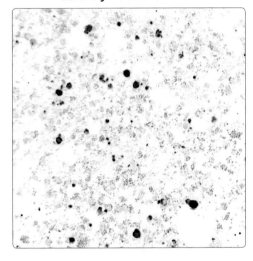

Fetal Heart in Parvovirus

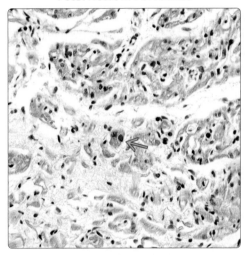

(Left) The same fetal liver is positive with immunohistochemistry for parvovirus. The diagnosis can be made even in the setting of severe tissue maceration. (Right) This section of the fetal heart shows frequent enlarged nuclei, including some that appear to contain viral inclusions. Cardiac myocytes do express P antigen required for parvovirus infection; however, whether the parvovirus inclusions in the myocardium are in myocytes or capillaries is difficult to prove ➡️.

Fetal Bone Marrow in Parvovirus

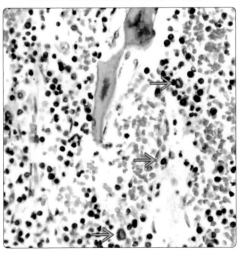

Fetal Adrenal Gland

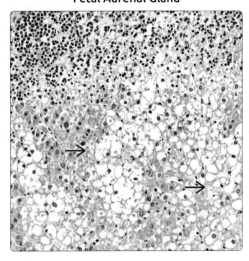

(Left) The 2nd-trimester bone marrow is often hypocellular, as hematopoiesis is still transitioning from the liver to bone marrow. This stain shows a predominance of erythroid precursors with intranuclear parvovirus inclusions ➡️. (Right) This adrenal gland shows massive accumulation of lipid in the fetal cortex ➡️. This feature of in utero hypoxic stress was noted in all cases of parvovirus that were examined. It likely reflects hypoxia due to the severe fetal anemia.

Herpes Simplex Virus

ETIOLOGY/PATHOGENESIS

- Herpes simplex virus (HSV) common, but vertical transmission is rare, may be in utero, peripartum, or after birth
- Majority of women who transmit virus to infant are asymptomatic

CLINICAL ISSUES

- 3 forms of neonatal HSV present after 1 week of age: Disseminated, CNS limited, mucocutaneous
- "In utero" transmission rare, diagnosed within 48 hours of life with microcephaly, eye defects, and rash
- Recognition of HSV on placental exam should prompt immediate communication to pediatrician
- Prompt antiviral treatment required to save organ function and life

MICROSCOPIC

- Ascending HSV infection
  - Zone of necrotic cells with viral cytopathic effects in cord stroma, connective tissue of amnion, and chorionic plate
  - Chronic maternal and fetal inflammatory responses ± plasma cells
  - Amnion may be necrotic and show viable or nonviable multinucleate cells
- Chronic villitis rare with HSV, may see necrosis of villous stromal cells, lymphoplasmacytic villitis with in utero transmission

DIAGNOSTIC CHECKLIST

- Rule out HSV whenever following are seen in placenta
  - Zones of individual necrotic cells in cord stroma, membranes, and chorionic plate
  - Plasma cell funisitis or fetal chronic inflammatory response without eosinophils
  - Lymphoplasmacytic chorioamnionitis with necrotic amnion ± multinucleation

Zone of Necrosis in Ascending HSV Infection

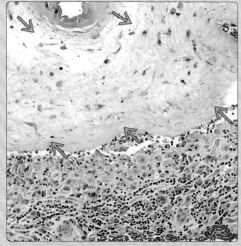

HSV Infection of Villous Stromal Cells

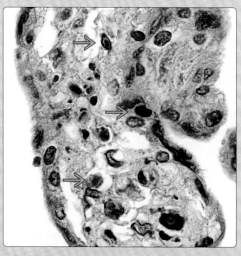

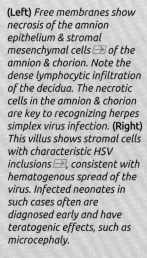

(Left) Free membranes show necrosis of the amnion epithelium & stromal mesenchymal cells ⊟ of the amnion & chorion. Note the dense lymphocytic infiltration of the decidua. The necrotic cells in the amnion & chorion are key to recognizing herpes simplex virus infection. (Right) This villus shows stromal cells with characteristic HSV inclusions ⊡, consistent with hematogenous spread of the virus. Infected neonates in such cases often are diagnosed early and have teratogenic effects, such as microcephaly.

Chronic Fetal Inflammatory Response in HSV

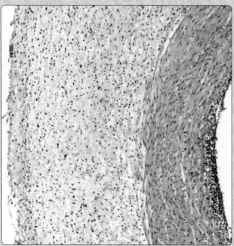

Viral Cytopathic Effects in Cord Stroma

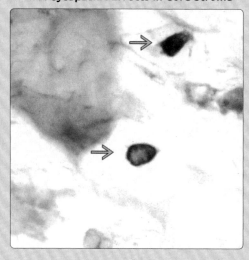

(Left) Lymphocytic and plasmacytic fetal inflammatory responses in the cord are important clues to HSV in what may otherwise appear to be a routine case of chorioamnionitis. The cord stroma shows a zone of necrosis with individually necrotic cells and stromal cells with viral cytopathic effects. (Right) The Cowdry type B intranuclear inclusion ⊡ causes a ground-glass appearance and thickening of the nuclear membrane.

TERMINOLOGY

Abbreviations

- Herpes simplex virus (HSV)
- Skin, eyes, mouth (SEM): Mucocutaneous type of neonatal HSV infection

Types

- HSV type 1 (HSV1)
- Herpes simplex virus type 2 (HSV2)

ETIOLOGY/PATHOGENESIS

Infectious Agents

- HSV1 and HSV2
  - HSV is double-stranded DNA, enveloped virus

Mechanism of Vertical Transmission

- Ascending infection from asymptomatic cervical shedding
  - Most reported cases of placental pathology depict involvement of cord, membranes, and chorionic plate
- Potential hematogenous spread from maternal viremia
  - Rare reported chronic villitis with viral cytopathic effects in villous stroma, could be secondary to fetal viremia
  - Syncytiotrophoblast is barrier to HSV entry
- During parturition with exposure to cervicovaginal lesions, most common mechanism
- After birth exposed to virus from close contacts

Placental Cells Susceptible to Herpes Simplex Virus Infection

- HSV entry mediators not expressed on syncytiotrophoblast
- Villous stromal cells, endothelium, and mast cells are permissive to infection
- Cord, membrane, and chorionic plate mesenchymal stromal cells permissive to infection

Timing of Vertical Transmission

- Data based upon clinical presentation, not from comprehensive placental exam
- 5% in utero
  - HSV very rare in stillbirth, < 1% virus-associated intrauterine fetal demise/stillbirth
- 85% peripartum
- 10% postnatal
  - Postnatal exposure to herpetic lesions, often from family members
  - Direct orogenital suction of bleeding penile wound at time of circumcision (Orthodox Jewish practice) associated with neonatal infection

CLINICAL ISSUES

Epidemiology

- HSV most common sexually transmitted infection in women worldwide
  - 20-30% of pregnant women HSV2 seropositive
  - 10% of seronegative pregnant women have seropositive partner
    - 3.7% of HSV1- and HSV2-seronegative pregnant women will seroconvert if partner is seropositive
    - 1.7% of HSV1-positive pregnant women will seroconvert to HSV2 positive during pregnancy if partner is seropositive
  - HSV1 now causes most genital lesions in USA
- Incidence of neonatal HSV is 5-33 per 100,000 live births in USA, 10 per 100,000 live births globally
- Risk factors for neonatal transmission
  - Type of maternal infection
    - 57% with 1st-episode primary infection (HSV1 and HSV2 seronegative)
    - 25% with 1st-episode nonprimary infection (e.g., seropositive for HSV1, acquire HSV2)
      - Majority of women who transmit virus to infant are asymptomatic
    - 2% with recurrent genital infection
  - Mode of delivery (vaginal delivery > C-section)
  - Prolonged rupture of membranes
  - Disruption of cutaneous barrier (i.e., fetal scalp electrodes, instrumentation)
  - HSV serotype (HSV1 > HSV2)

Presentation

- "In utero" vertical transmission
  - Based upon neonatal diagnosis within 48 hours of life, not necessarily placental involvement
  - Classic triad: Skin vesicles or scarring, eye lesions (microphthalmia, retinal dysplasia), and neurologic damage (intracranial calcifications, microcephaly, hydrencephaly)
- Neonatal HSV-mucocutaneous infection (SEM)
  - 45% of neonatal HSV in era of antiviral therapy
  - Infection confined to skin, eye, &/or mouth with no involvement of CNS or viscera
    - 80% have rash
      - Clustered vesicles with erythematous base, bullae, pustules, erythematous macular exanthem
    - Keratoconjunctivitis, can progress to chorioretinitis
    - Only 10% have mouth lesions
  - Presents at 10-12 days of life
- Neonatal HSV: CNS disease form
  - ~ 35% of neonatal HSV
  - Present as encephalitis
    - Focal/generalized seizures, lethargy, irritability, poor feeding, temperature instability, bulging fontanel
  - 60-70% will have rash at some point during illness
  - Presents later at 16-19 days of life
- Neonatal HSV: Disseminated infection
  - Most common clinical presentation with reported cases of placental involvement
  - ~ 25 % of neonatal HSV in era of antiviral therapy
  - Multisystem involvement, present with respiratory and hepatic failure, disseminated intravascular coagulation (DIC)
    - CNS, lungs, liver, adrenal, skin, eye, &/or mouth involved
    - 66% have encephalitis (hepatic encephalitis due to liver failure)
    - 40% never develop rash
  - Presents at 10-12 days of life

Treatment

- Drugs
  - Acyclovir suppressive therapy after 36 weeks recommended for women with known genital HSV
  - Treatment for neonatal HSV is parenteral acyclovir, sometimes followed by oral acyclovir

Prognosis

- Disseminated disease
  - 29% mortality in 1st year of life when treated with higher dose acyclovir, 85% before era of antiviral therapy
    - DIC, prematurity, pneumonitis associated with increased mortality
    - Seizures associated with increased long-term neurodevelopmental morbidity
- Encephalitic form of disease
  - 15% mortality in 1st year of life with higher dose acyclovir, 50% before era of antiviral therapy
  - ~ 64% of survivors have long-term neurodevelopmental sequelae, especially if seizures prior to therapy
- SEM disease
  - 0% mortality and no developmental disabilities at 1 year if treated with higher dose acyclovir
  - Risk for multiple skin recurrences, can progress to CNS or disseminated disease if not treated
- HSV2 has worse prognosis

MACROSCOPIC

General Features

- Cord may show necrotizing funisitis in cases of ascending infection
- Placenta may be normal in cases of transmission at or after birth

MICROSCOPIC

Histologic Features

- Placenta may be normal in cases with HSV transmission at or after delivery
- Ascending HSV infection
  - Cord
    - Zone of necrotic cells and debris in stroma
    - Viral cytopathic effects in amnion and stromal cells
    - Inflammation ranges from mild lymphocytic and neutrophilic infiltrates to numerous plasma cells
  - Membranes
    - Necrosis and viral cytopathic effects in amnion
    - Lymphocytic chorioamnionitis
  - Chorionic plate
    - Zone of necrosis and viral cytopathic effects in amnion and chorionic plate stroma
    - Chronic inflammatory cells in fetal vasculitis
- Hematogenous transplacental infection
  - Necrotizing lymphoplasmacytic villitis
  - Chronic inflammation around fetal vessels, variably rich in plasma cells
  - HSV inclusions in stromal cells, individually necrotic cells

Cytologic Features

- HSV cytopathic effects

- Multinucleated giant cells, nuclear molding, ground-glass chromatin with thickened nuclear membrane
- Cowdry type B inclusions
  - Intranuclear eosinophilic inclusion that pushes chromatin to nuclear membrane without halo
  - Smudged nuclei
  - Usually found in early or primary infections
- Cowdry type A inclusions
  - Large eosinophilic intranuclear inclusion surrounded by halo "owl eye"
  - Usually found in recurrent or older lesions

ANCILLARY TESTS

Immunohistochemistry

- Immunohistochemical confirmation of HSV useful
  - Be wary of nonspecific reactivity in decidual glands with Arias-Stella effect

DIFFERENTIAL DIAGNOSIS

Other Infectious Villitides

- Other herpesviruses have similar intranuclear inclusions and cause tissue necrosis
  - Cytomegalovirus, varicella-zoster virus, adenovirus

Ascending Amniotic Fluid Infection

- See chronic inflammatory cells in maternal and fetal responses with ascending HSV infection
- Zone of necrosis in cord, amnion, and chorion with viral cytopathic effects in HSV

Congenital Syphilis

- Also demonstrates necrotizing funisitis with plasma cells, lacks individually necrotic cells with viral cytopathic effects
- May show similar villitis but lacks individually necrotic cells
- Lacks zone of necrosis in membranes and chorionic plate

DIAGNOSTIC CHECKLIST

Pathologic Interpretation Pearls

- Rule out HSV whenever following are seen
  - Zone of individually necrotic cells in cord stroma, membranes, and chorionic plate
  - Plasma cell funisitis or fetal chronic inflammatory response without eosinophils
  - Lymphoplasmacytic chorioamnionitis with necrotic amnion ± multinucleation

SELECTED REFERENCES

1. Pinninti SG et al: Neonatal herpes simplex virus infections. Semin Perinatol. ePub, 2018
2. Looker KJ et al: First estimates of the global and regional incidence of neonatal herpes infection. Lancet Glob Health. 5(3):e300-e309, 2017
3. Edwards MS et al: Ascending in utero herpes simplex virus infection in an initially healthy-appearing premature infant. Pediatr Dev Pathol. 18(2):155-8, 2015
4. Finger-Jardim F et al: Herpes simplex virus: prevalence in placental tissue and incidence in neonatal cord blood samples. J Med Virol. 86(3):519-24, 2014
5. Avanzi S et al: Susceptibility of human placenta derived mesenchymal stromal/stem cells to human herpesviruses infection. PLoS One. 8(8):e71412, 2013
6. Chatterjee A et al: Severe intrauterine herpes simplex disease with placentitis in a newborn of a mother with recurrent genital infection at delivery. J Perinatol. 21(8):559-64, 2001

HSV Villitis

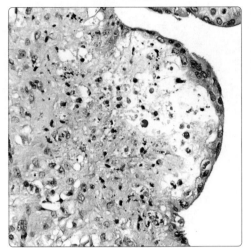

HSV Villitis

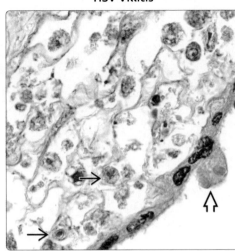

(Left) Transplacental infection may show active necrotizing villitis, usually lymphoplasmacytic. The inflammation may be subtle, but necrotic cells are abundant. (Right) Villitis with numerous necrotic Hofbauer cells ⊟ and syncytiotrophoblast ⊡ with possible inclusions are consistent with hematogenous transplacental HSV infection.

Chronic Chorioamnionitis

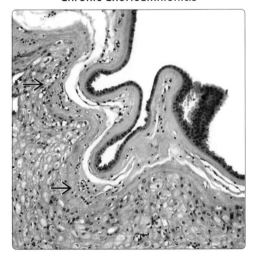

Ascending HSV-Chorionic Plate

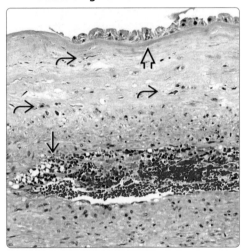

(Left) Chronic chorioamnionitis ⊟ is a common finding, and ascending HSV infection is rare. The differential diagnosis should be kept in mind with attention to foci of cell necrosis and viral cytopathic effects. (Right) This stain shows a chronic, amniotropic, fetal inflammatory response ⊟ in a chorionic plate vessel, viral cytopathic effects in the amnion epithelium ⊡, and a zone of necrosis with individually necrotic cells in the stroma ⊟ of the amnion and chorionic plate.

Ascending HSV

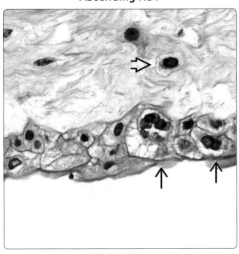

Ascending HSV

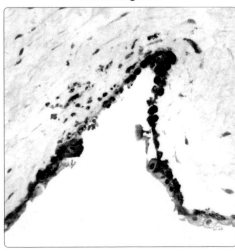

(Left) The amniotic surface epithelium of the umbilical cord shows multinucleated cells ⊟, and stromal cells with intranuclear inclusions ⊡ are seen in Wharton substance. (Right) An immunostain for HSV shows extensive infection of amniocytes on the surface of the umbilical cord as well as subamniotic stromal cells.

Neonatal HSV Pneumonitis

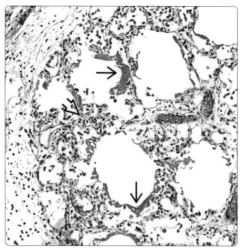

Neonatal HSV Pneumonitis

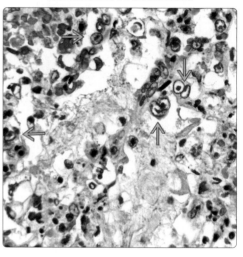

(Left) *H&E of lung shows diffuse alveolar damage with hyaline membranes ➡ and chronic pneumonitis ➡ from ascending HSV.* **(Right)** *High-power examination shows intraalveolar fibrin, chronic inflammation, hyaline membranes, and numerous HSV inclusions ➡ in alveolar epithelial cells.*

Adrenal Pathology in Neonatal HSV

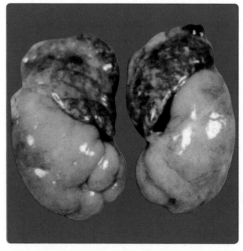

Adrenal Pathology in Neonatal HSV

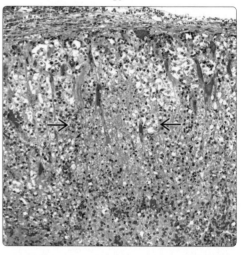

(Left) *In utero transmission neonatal HSV and disseminated neonatal HSV may cause adrenal necrosis. Multiple pinpoint areas of necrosis and calcification within the adrenal cortex are seen.* **(Right)** *Histologic section of the adrenal cortex shows focal necrosis ➡ that contains abundant virus on immunohistochemistry.*

Skin Findings in Neonatal HSV

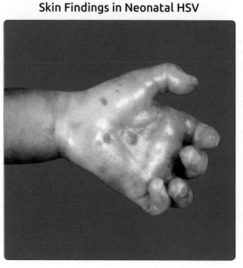

In Utero HSV With Cerebral Necrosis

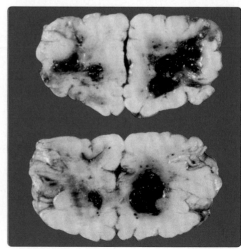

(Left) *Congenital disseminated HSV is shown with skin lesions present at birth. The eroded erythematous macules contain numerous organisms, which would be highly infectious.* **(Right)** *Transplacental HSV infection results in marked necrosis of the brain, which is not the typical temporal lobe involvement seen in older children and adults.*

Liver in Neonatal HSV

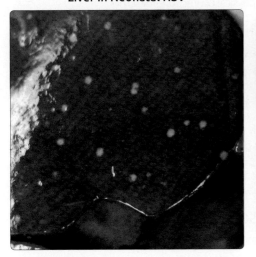

Liver in Disseminated Neonatal HSV

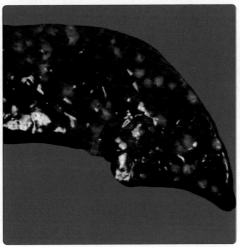

(Left) *This liver has multiple yellow-white, slightly depressed necrotic lesions, the classic appearance of hepatic involvement with disseminated neonatal HSV.* (Right) *Cut surface of the liver demonstrates multifocal necrosis. The central yellow-white areas of necrosis are surrounded by hyperemia.*

Liver in Disseminated Neonatal HSV

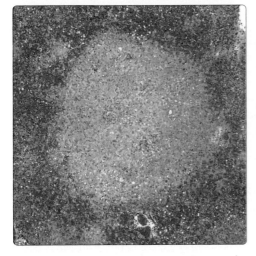

Liver in Disseminated Neonatal HSV

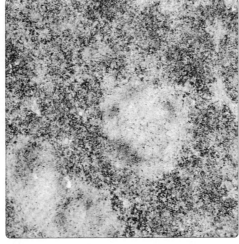

(Left) *Disseminated neonatal HSV shows an area of coagulative necrosis with acute hemorrhage at the interface.* (Right) *Immunohistochemistry for HSV is diffusely positive in the residual hepatic parenchyma but negative in the central area of necrosis.*

HSV Intranuclear Inclusions

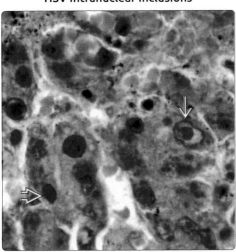

HSV Immunoreactivity

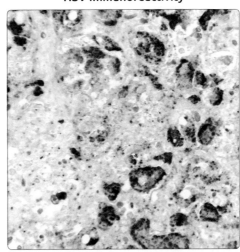

(Left) *These hepatocytes demonstrate both Cowdry type A ➡ and Cowdry type B ⮞ intranuclear inclusions of HSV.* (Right) *Immunohistochemistry for HSV may be positive within nuclei of the hepatocytes. Necrosis often results in leaky nuclear membranes, resulting in diffuse positivity in the cytoplasm of the hepatocytes.*

TERMINOLOGY

Abbreviations

- Human herpesvirus (HHV)
  - Varicella-zoster virus (VZV)
  - Epstein-Barr virus (EBV)
  - HHV types 6-8 (HHV-6, HHV-7, HHV-8)
- Human papillomavirus (HPV)
- HIV type 1 (HIV-1)

Definitions

- Vertical transmission: Transmission of virus from mother to fetus
- Villitis: Inflammation of chorionic villi may be lymphocytic ± plasma cells and histiocytes, granulomatous, or, rarely, neutrophilic
  - Inflammatory cells are predominately maternal T lymphocytes invading villous stroma
- Fetal inflammatory response: Usually acute and rarely chronic inflammation emanating from fetal vessels of chorionic plate or umbilical cord
  - Usually neutrophils
    - Lymphocytes, histiocytes, or plasma cells more common in viral infections

ROUTES OF VERTICAL TRANSMISSION

Intrauterine, Transplacental, or Ascending

- Virus must traverse several barriers to infect fetus from maternal viremia
  - Trophoblast, villous stroma, capillaries
- Trophoblast cells are highly resistant to viral infection
  - Attenuate viral replication by induction of autophagy
- Viruses may infect placenta from implantation site endometrium
- Virus present within vagina or cervix may ascend to infect amniotic fluid

Intrapartum

- Via exposure to infected blood or secretions during delivery

Postnatal

- Through physical contact or breast milk

CLINICAL IMPLICATIONS

Clinical Presentation

- Intrauterine viral infection may result in spontaneous abortion, stillbirth, prematurity, growth restriction, and malformations
  - Direct cell injury may result in tissue necrosis and is possibly responsible for congenital malformations
  - Infants often have persistent infection after birth and prolonged viral shedding
  - Infection of placenta may or may not be associated with fetal infection

MACROSCOPIC

General Features

- Villitis is rarely gross diagnosis
  - Placenta may have pale, granular or coarse appearance
  - Small, yellow-white areas of agglutinated villi or regions of villous atrophy may be present
  - Thickened layer of fibrinoid is frequently noted at maternal surface associated with villitis
- Hydrops may be present with pale, spongy, thickened placental parenchyma
  - Usually associated with fetal viral infection and anemia
- Rare infections associated with massive perivillous fibrin deposition (MPVFD)
  - Extensive replacement of parenchyma by firm, tan-white fibrin surrounding smaller foci of preserved villous texture

MICROSCOPIC

Histologic Features

- Normal placenta
- Nonspecific lymphohistiocytic villitis; similar if not identical to histology of villitis of undetermined etiology (VUE)

Varicella-Zoster Virus Placentitis

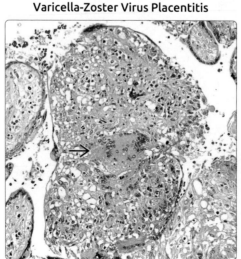

Lymphoplasmacytic Deciduitis

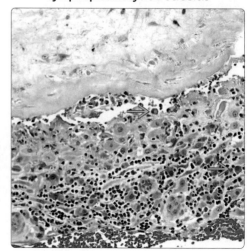

(Left) Granulomatous villitis with lymphocytes and Langhans-type multinucleated giant cells ⇨ is seen in this case of congenital varicella-zoster virus (VZV) infection occurring in the 1st trimester. (Right) A significant lymphocytic or lymphoplasmacytic deciduitis may be seen in women with viral syndrome. The membranous chorion and decidua are intensely inflamed with plasma cells ⇨ in this case of ascending herpes simplex virus.

- Villous enlargement with Hofbauer cell hyperplasia resembling villous immaturity
- Lymphoplasmacytic choriodeciduitis
- MPVFD with mixed acute and chronic intervillositis

HERPESVIRUSES

Varicella-Zoster Virus

- Etiology
  - Infection during pregnancy has incidence of 0.8-7.0 per 10,000 deliveries
  - Infection is most common in children < 14 years of age; most women of childbearing age are immune
  - Herpes zoster virus (shingles) is infectious to individuals who are not immune
- Clinical presentation
  - Congenital varicella syndrome: Seen in 1-12% of infections in 1st and 2nd trimesters
    - Stillbirth
    - Destructive skin lesions (cicatricial scars) in dermatomal distribution, associated with limb reduction and segmental dysfunction of somatic &/or autonomic nervous system
    - Microphthalmia, optic atrophy, chorioretinitis, cataract, nystagmus, anisocoria, Horner syndrome
    - Microcephaly, cortical atrophy, spinal cord atrophy, seizures, developmental delay
    - GI and GU abnormalities reported in 10-20%
  - Neonatal varicella
    - Occurs when maternal infection occurs 5 days before or 2 days after delivery
    - 50-62% of babies infected; most demonstrate giant cell pneumonia
  - VZV pneumonia develops in up to 33% of infected pregnant women
- Prognosis
  - Infection early in gestation results in spontaneous abortion in 7.5% of cases
  - Congenital varicella syndrome has 30% neonatal mortality rate
  - Neonatal varicella is associated with giant cell pneumonia and 23-30% neonatal mortality rate
  - Herpes zoster occurs during first 2 years of life in 20% of exposed neonates
  - Maternal VZV pneumonia has up to 45% mortality rate
- Histologic features
  - Granulomatous villitis with extensive necrosis and eosinophilic intranuclear inclusions
  - Multinucleated giant cells (histiocytic)
  - Infection occurring later in gestation may have nonspecific chronic villitis

Human Herpesvirus-6

- Agent of roseola infantum (exanthem subitum)
- Etiology
  - Most children are infected by 2-3 years of age
  - Congenital infection may occur
    - Virus has been found in cervical secretions and placenta
    - Maternal HIV coinfection leads to increased rate of vertical transmission

- Clinical presentation
  - Fever
- Prognosis
  - Acute infection is associated with severe CNS complications

Human Herpesvirus-7

- Etiology
  - Most children are infected by 7-10 years of age
  - Congenital infection may occur
    - Virus has been found in cervical secretions and placenta
    - Associated with early and late fetal loss

Human Herpesvirus-8 (Kaposi Sarcoma Virus)

- Etiology
  - Vertical transmission in 1 per 2,000-5,000 births
  - Present in saliva and breast milk
- Prognosis
  - Postnatal course after congenital infection is not known

Epstein-Barr Virus

- Etiology
  - Transplacental vertical transmission is extremely rare and may occur during either primary infection or reactivation
- Clinical presentation
  - Possibly associated with congenital cataracts
- Histologic features
  - Lymphoplasmacytic villitis and necrotizing deciduitis noted after 1st-trimester infection
  - Reactive lymphs in maternal circulation of intervillous space, EBV(+)
  - EBV latent genes expressed in decidual glands with Arias-Stella effect but not in nonpregnant endometrium

ENTEROVIRUSES

Clinical Presentation

- Most infections are acquired after birth and are associated with myocarditis and meningitis
- Seasonal infection: Summer and fall
- No evidence that enteroviruses are associated with cerebral palsy

Prognosis

- 25% have mild disease lasting 1-5 days with fever, rash, pneumonitis, GI symptoms
- 75% have severe disseminated disease with fever, coryza, poor feeding, diarrhea, meningitis, myocarditis, and hepatitis
  - 1% mortality
    - Highest for coxsackievirus B
    - Intermediate for echovirus
    - Lowest for coxsackievirus A

Histologic Features

- Possibly associated with chronic vasculitis of stem vessels, but this is also feature of cases attributed to VUE

Coxsackievirus

- Etiology
  - Rare congenital cases have been reported
- Clinical presentation

- ○ Rare cause of malformations, early fetal loss, hydrops, myocarditis, and ventriculitis with poor prognosis
- ○ Coxsackie A virus infections associated with in utero fetal demise and placental involvement
  - – Syncytiotrophoblast injury and necrosis
  - – MPVFD
  - – Intervillous acute and chronic inflammation
  - – Unlike cases of MPVFD with chronic histiocytic intervillositis commonly associated with intrauterine growth restriction (IUGR), placentas and affected fetuses from coxsackievirus-associated MPVFD were appropriate for gestational age weight

Echovirus

- Etiology
  - ○ Congenital infection has been reported
- Clinical presentation
  - ○ Associated with massive neonatal hepatic hemorrhage and necrosis

Enterovirus

- Etiology
  - ○ Most cases are acquired postnatally

HUMAN PAPILLOMAVIRUS

Etiology

- Most infants are infected at birth by contact with cervical or perineal lesions
  - ○ Transmission to infant may only be transitory
  - ○ Viral DNA has been recovered from placenta
- Rarely occurs with C-section
- Rarely identified in amniotic fluid

Clinical Presentation

- Respiratory papillomatosis of larynx, trachea, bronchi, and lungs is due to HPV-6 and HPV-11
  - ○ Incidence of respiratory papillomatosis: 0.6-4.3 per 100,000
- 25% present before 1 year of age

Prognosis

- Recurrent respiratory papillomatosis and juvenile-onset respiratory papillomatosis
- 2-3% progress to invasive papillomatosis or, rarely, to squamous cell carcinoma

Histologic Features

- No specific placental lesions have been described

INFLUENZA

Clinical Presentation

- Severe maternal illness is associated with poor fetal outcome, especially noted with H1N1 pandemic

Prognosis

- Infants are more likely to have IUGR and be preterm
  - ○ 0.5% fetal mortality most likely related to prematurity and severity of maternal illness
- Vaccination is safe during 2nd and 3rd trimesters of pregnancy and associated with better fetal outcome

Histologic Features

- Influenza A and B associated with injury of trophoblasts, amnion, decidua, and vascular endothelium
- Lymphocytes with eosinophilic cytoplasmic inclusions have been reported

Influenza A (H1N1)

- Etiology
  - ○ Unclear if congenital infection occurs
  - ○ Maternal fever with influenza associated with congenital anomalies, especially neural tube defects
- Prognosis
  - ○ H1N1 pandemic is associated with severe illness in pregnant women and 8% mortality
  - ○ Gestational influenza is associated with development of schizophrenia and bipolar disease in offspring

HIV

Etiology

- In utero vertical transmission occurs in 7% of untreated infected pregnant women
  - ○ CD4(+) endothelium, Hofbauer cells, and trophoblasts are permissive to infection
  - ○ Increased incidence of spontaneous abortion
- Most infections are acquired at time of delivery by exposure to maternal blood
  - ○ Transplacental transmission in utero is rare
- CMV viremia associated with increased rates of in utero HIV transmission

Clinical Presentation

- HIV-1
  - ○ Infected infants are rarely symptomatic at birth
    - – Transmission is noted with high viral load, low CD4, and lack of antiretroviral therapy
  - ○ Increased incidence of chorioamnionitis in HIV-infected women
    - – Transmission is associated with chorioamnionitis in some but not all studies
  - ○ Increased reactivation of CMV during pregnancy
    - – CMV viremia associated with increased risk of transmission
  - ○ Increased frequency of tuberculosis
  - ○ Increased rates of hepatitis C virus vertical transmission in HIV-infected women

Prognosis

- Long-term survival with antiretroviral therapy
  - ○ Zidovudine chemoprophylaxis has reduced vertical transmission from 15-39% to < 2%

Histologic Features

- No characteristic features of HIV infection or indication of which babies will be infected
- Identification of HIV within placental tissues is not always associated with fetal infection
  - ○ Hofbauer cells may sequester virus from fetal lymphocytes
- Placentas have been reported to be both smaller and larger than expected
- Increased incidence of chorioamnionitis

- Reported associated features are numerous, but none are specific
  o Proliferation of villous cytotrophoblasts, increased syncytial knots, fibrinoid changes, villous edema/immaturity, stromal fibrosis, increased calcifications

HEPATITIS

Clinical Presentation

- Associated with neonatal liver disease for some subtypes

Hepatitis A

- Etiology
  o Intrauterine transmission in 5-15% of infected pregnant women, but infection is not clinically significant

Hepatitis B

- Etiology
  o Intrauterine transmission in 5% of infected pregnant women
    - Most transmission occurs at delivery with exposure to maternal blood
    - Immunoglobulin at birth is protective for 90% of cases
- Prognosis
  o Chronic hepatitis B virus (HBV) infection leads to cirrhosis, hepatocellular carcinoma
- Histologic features
  o Increased bilirubin pigment within villous Hofbauer cells and macrophages in membranes
  o Carrier status is associated with positive immunohistochemistry staining for HBV antigen within maternal serum

Hepatitis C

- Etiology
  o Intrauterine or intrapartum transmission in 2-12% and increases to 15-25% with maternal HIV coinfection
- Prognosis
  o Neonates may have mild elevation of transaminases
  o Risk of cirrhosis, hepatocellular carcinoma later in childhood

RUBELLA

Etiology

- Risk for vertical transmission with maternal primary infection varies throughout gestation
  o 1st-trimester primary infection has 80-90% rate of vertical transmission
    - Increased fetal loss
  o 2nd-trimester primary infection has 25-30% rate of vertical transmission
  o 3rd-trimester primary infection has 60% rate of vertical transmission
  o Primary infection during final weeks of pregnancy has nearly 100% rate of vertical transmission
- Vaccination during pregnancy is associated with rare cases of subclinical fetal infection
- Most cases currently occur in women from outside USA
  o Highest number of cases reported in Southeast Asia

Clinical Presentation

- Congenital rubella syndrome occurs after maternal infection at < 16-weeks gestation
  o IUGR
  o Microcephaly, meningoencephalitis, developmental delay
  o Cataracts, glaucoma, pigmentary retinopathy
  o Hearing loss
  o Purpura, jaundice
  o Hepatosplenomegaly
  o Radiolucent bone disease
  o Congenital heart disease
    - Patent ductus arteriosus
    - Peripheral pulmonary artery stenosis
- Childhood or adult infection
  o Mild infection with tender occipital or postauricular lymphadenopathy
  o Nonspecific rash beginning on face and neck; small, irregular, pink maculopapules
  o Mild pharyngeal injection and small red spots (Forchheimer spots) on soft palate
  o Adults may have
    - Low-grade fever
    - Headache
    - Malaise
    - Coryza and conjunctivitis
    - Arthralgia or arthritis

Prognosis

- Teratogenic with disturbed organogenesis
- 85% of fetuses with 1st-trimester infection have sequelae, particularly deafness
- 35% mortality during 1st year of life

Histologic Features

- Damage to trophoblasts and endothelium, Hofbauer cell hyperplasia and eosinophilic inclusions, nonspecific villitis

ADENOVIRUS

Etiology

- Virus detected in amniotic fluid is associated with congenital infection and acute neonatal disease

Clinical Presentation

- Possibly associated with abortion and stillbirth
- May cause premature birth
- May cause fetal tachyarrhythmias and myocarditis, nonimmune hydrops
- Neonatal pneumonitis

Prognosis

- Fatalities associated with prematurity and pneumonitis

LYMPHOCYTIC CHORIOMENINGITIS VIRUS

Etiology

- Maternal infection is acquired by exposure to infected mice, hamsters, and gerbils as pets, in wild or in workplace
- Congenital infection may be more common than currently reported

Clinical Presentation

- Congenital infection
  - Microcephaly
  - Hydrocephalus and macrocephaly
  - Abnormal corpus callosum
  - Cerebellar hypoplasia
  - CNS calcifications
  - Chorioretinitis
- Adults and children
  - Nonspecific febrile illness
  - Aseptic meningitis and encephalitis
- Adults
  - Orchitis
  - Parotitis
  - Sudden-onset deafness

Prognosis

- Severe disease in subset of infected neonates with 33% mortality
- Neonatal survivors have severe neurologic sequelae, including cerebral palsy, intellectual disability, seizures, and visual impairment

FLAVIVIRUS

Dengue Virus

- Etiology
  - Mosquito vector
  - Vertical transmission reported
- Clinical presentation
  - Acute febrile illness and hemorrhagic fever due to vascular permeability and abnormal hemostasis
  - Associated with spontaneous abortion, intrauterine fetal death, prematurity, and perinatal infection
- Placenta, choriodeciduitis, villitis, and intervillositis

West Nile Virus

- Etiology
  - Mosquito vector
  - Infection during summer months
- Clinical presentation
  - Causes severe disease in pregnant women
  - Associated with spontaneous abortion
  - < 5% of infants infected
    - Most are asymptomatic
    - Severe disease in subset of infants
      - □ Viral infection of brain through choroid plexus, infection of ependyma and germinal matrix
      - □ Associated with chorioretinitis, encephalitis, periventricular calcifications
      - □ 92% have chorioretinitis
- Placenta, no specific changes described

Zika Virus

- Etiology
  - Aedes mosquito vector
- Clinical presentation
  - Adult: Asymptomatic, fever, rash, arthralgia, conjunctivitis, rare severe neurologic phenotype
  - Fetal infection
    - 6% of babies have birth defects

- 10-15% incidence of fetal demise or stillbirth
- Microcephaly, dilated ventricles, malformations of cortex, and calcifications
- Retinal atrophy
- Placenta
  - Nonspecific changes of villous enlargement with appearance of relative immaturity and Hofbauer cell hyperplasia
  - Zika virus localized to Hofbauer cells with in situ hybridization
  - No significant villitis or viral cytopathic effects seen

DIAGNOSTIC CHECKLIST

Pathologic Interpretation Pearls

- Chronic villitis in 1st and 2nd trimesters should raise concern for viral infection
- Placental infection is not always associated with fetal infection
- With exception of VZV, most of these agents show nonspecific villitis or no changes on placental exam

SELECTED REFERENCES

1. Kim Y et al: Identification of Epstein-Barr virus in the human placenta and its pathologic characteristics. J Korean Med Sci. 32(12):1959-1966, 2017
2. Schwartz DA: Viral infection, proliferation, and hyperplasia of Hofbauer cells and absence of inflammation characterize the placental pathology of fetuses with congenital Zika virus infection. Arch Gynecol Obstet. 295(6):1361-1368, 2017
3. Heller DS et al: Placental massive perivillous fibrinoid deposition associated with coxsackievirus A16-report of a case, and review of the literature. Pediatr Dev Pathol. 19(5):421-423, 2016
4. Johnson EL et al: HIV-1 at the placenta: immune correlates of protection and infection. Curr Opin Infect Dis. 29(3):248-55, 2016
5. Meijer WJ et al: High rate of chronic villitis in placentas of pregnancies complicated by influenza A/H1N1 infection. Infect Dis Obstet Gynecol. 2014:768380, 2014
6. Delorme-Axford E et al: Human placental trophoblasts confer viral resistance to recipient cells. Proc Natl Acad Sci U S A. 110(29):12048-53, 2013
7. Ribeiro CF et al: Perinatal transmission of dengue: a report of 7 cases. J Pediatr. 163(5):1514-6, 2013
8. Park H et al: Rate of vertical transmission of human papillomavirus from mothers to infants: relationship between infection rate and mode of delivery. Virol J. 9:80, 2012
9. Cardenas I et al: Viral infection of the placenta leads to fetal inflammation and sensitization to bacterial products predisposing to preterm labor. J Immunol. 2010 Jul 15;185(2):1248-57. Erratum in: J Immunol. 187(5):2835, 2011
10. Centers for Disease Control and Prevention (CDC): Maternal and infant outcomes among severely ill pregnant and postpartum women with 2009 pandemic influenza A (H1N1)--United States, April 2009-August 2010. MMWR Morb Mortal Wkly Rep. 60(35):1193-6, 2011
11. Mor G et al: Inflammation and pregnancy: the role of the immune system at the implantation site. Ann N Y Acad Sci. 1221:80-7, 2011
12. Al-Husaini AM: Role of placenta in the vertical transmission of human immunodeficiency virus. J Perinatol. 29(5):331-6, 2009
13. Cover J et al: Enterovirus is not present in placentas from cases of perinatal depression using polymerase chain reaction analysis. Pediatr Dev Pathol. 12(3):177-9, 2009
14. Caserta MT et al: Human herpesvirus (HHV)-6 and HHV-7 infections in pregnant women. J Infect Dis. 196(9):1296-303, 2007
15. D'costa GF et al: Pathology of placenta in HIV infection. Indian J Pathol Microbiol. 50(3):515-9, 2007

Chronic Villitis With Increased Fibrinoid

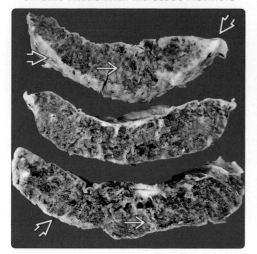

Chronic Villitis

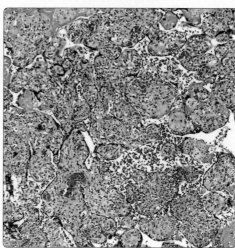

(Left) *Diffuse chronic villitis may be associated with a granular cut surface. There is increased fibrinoid deposition with the parenchyma ➡ and on the maternal surface ⇥ at the basal plate and margin.* **(Right)** *Most viral infections are spread to the placenta during maternal viremia. The villi may have neutrophilic, lymphocytic, histiocytic, granulomatous, or plasmacytic inflammation. This case of villitis of undetermined etiology (VUE) is similar to infectious villitis but is usually only lymphohistiocytic.*

Necrotizing Villitis

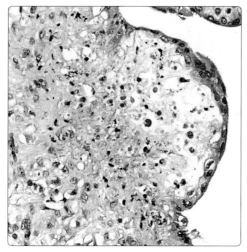

Plasma Cell Villitis

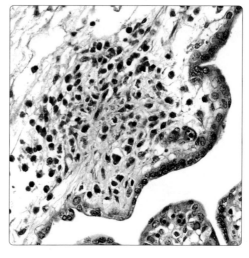

(Left) *Necrotizing villitis is shown here in a case of transplacentally acquired herpes simplex virus.* **(Right)** *Lymphoplasmacytic villitis is characteristic of CMV infection. If no inclusions are identified, an immunohistochemistry stain for CMV or PCR for the virus from formalin-fixed, paraffin-embedded tissue may be useful to confirm the infection.*

Intervillous Reactive Lymphocytes

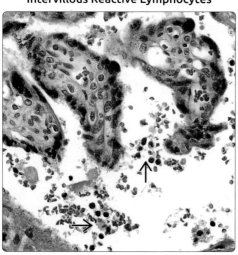

Epstein-Barr Virus

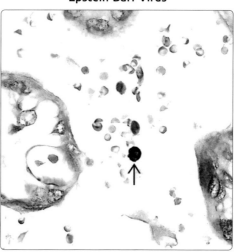

(Left) *The placenta from a case wherein Epstein-Barr virus (EBV) was suspected to have been vertically transmitted to the fetus has an increase in mononuclear cells ➡ within the intervillous maternal blood space.* **(Right)** *This in situ hybridization study for EBV [EBV-encoded RNA1 (EBER)] shows a rare positive lymphocyte ➡ in the maternal intervillous space. Finding EBV in the placenta does not necessarily indicate fetal infection.*

(Left) In this case, VZV infection is the etiology of fetal demise at 17-weeks gestation. The villi have diffuse granulomatous, necrotizing villitis with Langhans-type multinucleated giant cells ➡. (Right) H&E shows VZV infection with eosinophilic inclusions ➡ in Hofbauer cells. Syncytiotrophoblasts ➡ are usually easily distinguished from Langhans-type multinucleated histiocytic giant cells ➡.

Varicella-Zoster Virus Placentitis

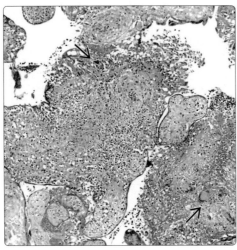

Varicella-Zoster Virus Placentitis

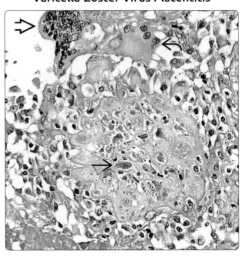

(Left) H&E of a villus shows an infected Hofbauer cell ➡ with a classic eosinophilic intranuclear viral inclusion and peripheral condensed nuclear chromatin. These viral cytopathic effects are common to herpes viruses, including VZV. (Right) Immunohistochemistry for VZV is strongly positive within the necrotic villous stromal cells.

Varicella-Zoster Virus Placentitis

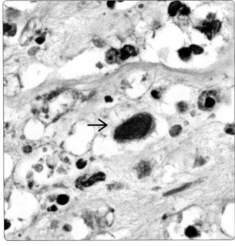

Varicella-Zoster Virus Placentitis

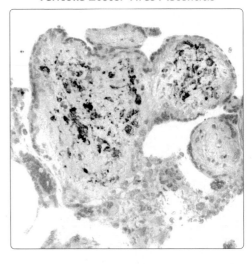

(Left) In this case, VZV infection in the 1st trimester resulted in fetal demise. Even though markedly macerated, the skin shows cellular changes that are suggestive of herpes infection. This same section was strongly positive with immunohistochemistry. (Right) Tzanck preparation from a skin lesion of herpes zoster virus (shingles) has multinucleated viral infected cells indistinguishable from other herpesviruses. The skin lesions of shingles are infectious to those who are not immune.

Varicella-Zoster Virus Infection of Fetal Skin

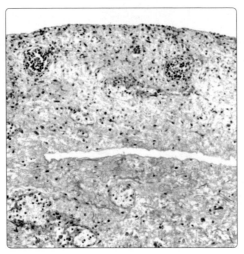

Varicella-Zoster Virus Cytopathic Effects

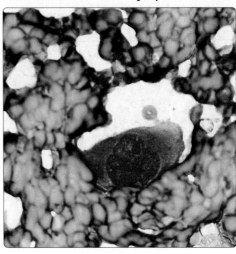

Chronic Villitis

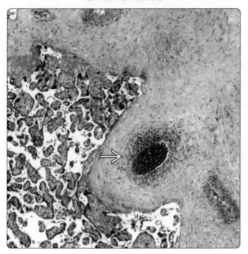

HIV-Infected Hofbauer Cell

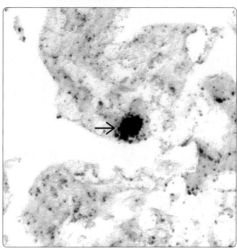

(Left) *This placenta from a case of vertical HIV transmission in utero shows a single focus of chronic vasculitis ➡ noted within a large stem villus. Whether or not this reflects a fetal response to infection or is a nonspecific change of chronic villitis is unclear.* (Right) *This image shows an in situ hybridization study for HIV p24 messenger RNA in the placenta from an HIV-infected mother. A placental Hofbauer cell ➡ is positive. Hofbauer cells are known to sequester HIV.*

CMV Placentitis in HIV Infection

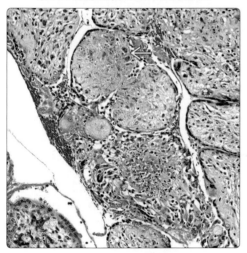

CMV Placentitis in HIV Infection

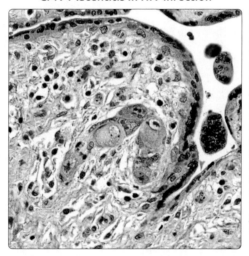

(Left) *Granulomatous and necrotizing villitis is present in this case of reactivation of CMV infection in the presence of HIV coinfection. Multiple eosinophilic cells ➡ suspicious for CMV inclusions are present. There is a strong association between maternal CMV viremia and in utero transmission of HIV from mother to fetus. Villous damage may be a mechanism of transmission.* (Right) *A large number of CMV inclusions are noted in this villus from a patient with coinfection of HIV and CMV.*

Influenza and Chronic Villitis

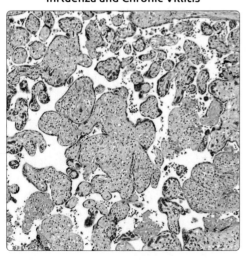

Congenital Zika Virus Infection

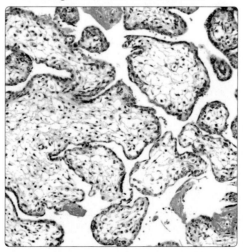

(Left) *This placenta is from a mother with H1N1 infection and shows high-grade chronic villitis. It is not known if the maternal lymphocytes are responding to flu virus in the villi or trophoblastic/fetal antigens (VUE).* (Right) *This 21-weeks-gestation fetus had Zika virus infection and brain abnormalities. The villi appear edematous with frequent Hofbauer cells. Zika can be localized to Hofbauer cells with special studies. Necrosis, villitis, or intervillositis are not features of transplacental Zika infection. (Courtesy D. A. Schwartz, MD.)*

Syphilis

KEY FACTS

ETIOLOGY/PATHOGENESIS

- Most cases result of no or inadequate treatment during pregnancy

CLINICAL ISSUES

- High incidence of intrauterine fetal demise
- Transmission occurs during all trimesters of pregnancy and at all stages of disease

MACROSCOPIC

- Umbilical cord has characteristic barber pole appearance due to chalky white necrotic debris that partially surrounds vessels in amniotropic fashion

MICROSCOPIC

- Severe necrotizing funisitis is seen in 50% of cases
  - More common in intrauterine fetal demise
- Spirochetes present in cases that have not received antibiotics during gestation or labor or in fetuses that are stillborn prior to antibiotic therapy

- Rarely has chronic lymphoplasmacytic villitis
- Villous edema, increased Hofbauer cells
- Proliferative vasculitis of fetal stem vessels useful in diagnosis
- Increased nucleated red blood cells in fetal circulation
- Commonly has increased lymphocytes and plasma cells in decidua
- Organisms are disseminated to nearly all fetal organs
- Inflammatory response occurs in perivascular connective tissue rather than parenchyma

DIAGNOSTIC CHECKLIST

- "Classic" triad
  - Enlarged, immature-appearing, hypercellular villi with numerous Hofbauer cells
  - Thickened villous vessels
  - Perivillitis

Barber Pole Gross Appearance of Umbilical Cord in Syphilis

(Left) The umbilical cord shows a barber pole appearance due to accumulation of calcified necrotic debris around the vessels. (Right) Necrotizing funisitis shows intense amniotropic inflammation ➡ emanating from the fetal vessels. These changes may be focal, often at the placental end, when associated with syphilis.

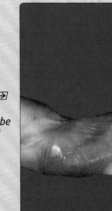

Necrotizing Funisitis

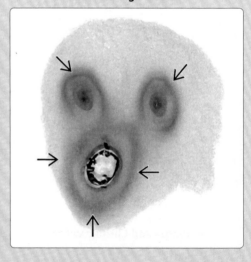

(Left) Prolonged, severe inflammation leads to degeneration of the vessel smooth muscle ➡. The inflammatory cells become necrotic ➡ with stippled calcification in the cord substance. (Right) The villi in syphilis will rarely show chronic lymphoplasmacytic villitis with intervillositis and mixture of necrotic debris and perivillous fibrinoid.

Necrotizing Funisitis With Calcified Debris

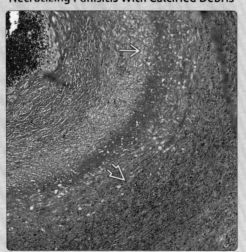

Syphilis With Villitis and Intervillositis

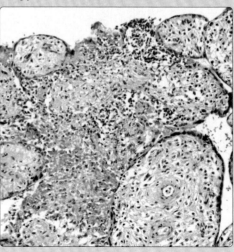

ETIOLOGY/PATHOGENESIS

Infectious Agents

- *Treponema pallidum*

Timing of transmission

- Usually acquired in utero during maternal spirochetemia
- Rarely acquired during delivery through contact with maternal blood or genital lesions

CLINICAL ISSUES

Epidemiology

- Incidence, 10 per 100,000 live births
  - Increasing in USA since 2012
  - Higher incidence in southern USA
  - More common in women < 19 years of age

Presentation

- Transmission usually occurs in untreated or inadequately treated mothers
- Transmission occurs during all trimesters of pregnancy and at all stages of disease
  - May not see significant inflammatory response early in gestation
  - 50% in primary and secondary syphilis
    - 40-80% in early latent syphilis
    - 30% in late syphilis
- 2/3 of infected infants are asymptomatic at birth
  - Early signs include characteristic vesiculobullous or erythematous maculopapular rash on hands and feet
- 30-40% of infected infants are stillborn
- High incidence of prematurity and intrauterine growth restriction

MACROSCOPIC

General Features

- Placenta is thick, friable, and frequently pale
- Umbilical cord has characteristic barber pole appearance due to chalky white necrotic debris that partially surrounds vessels in amniotropic fashion

MICROSCOPIC

Histologic Features

- Umbilical cord
  - Severe necrotizing funisitis is seen in 50% of cases
    - More common in intrauterine fetal demise
  - Degeneration of inflammatory cells (neutrophils, lymphocytes, plasma cells, and macrophages) in Wharton substance
  - Spirochetes present in cases that have not received antibiotics during gestation or labor or in fetuses that are stillborn prior to antibiotic therapy
- Villi
  - Villous edema, increased Hofbauer cells
  - Rarely has chronic lymphoplasmacytic villitis
  - May see focal acute villitis
  - Proliferative vasculitis similar to vascular pathology elsewhere in syphilis
    - Inflammation and thickening of vessel wall with loose perivascular fibrosis
    - Septation of lumen, distinguish from changes of demise
  - Increased nucleated red blood cells in fetal circulation
  - Spirochetes more often seen in fibrin, not sites of active inflammation
- Membranes
  - Rarely associated with acute &/or chronic chorioamnionitis
- Decidua
  - Commonly has increased lymphocytes and plasma cells
- Fetal organs
  - Organisms are disseminated to nearly all organs
  - Inflammatory response occurs in perivascular connective tissue rather than parenchyma
  - Lung, bone, liver, pancreas, small bowel, kidney, and spleen are most severely affected
  - There is diffuse extramedullary hematopoiesis

ANCILLARY TESTS

Histochemistry

- Warthin-Starry stain, often difficult to interpret
  - Organisms found in fibrin, necrotic debris

Immunohistochemistry

- *T. pallidum* antibodies available

DIFFERENTIAL DIAGNOSIS

Other Forms of Villitis and Necrotizing funisitis

- Cytomegalovirus
  - Usually associated with lymphoplasmacytic villitis, rarely with funisitis
- Herpes simplex virus
  - May have plasma cell-rich infiltrates in membranes or umbilical cord, rare villitis
- Villitis of undetermined etiology
  - Usually associated with lymphohistiocytic villitis, no funisitis

DIAGNOSTIC CHECKLIST

Clinically Relevant Pathologic Features

- Necrotizing funisitis
- Classic triad: Enlarged hypercellular villi, thickened fetal vessels, villitis with perivillitis

Pathologic Interpretation Pearls

- All cases of necrotizing funisitis need to be correlated with maternal syphilis serology

SELECTED REFERENCES

1. Cooper JM et al: Congenital syphilis. Semin Perinatol. ePub, 2018
2. Akahira-Azuma M et al: Republication: two premature neonates of congenital syphilis with severe clinical manifestations. Trop Med Health. 43(3):165-70, 2015
3. Sheffield JS et al: Placental histopathology of congenital syphilis. Obstet Gynecol. 100(1):126-33, 2002
4. Genest DR et al: Diagnosis of congenital syphilis from placental examination: comparison of histopathology, Steiner stain, and polymerase chain reaction for Treponema pallidum DNA. Hum Pathol. 27(4):366-72, 1996

Pale Edematous Placenta in Congenital Syphilis

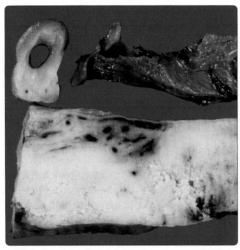

Perivascular White Necrotic Debris in Umbilical Cord Substance

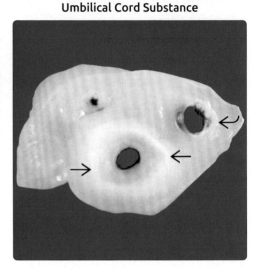

(Left) *The placental disc is often bulky, friable, and very pale due to severe fetal anemia in congenital syphilis. This segment of umbilical cord does not have necrotizing funisitis.* (Right) *This section of the cord shows chalky necrotic debris ⊳ surrounding the umbilical vein and adjacent to an artery ⊡.*

Thrombosed Umbilical Vessel With Necrotizing Funisitis

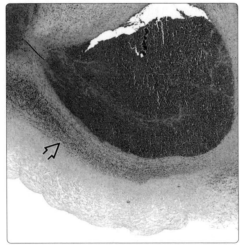

Fetal Normoblastemia

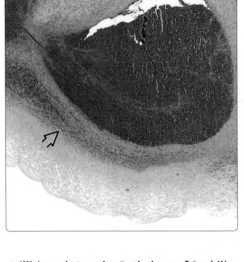

(Left) *The necrotic debris ⊳ is seen outside the vessel wall in Wharton substance. The vessel may thrombose due to the severe inflammation and become devitalized.* (Right) *There may be a marked increase in nucleated red blood cells within the fetal circulation ⊳ in congenital syphilis. This finding is more common in cases with fetal demise.*

Villitis and Vascular Pathology of Syphilis

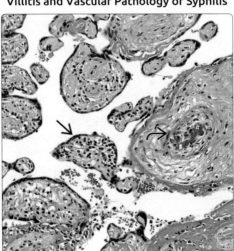

Chronic Villitis With Proliferative Vasculitis

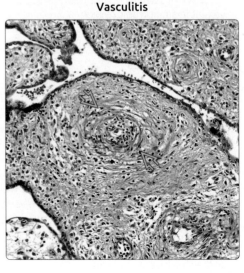

(Left) *Lymphoplasmacytic villitis ⊳ is an uncommon finding in syphilis. Proliferative vasculitis ⊳ is characteristic in congenital syphilis but can be difficult to distinguish from the fibrointimal ingrowth seen after fetal demise. Note pallor of the intimal proliferation and presence of inflammatory cells, a change not seen in the vascular involution of fetal demise.* (Right) *Proliferative vasculitis ⊳ shows thickening and disruption of the vessel wall with an increase in nuclei. Prominent perivascular connective tissue is also termed concentric fibrosis.*

Spirochetes Warthin-Starry

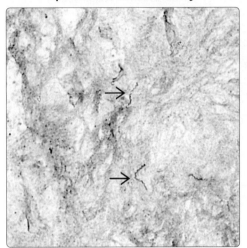

Spirochete Immunohistochemistry

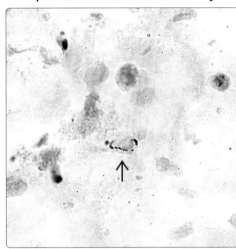

(Left) *Warthin-Starry staining shows several spirochetes ➡ from the umbilical cord of a stillborn. The spirochetes are found within the band of necrotic debris, which makes interpretation of the stain difficult.* (Right) *Immunohistochemistry for Treponema pallidum may be useful in identifying rare organisms ➡ and is less difficult to interpret than the Warthin-Starry stain, which often has a dirty background.*

Radiographs in Congenital Syphilis

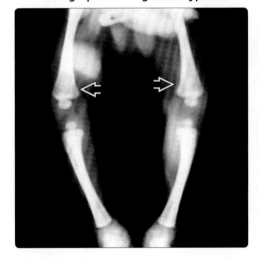

Osteochondritis

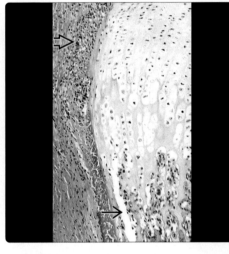

(Left) *Marked flaring of the epiphyses ➡ is noted in this case of congenital syphilis. Osteochondritis is a common complication of untreated congenital syphilis and may present with symptoms of osteomyelitis.* (Right) *A decalcified section from the femoral epiphysis from a fetus with congenital syphilis shows growth disturbance with loss of the marrow free zone ➡. A large number of plasma cells ➡ is seen in the periosteum.*

Pneumonia Alba

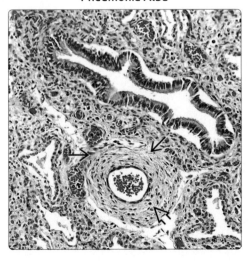

Fetal Pancreas in Congenital Syphilis

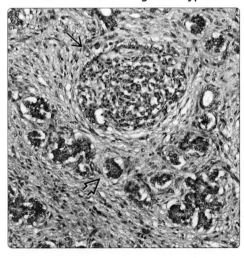

(Left) *Pneumonia alba is characteristic of congenital syphilis. Vessels in syphilis, including those of stem villi, show prominence of perivascular tissue with loosening and inflammation of the vessel wall ➡ and eventual perivascular fibrosis. A rare plasma cell ➡ is present.* (Right) *Another characteristic feature of congenital syphilis is marked loose fibrosis within the pancreas involving both islets ➡ and acinar ➡ components. Extramedullary hematopoiesis may also be a prominent feature in this location.*

KEY FACTS

CLINICAL ISSUES

- Disseminated *Coccidioides immitis* infection in pregnant mother
- Diagnosis usually clinically obvious in endemic areas
- Transmission to fetus uncommon despite massive placental burden
  - Transplacental spread reported in premature births

MACROSCOPIC

- Tan lesions resembling infarcts
- Increased fibrin

MICROSCOPIC

- Intervillous and perivillous foci of infection with numerous large fungal spherules
  - Endospore-containing spherules of *Coccidioides immitis* (10-100 μm in size) visible on H&E stain
- Chronic lymphocytic villitis with increased perivillous fibrin, avascular villi

- Acute and chronic intervillositis with foreign body giant cell reaction to spherules
- Intervillous neutrophilic exudate with necrosis, perivillous fibrin deposition

ANCILLARY TESTS

- Spherules visible on H&E
- Also reactive on GMS stains

TOP DIFFERENTIAL DIAGNOSES

- *Paracoccidioides brasiliensis*
- *Blastomyces dermatidis*
- *Cryptococcus neoformans*
- *Histoplasma capsulatum*
- *Tuberculosis*
- *Listeriosis*

(Left) Coccidioides immitis is spread hematogenously to the placenta. Infection is confined to the intervillous space accompanied by chronic villitis ⊡. Note the absence of any amniotropic maternal inflammatory response ⊡. (Right) Intervillous fibrin and a maternal foreign body giant cell reaction encases foci with spherules of Coccidioides immitis ⊡.

Chorionic Plate in Coccidioidomycosis

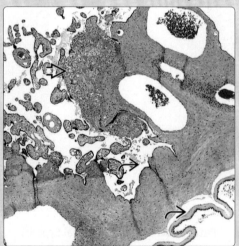

Coccidioides Immitis Spherules

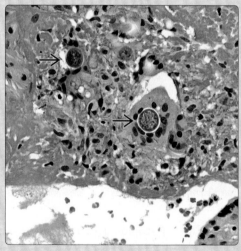

(Left) Areas resembling infarcts on gross exam show masses of chronic villitis ⊡, perivillitis and perivillous fibrin deposition with necrotic debris ⊡, progressive infarction of encased villi ⊡, and fungal spherules ⊡. (Right) Numerous fungal spherules ⊡ are accompanied by a histiocytic response ⊡ and neutrophilic exudate ⊡. Despite heavy fungal burden, transplacental transmission to the fetus is very rare.

Chronic Villitis and Perivillitis

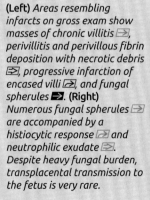
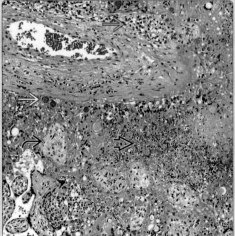

Heavy Fungal Load in Intervillous Space

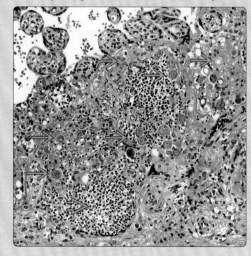

Coccidioidomycosis

TERMINOLOGY

Synonyms

- *Coccidioides immitis*, valley fever

Definitions

- Soil-borne fungus found mostly in southwestern United States and northern Mexico

CLINICAL ISSUES

Presentation

- Disseminated infection in pregnant mother
- Diagnosis usually clinically obvious in endemic areas

Prognosis

- Despite massive placental burden, transmission to fetus is uncommon

MACROSCOPIC

General Features

- Numerous parenchymal tan lesions on cut section
- Variably increased parenchymal fibrin

MICROSCOPIC

Histologic Features

- Umbilical cord
  - No fetal inflammatory response
  - Fetal inflammatory response suggests concomitant ascending infection and chorioamnionitis
- Membranes
  - No significant inflammation of chorion or amnion
  - Chorioamnionitis suggests concomitant infection with ascending organism
- Villous parenchyma
  - Multiple intervillous and perivillous foci of infection
    - Increased fibrin
    - Abscesses rich in neutrophils and purulent debris
    - Acute villitis not common
    - Endospore-containing spherules (10-100 μm in size) of *Coccidioides immitis* visible on H&E stain
    - Foreign body giant cell reaction to spherules
    - Lymphohistiocytic chronic villitis with involution of fetal vasculature in adjacent villi
    - Stainable organisms may be absent if mother treated with antifungal drugs during pregnancy
- Decidua
  - Variable inflammation
  - Abscesses not commonly seen

DIFFERENTIAL DIAGNOSIS

Other Fungal Infections

- *Candida albicans*
  - Most common fungal infection of placenta
  - Ascending chorioamnionitis pattern with peripheral funisitis; does not have villitis or intervillositis component
- *Cryptococcus neoformans*
  - Opportunistic infection occurs in severely immunocompromised patients
  - Yeast buds 5-10 μm, smaller than spherules of *Coccidioides*
  - Rare reported cases of placental involvement describe intervillous yeasts with minimal inflammation
- *Blastomyces dermatitidis*
  - Rarely seen in placenta, transplacental infection described in ~ 10% of cases with high infant mortality
  - Broad-based budding yeasts 10-15 μm in size, smaller than spherules of *Coccidioides*
  - Reported cases describe chronic villitis and intervillous granulomatous inflammation in subset of infected mothers
- *Paracoccidioides brasiliensis*
  - Budding yeast, 4-60 μm, similar size but different appearance than round spherules of *Coccidioides*
  - Similar pattern of intervillositis with neutrophils and histiocytic response
- *Histoplasma capsulatum*
  - Budding small yeast, 3-5 μm in size
  - Rare case reported of vertical transmission in setting of maternal HIV with yeasts in terminal villi and perivillous fibrin, no significant inflammation

Other Infections With Hematogenous Spread

- Tuberculosis
  - Villous and intervillous granulomas, bacilli may be hard to find
- Listeriosis
  - Can be ascending &/or hematogenous, intervillous abscesses often with chorioamnionitis
- Toxoplasmosis
  - Histiocytic and lymphoplasmacytic villitis with *Toxoplasma* cysts beneath amnion and in cord stroma

DIAGNOSTIC CHECKLIST

Clinically Relevant Pathologic Features

- Fetal inflammatory response (umbilical or chorionic acute vasculitis) uncommon
  - If present, suggests possible exposure of fetus to *Coccidioides* in amniotic fluid, or concomitant ascending chorioamnionitis

Pathologic Interpretation Pearls

- Large intervillous abscesses with foreign body giant cell reaction, numerous large fungal spherules and excess fibrin deposition

SELECTED REFERENCES

1. Youssef D et al: Pulmonary blastomycosis during pregnancy: case report and review of the literature. Tenn Med. 106(3):37-9, 2013
2. Patel M et al: Transplacental transmission of Cryptococcus neoformans to an HIV-exposed premature neonate. J Perinatol. 32(3):235-7, 2012
3. Hooper JE et al: Disseminated coccidioidomycosis in pregnancy. Arch Pathol Lab Med. 131(4):652-5, 2007
4. Crum NF et al: Coccidioidomycosis in pregnancy: case report and review of the literature. Am J Med. 119(11):993, 2006
5. Charlton V et al: Intrauterine transmission of coccidioidomycosis. Pediatr Infect Dis J. 18(6):561-3, 1999
6. Linsangan LC et al: Coccidioides immitis infection of the neonate: two routes of infection. Pediatr Infect Dis J. 18(2):171-3, 1999

TERMINOLOGY

Definitions

- Hematogenous infection: Parasitemia spreads from maternal bloodstream into placental villi
  - Trophoblast epithelium, basal laminae, villous stroma, fetal capillary endothelium are crossed to infect fetal bloodstream
- Vertical transmission: Transmission from mother to child in utero, during delivery from cervical secretions, or postpartum through breast milk

TOXOPLASMOSIS

Toxoplasma gondii

- Ubiquitous obligate intracellular coccidian protozoan
  - 3 genotypes: Type II is most common; type I has higher pathogenicity
- Definitive host is cats; kittens are particularly infectious
- Intermediate hosts are humans, cows, pigs, sheep, rabbit, goat, poultry
- Human infection
  - Transplacental congenital infection
  - Eating raw vegetables or water containing oocytes contaminated with feline feces
  - Ingesting oocysts from hands contaminated with feline feces
  - Eating undercooked meat containing cysts
- Seroconversion risk is 3-5% per year; immunity is protective against vertical transmission
  - High incidence of false-positive IgM serology

Presentation

- Usually asymptomatic infection in normal host or mild viral-like illness in immunoincompetent host, reactivation possible in immunoincompetent host
- Parasitemic stage occurs 1-2 weeks after ingestion of oocytes or cysts
- Congenital toxoplasmosis occurs in 33-50% of parasitemic pregnant women
  - Risk for transmission varies with gestational age
    - 17% in 1st trimester, 25% in 2nd trimester, and 63% in 3rd trimester
  - Long delay between maternal infection and transmission may occur
  - Most cases are asymptomatic but increased risk of intrauterine growth restriction and prematurity
  - 5-15% of cases are stillbirths, usually after infection early in pregnancy
  - Symptomatic infants may show hydrops, sepsis, hepatosplenomegaly, jaundice, petechiae, eye and CNS abnormalities

Treatment

- Spiramycin treatment during pregnancy has questionable impact on outcome, poor placental transfer but may prevent spread across placenta
- Pyrimethamine plus sulfadiazine, during pregnancy for confirmed fetal infection
- Neonatal treatment with pyrimethamine plus sulfadiazine, recommended, even when asymptomatic

Prognosis of Congenital Infection

- Stillbirth in 5-15%, rarely associated with abortion
- 85-95% of survivors have chorioretinitis and may develop unilateral or bilateral blindness
- 10-20% of survivors have hydrocephalus with diffuse intracranial calcifications, learning disorders, or severe intellectual disability

Macroscopic Features

- No specific features

Histologic Features

- Organisms are intracellular in amnion epithelial cells, stromal cells between amnion and chorion, and villous Hofbauer cells
- Pseudocysts contain many tachyzoites, appear round in section, 2 x 6 μm, central nucleus
- True cysts are round to oval in section and may contain hundreds of crescentic bradyzoites that are periodic acid-Schiff positive

Toxoplasma gondii

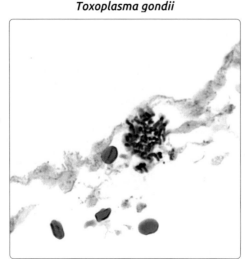

Trypanosoma cruzi

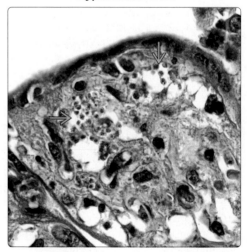

(Left) Crescent-shaped toxoplasmosis tachyzoites are present within the connective tissue of the placental membranes. (Right) Chagas disease villitis shows numerous intracellular, 3- to 5-μm amastigotes ➡ that have a kinetoplast on one end of the organism that stains darkly on routine H&E.

- *Toxoplasma* organisms in placenta are considered diagnostic of congenital toxoplasmosis but have low sensitivity
  - 91% positive in symptomatic and 11-25% in asymptomatic infants
- May see nonspecific villous enlargement with numerous Hofbauer cells
- Lymphohistiocytic or granulomatous villitis with Langhans-type multinucleated giant cells, necrosis
  - Rupture of cysts results in inflammation and release of tachyzoites or bradyzoites

Immunohistochemistry

- *Toxoplasma* immunohistochemistry is available but is rarely needed for identification of cysts or pseudocysts; identifies tachyzoites after cyst rupture
- Cysts are positive with silver stains and periodic acid-Schiff

CHAGAS DISEASE

Trypanosoma cruzi

- Hemoflagellate protozoan, endemic in Latin America and 1st reported in Mexico in 1998
  - Chagas transmitted through feces of triatomid bug (reduviid or kissing bug) that contains trypomastigotes, contaminated food or water, blood transfusion, or organ transplantation

Presentation

- Parasitemia occurs 3 weeks after ingestion
  - Acute infection lasts 4-8 weeks
  - Only 1% of individuals are symptomatic
  - Peripheral blood smear will be positive for trypomastigotes
- Congenital Chagas results from transplacental transmission in 1-19% and rarely through breast milk
  - Transmission occurs at all stages of disease and is directly related to level or parasitemia
    - Primary infection has high parasitemia; chronic, latent, or indeterminate phases have intermittent parasitemia
  - Can recur in subsequent pregnancies
  - Most babies are asymptomatic with increased incidence of prematurity and low birth weight
  - Symptomatic infants may be stillborn, have hydrops, hepatosplenomegaly, anemia, jaundice, petechiae, seizures
  - Congenital Chagas accounts for 22% of new cases

Treatment

- No in utero treatment due to teratogenic risks of available medicines
- Benznidazole and nifurtimox are recommended for treatment as soon as diagnosis is confirmed after birth
  - Early detection and treatment is highly successful, < 50% are diagnosed early

Prognosis

- Early pregnancy loss or stillbirth in 25% of cases
- Live born
  - Most are asymptomatic at birth with good prognosis
  - Low birth weight and respiratory distress
  - Symptomatic infants have high mortality

- 20-30% lifetime risk for cardiac or gastrointestinal dysfunction

Macroscopic Features

- No specific features

Histologic Features

- Trypomastigotes penetrate villous trophoblast or chorionic plate
  - Trypomastigotes are C- or U-shaped with posterior kinetoplast
  - Sloughing of syncytiotrophoblast may help prevent congenital infection
- Organisms infect Hofbauer, cytotrophoblasts, and stromal cells, then transform into amastigotes
  - Amastigotes may be found in villi, umbilical cord, chorionic plate, and decidua
  - Amastigotes are 3-5 μm, have kinetoplast, prominent bar, and deep staining with H&E
  - Pseudocysts may form through confluence of many organisms
- Villitis occurs with rupture of parasitized macrophage
  - Lymphocytic, histiocytic, granulomatous, or necrotizing villitis
  - Maternal lymphohistiocytic intervillositis occurs in areas of necrosis
- Stillborns have heavy parasitemia with diffuse villitis
- Asymptomatic newborns may have rare foci of villitis, intervillositis, and low to no parasitemia
- Separation of syncytiotrophoblast and disorganization of basal lamina without parasites or inflammation
- Rare villous stromal nucleomegalic cells contain large numbers of parasites and are hypertetraploid or aneuploid

Ancillary Tests

- Immunofluorescence or PCR on formalin-fixed, paraffin-embedded tissues available in reference labs

MALARIA

Infectious Agents

- *Plasmodium falciparum* (most common) found exclusively in tropical climates, *Plasmodium vivax* (higher frequency in South America) found in more temperate climates, *Plasmodium malariae*, *Plasmodium ovale* are uncommon
  - Sporozoite is transmitted by bite of infected female *Anopheles* mosquito or infected blood products
  - Sporozoite enters liver and replicates; rupture of hepatocytes releases merozoites that invade red blood cells
  - *P. falciparum*-infected red blood cells accumulate in placenta due to adhesion to molecules, such as chondroitin sulphate A on villus
    - Immunity from prior infection produces blocking antibodies that prevent this binding
  - Peripheral blood smears, antigen capture dipstick, PCR, DNA probe used for diagnosis

Presentation

- Parasitemia occurs 6-12 days after infection
- 4-10x increased risk for pregnant women to contract malaria; especially during 1st or 2nd pregnancy
  - Highest risk in primigravidas without immunity

- Highest risk for maternal infection occurs between 13-16 weeks with decreasing incidence after 24 weeks

Treatment

- Prevention and treatment during pregnancy with chloroquine and mefloquine during 2nd and 3rd trimesters

Prognosis

- Associated with maternal anemia, preterm, and low-birth-weight infants
  - Accounts for up to 20% maternal deaths in endemic areas
- 2.4% incidence of stillbirth, usually with placental parasitemia
  - Placental parasitemia is associated with increased risk of malaria during 1st year of life
- Transmission to fetus is rare: 3-7% incidence of umbilical cord parasitemia, rapidly eliminated without treatment
- Coinfection with HIV associated with increased prevalence and intensity of parasitemia; HIV viral load is also higher

Macroscopic Features

- Reduced weight of placenta

Histologic Features

- Histiocytic intervillositis with hemozoin pigment and parasites in maternal red blood cells
  - 25% of placentas from women with malaria contain trophozoite ring forms within maternal red blood cells
  - Hemozoin pigment is birefringent and may be in parasites, erythrocytes, histiocytes, and fibrin in intervillous space; product of hemoglobin digestion
  - Placental sequestration results in much higher parasitemia in intervillous space than in peripheral blood
  - Intervillous maternal blood space contains
    - Parasites in erythrocytes in acute infection
    - Parasites in erythrocytes and hemozoin pigment in histiocytes in chronic infection
    - Hematoidin pigment in nodules of intervillous fibrin and some histiocytes in past infection
      - Formalin pigment and hematoidin appear similar
- *P. falciparum*: Heavy parasitemia, multiple parasites per red blood cell, prominent mononuclear cell intervillositis, abundant, brown to black hemozoin pigment
- *P. vivax*: Rarely has parasitemia, fewer intervillous mononuclear cells, and less yellow to brown hemozoin pigment
- Nonspecific changes include increased syncytial knots, injury of syncytiotrophoblast, thickened trophoblast basement membrane, villous necrosis

Ancillary Tests

- Organisms are usually visible on routine H&E stains; special stains (Giemsa, Thomas) are useful with low parasitemia

DIFFERENTIAL DIAGNOSIS

Toxoplasmosis vs. Chagas vs. Leishmaniasis

- *Toxoplasma* trophozoites distinguished from Chagas amastigotes by dark-staining kinetoplast in latter
- *Leishmania* concentrates in macrophages in skin, mouth, nose, or lymphoid organs, has smaller kinetoplast; human placental involvement has not been described

Malaria vs. Chronic Histiocytic Intervillositis

- Identification of hematoidin pigment may be useful to rule in malaria

SELECTED REFERENCES

1. Juiz NA et al: Different genotypes of Trypanosoma cruzi produce distinctive placental environment genetic response in chronic experimental infection. PLoS Negl Trop Dis. 11(3):e0005436, 2017
2. Sharma L et al: Placental malaria: a new insight into the pathophysiology. Front Med (Lausanne). 4:117, 2017
3. Singh S: Congenital toxoplasmosis: clinical features, outcomes, treatment, and prevention. Trop Parasitol. 6(2):113-122, 2016
4. Asante KP et al: Placental malaria and the risk of malaria in infants in a high malaria transmission area in ghana: a prospective cohort study. J Infect Dis. 208(9):1504-13, 2013
5. Carmona-Fonseca J et al: Placental malaria in Colombia: histopathologic findings in Plasmodium vivax and P. falciparum infections. Am J Trop Med Hyg. 88(6):1093-101, 2013
6. Cullen KA et al: Malaria surveillance--United States, 2011. MMWR Surveill Summ. 62(5):1-17, 2013
7. Kalilani-Phiri L et al: Timing of malaria infection during pregnancy has characteristic maternal, infant and placental outcomes. PLoS One. 8(9):e74643, 2013
8. Paquet C et al: Toxoplasmosis in pregnancy: prevention, screening, and treatment. J Obstet Gynaecol Can. 35(1):78-9, 2013
9. Souza RM et al: Placental histopathological changes associated with Plasmodium vivax infection during pregnancy. PLoS Negl Trop Dis. 2013;7(2):e2071. Epub 2013 Feb 14. Erratum in: PLoS Negl Trop Dis. 7(4), 2013
10. Centers for Disease Control and Prevention (CDC): congenital transmission of Chagas disease - Virginia, 2010. MMWR Morb Mortal Wkly Rep. 61(26):477-9, 2012
11. Duaso J et al: Reorganization of extracellular matrix in placentas from women with asymptomatic chagas disease: mechanism of parasite invasion or local placental defense? J Trop Med. 2012:758357, 2012
12. Robbins JR et al: Tissue barriers of the human placenta to infection with Toxoplasma gondii. Infect Immun. 80(1):418-28, 2012
13. Carlier Y et al: Congenital Chagas disease: recommendations for diagnosis, treatment and control of newborns, siblings and pregnant women. PLoS Negl Trop Dis. 5(10):e1250, 2011
14. Filisetti D et al: Placental testing for Toxoplasma gondii is not useful to diagnose congenital toxoplasmosis. Pediatr Infect Dis J. 29(7):665-7, 2010
15. Robert-Gangneux F et al: Clinical relevance of placenta examination for the diagnosis of congenital toxoplasmosis. Pediatr Infect Dis J. 29(1):33-8, 2010
16. Fricker-Hidalgo H et al: Value of Toxoplasma gondii detection in one hundred thirty-three placentas for the diagnosis of congenital toxoplasmosis. Pediatr Infect Dis J. 26(9):845-6, 2007
17. Bittencourt AL et al: The placenta in hematogenous infections. Pediatr Pathol Mol Med. 21(4):401-32, 2002
18. Drut R et al: Image analysis of nucleomegalic cells in Chagas' disease placentitis. Placenta. 21(2-3):280-2, 2000
19. Ismail MR et al: Placental pathology in malaria: a histological, immunohistochemical, and quantitative study. Hum Pathol. 31(1):85-93, 2000
20. Bulmer JN et al: Placental malaria. I. Pathological classification. Histopathology. 22(3):211-8, 1993
21. Bulmer JN et al: Placental malaria. II. A semi-quantitative investigation of the pathological features. Histopathology. 22(3):219-25, 1993
22. Popek EJ: Granulomatous villitis due to Toxoplasma gondii. Pediatr Pathol. 12(2):281-8, 1992
23. Lawrence C et al: Birefringent hemozoin identifies malaria. Am J Clin Pathol. 86(3):360-3, 1986

T. gondii, Granulomatous Villitis

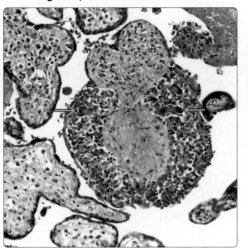

Chronic Villitis in Toxoplasmosis

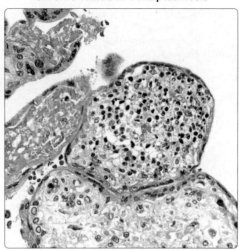

(Left) *Toxoplasmosis often shows granulomatous villitis with Langhans-type multinucleated giant cells* ➡.
(Right) *This case of toxoplasmosis displays only a nonspecific lymphocytic villitis. Careful inspection of the cord and membranes for Toxoplasma cysts is needed.*

True Cyst of *T. gondii*, PAS

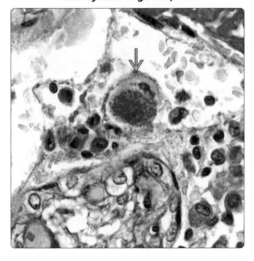

T. gondii Bradyzoites

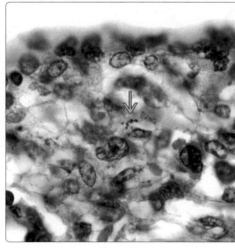

(Left) *True toxoplasmosis cysts show periodic acid-Schiff-positive bradyzoites* ➡.
(Right) *Bradyzoites of toxoplasmosis* ➡ *are present within a Hofbauer cell. The organisms can resemble karyorrhectic debris. Their location in a Hofbauer cell, not among the remnants of involuting fetal vessels, is key.*

True *T. gondii*

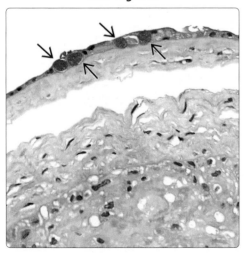

T. gondii

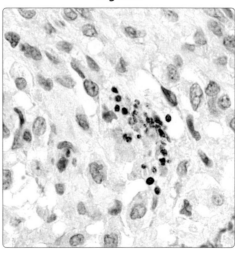

(Left) *Multiple true toxoplasmosis cysts* ➡ *are present in the amnion epithelium, which is why the amniotic fluid is a good source of organisms for diagnosis.*
(Right) *Bradyzoites in the villous stroma are more easily seen when stained with immunohistochemistry.*

T. cruzi

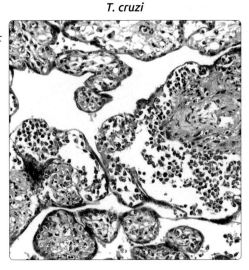

Histiocytic Intervillositis With _T. cruzi_

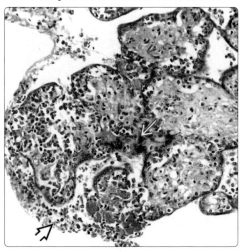

(Left) Chagas disease may feature a prominent histiocytic villitis at the periphery of the villus. (Right) The histiocytic villitis of Chagas disease may include Langhans-type multinucleated giant cells ➡. There is also a moderate maternal histiocytic intervillositis ⊟.

Amastigotes of _T. cruzi_

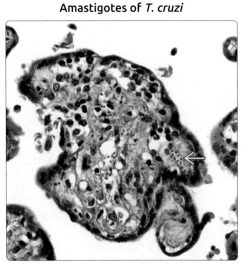

Amastigotes of _T. cruzi_

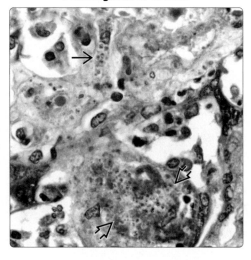

(Left) The villitis in this case of Chagas disease is mostly lymphocytic. Amastigotes are focally present ➡. (Right) Large numbers of extracellular Chagas amastigotes ⊟ are present in this villus. Organisms are intracellular ➡ within a Hofbauer cell.

T. cruzi in Hofbauer Cells of Membranes

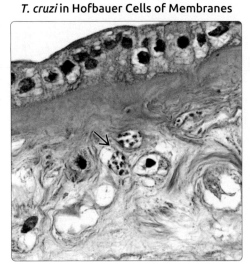

Chronic Chorionitis and _T. cruzi_

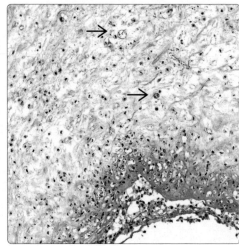

(Left) The amnion displays intracellular Chagas organisms ⊟ beneath the amnion basement membrane. (Right) This case of Chagas disease shows chronic chorionitis with lymphocytes and plasma cells infiltrating the chorionic plate from the maternal intervillous space. Hofbauer cells are present, containing amastigotes ⊟.

Acute Malaria in Red Blood Cells

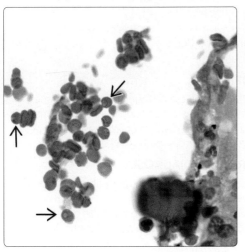

Heavy Malaria With Giemsa Staining

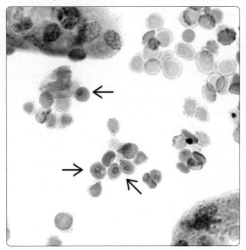

(Left) *Placental intervillous space in acute malaria shows only infected red blood cells. The organisms are difficult to see on an H&E stain and may appear only as vacuoles* ⊟. (Right) *Thomas staining (Giemsa) of the slide highlights the heavy parasitemia* ⊟ *of this case of primary falciparum malaria in a primigravida.*

Chronic Malaria With Hemozoin

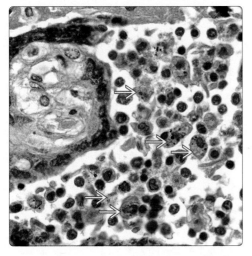

Chronic Malaria With Sickled Cells

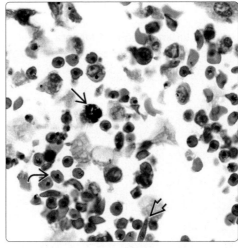

(Left) *Chronic malaria is usually associated with histiocytic intervillositis. The macrophages/histiocytes contain hemozoin pigment* ⊟. (Right) *Chronic malaria may show parasites* ⊟ *and hemozoin pigment in red blood cells and, to a lesser degree, within histiocytes* ⊟. *Note that there are sickled red blood cells* ⊟ *also present.*

Chronic Malaria With Massive Histiocytic Intervillositis

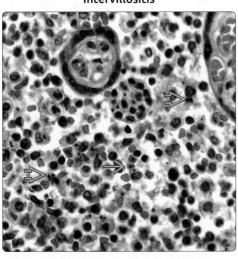

Past Malarial Infection

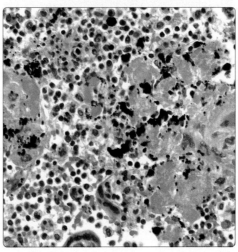

(Left) *Chronic or past infection often displays no parasites in red blood cells, but there may be massive histiocytic intervillositis. Hemozoin pigment is seen within red blood cells* ⊟ *and histiocytes* ⊟. (Right) *This case of past malarial infection shows massive histiocytic intervillositis and abundant hemozoin pigment, mostly within histiocytes.*

Cellular Composition of Chronic Inflammatory Lesions

TERMINOLOGY

- Infiltrates of lymphocytes, histiocytes, plasma cells, and eosinophils in various compartments of placenta

ETIOLOGY/PATHOGENESIS

- Majority of chronic inflammation believed to be maternal alloimmune reaction
  - Elevated levels of inflammatory-related cytokines in placentas with chronic inflammation
  - Fetus is semiallograft to maternal host
- Rule out infectious etiology, particularly early in gestation

CLINICAL ISSUES

- Severe chronic inflammatory lesions may recur in subsequent pregnancies
  - Associated with poor fetal/neonatal outcome
    - Preterm premature rupture of membranes and preterm delivery
    - Intrauterine growth restriction

- Increased risk for neurodevelopmental abnormalities
- Intrauterine fetal demise
  - Associated with maternal complications
    - Recurrent abortions
    - Preeclampsia

MICROSCOPIC

- Chronic inflammation can be found in villi, membranes, chorionic plate, fetal vessels, decidua, and intervillous space
- Can be associated with features of fetal vascular malperfusion and uteroplacental malperfusion

TOP DIFFERENTIAL DIAGNOSES

- Some patterns suggest infectious placentitis, prompting further investigation
- Acute chorioamnionitis and acute villitis can occur concurrently with chronic inflammatory lesions

---

Cellular Components of Chronic Inflammation in Placenta

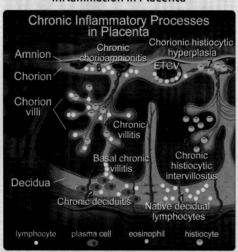

(Left) Chronic inflammatory cells occupy compartments of the placenta, including decidua (1 & 2), basal chorionic villi (3), chorionic villi (4), intervillous space (5), chorioamnion (6 & 7), and chorionic vessel (8). (Right) This case of congenital CMV infection has chronic villitis with mixed chronic inflammatory cells: Lymphocytes ➡, histiocytes ➡, and plasma cells ➡. Plasma cell villitis should always suggest a work-up for CMV infection.

CMV Chronic Villitis

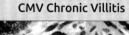
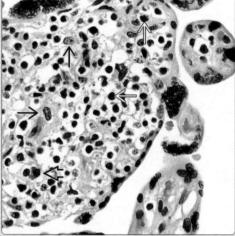

Chronic Chorioamnionitis

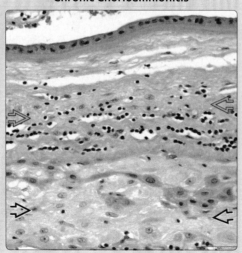

(Left) Chronic chorioamnionitis can be present in both the chorionic plate and free membranes ➡. The decidua ➡ has only a few deep lymphocytes. Lymphocytes are more common in the decidua and hug the cellular chorion. Plasma cells are uncommon in the free membranes. (Right) In chronic basal deciduitis, lymphocytes usually predominate. When lymphocytes become moderate to severe, there are almost always plasma cells ➡, as seen in this case. Some inflammatory cells may extend into the basal villi ➡.

Lymphoplasmacytic Deciduitis

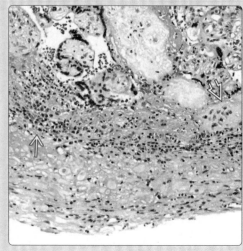

Cellular Composition of Chronic Inflammatory Lesions

TERMINOLOGY

Definitions

- Chronic inflammation in free membranes, decidua, chorionic plate, fetal vessels, villi, maternal intervillous space, and basal plate

ETIOLOGY/PATHOGENESIS

Infectious Agents

- Chronic inflammation may be reaction to infection
  - Cytomegalovirus, herpes simplex virus, syphilis, and toxoplasmosis may be associated with chronic inflammation

Maternal Alloimmune Reaction

- Most chronic inflammation believed to be maternal alloimmune reaction
  - Fetus is semiallograft to maternal host
  - Elevated levels of inflammatory-related cytokines are present in placentas with chronic inflammation

CLINICAL ISSUES

Presentation

- Chronic inflammation is associated with significant fetal/neonatal morbidity
  - Preterm premature rupture of membranes and preterm delivery
  - Intrauterine growth restriction
  - Increased risk for neurodevelopmental abnormalities
  - Intrauterine fetal demise
- Chronic inflammation is associated with maternal conditions
  - Recurrent abortion
  - Preeclampsia

Treatment

- No treatment is recognized for chronic inflammatory lesions of placenta
  - Identification of infectious etiology may result in specific therapies

Prognosis

- Chronic inflammatory lesions may recur in subsequent pregnancies
  - Preterm birth associated with chronic inflammation has 23% recurrence risk

MICROSCOPIC

Histologic Features

- Chronic inflammatory cells involved in various lesions include
  - Maternal lymphocytes, macrophages/histiocytes
  - Fetal histiocytes (Hofbauer cells)
  - Eosinophils, usually fetal
  - Plasma cells, may be either fetal or maternal
- Placental compartments that may contain chronic inflammatory cell infiltrates include
  - Villi
  - Maternal intervillous space
  - Amnion and chorion of extraplacental membranes
  - Maternal decidua, basal and parietalis
  - Fetal vessels of umbilical cord and chorionic plate
- Very common for chronic inflammation to be present in more than one compartment
- Associated with features of fetal vascular malperfusion (fetal thrombotic vasculopathy) and uteroplacental malperfusion

ANCILLARY TESTS

Immunohistochemistry

- CD3(+) T cells or CD8(+) cytotoxic T cells
- CD68(+) histiocytes, macrophages, and Hofbauer cells

DIFFERENTIAL DIAGNOSIS

Infectious Placentitis

- Cytomegalovirus, herpes simplex virus, syphilis, and toxoplasmosis all may have chronic inflammatory lesions

Acute Inflammatory Lesions

- Acute chorioamnionitis
  - Maternal response to ascending intrauterine infection
  - Neutrophils compose majority of inflammatory cells
  - Eosinophils can be seen in small numbers
- Acute villitis
  - Often accompanied by acute chorioamnionitis
  - Fetal sepsis, neutrophils in villous capillaries, ± bacteria
- Can occur concurrently with chronic inflammatory lesions

DIAGNOSTIC CHECKLIST

Pathologic Interpretation Pearls

- Villi normally contain fetal histiocytes (Hofbauer cells)
  - Lymphocytes and plasma cells are not normal components of villous stroma
  - Do not overcall normal, more cellular stroma of immature villi as inflammatory infiltrate
    - Cellularity is homogeneous in immature villi; vessels are intact
    - Cellularity is patchy or focal in chronic inflammatory lesions; vessels often involved

SELECTED REFERENCES

1. Maymon E et al: Chronic inflammatory lesions of the placenta are associated with an up-regulation of amniotic fluid CXCR3: a marker of allograft rejection. J Perinat Med. 46(2):123-137, 2018
2. Keenan-Devlin LS et al: Maternal income during pregnancy is associated with chronic placental inflammation at birth. Am J Perinatol. 34(10):1003-1010, 2017
3. Kim CJ et al: Chronic inflammation of the placenta: definition, classification, pathogenesis, and clinical significance. Am J Obstet Gynecol. 213(4 Suppl):S53-69, 2015
4. Raman K et al: Overlap chronic placental inflammation is associated with a unique gene expression pattern. PLoS One. 10(7):e0133738, 2015
5. Katzman PJ et al: Immunohistochemical analysis reveals an influx of regulatory T cells and focal trophoblastic STAT-1 phosphorylation in chronic villitis of unknown etiology. Pediatr Dev Pathol. 14(4):284-93, 2011
6. Kim CJ et al: The frequency, clinical significance, and pathological features of chronic chorioamnionitis: a lesion associated with spontaneous preterm birth. Mod Pathol. 23(7):1000-11, 2010
7. Khong TY et al: Chronic deciduitis in the placental basal plate: definition and interobserver reliability. Hum Pathol. 31(3):292-5, 2000

Placental Diagnoses

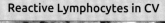
KEY FACTS

ETIOLOGY/PATHOGENESIS

- Only 5% of villitis is due to infection
- Chronic villitis (CV) of unknown etiology (CVUE) is considered aberrant maternal immune response against antigens expressed in villi

CLINICAL ISSUES

- CVUE: Fairly common, 2-34% of term placentas, more common in 3rd trimester
- Associated with intrauterine growth restriction, prematurity, intrauterine fetal demise, and recurrent pregnancy loss
  - Severity of conditions related to extent of placental involvement

MICROSCOPIC

- CVUE (95%)
  - Maternal CD3(+) CD8(+) T cells infiltrate villous stroma

- Proximal CV may obliterate stem vessels with avascular distal villi
- May involve subchorionic, basal, or midparenchymal distribution
- Low-grade CV, clusters of < 10 contiguous inflamed villi per focus (in > 1 focus)
  - Focal: All foci present on one slide
  - Multifocal: Foci present on multiple slides
- High-grade CV, 10 or more inflamed villi in multiple foci per slide
  - Patchy: Involves < 30% of parenchyma (involvement of > 5% is uncommon and suggests severe disease)
  - Diffuse: > 30% of villi involved
- Infectious villitis (5%)
  - Plasma cells are common in CMV, HSV, and syphilis
  - Always carefully examine for viral inclusions; perform special studies as indicated

---

(Left) Maternal T lymphocytes diffusely infiltrate the stroma, sparing the syncytiotrophoblast in this villus. (Right) Maternal lymphocytes in chronic villitis (CV) can resemble immunoblasts ⟶ in their reactive state with large nuclei, prominent nucleoli, and mitoses.

Lymphoid Infiltrates

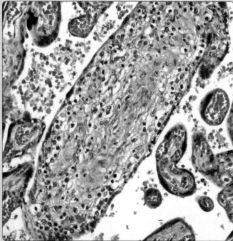

Reactive Lymphocytes in CV

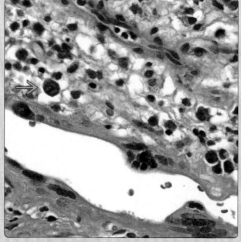

(Left) Multinucleated Langhans-type giant cells ⟶ are variably present in CV of unknown etiology (CVUE). They may also be seen in infectious villitides such as toxoplasmosis. (Right) Plasma cells are not a normal component of CVUE in the midparenchyma. Their presence should prompt exclusion of CMV infection. Hemosiderin ⟶ is usually present secondary to vascular injury. Viral inclusions may be inconspicuous.

Multinucleated Giant Cells in CV

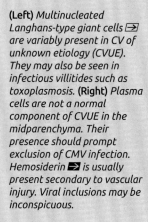
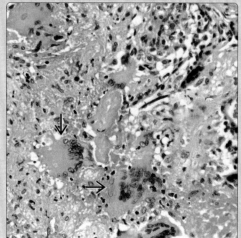

Plasmacytic Villitis With CMV

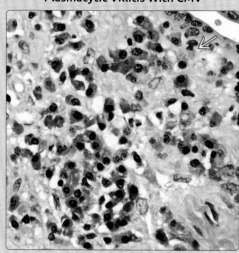

TERMINOLOGY

Abbreviations

- Chronic villitis (CV)
- Chronic villitis of unknown etiology (CVUE)

Synonyms

- CVUE, villitis of unknown etiology (VUE)

Definitions

- CV
  - Microscopic pattern of lymphocytes, histiocytes, and, in some cases, plasma cells within villous stroma
- CVUE
  - CV with no identifiable infectious etiology
  - Because of similarities in inflammatory infiltrate in infectious and CVUE, some have proposed an infection as yet unidentified
- Proximal CV
  - 10-30% involve stem villi, usually also with involvement of terminal villi
  - More likely also to have stem vessel obliteration and avascular villi
- Distal CV
  - 50% only involve terminal and mature intermediate villi
- Basal chronic villitis (BCV)
  - CV affecting villi near maternal floor
- Low-grade CV: < 10 contiguous inflamed villi in any one focus with > 1 focus required
  - Focal low-grade CV: Only one slide involved
  - Multifocal low-grade CV: Multiple slides involved
- High-grade CV: 10 or more villi inflamed per focus
  - Patchy high-grade CV: Foci of high-grade seen on multiple slides
  - Diffuse high-grade CV: > 30% of villi involved
- Single foci of CV are termed "ungradable"
  - Ungradable-possible low grade: Only single focus with < 10 villi
  - Ungradable-possible high grade: Only single focus with ≥ 10 villi
- CV with stem vessel obliteration: Infiltrates associated with muscular vessel damage/involution
- CV with avascular villi: Large foci (> 10 villi) of contiguous avascular villi associated with CV in adjacent regions

ETIOLOGY/PATHOGENESIS

Infectious Agents

- Infectious villitis accounts for 5% of villitis cases, usually TORCH organisms

Chronic Villitis of Unknown Etiology

- Maternal alloimmune response, similar to rejection of organ transplant
  - Fetal-maternal syncytiotrophoblast barrier may be breached, exposing stromal HLA antigens
  - Balance of antiinflammatory and proinflammatory cytokines in CVUE is altered
  - Placentas with CVUE have enrichment of genes involved in antigen presentation and immune rejection
  - C4d(+) staining of syncytiotrophoblasts and villous endothelial cells indicates complement activation due to humoral antibody and supports host vs. graft situation
- Infiltrate of maternal CD8(+) cytotoxic T cells that express receptor for T-cell chemokines CXCR3(+) and include subset of FOXP3(+) T-regulatory cells
- Inflamed villi express intercellular adhesion molecule-1 (ICAM-1) in syncytiotrophoblasts and maternal lymphocytes and facilitate maternal T-cell infiltration
- Hofbauer cells become activated, becoming CD14(+); proinflammatory marker
- Focal CV may be seen at edges of perivillous fibrinoid deposition, infarctions, and intervillous thrombi
  - MHC class II expression turned on at these sites with parenchymal injury; may facilitate CV

CLINICAL ISSUES

Epidemiology

- Incidence
  - Infectious villitis: 5% of villitis cases, more common in 2nd trimester
  - CVUE: Fairly common, 2-34% of term placentas
    - Variation may be due to amount of parenchyma sampled; for example, more BCV will be identified if basal plate wedge sections are routinely examined
    - This lesion is frequently missed by general pathologists examining placenta

Presentation

- CVUE is more common in 3rd trimester
- CV may have elevated maternal serum α-fetoprotein, indicating villus injury

Prognosis

- CV is associated with intrauterine growth restriction (IUGR), prematurity, intrauterine fetal demise (IUFD), and recurrent pregnancy loss
  - More extensive involvement associated with IUGR and IUFD; outcome studies did not utilize Amsterdam grading criteria
- CV can recur with subsequent pregnancies; grade may escalate; can recur as chronic histiocytic intervillositis
- Proximal CV with stem vessel obliteration may be associated with neurologic impairment in some neonates
- Chronic inflammation may produce systemic fetal inflammatory response, accounting for increased incidence of neurodevelopmental problems

MACROSCOPIC

General Features

- CV
  - Focal lesions are microscopic diagnosis only
  - More extensive involvement may be seen grossly as pale areas or increased granularity of cut surface

MICROSCOPIC

Histologic Features

- Location
  - Location of CV may be described as basal/paraseptal, midparenchymal, or subchorionic

○ Inflamed villi generally will appear more blue on low power due to increased stromal cellularity and decreased vascularity

- Inflammatory cells
  ○ Maternal lymphocytes infiltrate villus stroma
    – Lymphoid infiltrates may be dense or more subtle
    – Lymphoid infiltrates can be highly reactive, mitotically active with enlarged, blast-like nuclei
    – May see proliferation of fetal Hofbauer cells
    – Eosinophils can rarely mix with lymphocytes and histiocytes in CV
    – May see granulomatous inflammation with Langhans type multinucleated giant cells
    – May see perivillitis with histiocyte-rich inflammation tethered to villous surface
      □ Distinguish from chronic histiocytic intervillositis where histiocytes are free floating in intervillous space
    – Some lesions may have small foci of admixed neutrophils
      □ Not common pattern of CV; make sure infection is excluded
- Associated features
  ○ Some lesions are intensely destructive with necrosis of entire villi
  ○ CV with stem vessel obliteration
    – Involvement of proximal stem villus, close to chorionic plate, associated with more severe effects because of larger number of downstream villi with impaired perfusion
  ○ CV with avascular villi
    – Villi may be completely avascular or show residual villous stromal-vascular karyorrhexis
    – Hemosiderin may be present as result of vascular injury
    – Distinct from loss of vessels due to inflammation of villi themselves
  ○ CV with increased perivillous fibrin deposition
    – Syncytiotrophoblast injury leads to deposition of fibrin around inflamed villi
  ○ BCV may have associated plasma cell deciduitis

ANCILLARY TESTS

Immunohistochemistry

- CD3 staining highlights T-cell infiltrates of CV, helps delineate extent of involvement if in doubt
  ○ Only stromal T cells count, not those in villous vessels or maternal blood space

DIFFERENTIAL DIAGNOSIS

Massive Perivillous Fibrin Deposition

- CV with increased perivillous fibrin may resemble this entity
- Some cases may be due to maternal immune-mediated injury of parenchyma
  ○ Diagnosis reserved for cases with extensive fibrin deposition (50% of parenchyma)

Fetal Vascular Malperfusion

- CV with stem vessel obliteration and CV with avascular villi resemble this entity

○ Mechanism of malperfusion is secondary to CV, not termed fetal vascular malperfusion
- When true thrombi are seen, or avascular villi are remote from areas of CV, fetal vascular malperfusion is also diagnosed

2nd-Trimester Placenta

- Large number of stromal cells in 2nd-trimester villi can mimic CV
  ○ Stromal cells are uniformly increased within villi, while CV usually has patchy distribution of inflammatory cells in stroma

Infectious Placentitis

- CV: Exclude TORCH infections
  ○ Plasma cells should prompt search for viral inclusions of CMV or HSV
  ○ Infection more common in 2nd trimester
  ○ Infection is often associated with funisitis

Chronic Histiocytic Intervillositis

- CV with perivillitis can mimic chronic histiocytic intervillositis
  ○ Presence of stromal lymphoid infiltrates and tethering of perivillous histiocytes to villous surface distinguishes CV from chronic histiocytic intervillositis

DIAGNOSTIC CHECKLIST

Pathologic Interpretation Pearls

- Increased villous stromal lymphocytes in CV are often patchy, best seen on low-power objective
- Identification of CV may be associated with chronic inflammation in additional placental compartments
- Infectious villitis should be excluded in high-grade cases by examining for viral inclusions and performing appropriate immunostains, histochemical stains, or molecular studies
- Homogeneously highly cellular stroma in 2nd-trimester placentas can mimic CV

SELECTED REFERENCES

1. Khong TY et al: Sampling and definitions of placental lesions: Amsterdam Placental Workshop Group consensus statement. Arch Pathol Lab Med. 140(7):698-713, 2016
2. Nowak C et al: Perinatal prognosis of pregnancies complicated by placental chronic villitis or intervillositis of unknown etiology and combined lesions: about a series of 178 cases. Placenta. 44:104-8, 2016
3. Katzman PJ: Chronic inflammatory lesions of the placenta. Semin Perinatol. 39(1):20-6, 2015
4. Kim CJ et al: Chronic inflammation of the placenta: definition, classification, pathogenesis, and clinical significance. Am J Obstet Gynecol. 213(4 Suppl):S53-69, 2015
5. Katzman PJ et al: Eosinophilic/T-cell chorionic vasculitis and chronic villitis involve regulatory T cells and often occur together. Pediatr Dev Pathol. 16(4):278-91, 2013
6. Rudzinski E et al: Positive C4d immunostaining of placental villous syncytiotrophoblasts supports host-versus-graft rejection in villitis of unknown etiology. Pediatr Dev Pathol. 16(1):7-13, 2013
7. Katzman PJ et al: Immunohistochemical analysis reveals an influx of regulatory T cells and focal trophoblastic STAT-1 phosphorylation in chronic villitis of unknown etiology. Pediatr Dev Pathol. 14(4):284-93, 2011
8. Kim JS et al: Involvement of Hofbauer cells and maternal T cells in villitis of unknown aetiology. Histopathology. 52(4):457-64, 2008
9. Redline RW: Villitis of unknown etiology: noninfectious chronic villitis in the placenta. Hum Pathol. 38(10):1439-46, 2007

Basal CV

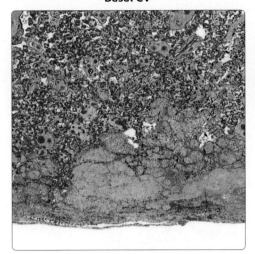

Chronic Chorionitis and Subchorionic CV

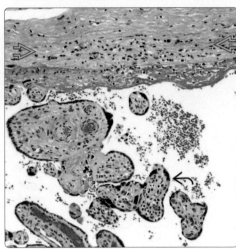

(Left) *Villitis may be restricted to the basal villi. In some cases, such as this one, there is a relatively uniform band of inflamed villi. There is often chronic inflammation within the decidua basalis as well, including plasma cells.* (Right) *The lymphoid infiltrates of CV* ⇗ *may also involve the chorionic plate* ⇘. *The cells in the chorion are T cells of maternal origin, as are the lymphocytes in the villi. It is very common for chronic inflammation to be found in multiple placental compartments.*

Low-Grade CV

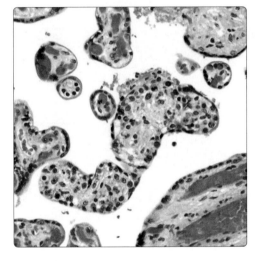

High-Grade CV

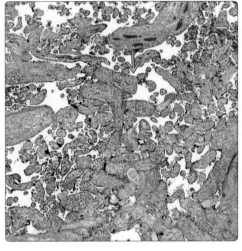

(Left) *Involvement of < 10 contiguous villi is termed "low grade." At least 2 foci are required to make the diagnosis. If low-grade CV is found on only 1 slide, the diagnosis is focal low-grade CV. If it involves ≥ 2 slides, the diagnosis is multifocal low-grade CV.* (Right) *Involvement of ≥ 10 contiguous villi in any one focus is high grade* ⇘. *When > 30% of the parenchyma is affected, diffuse high-grade CV is diagnosed.*

CV and Stem Vessel Obliteration

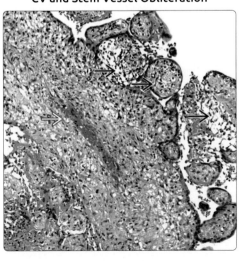

Proximal CV With Stem Vessel Obliteration

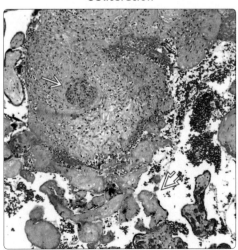

(Left) *Proximal CV with associated stem vessel obliteration is shown. Inflammation involves the distal* ⇘ *and stem villi with vascular involutional changes* ⇨ *evidenced by the disrupted endothelium.* (Right) *There is inflammation of the stem villus with obliteration of the stem vessel* ⇨. *Some of the associated distal villi are avascular* ⇨.

CV With Villous Agglutination

CV With Avascular Villi

(Left) *The villitis can be necrotizing with villous agglutination.* (Right) *CV* ➡ *may have avascular villi* ➡*. The presence of true thrombi suggests an unrelated process of fetal vascular malperfusion.*

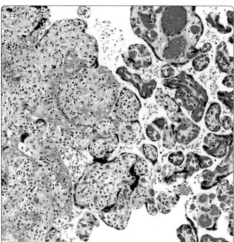

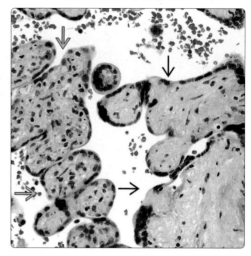

CV With Perivillitis and Eosinophils

Basal CV With Plasma Cell Deciduitis

(Left) *This is an unusual mixed cellular infiltrate of lymphocytes, histiocytes, and eosinophils* ➡ *in the villous and perivillous regions.* (Right) *Plasma cells may extend into foci of basal CV, overlying plasma cell deciduitis. This pattern is not usually associated with CMV infection.*

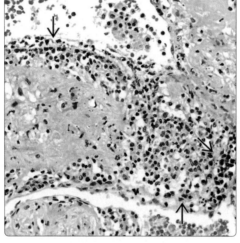

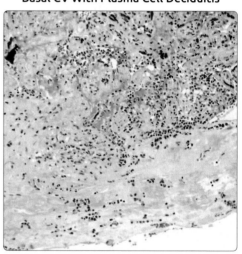

Plasmacytic Villitis and CMV

CV With CMV Immunostain

(Left) *The presence of plasma cells in CV* ➡ *should prompt a search for viral inclusions* ➡*, which are often very rare. There is also hemosiderin* ➡*, which is due to viral involvement of endothelial cells.* (Right) *CMV immunostain highlights infected cells in a villus that contains both nuclear* ➡ *and cytoplasmic* ➡ *inclusions. Viral inclusions may be difficult to identify on hematoxylin & eosin stains alone.*

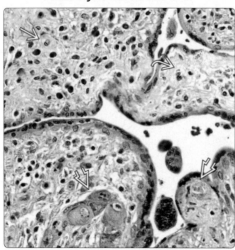

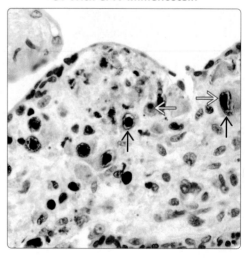

Acute Villitis

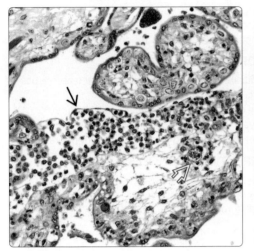

High-Grade CV With Neutrophils

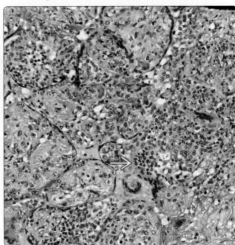

(Left) *This 2nd-trimester placenta shows acute villitis due to intrauterine E. coli sepsis. Neutrophils are first seen just beneath the trophoblast lining ➡. Bacteria can be seen in the villous vessels ➡.* (Right) *In some cases of high-grade CV, there may be a minor component of neutrophils ➡. They are most likely a reaction to the extensive villous injury. Such lesions have also been termed "active" CV.*

Perivillous Fibrin Deposition

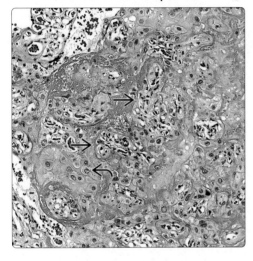

CV With Perivillous Fibrin Deposition

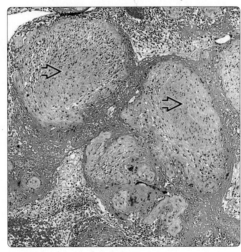

(Left) *Identifying CV in areas of perivillous fibrin deposition can be difficult. These villi ➡ are surrounded by fibrin with focal extravillous trophoblasts ➡. Compression makes the villi appear more cellular, but no CV is identified.* (Right) *This is CV with increased perivillous fibrin. Prolonged damage to the syncytiotrophoblast layer leads to perivillous fibrin deposition. The vessels ➡ of these stem villi are fully obliterated. There is significant perivillitis as well.*

Normal 2nd-Trimester Villi

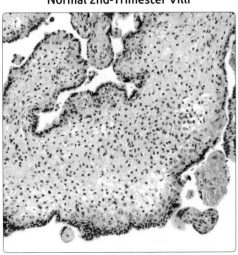

CV

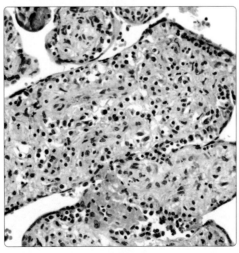

(Left) *Immature villi can have homogeneously cellular stroma that can mimic CV. Also note that the syncytiotrophoblast layer is uniform along the entire villous circumference. CVUE is seen primarily in the 3rd trimester. If in doubt, an immunostain for CD3 shows the presence or absence of T cells.* (Right) *In contrast, the cellularity of the inflamed villus in CV is not evenly distributed, and there is variation in cell size and shape.*

TERMINOLOGY

- Chronic histiocytic intervillositis (CHI): Monomorphic infiltrate of histiocytes (mononuclear phagocytes) in intervillous space; variable amount of perivillous fibrin

ETIOLOGY/PATHOGENESIS

- Aberrant maternal immune response is proposed in CHI
- ~ 20-30% of women with CHI have autoimmune disease (e.g., autoimmune thyroiditis, mixed connective tissue disease, systemic lupus erythematosus) or autoantibodies detected

CLINICAL ISSUES

- Very rare (0.6% of 2nd- or 3rd-trimester placentas); may be higher in 1st-trimester spontaneous abortions, but unknown
- Elevated maternal alkaline phosphatase levels noted in 55% of cases in 1st and 2nd trimester
- High recurrence rate (50-70% at any gestational age)

- History of pregnancy loss with CHI is strongest predictor of future pregnancy loss with CHI
- Intrauterine growth restriction in 80%; correlated with extent of perivillous fibrin deposition

MICROSCOPIC

- Dense infiltrates of histiocytes comprising at least 5% of intervillous space volume
  - Exclude cases with polymorphous infiltrates (<80% histiocytes)
- Associated with increased perivillous fibrin deposition

TOP DIFFERENTIAL DIAGNOSES

- Massive perivillous fibrin deposition
- Placental malaria, other infections
- Chronic villitis with perivillitis

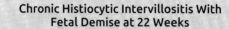

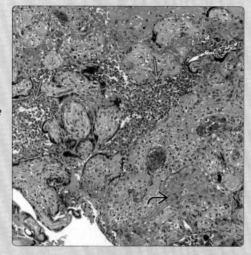

Chronic Histiocytic Intervillositis With Fetal Demise at 22 Weeks

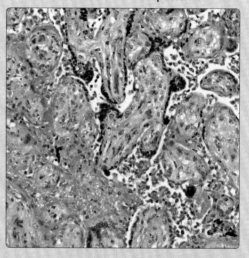

Chronic Histiocytic Intervillositis With Perivillous Fibrin Deposition

(Left) The intervillous space here is effaced by sheets of histiocytes ⊡. Elsewhere, perivillous fibrin accumulates and extravillous trophoblast ⊡ proliferates within the fibrin. (Right) The placenta shown here was delivered at 30-weeks gestation for severe intrauterine growth restriction. The mother has had recurrent pregnancy loss.

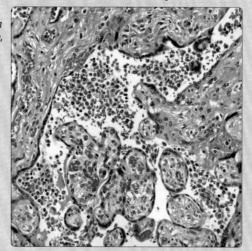

Intervillous Histiocytes

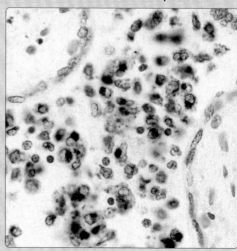

Chronic Intervillositis, CD68

(Left) The intervillous histiocytes can be small with a high nuclear:cytoplasmic ratio, as seen here. The infiltrates are free floating in the intervillous space. (Right) The intervillous cells are positive for histiocytic/macrophage markers, as in this case with CD68.

TERMINOLOGY

Abbreviations
- Chronic histiocytic intervillositis (CHI)
- Chronic villitis (CV)

Synonyms
- Chronic histiocytic intervillositis, massive chronic intervillositis, chronic intervillositis, nonspecific chronic histiocytic intervillositis

Definitions
- CHI
  - Monomorphic infiltrate of histiocytes (mononuclear phagocytes) in intervillous space (> 80% histiocytes) comprising at least 5% of intervillous space
    - Polymorphous infiltrate of histiocytes with neutrophils; lymphocytes and eosinophils are not termed CHI
    - Chronic villitis with perivillitis (usually lymphocytes, histiocytes, and occasional neutrophils) is distinct from CHI
  - Variable association with perivillous fibrin deposition and chronic villitis

ETIOLOGY/PATHOGENESIS

Auto/Alloimmunity
- Aberrant maternal immune response is proposed in CHI
  - ~ 20-30% of women with CHI have autoimmune disease (e.g., autoimmune thyroiditis, mixed connective tissue disease, systemic lupus erythematosus) or autoantibodies detected

CLINICAL ISSUES

Epidemiology
- Incidence
  - Very rare (0.6% of 2nd- or 3rd-trimester placentas); true incidence in 1st-trimester spontaneous abortions unknown

Presentation
- Early and late spontaneous abortion, recurrent pregnancy loss, prematurity, intrauterine growth restriction (IUGR) (80%)
  - Frequent abnormal bleeding in 1st trimester
- Elevated alkaline phosphatase levels have been noted in 55% of cases in 1st and 2nd trimester

Treatment
- Therapies to prevent recurrent pregnancy loss include aspirin, low-molecular weight heparin, prednisone, and hydroxychloroquine
- Combined regimens may be helpful for patients with history of recurrent fetal loss with CHI

Prognosis
- High recurrence rate of 50-70% at any gestational age; recurrences do not necessarily escalate in severity of outcome
- History of pregnancy loss with CHI is strongest predictor of future pregnancy loss with CHI

MACROSCOPIC

General Features
- May see firm, tan-white strands of perivillous fibrin deposition

MICROSCOPIC

Histologic Features
- Dense infiltrates of histiocytes comprising at least 5% of intervillous space volume
  - Has been recognized on chorionic villus sampling
  - May be patchy or diffuse
- Literature varies on how much CV is allowed in diagnosis of CHI

ANCILLARY TESTS

Immunohistochemistry
- Intervillous histiocytes are CD68(+), CD163(+), CD1a(-)

DIFFERENTIAL DIAGNOSIS

Massive Perivillous Fibrin Deposition
- CHI may have intense perivillous fibrin deposition over time with prolonged syncytiotrophoblast injury
- Important to recognize cases of extensive perivillous fibrin deposition that have CHI, as causes of massive perivillous fibrin deposition are diverse

Placental Malaria
- Malaria organisms, hemozoin pigment in maternal red cells and histiocytes
- Infiltrate often histiocyte rich, but polymorphous

Other Infections
- Polymorphous intervillositis seen with *Listeria monocytogenes*, *Campylobacter fetus*, *Francisella tularensis*, and *Coccidioides immitis*
- Histiocyte-rich polymorphous intervillositis with associated perivillous fibrin deposition reported in cases of Coxsackievirus infection

Chronic Villitis With Perivillitis
- Cases of CV with lymphohistiocytic infiltrates tethered to villus surface are not considered CHI

DIAGNOSTIC CHECKLIST

Pathologic Interpretation Pearls
- Chronic histiocytic intervillositis may be focal in early pregnancy loss; important not to miss diagnosis due to potential for recurrent pregnancy loss

SELECTED REFERENCES

1. Bos M et al: Towards standardized criteria for diagnosing chronic intervillositis of unknown etiology: A systematic review. Placenta. 61:80-88, 2018
2. Koby L et al: Chronic histiocytic intervillositis - clinical, biochemical and radiological findings: an observational study. Placenta. 64:1-6, 2018
3. Mekinian A et al: Chronic histiocytic intervillositis: outcome, associated diseases and treatment in a multicenter prospective study. Autoimmunity. 48(1):40-5, 2015
4. Marchaudon V et al: Chronic histiocytic intervillositis of unknown etiology: clinical features in a consecutive series of 69 cases. Placenta. 32(2):140-5, 2011

TERMINOLOGY

- Basal chronic villitis: Chronic inflammation restricted to villi at maternal floor
- Chronic deciduitis: Presence of dense lymphocytic infiltrates, or plasma cells in basal or membranous decidua

CLINICAL ISSUES

- Chronic villitis and chronic deciduitis frequently occur together
  o More frequent in late preterm birth and may be associated with recurrent preterm birth

MICROSCOPIC

- Basal chronic villitis is graded and staged as in other locations
  o Focal (1 slide) or multifocal (> 1 slide), low grade (< 10 villi involved per focus)
  o Patchy (< 30%) or diffuse (> 30%) high grade (> 10 villi per focus)

- Chronic deciduitis defined as ≥ 50 lymphocytes/HPF; some authors require plasma cells
  o Extent: Focal, multifocal, diffuse
  o Severity: Mild, moderate, or severe
  o While scattered lymphocytes are normal in decidua, plasma cells are not normal component; their presence is diagnostic of chronic deciduitis

TOP DIFFERENTIAL DIAGNOSES

- Acute deciduitis, associated with acute chorioamnionitis

DIAGNOSTIC CHECKLIST

- Any plasma cells in basal plate or free membranes consistent with chronic deciduitis
- Lymphoplasmacytic infiltrate in basal chorionic villi may be focal or diffuse
- Look for concurrent basal chronic villitis and chronic deciduitis

Basal Chronic Villitis and Chronic Deciduitis

(Left) *Basal chronic villitis (BCV) involves villi along the maternal floor ➡. Chronic deciduitis (CD) is often present concurrently in the subjacent decidua basalis ➡. (Right) Plasma cells ➡, characterized by their eccentric nucleus and perinuclear hof ➡, are diagnostic for CD in either the basal or membranous decidua. Plasma cells rarely occur alone, as lymphocytes ➡ make up most of the cellularity.*

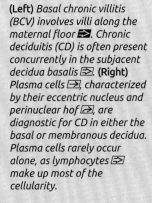
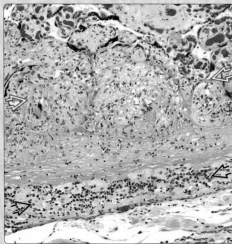

Plasma Cells in Chronic Deciduitis

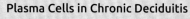
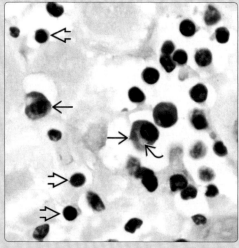

Membranous Decidua

(Left) *Focally increased numbers (> 50) of lymphocytes are present in the membranous decidua of this high-power field with a rare plasma cell ➡. Some authors require plasma cells, as lymphocytes are a normal part of the decidua. (Right) Plasma cell deciduitis ➡ is a reported association with recurrent preterm birth. This case was associated with prematurity and remote retromembranous hemorrhage. There are a few hemosiderin laden macrophages present ➡.*

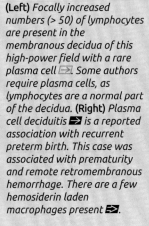
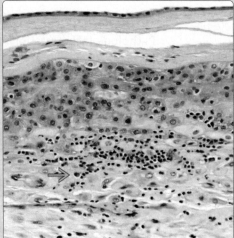

Chronic Deciduitis With Plasma Cells

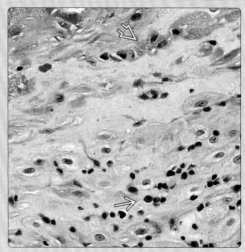

TERMINOLOGY

Definitions

- Basal chronic villitis (BCV)
  - Chronic inflammation restricted to villi at maternal floor
- Chronic deciduitis (CD)
  - Presence of plasma cells, or dense lymphoid infiltrates (≥ 50 lymphocytes/HPF) in decidua basalis or membranous decidua

ETIOLOGY/PATHOGENESIS

Infectious Agents

- Possible association of plasma cell deciduitis with subclinical chronic infection of endometrium
  - *Mycoplasma hominis*, *Ureaplasma urealyticum*, *Streptococcus agalactiae*, and *Chlamydia trachomatis*
- Relationship of CD to chronic endometritis is not defined

Abnormal Maternal Alloimmune Response

- BCV may be alloimmune response of maternal lymphocytes to fetal antigens; graft-vs.-host reaction
  - Basal plate represents unique site where maternal and fetal cells interface without syncytiotrophoblast
  - Immune status in basal plate may be perturbed in preeclampsia and placenta accreta
- Function of plasma cells in CD is unknown

CLINICAL ISSUES

Presentation

- BCV
  - Common finding in term placenta, increased incidence in preeclampsia, intrauterine growth restriction (IUGR), and preterm delivery
  - Seen at least focally in nearly all cases of placenta accreta
  - Associated with neonatal alloimmune thrombocytopenia
- CD
  - Recognized in 1-2% of 3rd-trimester placentas
    - Incidence varies depending upon definition used (± plasma cells)
  - In ~ 10% of placentas from spontaneous abortions and preterm deliveries
  - In ~ 40% of cases of preterm labor without chorioamnionitis
  - Increased in pregnancies utilizing donor eggs (completely allogeneic fetus)
    - Also associated with chronic villitis, chronic intervillositis, and plasma cells
    - Increased numbers of T helper cells, natural killer cells, and macrophages
  - Associated with maternal autoimmune disorders
  - Associated with intrauterine fetal demise, prematurity, IUGR, admission to neonatal intensive care unit

Prognosis

- Both BCV and CD can recur in subsequent pregnancies
- Neurologic abnormalities have been associated with BCV and CD, but this may only be related to prematurity

MACROSCOPIC

Gross Examination

- BCV and CD when severe may show mild thickening of maternal surface of disc

MICROSCOPIC

Histologic Features

- BCV
  - Lymphocytic and histiocytic inflammation of basal and anchoring villi
  - Rarely plasma cells infiltrate into basal villi from basal decidua
  - Commonly associated with non-BCV and CD
  - Graded according to Amsterdam consensus criteria as is CVUE in other locations
    - Focal (1 slide) or multifocal (> 1 slide), low grade (< 10 villi involved per focus)
    - Patchy (< 30%) or diffuse (> 30%) high grade (> 10 villi per focus)
- CD
  - Defined as ≥ 50 lymphocytes/HPF on at least 1 slide; some authors require plasma cells
    - Suggested scoring criteria
      - □ Extent: Focal-1, multifocal-2, or diffuse-3
      - □ Severity: Mild-1, moderate-2, severe-3
    - Presence of plasma cells defines plasma cell deciduitis
  - Chronic inflammation of membranous decidua, even when severe, rarely includes plasma cells
  - Chronic inflammation of decidua basalis when severe, usually includes plasma cells

DIFFERENTIAL DIAGNOSIS

Acute Deciduitis

- Mimics CD on low power
- Neutrophils are abundant, contain multilobated nuclei, and are often associated with necrosis and karyorrhectic debris and acute chorioamnionitis

Herpes Simplex Virus, CMV, and Syphilis Infections

- Lymphoplasmacytic deciduitis with numerous plasma cells
- May see necrosis of amnion, chorion, and villi

SELECTED REFERENCES

1. Dubruc E et al: Placental histological lesions in fetal and neonatal alloimmune thrombocytopenia: a retrospective cohort study of 21 cases. Placenta. 48:104-109, 2016
2. Ernst LM et al: Placental pathologic associations with morbidly adherent placenta: potential insights into pathogenesis. Pediatr Dev Pathol. ePub, 2016
3. Khong TY et al: Sampling and definitions of placental lesions: Amsterdam placental workshop group consensus statement. Arch Pathol Lab Med. 140(7):698-713, 2016
4. Katzman PJ: Chronic inflammatory lesions of the placenta. Semin Perinatol. 39(1):20-6, 2015
5. Kim CJ et al: Chronic inflammation of the placenta: definition, classification, pathogenesis, and clinical significance. Am J Obstet Gynecol. 213(4 Suppl):S53-69, 2015

Normal Basal Plate With Anchoring Villus

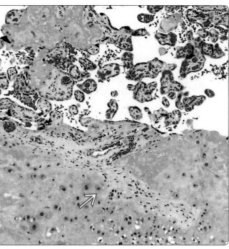

Basal Chronic Villitis

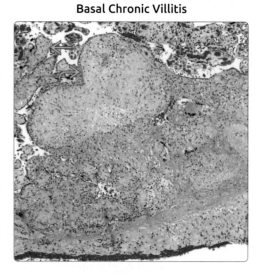

(Left) *Anchoring villi ➡ are surrounded by extravillous trophoblast and fibrinoid. Immunomodulatory syncytiotrophoblast are not present at this maternal/fetal interface. This may be why basal villi are more often involved by the maternal T-cell infiltrates of CVUE. Once inside anchoring villi, T cells can spread along the villous stroma.* **(Right)** *This large aggregate of inflamed villi is a focus of high-grade BCV. When stem villi are involved ➡, adjacent downstream villi may become avascular ➡.*

Basal Chronic Villitis and Chronic Deciduitis

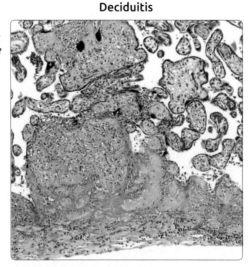

Basal Chronic Villitis With Giant Cells

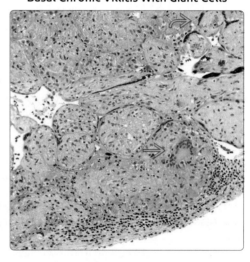

(Left) *This preterm placenta had band-like near contiguous involvement of the basal plate by chronic inflammation (BCV and CD).* **(Right)** *This slide of BCV shows a focal Langhans giant cell ➡. Note the CD deep to the villus. Adjacent villi ➡ are becoming avascular. CVUE with many giant cells should raise consideration for Toxoplasma infection.*

Basal Chronic Villitis, Chronic Deciduitis With Intervillous Fibrin

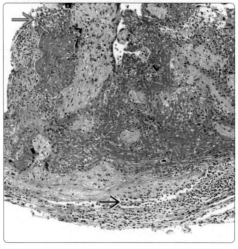

Concurrent Basal Chronic Villitis and Chronic Deciduitis

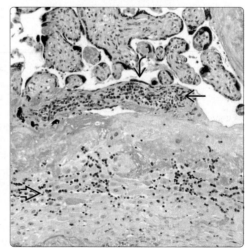

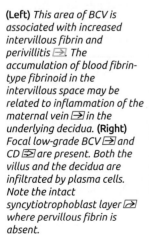

(Left) *This area of BCV is associated with increased intervillous fibrin and perivillitis ➡. The accumulation of blood fibrin-type fibrinoid in the intervillous space may be related to inflammation of the maternal vein ➡ in the underlying decidua.* **(Right)** *Focal low-grade BCV ➡ and CD ➡ are present. Both the villus and the decidua are infiltrated by plasma cells. Note the intact syncytiotrophoblast layer ➡ where pervillous fibrin is absent.*

Basal Chronic Villitis With Plasma Cells

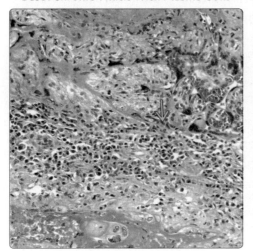

Placenta Accreta With Basal Chronic Villitis

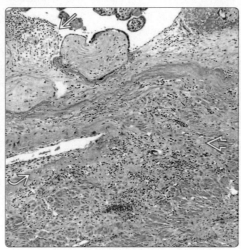

(Left) *Plasma cell villitis* ➡ *raises concern for infection, especially CMV. Stains are usually negative when limited to BCV with plasma cell deciduitis.* (Right) *Placenta accreta is almost always associated with chronic inflammation. In this case, there is BCV* ➡ *and extensive chronic inflammation is in the myometrium* ➡. *One maternal spiral artery has subendothelial lymphocytes* ➡. *Maternal vasculopathy is also often seen in accreta.*

Plasma Cell Deciduitis in Membranes

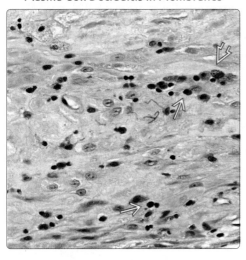

Large Plasma Cell Infiltrate in Chronic Deciduitis

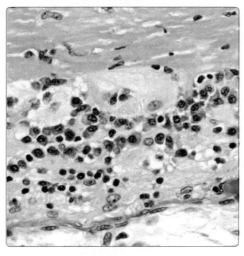

(Left) *Compared to the more dense infiltrates seen in the decidua basalis, plasma cell infiltrates in the membranous decidua tend to be sparse* ➡. *This case also had significant remote retromembranous hemorrhage with hemosiderin-laden macrophages* ➡. (Right) *Occasionally, large numbers of plasma cells are present in CD, which can be seen easily at low power. This focus has admixed eosinophils.*

Eosinophils in Chronic Deciduitis

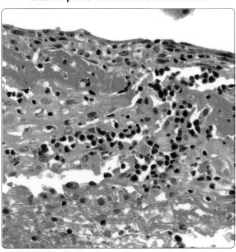

Granulomatous Chronic Deciduitis in Membranes

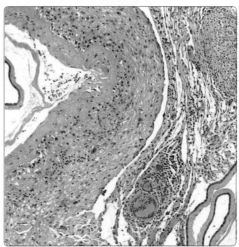

(Left) *The decidua basalis of this case had eosinophils accompanying the lymphoid infiltrates, an uncommon finding.* (Right) *In this case, granulomas are localized to the deep decidua. AFB and GMS stains are warranted to rule out infection. Rarely Enterobius vermicularis (pinworm) infection can involve the endometrium.*

Chronic Chorioamnionitis and Chorionic Histiocytic Hyperplasia

TERMINOLOGY

- Chronic chorioamnionitis (CCA): Lymphoid infiltrate centered on extravillous trophoblast of extraplacental membranes
- Chronic histiocytic hyperplasia (CHH): Diffuse lichenoid infiltrate of spindled histiocytes in deep chorionic plate

ETIOLOGY/PATHOGENESIS

- CCA is attributed to maternal alloimmune response; lymphocytes are of maternal origin
  - Rare cases of CCA associated with HSV, CMV, and syphilis
- CHH is reactive process where fetal histiocytes are predominant cell population, often in setting of chronic villitis

CLINICAL ISSUES

- CCA is associated with preterm premature rupture of membranes (PPROM) and preterm labor (PTL), intrauterine growth restriction (IUGR), and spontaneous abortion

- Most frequent pathologic change in late preterm birth

MICROSCOPIC

- CCA
  - Predominantly CD3(+) lymphocytic infiltrate centered on cellular chorion of membranes
  - Grade 1 = patchy, grade 2 = diffuse; stage 1 = confined to cellular chorion, stage 2 = above cellular chorion
- CHH
  - CD68(+) and vimentin (+) histiocytes, diffuse infiltrate in deep chorionic plate, rarely involves free membranes

DIAGNOSTIC CHECKLIST

- Chronic chorioamnionitis often presents concurrently with chronic villitis elsewhere in placenta
- Do not mistake lymphocytic aggregates in decidua for chronic chorioamnionitis

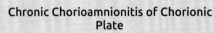

Chronic Chorioamnionitis of Chorionic Plate

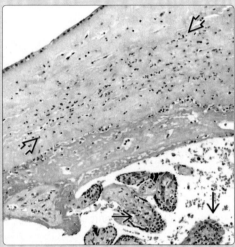

Chronic Chorioamnionitis: CD3

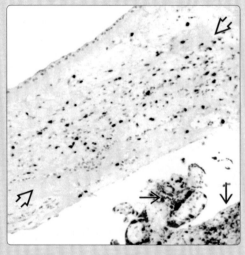

(Left) *Chronic chorioamnionitis may involve the extraplacental membranes or chorionic plate. The infiltrate is predominantly lymphoid, with fewer numbers of histiocytes ➡. It is uncommon for the lymphocytes to extend into the amnion, as is seen here. Chronic villitis is also present ➡.* (Right) *CD3 immunostain of the same area highlights the T-cell infiltrate in the chorionic plate ➡ and subchorionic villi ➡.*

Chronic Inflammation of Chorionic Plate

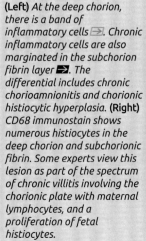
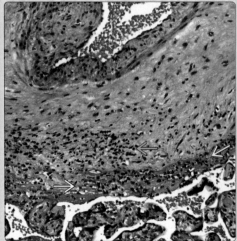

Chronic Histiocytic Hyperplasia

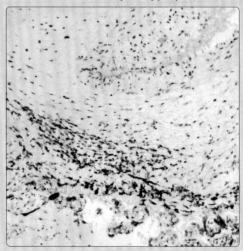

(Left) *At the deep chorion, there is a band of inflammatory cells ➡. Chronic inflammatory cells are also marginated in the subchorion fibrin layer ➡. The differential includes chronic chorioamnionitis and chorionic histiocytic hyperplasia.* (Right) *CD68 immunostain shows numerous histiocytes in the deep chorion and subchorionic fibrin. Some experts view this lesion as part of the spectrum of chronic villitis involving the chorionic plate with maternal lymphocytes, and a proliferation of fetal histiocytes.*

Chronic Chorioamnionitis and Chorionic Histiocytic Hyperplasia

TERMINOLOGY

Definitions

- Chronic chorioamnionitis (CCA)
  - Lymphocytic infiltrate centered on chorionic extravillous trophoblast cells
  - May involve chorionic plate, usually with chronic villitis of unknown etiology (CVUE)
- Chorionic histiocytic hyperplasia (CHH)
  - Spindled histiocytes in deep chorionic plate, less common in free membranes
- Subacute necrotizing chorioamnionitis
  - Infiltrate of rare histiocytes and lymphocytes in chorion in cases of longstanding amniotic fluid infection, associated with necrotizing chorioamnionitis

ETIOLOGY/PATHOGENESIS

Chronic Chorioamnionitis

- Infection
  - May be seen with ascending herpes simplex virus (HSV), cytomegalovirus (CMV), or syphilis
- Maternal alloimmune reaction
  - Infiltrating lymphocytes are of maternal origin
  - Often associated with chronic villitis and chronic deciduitis

Chorionic Histiocytic Hyperplasia

- Unknown etiology
- Histiocytes are of fetal origin, suggesting reactive process
- Increased incidence of meconium (41%)
- Often associated with chronic villitis, chronic deciduitis, or chronic chorioamnionitis

CLINICAL ISSUES

Epidemiology

- Chronic chorioamnionitis
  - Present in 14% of term and 39% of preterm placentas
- Chorionic histiocytic hyperplasia
  - Occurs in 1.3% of 3rd-trimester placentas
- CCA and CHH may occur together

Presentation

- CCA is associated with preterm premature rupture of membranes (PPROM) and preterm labor (PTL), intrauterine growth restriction (IUGR), and spontaneous abortion
  - Most frequent pathologic change in late preterm birth
- CHH is seen more commonly in late 3rd trimester

Prognosis

- CCA can be recurrent in subsequent pregnancies

MICROSCOPIC

Histologic Features

- Chronic chorioamnionitis
  - Maternal chronic inflammatory infiltrate
    - Lymphoid infiltrates in extraplacental membranes centered on cellular chorion (extravillous trophoblast cells) often associated with trophoblast cell dropout
    - Unlike maternal neutrophils in amniotic fluid infection, lymphocytes rarely reach amnion

- CD3 staining confirms T-cell lineage, usually not necessary for diagnosis
  - Grading and staging system
    - Grade 0: No inflammation or only single small focus
    - Grade 1: Patchy inflammation involving > 2 foci
    - Grade 2: Diffuse inflammation
    - Stage 1: Infiltrate confined to cellular chorion (chorionic extravillous trophoblast cells)
    - Stage 2: Infiltrate extends above cellular chorion into chorioamnionic connective tissue layers
  - Associated with chronic villitis (30-40%) and chronic deciduitis (14-25%)
  - Rare cases will contain predominant plasma cell infiltrate (rule out infection), may have granulomatous component
- Chorionic histiocytic hyperplasia
  - Diffuse lichenoid infiltrate of spindled histiocytes in deep chorionic plate, less commonly involves free membranes
  - Cells are CD68(+) and vimentin (+) histiocytes
  - Associated with chronic villitis (67%), chronic deciduitis (40%), and chronic chorioamnionitis (31%)

ANCILLARY TESTS

Immunohistochemistry

- CD3 will confirm presence of diagnostic T lymphocytes
- CD68 and vimentin stain will identify histiocytes

DIFFERENTIAL DIAGNOSIS

Acute Chorioamnionitis

- Maternal neutrophils extend from decidual vessels or intervillous space into chorion and amnion
- Mixed acute and chronic chorioamnionitis implies chronicity of amniotic fluid infection, as in subacute necrotizing chorioamnionitis

Chronic Deciduitis

- Dense lymphoid infiltrates or lymphocytes with plasma cells in membranous decidua, sparing trophoblast cells of cellular chorion

DIAGNOSTIC CHECKLIST

Pathologic Interpretation Pearls

- Chronic chorioamnionitis is often present concurrently with chronic villitis and chronic deciduitis elsewhere in placenta
- Most cases are not associated with recognizable infection

SELECTED REFERENCES

1. Katzman PJ et al: Chorionic histiocytic hyperplasia is associated with chronic inflammatory lesions in the placenta. Pediatr Dev Pathol. 20(3):197-205, 2017
2. Lee J et al: Chronic chorioamnionitis is the most common placental lesion in late preterm birth. Placenta. 34(8):681-9, 2013
3. Lee J et al: A signature of maternal anti-fetal rejection in spontaneous preterm birth: chronic chorioamnionitis, anti-human leukocyte antigen antibodies, and C4d. PLoS One. 6(2):e16806, 2011
4. Kim CJ et al: The frequency, clinical significance, and pathological features of chronic chorioamnionitis: a lesion associated with spontaneous preterm birth. Mod Pathol. 23(7):1000-11, 2010
5. Jacques SM et al: Chronic chorioamnionitis: a clinicopathologic and immunohistochemical study. Hum Pathol. 29(12):1457-61, 1998
6. Gersell DJ et al: Chronic chorioamnionitis: a clinicopathologic study of 17 cases. Int J Gynecol Pathol. 10(3):217-29, 1991

(Left) *In the normal free membranes, there is often a mild lymphocytic infiltrate in the decidua* ⇥ *but not in the amnion* ⇥*, fibroblastic chorion* ⇥*, or chorion laeve* ⇥*. (Right) This dense lymphocytic infiltrate is centered on the extravillous trophoblast layer* ⇥ *of the cellular chorion. The infiltrate was diffusely present in the membranes (grade 2), but limited to the cellular chorion (stage 1). The lichenoid infiltrate with dropout of extravillous trophoblast is similar to a graft-vs.-host reaction seen in the skin.*

Normal Free Membranes

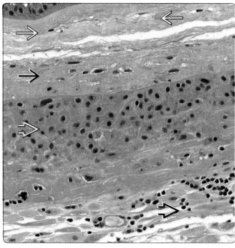

Chronic Chorioamnionitis

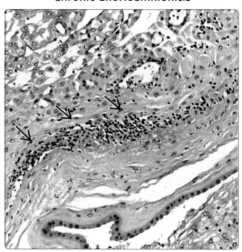

(Left) *These membranes were delivered with a 31-weeks-gestation placenta, showing grade 1, stage 2 inflammation. Multifocal low-grade basal chronic villitis was also present in the placenta.* **(Right)** *This image demonstrates both acute chorionitis* ⇥ *on the amniotic side of the cellular chorion and chronic chorionitis, with a band-like infiltrate of mononuclear cells beneath the cellular chorion. There is focal necrosis of trophoblasts* ⇥*.*

Chronic Chorioamnionitis

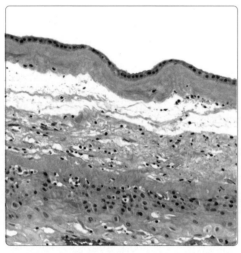

Mixed AC and CC in Free Membranes

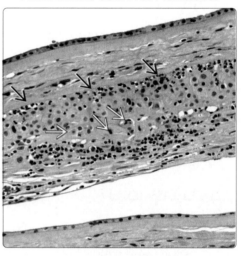

(Left) *Most of the inflammation is in the amnion and shows significant degeneration* ⇥*. There are lymphocytes and macrophages within the chorionic plate* ⇥*. If the amnion were stripped off of the section, this could be mistaken for CCA or diffuse histiocytic hyperplasia.* **(Right)** *Ascending HSV infection is associated with chronic inflammation* ⇥ *in the membranes. Viral inclusions are hypereosinophilic and infected cells appear necrotic* ⇥*.*

Subacute Necrotizing Chorioamnionitis

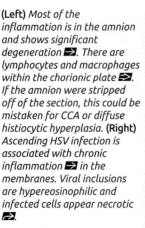

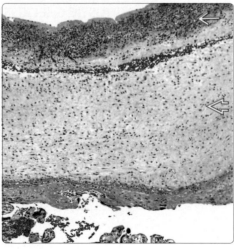

HSV Infection With Chronic Chorioamnionitis

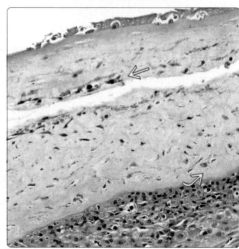

Chorionic Histiocytic Hyperplasia in Chorionic Plate

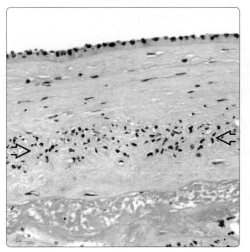

Chronic Histiocytic Hyperplasia With a Few CD3(+) Lymphocytes

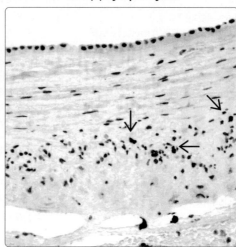

(Left) A lichenoid pattern of chronic inflammatory cells ⇾ are described in chorionic histiocytic hyperplasia. The cells do not resemble the usual chorionic trophoblast population or lymphocytes. (Right) CD3 immunostain shows only a few positive T cells ⇾ in the chorion, while most of the cells are negative.

Chorionic Histiocytic Hyperplasia

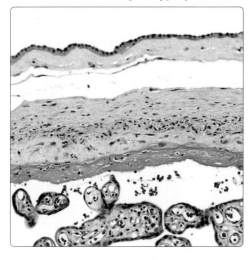

Chorionic Histiocytic Hyperplasia: CD3

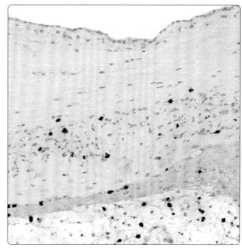

(Left) Lichenoid band of cells is present in the deep chorionic plate. Note the paucity of extravillous trophoblast. (Right) A minor component of the inflammatory infiltrate is CD3(+) T cells.

Histiocytic Hyperplasia: CD68

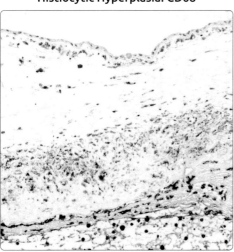

Chorionic Histiocytic Hyperplasia

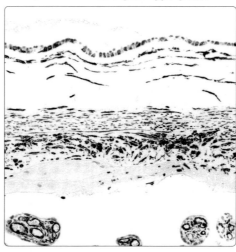

(Left) The majority of the cells in the infiltrate are CD68(+) histiocytes/macrophages. (Right) The increased cellularity in the chorionic plate is vimentin positive.

ETIOLOGY/PATHOGENESIS

- Eosinophilic/T-cell chorionic vasculitis (ETCV)
  - Inflammation of chorionic plate vessel with mixture of T cells and eosinophils
  - Most are 3rd trimester, > 35 weeks
- Inflammatory process vs. thrombotic process
  - Thrombus seen in many cases of ETCV may be response to inflammation
- Lymphocytes and eosinophils are of fetal origin
- ETCV has not been associated with
  - Infection
  - any particular maternal or fetal condition
  - adverse outcome
- ETCV is rare lesion (< 0.2% incidence) when compared to acute chorionic vasculitis, seen in fetal acute inflammatory response

MICROSCOPIC

- Usually involves single chorionic plate vessel, may be multiple
- In most cases, inflammation is oriented in vessel toward intervillous space
  - Inflammation can be oriented to one side or other and in some cases; it is circumferential
- Fetal T cells and eosinophils are major inflammatory components, although eosinophils may be sparse
- Cushion lesions and thrombus may be present in vessel affected by ETCV
- Chronic villitis often seen elsewhere in placenta
- ETCV can affect only one or both twin placentas, whether dichorionic or monochorionic

TOP DIFFERENTIAL DIAGNOSES

- Amniotic fluid infection sequence with acute chorionic vasculitis
- Fetal thrombotic vasculopathy

ETCV With Circumferential Inflammation and Thrombus

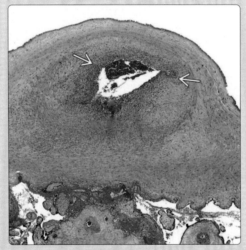

ETCV With Thrombus

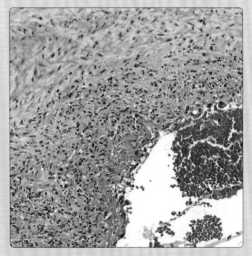

(Left) *This chorionic plate vessel has as much inflammation on the placental side as on the amnion side of the vessel. There is a thin fibrin thrombus ➡ covering much of the endothelium.* (Right) *A higher magnification of the vessel shows thrombus overlying the inflamed portion of the vessel wall. Eosinophils are inconspicuous in this field.*

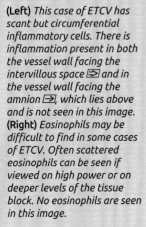

ETCV With Circumferential Inflammation

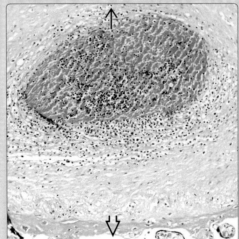

Lymphocytes in ETCV

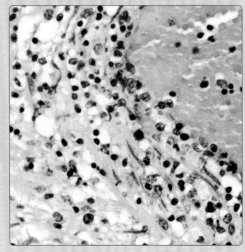

(Left) *This case of ETCV has scant but circumferential inflammatory cells. There is inflammation present in both the vessel wall facing the intervillous space ➡ and in the vessel wall facing the amnion ➡, which lies above and is not seen in this image.* (Right) *Eosinophils may be difficult to find in some cases of ETCV. Often scattered eosinophils can be seen if viewed on high power or on deeper levels of the tissue block. No eosinophils are seen in this image.*

TERMINOLOGY

Abbreviations

- Eosinophilic/T-cell chorionic vasculitis (ETCV)

ETIOLOGY/PATHOGENESIS

Inflammatory vs. Thrombotic

- Many cases have thrombus in vessel affected by ETCV
  - Inflammation may be reaction to thrombus
  - Or thrombus may be reaction to inflammation
- Inflammatory cells are of fetal origin, suggesting fetal reaction to unknown stimulus
- ETCV has not been associated with infection

Alloimmunity

- Chronic villitis of unknown etiology (CVUE) present in many cases of ETCV

Environmental

- In monozygotic and dizygotic twin pregnancies, ETCV is seen preferentially in 1 of 2 twin placentas, suggesting nongenetic stimulus

CLINICAL ISSUES

Epidemiology

- Incidence
  - Uncommon lesion, < 0.2% of placentas

Presentation

- No known clinical presentation or associations
- No known adverse neonatal outcome
- Most are 3rd trimester, > 35 weeks

MICROSCOPIC

Histologic Features

- Eosinophilic and T-cell infiltrate present in chorionic vessel wall, usually toward intervillous space
  - Infiltrate can be oriented toward amniotic cavity or circumferential
  - ETCV usually affects only 1 chorionic vessel in any given case
  - Inflammatory cells in ETCV are of fetal origin
- Rarely similar features are seen in stem vessels and even umbilical cord vessels
- Eosinophils can be sparse and T cells may predominate
  - Regulatory T cells are component of lymphocytic infiltrate in ETCV
    - Role of regulatory T cells unclear in ETCV, but they are known to modulate immune response
  - Role of eosinophils in ETCV is unclear but likely recruited by cytokines released by lymphocytes
- 25-42% of ETCV have thrombus in affected vessel
  - Usually small, nonocclusive
  - Less common in very mild infiltrates of ETCV
- Chronic villitis accompanies ETCV in 32-43% of cases
- Chronic deciduitis and chronic chorioamnionitis may also accompany ETCV

ANCILLARY TESTS

Immunohistochemistry

- CD3 T-cell immunostain helpful to confirm presence of lymphocytes in vessel wall and will also identify concurrent chronic villitis
- Subset of CD3(+) T cells, regulatory T cells, FOXP3(+), and CD25(+) are present

DIFFERENTIAL DIAGNOSIS

Amniotic Fluid Infection Sequence With Acute Chorionic Vasculitis

- Most of neutrophils are in wall of vessel facing amniotic cavity, amniotropic
- Eosinophils can be minor component of inflammation in acute chorionic vasculitis
  - Preterm fetus may have limited pool of myeloid cells; eosinophils act more like acute reaction

Fetal Thrombotic Vasculopathy

- True thrombi in chorionic vessel affected by ETCV should prompt search for other features of fetal thrombotic vasculopathy, including avascular villi and villous stromal karyorrhexis

Viral Infection

- Rarely transplacental or ascending HSV infection associated with lymphocytic or lymphoplasmacytic chorionic plate vasculitis

DIAGNOSTIC CHECKLIST

Pathologic Interpretation Pearls

- Inflamed fetal chorionic plate vessels may be either ETCV or acute vasculitis
  - Eosinophils can be present in both
  - Both changes can be concurrent
- Inflammation in ETCV may be circumferential or on placental side of vessel
- Acute vasculitis associated with chorioamnionitis is amniotropic, on amnion side
- Both may be associated with fibrin thrombi

SELECTED REFERENCES

1. Cheek B et al: Eosinophilic/T-cell chorionic vasculitis: histological and clinical correlations. Fetal Pediatr Pathol. 34(2):73-9, 2015
2. Katzman PJ et al: Identification of fetal inflammatory cells in eosinophilic/T-cell chorionic vasculitis using fluorescent in situ hybridization. Pediatr Dev Pathol. 18(4):305-9, 2015
3. Katzman PJ et al: Eosinophilic/T-cell chorionic vasculitis and chronic villitis involve regulatory T cells and often occur together. Pediatr Dev Pathol. 16(4):278-91, 2013
4. Jacques SM et al: Eosinophilic/T-cell chorionic vasculitis: a clinicopathologic and immunohistochemical study of 51 cases. Pediatr Dev Pathol. 14(3):198-205, 2011
5. Jaiman S et al: Eosinophilic/T-cell chorionic vasculitis and intrauterine fetal demise at 34 weeks: case report and review of the literature. Pediatr Dev Pathol. 13(5):393-6, 2010
6. Fraser RB et al: Eosinophilic/T-cell chorionic vasculitis. Pediatr Dev Pathol. 5(4):350-5, 2002
7. Nohr EW et al. Discordance of twin placentas for multifocal eosinophilic/T-cell chorionic vasculitis. Pediatr Develop Pathol. accepted for publication

(Left) *This large cushion lesion has fibrinoid necrosis on the surface and very minimal lymphocytic and eosinophilic inflammation on the surface of the cushion.* **(Right)** *There are a few lymphocytes ➡ and eosinophils ⮕ overlying the fibrinoid necrosis on this cushion lesion.*

Cushion Lesion With ETCV

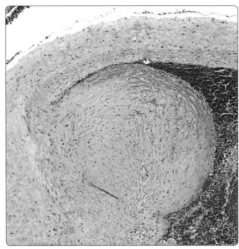

Cushion Lesion With Minimal Inflammation

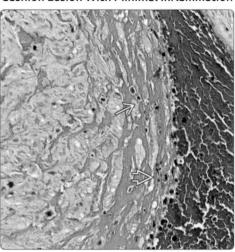

(Left) *Eosinophils can vary from very few to prominent, as in this case.* **(Right)** *CD3 immunostain highlights the T-cell infiltrate in this case of ETCV.*

ETCV With Abundant Eosinophils

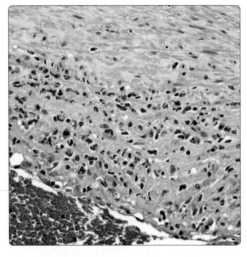

ETCV T Cells, CD3

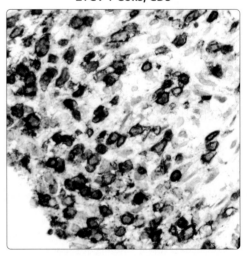

(Left) *A subset of lymphocytes in ETCV are CD25(+), consistent with regulatory T cells. The role of the regulatory T cells in ETCV is unknown, but they are also present in larger numbers in chronic villitis, a lesion often seen concurrently with ETCV.* **(Right)** *A double immunostain of CD3 (brown) ➡ and FOXP3 (blue) ⮕ highlights a subset of regulatory T cells within the lymphocytic infiltrate.*

ETCV With CD25(+) T Cells

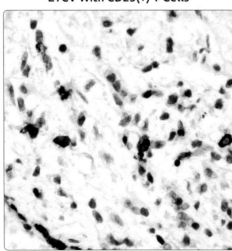

ETCV CD3 and FOXP3 Staining

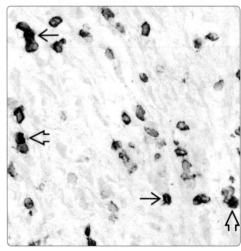

Sparse Infiltrate in ETCV

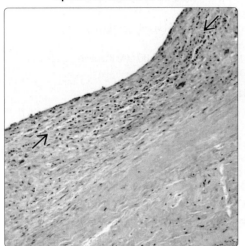

CD3 T Cells in ETCV

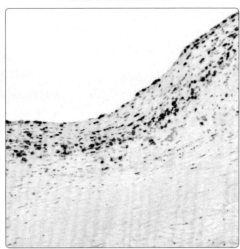

(Left) *Some cases of ETCV have very sparse infiltrates ⇨. Eosinophils may be rare. This could be easily overlooked on low-power examination.* **(Right)** *A CD3 immunostain highlights the presence of lymphocytes in this case.*

Circumferential Inflammation in ETCV

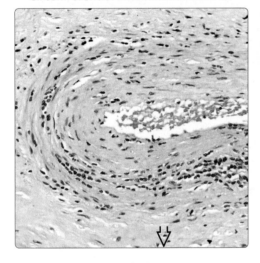

Abundant Eosinophils in ETCV

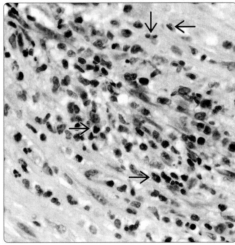

(Left) *Perivascular lymphocytic and eosinophilic inflammation is distributed around this chorionic vessel but is largely concentrated in the vessel wall facing the intervillous space ⇨, out of view on this section.* **(Right)** *In other cases of ETCV, eosinophils ⇨ are abundant and intermixed with lymphocytes. Their role in ETCV is not clear, but they are likely attracted by cytokines released by lymphocytes.*

Acute Vasculitis With Amniotropic Infiltrate

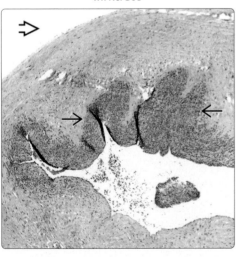

Acute Vasculitis With Eosinophils

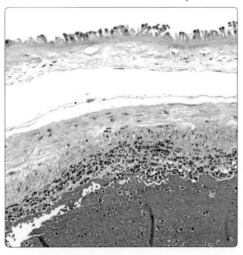

(Left) *In contrast to ETCV, the acute inflammatory infiltrate in acute chorionic vasculitis ⇨ is mainly amniotropic, located in the vessel wall adjacent to the amniotic cavity ⇨.* **(Right)** *A chorionic plate vessel with acute vasculitis that also has a large number of eosinophils is shown. This is associated with prematurity due to the limited pool of myeloid cells and group B Streptococcus infection, for unknown reasons.*

KEY FACTS

TERMINOLOGY

- Massive perivillous fibrin deposition (MPVFD) and maternal floor infarction (MFI) have often been used interchangeably
- Diagnosis of MPVFD requires 50% of parenchyma to be involved on gross exam &/or slides
  - Perivillous fibrin extending from maternal to fetal surface and encasing ≥ 50% of villi on ≥ 1 slide or grossly involving ≥ 50% of parenchyma
- Diagnosis of MFI requires at least 25% of basal plate involved on gross exam
  - Basal villi of entire maternal floor encased by fibrin ≥ 3 mm thick on ≥ 1 slide, or gross involvement of basal plate, measuring 0.3-2.0 cm thick
- Lesser amounts of perivillous fibrin may be called borderline MPVFD, unclear clinical significance
  - Involvement of 25-50% of villi on ≥ 1 slide in transmural or nearly transmural distribution, mild > 5% but < 20% of total villi involved

ETIOLOGY/PATHOGENESIS

- MPVFD may be endstage of several different disorders of pregnancy
- Several mechanisms of formation of abnormal perivillous fibrin have been proposed, including strong association with auto-/alloimmune disorders and thrombophilia
- Any mechanism leading to excessive syncytiotrophoblast injury may cause perivillous fibrin deposition

CLINICAL ISSUES

- Rare placental lesion with incidence between 0.028-0.500% of placentas
- High recurrence rates of 12-78%
- Poor obstetrical and neonatal outcomes common

MACROSCOPIC

- Diffusely distributed pattern of firm, tan-white, vertically oriented trabeculae and lattice-like appearance extending to chorionic plate (MPVFD)
  - Involving ≥ 50% of parenchyma

  - Associated with chorionic cysts, septal cysts, and intervillous thrombi
- Dense, firm placenta with basally located "orange rind" of fibrin (MFI)
  - Thick layer of fibrin (0.03-2.00 cm) involving ≥ 25% of maternal surface

MICROSCOPIC

- Chorionic villi encased in amorphous, eosinophilic fibrin that obliterates intervillous space
- Chronic lesions may have proliferation of extravillous trophoblasts
- Villi show spectrum of changes from atrophy of syncytiotrophoblast to frank avascularity
- Decidual arteriopathy not typically present in MPVFD

TOP DIFFERENTIAL DIAGNOSES

- Ischemic infarction of chorionic villi
- Chronic histiocytic intervillositis with increased perivillous fibrin deposition
- Extensive chronic villitis with increased perivillous fibrin deposition
- Increased perivillous fibrin deposition or localized perivillous fibrin deposition not meeting gross threshold for involvement

REPORTING

- Avoid use of gross terms, such as "fibrotic" or "infarcted" parenchyma
- Describe pattern of parenchymal involvement (predominantly basal, transmural, or irregular)
- Describe amount of maternal surface and parenchymal involvement
- MPVFD terminology used for transmural involvement, MFI for predominantly basal involvement
- Include comment about high risk of recurrence

Gross Appearance of MPVFD

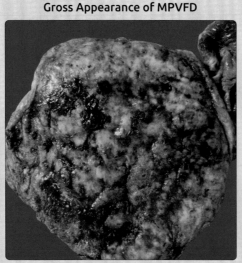

Gross Appearance of MPVFD

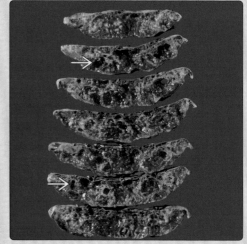

(Left) *The maternal surface may show diffuse, yellow-tan discoloration and thickening in massive perivillous fibrin deposition (MPVFD)/maternal floor infarction (MFI). The individual cotyledons lose their demarcation.* (Right) *Cut sections of placenta with MPVFD show vertically oriented, firm trabeculae and a lattice-like deposition of fibrin. Intervillous thrombi are also seen* ➔.

TERMINOLOGY

Abbreviations

- Massive perivillous fibrin deposition (MPVFD)
- Maternal floor infarction (MFI)

Synonyms

- MPVFD and MFI often used interchangeably
  o May represent spectrum of same disease process
- "Gitterinfarkt" another older term used to describe MPVFD

Definitions

- MPVFD
  o Excessive fibrin deposition entrapping villi and completely obliterating intervillous space, grossly involving ≥ 50% of parenchyma
  o Involves but not necessarily confined to basal plate
  o Perivillous fibrin deposition extends vertically toward chorionic plate
- MFI
  o Gross finding of rind-like, yellow thickening of basal, maternal surface, measuring 0.5-2.0 cm in thickness, involving ≥ 25% of basal plate
  o Basal villi encased in excessive fibrin deposition
  o "Infarct" is misnomer since deposition of fibrin and villous injury does not display pattern seen in ischemic injury
- Proposed microscopic diagnostic terminology may be misleading if sections specifically taken from focal lesions
  o Transmural MPVFD
    – Perivillous fibrin extending from maternal to fetal surface and encasing ≥ 50% of villi on ≥ 1 slide
  o Borderline MPVFD
    – Involvement of 25-50% of villi on ≥ 1 slide in transmural or nearly transmural distribution
    – Mild has been described as > 5% but < 20% of terminal villi
  o Classic MFI
    – Basal villi of entire maternal floor encased by fibrinoid ≥ 3 mm thick on ≥ 1 slide

Fibrin vs. Fibrinoid

- Both terms frequently used interchangeably in literature
  o Fibrin of MPVFD includes mixture of 2 types
    – Fibrin-like fibrinoid; combination of maternal and fetal serum fibrin, cellular fibronectin, and other molecules derived from blood clotting
    – Matrix-type fibrinoid; trophoblast-derived extracellular matrix product, includes oncofetal fibronectin, basement membrane collagen IV, laminin and supports X-cell proliferation

ETIOLOGY/PATHOGENESIS

Etiology

- Uncertain if MPVFD single entity or endstage of several different disorders of pregnancy
- Several mechanisms of formation of abnormal perivillous fibrin have been proposed
  o Maternal blood flow abnormalities
    – Stasis of blood in intervillous space
    – Inadequate drainage of intervillous space

    – Increase in intervillous thrombi/hematomas may reflect abnormal blood flow
  o Abnormal procoagulant properties of intervillous blood or trophoblast
    – Increase in intervillous thrombi/hematomas
  o Intrinsic abnormality of extravillous trophoblast differentiation leading to excess secretion of extracellular matrix
  o Auto-/alloimmune mechanisms that directly damage syncytiotrophoblast
- Any mechanism leading to excessive syncytiotrophoblast injury may cause perivillous fibrin deposition
  o Intrinsic vulnerability of syncytiotrophoblast to injury or diminished capability for regeneration from cytotrophoblast
  o Villous damage from infection
  o Villous damage from inflammatory infiltrates, chronic villitis, histiocytic intervillositis
  o Ischemic injury

Pathogenesis

- Normal perivillous fibrin deposition
  o By-product of turbulence and eddying of intervillous blood flow, aging of villi
    – Cytotrophoblasts (cells that replenish syncytiotrophoblast when injured) become fewer in number with villus maturation
  o Present at interface between maternal and fetal tissues
  o Response to localized syncytiotrophoblast injury
  o Increases with gestational age
  o Typically does not have significant effect on maternofetal exchange
- MPVFD
  o Altered pattern of increased perivillous deposition, more prominent basally but more often full-thickness distribution
    – Fills and obliterates intervillous space
    – Surrounds and chokes off affected chorionic villi
    – Progressive involvement of more and more villi
    – Chorionic villi become avascular over time
  o Ultimately leads to impaired exchange of gases and nutrients
    – Can lead to fetal morbidity (growth restriction, prematurity) and mortality

CLINICAL ISSUES

Epidemiology

- Incidence
  o Rare placental lesion with incidence 0.028-0.500% of placentas
  o Transmural form more common than cases limited to basal plate

Laboratory Tests

- Elevated maternal serum α-fetoprotein associated with MPVFD

Natural History

- Retrospective studies have reported recurrence rates of 12-78%

Treatment

- No randomized controlled trials exist of treatment of MPVFD
- Therapeutic interventions with case reports of favorable outcomes include
  o Low-dose aspirin
  o Pravastatin
  o Intravenous gamma globulin
  o Lovenox
- Placenta after treatment does not show significant improvement but may slightly prolong gestation

Clinical Associations

- Maternal
  o Hypertension, preeclampsia
  o Oligohydramnios
  o Poor past reproductive history with high rates of spontaneous abortion, fetal demise, intrauterine growth restriction, and neonatal death
  o Case reports associated with
    − Autoimmune disorders, antiphospholipid antibody syndrome, polymyositis
    − Inherited or acquired coagulopathies
- Fetal/neonatal
  o Fetal and neonatal death
  o Severe intrauterine growth restriction
  o Premature birth
  o Adverse neurodevelopmental outcomes
  o Case reports associated with
    − Kidney disorders, cystic renal dysplasia, renal tubular dysgenesis
    − Long-chain 3-hydroxyacyl-CoA dehydrogenase deficiency
- Placental
  o Discordant MFI/MPVFD in both dichorionic and monochorionic twin placentas has been reported
  o Concurrence of MPVFD with chronic histiocytic intervillositis and MPVFD with chronic villitis has been reported

Clinical Outcomes

- Preterm delivery (26-60%)
- Severe intrauterine growth restriction (24-100%)
- Adverse neurodevelopmental outcomes
- Spontaneous abortion, unknown incidence, may be underdiagnosed
- Stillbirth (13-50%)

IMAGING

Ultrasonographic Findings

- Increased placental echogenicity with cystic spaces, which are areas of normal placenta parenchyma
- Intrauterine growth restriction
  o Long bone growth may be very delayed, suggesting chondrodysplasia
  o Osteopenia
- Oligohydramnios
- Reduced or abnormal blood flow within placenta may also be seen

MACROSCOPIC

General Features

- Dense, firm placenta with basally located "orange rind" of fibrin (MFI)
  o Corrugated appearance that obliterates usual lobular pattern
  o Document thickness of fibrin layer and percentage of maternal surface involved
- Diffusely distributed pattern of vertically oriented, firm trabeculae of fibrin that may be concentrated along basal plate or extend to chorionic plate
  o Lattice- or net-like appearance of fibrin deposition, separated by areas of more normal-appearing villous tissue
  o Document percentage of placental parenchymal involvement
- Parenchyma may have pale, granular appearance
- Cut surface of fibrinoid tan-white, homogeneous, and shiny
- Increased numbers of chorionic cysts and septal cysts in some cases
- Increased numbers of intervillous thrombi

Size

- Placenta typically small for gestational age
- Placenta may be of normal or even increased weight due to presence of abundant fibrin and intervillous thrombi

Sections to Be Submitted

- Full-thickness sections essential to assess level of involvement, sample normal-appearing parenchyma as well as lesional

MICROSCOPIC

Histologic Features

- Chorionic villi encased in amorphous, eosinophilic fibrin
- Intervillous space filled in and obliterated by fibrin
- Patches of uninvolved intervillous space with villi usually intermixed within lesion
- Encased villi remain separated/individuated without collapse of intervillous space
- Villi show spectrum of changes from syncytiotrophoblast atrophy to frank avascularity
- Perivillous fibrin may contain proliferation of extravillous trophoblast cells, may be sign of chronicity
- May have multiple extravillous trophoblast cell-lined cysts containing eosinophilic, colloid-like fluid
- Intervillous thrombi common
- Some cases associated with chronic histiocytic intervillositis or chronic villitis; important to recognize and diagnose appropriately
- Very rare cases associated with mixed acute and chronic intervillositis due to Coxsackie virus infection

ANCILLARY TESTS

Serologic Testing

- Work-up for autoimmune disorders, genetic and acquired thrombophilia can be suggested

DIFFERENTIAL DIAGNOSIS

Infarction

- True infarcts show collapse of intervillous space **and** coagulative necrosis of villi
  - Marginal infarcts often associated with localized increase in perivillous fibrin
  - When histologic distinction difficult and > 50% of lesion comprised of villi, call it infarct
- Multiple infarcts usually of different ages and show variable appearance from red to white
- Decidual arteriopathy often present in cases with multiple infarcts, feature not typically seen in MPVFD

Diffuse Chronic Villitis of Unknown Etiology

- Diffuse chronic inflammatory infiltrates can lead to villous agglutination and perivillous fibrin deposition
- As lesions of chronic villitis age ("burnt-out villitis"), villi may become avascular and surrounded by bland fibrin
  - Residual chronic inflammation usually present

Chronic Histiocytic Intervillositis (CHI)

- Occasional histiocytes may be seen in foci of perivillous fibrin depositions
- Histiocytic infiltrates of CHI are dense, appear as mass of cells on low power
- Longstanding CHI associated with increased perivillous fibrin deposition

Fetal Vascular Malperfusion, Longstanding

- Typically, avascular villi show no significant surrounding perivillous fibrin, but with longstanding lesions, fibrin can fill in intervillous space
- In longstanding FVM, avascular villi not encased in fibrin are visible at edges of lesion
- Thrombi in chorionic plate or stem villous vessels may be present, features not typically seen in MPVFD

DIAGNOSTIC CHECKLIST

Clinically Relevant Pathologic Features

- MPVFD important to recognize due to high recurrence risk
- Check for history of pregnancy loss or other adverse outcomes

Pathologic Interpretation Pearls

- MPVFD is grossly recognizable lesion; extent of involvement on gross exam part of diagnosis
  - Trabecular and lattice-like deposition of fibrin concentrated along basal plate and extending vertically to chorionic plate, involving ≥ 50% of parenchyma
- MPVFD histology distinct from infarction
  - Chorionic villi surrounded by fibrinoid, which fill intervillous space without collapse of villous architecture
  - Coagulative necrosis absent
  - Decidual vasculopathy absent
  - Inflammation not typically present

REPORTING

Gross Description

- Avoid use of gross terms, such as "fibrotic" or "infarcted" parenchyma
- Use descriptors of color (tan-white), consistency (firm), and shape (linear, lace-like, lattice-like network) of parenchymal change
- Describe pattern of parenchymal involvement
  - Predominantly basal, transmural, or irregular
- Describe percentage of maternal floor &/or parenchymal involvement

Final Diagnosis

- MPVFD terminology used for transmural involvement involving ≥ 50% of parenchyma
- Include comment about high risk of recurrence

SELECTED REFERENCES

1. He M et al: Follow-up and management of recurrent pregnancy losses due to massive perivillous fibrinoid deposition. Obstet Med. 11(1):17-22, 2018
2. Kingdom JC et al: A placenta clinic approach to the diagnosis and management of fetal growth restriction. Am J Obstet Gynecol. 218(2S):S803-S817, 2018
3. Abdulghani S et al: Recurrent massive perivillous fibrin deposition and chronic intervillositis treated with heparin and intravenous immunoglobulin: A case report. J Obstet Gynaecol Can. 39(8):676-681, 2017
4. Heller DS et al: Placental massive perivillous fibrinoid deposition associated with Coxsackievirus A16-Report of a case, and review of the literature. Pediatr Dev Pathol. 19(5):421-423, 2016
5. Taweevisit M et al: Maternal floor infarction/massive perivillous fibrin deposition associated with hypercoiling of a single-artery umbilical cord: A case report. Pediatr Dev Pathol. 19(1):69-73, 2016
6. Faye-Petersen OM et al: Maternal floor infarction and massive perivillous fibrin deposition. Surg Pathol Clin. 6(1):101-14, 2013
7. Linn RL et al: Recurrent massive perivillous fibrin deposition in the placenta associated with fetal renal tubular dysgenesis: case report and literature review. Pediatr Dev Pathol. 16(5):378-86, 2013
8. Romero R et al: Maternal floor infarction/massive perivillous fibrin deposition: a manifestation of maternal antifetal rejection? Am J Reprod Immunol. 70(4):285-98, 2013
9. Griffin AC et al: Mutations in long-chain 3-hydroxyacyl coenzyme a dehydrogenase are associated with placental maternal floor infarction/massive perivillous fibrin deposition. Pediatr Dev Pathol. 15(5):368-74, 2012
10. Taweevisit M et al: Maternal floor infarction associated with oligohydramnios and cystic renal dysplasia: report of 2 cases. Pediatr Dev Pathol. 13(2):116-20, 2010
11. Uxa R et al: Genetic polymorphisms in the fibrinolytic system of placentas with massive perivillous fibrin deposition. Placenta. 31(6):499-505, 2010
12. Gogia N et al: Maternal thrombophilias are associated with specific placental lesions. Pediatr Dev Pathol. 11(6):424-9, 2008
13. Hung NA et al: Pregnancy-related polymyositis and massive perivillous fibrin deposition in the placenta: are they pathogenetically related? Arthritis Rheum. 55(1):154-6, 2006
14. Waters BL et al: Significance of perivillous fibrin/oid deposition in uterine evacuation specimens. Am J Surg Pathol. 30(6):760-5, 2006
15. Weber MA et al: Co-occurrence of massive perivillous fibrin deposition and chronic intervillositis: case report. Pediatr Dev Pathol. 9(3):234-8, 2006
16. Kaufmann P et al: The fibrinoids of the human placenta: origin, composition and functional relevance. Ann Anat. 178(6):485-501, 1996

(Left) This dichorionic twin placenta was discordant for MPVFD. Note the nearly complete involvement of parenchyma of twin A placenta with diffusely pale, tan, firm, and finely granular parenchyma ➡. Twin B has normal spongy, dark-red parenchyma ➡. (Right) Note the diffusely distributed pattern of vertically oriented, firm trabeculae and a lattice-like deposition of fibrin in this placenta with MPVFD. Intervillous hematomas are almost always present ➡.

Discordance for MPVFD in Twin Placenta

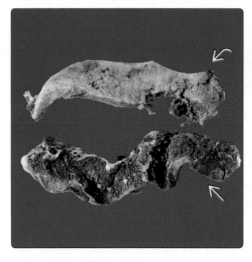

Intervillous Hematomas in MPVFD

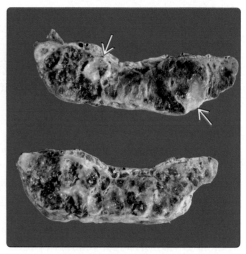

(Left) Close inspection of the parenchyma in MPVFD shows a trabecular, lacy or lattice-like appearance that is not typically seen in an ischemic infarct. (Right) Multiple chorionic cysts ➡, some with recent and remote hemorrhage, are frequently seen in association with MPVFD. These cysts often appear to be subamniotic, but you can see that the chorionic plate vessels overly the surface of the cyst ➡.

Lattice-Like Fibrin in MPVFD

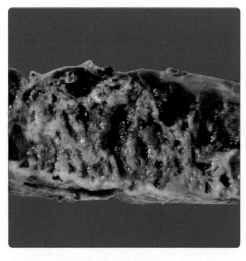

Chorionic Cysts With MPVFD

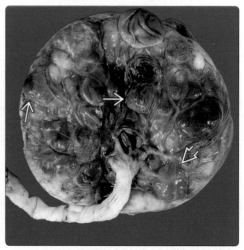

(Left) Gross photograph shows a septal cyst in an otherwise normal placenta. These are simple, nonseptate cysts lined by extravillous trophoblastic cells. They are found in increased numbers in cases of MPVFD. (Right) Low-power examination of MPVFD shows diffuse, nearly full-thickness encasement of the chorionic villi by eosinophilic, bland, noninflamed fibrin. The fibrin typically is most concentrated at the basal surface ➡ and extends toward the chorionic plate.

Septal Cyst

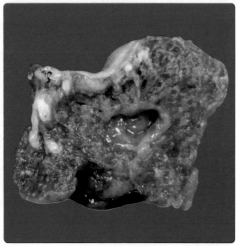

Histologic Appearance of MPVFD

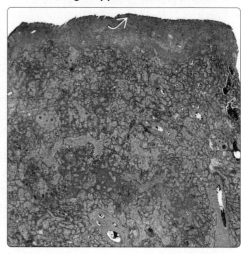

Histologic Appearance of MPVFD

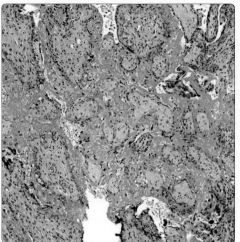

Maternal Floor Infarction/MPVFD

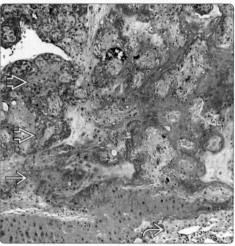

(Left) On higher power examination of chorionic villi encased by perivillous fibrin, there is still some preservation of the trophoblast layer and villous stroma, but villous capillaries are sparse. Over time, the villi become more devitalized. (Right) This section of the basal plate shows a thick layer of fibrin surrounding the basal villi ➡ and several layers additional layers of villi ➡. Normal decidua is focally present ➡.

Perivillous Fibrin With Extravillous Trophoblast Proliferation

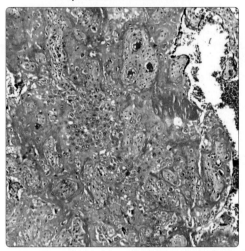

MPVFD Border

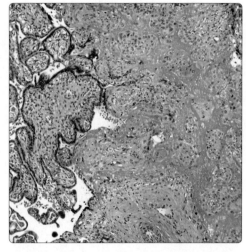

(Left) Extravillous trophoblast proliferation in the fibrin is a sign of chronicity. The cells likely produce the matrix-type of fibrin. (Right) The border between the normal tissue and the areas with perivillous fibrin is often abrupt and well defined, as shown here. Spared areas sometimes appeared to be within the lesion.

Differential Diagnosis: Infarction

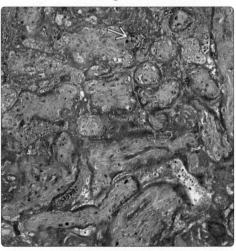

Differential Diagnosis: High-Grade Chronic Villitis

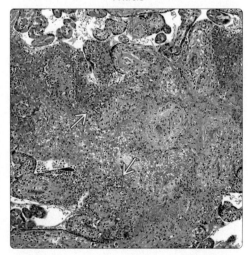

(Left) Remote infarction shows collapse of the intervillous space with villi touching each other and evidence of coagulative necrosis with karyorrhectic debris ➡. Infarcts are more circumscribed on gross exam than MPVFD. (Right) In high-grade necrotizing chronic villitis, there may be extensive perivillous fibrin deposition. The fibrin deposition in chronic villitis is more cellular than in MPVFD because of perivillitis ➡.

Large Vessel Fetal Vascular Malperfusion

TERMINOLOGY

- Occlusive changes in large fetal vessels are now considered changes of "fetal vascular malperfusion" (FVM)
- Large fetal vessels: Umbilical, chorionic plate, and stem villous vessels

CLINICAL ISSUES

- Thrombosis of chorionic plate or stem villous vessel occurs in ~ 4% of placentas submitted for pathologic evaluation; multiple thrombi occur in 3%
- Associated with fetal demise, growth restriction, neurologic injury, and thrombo/emboli in organs

MACROSCOPIC

- Vascular ectasia without thrombus
- Distension of vessel by slightly firm, red-tan thrombus
- Firm, variegated, layered, or white and calcified
- Extravasation of blood products and red cell lysis may discolor cord or chorionic plate

- Document whether involved vessel is artery or vein as this is difficult to do on histology
- Thrombosed vessel may be surrounded by pale villi

MICROSCOPIC

- Umbilical cord thrombi result in devitalization of muscle wall
- Thrombi in placental vessels rarely show classic lines of Zahn; vague layering may be present
- Mural/intramural thrombi consist of fibrin and platelets with few red or white cells
- True thrombi are adherent to vessel wall
- Acute thrombi consist mostly of red blood cells with some fibrin layering
- Subacute to remote thrombi may show mural calcification

Large Vessel Thrombosis

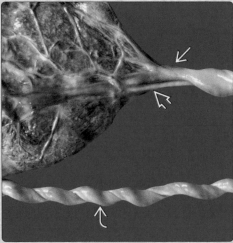

Intramural Fibrin Deposition With Calcification

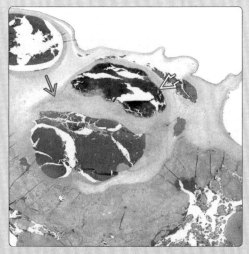

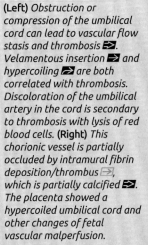

(Left) *Obstruction or compression of the umbilical cord can lead to vascular flow stasis and thrombosis* ➡️. *Velamentous insertion* ➡️ *and hypercoiling* ➡️ *are both correlated with thrombosis. Discoloration of the umbilical artery in the cord is secondary to thrombosis with lysis of red blood cells.* (Right) *This chorionic vessel is partially occluded by intramural fibrin deposition/thrombus* ➡️, *which is partially calcified* ➡️. *The placenta showed a hypercoiled umbilical cord and other changes of fetal vascular malperfusion.*

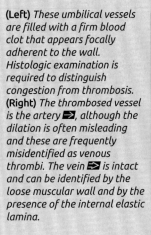

(Left) *These umbilical vessels are filled with a firm blood clot that appears focally adherent to the wall. Histologic examination is required to distinguish congestion from thrombosis.* (Right) *The thrombosed vessel is the artery* ➡️, *although the dilation is often misleading and these are frequently misidentified as venous thrombi. The vein* ➡️ *is intact and can be identified by the loose muscular wall and by the presence of the internal elastic lamina.*

Umbilical Vessel Thrombus

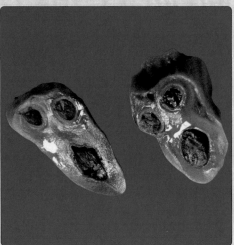

Old Umbilical Artery Thrombus

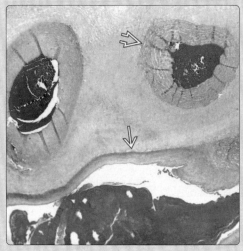

TERMINOLOGY

Synonyms

- Occlusive changes in large fetal vessels are now considered changes of fetal vascular malperfusion (FVM)
- Similar pathologic changes are encompassed by terms
  o Fetal thrombotic vasculopathy
    - No longer preferred terminology, but much of literature based on this diagnosis
  o Chronic obstructive fetal vasculopathy or changes
  o Vasoobliterative fetal vascular changes
  o Fetal vascular involutional changes
  o Hemorrhagic endovasculitis or endovasculosis
- Older terminology includes fibrinous vasculosis, thrombosclerosing placentitis, endarteritis obliterans, and fibromuscular sclerosis

Definitions

- Large fetal vessels of placenta includes umbilical, chorionic plate, and stem villous vessels
- Pathologic changes in large fetal vessels that indicate fetal vascular obstruction are now referred to as FVM
  o Findings consistent with FVM
    - Thrombosis; arterial or venous; occlusive or nonocclusive
      □ Includes organizing mural thrombi now termed "intramural fibrin deposition"
      □ Includes progressive changes of stem vessel obliteration ending with thickening of vascular wall and obliteration of lumen
    - Avascular villi or villous stromal-vascular karyorrhexis (VSVK)
      □ Small foci, 3 or more foci of 2-4 villi
      □ Intermediate foci, 5-10 villi
      □ Large foci, > 10 villi
    - Other possible markers
      □ Vascular ectasia; luminal diameter ≥ 4x compared to adjacent vessel
  o Grading FVM
    - Low grade (either of following)
      □ Avascular villi, ≥ 5 but < 45 villi involved
      □ Single chorionic plate or stem villous occlusive or nonocclusive thrombus
    - High grade (either of following)
      □ Avascular villi, 2 or more foci, totaling ≥ 45 villi over 3 sections or average of > 15 avascular villi per section ± thrombus
      □ 2 or more occlusive or nonocclusive thrombi in chorionic plate or major stem villous vessels **or** multiple nonocclusive thrombi
  o Pattern of FVM
    - Segmental
      □ Thrombotic occlusion of chorionic plate or stem villous vessel and large segmental area of avascular villi
      □ Regional abnormality that follows placental vascular pattern
      □ Results in complete obstruction of fetal blood flow to downstream villi
    - Global

      □ Vascular ectasia, intramural fibrin deposition in large fetal vessels, &/or multiple small foci (< 5 villi per focus) of avascular or karyorrhectic villi
      □ Suggest partially or intermittently obstructed umbilical blood flow

ETIOLOGY/PATHOGENESIS

Causes

- Cord compromise from kinking, tight knots, tight nuchal cords or limb/body entanglement, hypercoiling, stricture
- Compression of large fetal vessels not protected by Wharton substance in velamentous, furcate, or marginal umbilical cord insertion, vasa previa
- Amnion bands
- Trauma, such as in utero cordocentesis
- Vascular injury secondary to inflammation or meconium
- Fetal hypercoaguability
- Fetal heart failure
- Maternal diabetes associated with fetal polycythemia

Factors That Promote Thrombosis in Fetal Vasculature

- Stasis of fetal blood flow
  o Fetal heart failure, intraabdominal umbilical venous obstruction, polycythemia
  o Interruption of blood flow due to compression or kinking of umbilical or compression of chorionic plate vessels
- Vascular/endothelial cell injury
  o Severe acute inflammation of umbilical or chorionic plate vessels in fetal response to amniotic fluid infection
  o Chronic inflammation of stem villi in chronic villitis of unknown etiology or chronic villitis due to hematogenous infections
  o Meconium-associated vascular injury
- Hypercoagulability of fetal blood
  o Thrombophilia; genetic or acquired
    - Contribution of genetic thrombophilias is likely small

Thrombotic/Ischemic Complications in Fetus

- Systemic activation of coagulation system, disseminated intravascular coagulopathy, thrombocytopenia
- Potential for emboli from large placental vessels via umbilical vein to brain and viscera
- Reduced capacity for maternofetal gas and nutrient exchange due to downstream villous compromise

CLINICAL ISSUES

Epidemiology

- Incidence
  o Thrombosis of umbilical vessels in 1/3,000 deliveries and up to 1/250 high-risk pregnancies
    - Umbilical venous thrombi are reported as more common than umbilical artery thrombi
      □ Involved vessel may be markedly dilated and muscular wall degenerated
      □ Umbilical vein has internal elastic lamina, which is absent in artery
      □ Elastic stain may be helpful in defining type of vessel involved

o Thrombosis of chorionic plate or stem villous vessel occurs in ~ 4% of placentas submitted for pathologic evaluation; multiple thrombi occur in 3%

Prognosis

- Thrombosis of umbilical vessel is associated with significant fetal morbidity and mortality
  o Fetal death
  o Intrauterine growth restriction (IUGR)
  o Neurologic injury such as encephalopathy, seizures, or cerebral palsy
  o Thrombo/emboli in viscera
- Significance of chorionic plate or stem vessel thrombi is dependent upon other additional placental findings, including
  o Multiple chorionic plate or stem villous thrombi
  o Avascular villi
  o High-grade chronic villitis
  o Amniotic fluid infection sequence
  o Changes of maternal vascular malperfusion

Other Obstetric Complications Associated With High-Grade Fetal Vascular Malperfusion

- Preeclampsia
- Pregnancy-associated recurrent hemolytic-uremic syndrome
- IUGR
- Oligohydramnios
- Abnormal umbilical artery Doppler velocimetry
- Decrease in cord blood arterial and venous pH
- Stillbirth
- Single umbilical artery
- Decreased fetal movement

Neonatal Complications Associated With High-Grade Fetal Vascular Malperfusion

- Central nervous system injury; infarcts (stroke), neonatal encephalopathy, developmental delay, cerebral palsy
- Visceral ischemic disease; perinatal liver disease, Budd-Chiari syndrome, renal vein thrombosis, bowel atresia, myocardial infarction
- Transverse ischemic limb reduction defects
- Thrombocytopenia
- Increased nucleated erythrocytes
- Coagulopathy

MACROSCOPIC

Umbilical Vessels

- Document presence of gross umbilical cord abnormalities, such as abnormal insertion, hypercoiling, excessively long cord, or true knot
- Ectasia without thrombus
  o May indicate obstruction near dilated region
    – Dilated region is usually on placental side of lesion
  o Look for compression or maceration or discoloration of adjacent cord
- Acute intraluminal thrombus
  o Distension of vessel by slightly firm, red-tan thrombus
- Subacute to remote intraluminal thrombus
  o Firm, variegated, layered, or white

o Well-established thrombus has lysis of red blood cells that discolors surrounding umbilical cord or chorionic plate

Velamentous Vessels

- Higher risk of injury secondary to lack of protection by Wharton substance
- Distension, discoloration, or firmness of vessels raises suspicion for thrombosis

Chorionic Vessels

- Document grossly whether involved vessel is artery or vein as this is difficult to do on histology
  o Arteries cross over veins on placental surface
- Ectasia without thrombosis
  o Ectasia; diameter ≥ 4x diameter compared of adjacent vessel
- Acute intraluminal thrombus
  o Distension of vessel by slightly firm, red-tan thrombus
- Subacute to remote intraluminal thrombus
  o Firm
  o Variegated, layered, or white with chalky calcifications

Stem Vessels

- Dilated and filled with firm blood
- Thrombosed vessel may be surrounded by pale avascular villi

MICROSCOPIC

General Features

- Thrombosis, occlusive or nonocclusive
  o Thrombi in placental vessels rarely show classic lines of Zahn; vague layering may be present
  o Mural/intramural thrombi consist of fibrin and platelets with few red or white cells
  o True thrombi are densely eosinophilic and adherent to vessel wall
- Chronicity
  o Acute thrombi
    – Vessel is distended
    – Consist mostly of red blood cells with some fibrin layering
    – Focal attachment to vessel wall
    – Loose collections of fibrin and cells within vascular lumen are not true thrombi
  o Subacute to remote
    – Reduced red cell component; consists mostly of fibrin and platelets
    – Usually nonocclusive
    – May show incorporation into wall, often with mural calcification
- Thrombosis of umbilical vessels
  o Umbilical vessels lack vasa vasorum and received oxygenation from fetal circulation
    – Thrombosis of lumen will result in devitalization of smooth muscle wall
    – Compare vitality of smooth muscle of suspected thrombosed to nonthrombosed vessel
    – Recent thrombosis can be very subtle
- Other vasoobliterative changes of large vessels
  o Loss of endothelial integrity

- ○ Mural hemorrhage with red cell fragmentation
- ○ Fibroblastic proliferation with luminal septation/recanalization
- ○ Overlap with fetal vascular involutional changes after fetal demise
  - – True fibrin or layered thrombus and vascular ectasia of fetal vessels not part of involutional changes after fetal demise
  - – Premortem fetal vascular occlusion is usually variable and segmental; postmortem fetal vascular involution is uniform and diffuse
- ○ Rarely, thrombi of fetal vessels are associated with eosinophilic/T-cell vasculitis, acute chorionic vasculitis, or chronic villitis

DIFFERENTIAL DIAGNOSIS

Intimal Fibrin Cushion vs. Mural Thrombus

- Chorionic vessels and stem vessels often have asymmetric fibrointimal proliferations, which may protrude into lumen
- Some fibrointimal proliferations may have eosinophilic cap of fibrin
  - ○ Old term; "intimal fibrin cushion" now replaced with "intramural fibrin deposition"
  - ○ Intimal proliferations without any fibrin do not merit FVM diagnosis

Changes of Intrauterine Fetal Demise

- Obliterative changes of large chorionic and stem vessels are expected after fetal death due to cessation of fetal blood flow
  - ○ Features include karyorrhexis, red cell fragmentation, &/or fibroblastic luminal septation
  - ○ Changes should be uniform and diffuse within parenchyma
- True fibrin thrombi are not feature of intrauterine fetal demise
  - ○ Features to look for to indicate true antemortem thrombosis: Presence of mural or intraluminal fibrin, adherence of fibrin to wall, mural calcification, vascular ectasia
- Iron staining within Hofbauer cells may highlight vascular injury
  - ○ Premortem injury should be variable and segmental within parenchyma
  - ○ Postmortem involution should be uniform and diffuse within parenchyma

Refrigeration Artifact/Autolysis

- Endothelial cells degenerate and detach with prolonged refrigeration, resembling loss of endothelial integrity
- Mural hemorrhage, red cell fragmentation, or fibroblastic luminal septation of true vasoobliterative lesions are not present

REPORTING

Key Elements to Report

- Gross umbilical cord or chorionic plate vascular abnormalities (i.e., velamentous vessels, ectasia)
  - ○ Identify venous vs. arterial, if possible (arteries run over veins on chorionic plate)
- Microscopic vascular lesions

- ○ Number and type of vessels with thrombi
  - – Intraluminal vs. intramural fibrin deposition (occlusive vs. nonocclusive)
- ○ Other vascular features associated with thrombus formation
  - – Acute vasculitis
  - – Meconium
  - – High-grade chronic villitis
  - – Eosinophilic/T-cell vasculitis
  - – Changes of maternal vascular malperfusion
- Microscopic distal villous lesions of FVM
  - ○ Avascular villi
  - ○ VSVK
- Grade FVM: High or low
- Pattern FVM: Global or segmental

SELECTED REFERENCES

1. Bernson-Leung ME et al: Placental pathology in neonatal stroke: a retrospective case-control study. J Pediatr. 195:39-47.e5, 2018
2. Stanek J: Fetal vascular malperfusion. Arch Pathol Lab Med. 142(6):679-681, 2018
3. Battarbee AN et al: Placental abnormalities associated with isolated single umbilical artery in small-for-gestational-age births. Placenta. 59:9-12, 2017
4. Heider A: Fetal vascular malperfusion. Arch Pathol Lab Med. 141(11):1484-1489, 2017
5. Khong TY et al: Sampling and definitions of placental lesions: Amsterdam placental workshop group consensus statement. Arch Pathol Lab Med. 140(7):698-713, 2016
6. Chisholm KM et al: Fetal thrombotic vasculopathy: significance in liveborn children using proposed society for pediatric pathology diagnostic criteria. Am J Surg Pathol. 39(2):274-80, 2015
7. Redline RW: Classification of placental lesions. Am J Obstet Gynecol. 213(4 Suppl):S21-8, 2015
8. Ernst LM et al: Gross patterns of umbilical cord coiling: correlations with placental histology and stillbirth. Placenta. 34(7):583-8, 2013
9. Ryan WD et al: Placental histologic criteria for diagnosis of cord accident: sensitivity and specificity. Pediatr Dev Pathol. 15(4):275-80, 2012
10. Pathak S et al: Frequency and clinical significance of placental histological lesions in an unselected population at or near term. Virchows Arch. 459(6):565-72, 2011
11. Rogers BB et al: Avascular villi, increased syncytial knots, and hypervascular villi are associated with pregnancies complicated by factor V Leiden mutation. Pediatr Dev Pathol. 13(5):341-7, 2010
12. Saleemuddin A et al: Obstetric and perinatal complications in placentas with fetal thrombotic vasculopathy. Pediatr Dev Pathol. 13(6):459-64, 2010
13. Taweevisit M et al: Massive fetal thrombotic vasculopathy associated with excessively long umbilical cord and fetal demise: case report and literature review. Pediatr Dev Pathol. 13(2):112-5, 2010
14. Tantbirojn P et al: Gross abnormalities of the umbilical cord: related placental histology and clinical significance. Placenta. 30(12):1083-8, 2009
15. Parast MM et al: Placental histologic criteria for umbilical blood flow restriction in unexplained stillbirth. Hum Pathol. 39(6):948-53, 2008
16. Ariel I et al: Placental pathology in fetal thrombophilia. Hum Pathol. 35(6):729-33, 2004
17. Redline RW et al: Fetal vascular obstructive lesions: nosology and reproducibility of placental reaction patterns. Pediatr Dev Pathol. 7(5):443-52, 2004
18. Genest DR: Estimating the time of death in stillborn fetuses: II. Histologic evaluation of the placenta; a study of 71 stillborns. Obstet Gynecol. 80(4):585-92, 1992

Large Fetal Vessels of Placenta

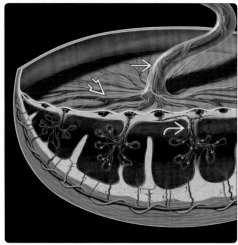

(Left) *Thrombi and other occlusive lesions of the large fetal vessels of the placenta can involve cord vessels ➡, chorionic plate vessels ➡, and stem villous vessels ➡. **(Right)** Umbilical cord abnormalities, such as hypercoiling and marginal insertion, are associated with large vessel thrombi. These chorionic plate vessels ➡ are distended and appear chalky. Histology revealed thrombosis. The thrombosed vessel appears to be a vein, as a small artery crosses over it.*

Hypercoiled, Marginally Inserted Umbilical Cord

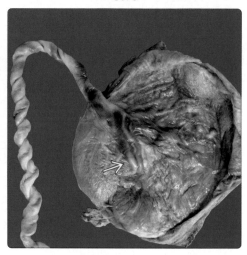

Recent Thrombosis of Umbilical Artery

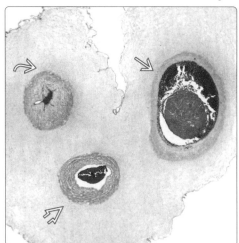

(Left) *Thrombosis of one umbilical artery ➡ is noted in this section of cord. The vessel is dilated, which can be misleading and may suggest that it is the vein. The vein ➡ and the other artery ➡ are normal. **(Right)** Once thrombosed, the vascular smooth muscle will become devitalized ➡. The umbilical vessels have no vasa vasorum; therefore, the vessel receives oxygen only through the blood within the lumen. Careful comparison of the normal ➡ and suspected abnormal vessel is necessary to identify early thrombi.*

Normal and Devitalized Umbilical Artery

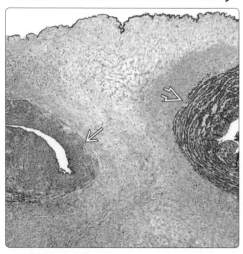

Remote Thrombosis Umbilical Artery

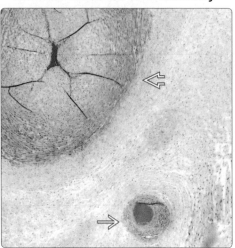

(Left) *This umbilical cord is functionally a single umbilical artery (SUA). The thrombosed artery is significantly smaller ➡ than the normal adjacent artery ➡. This is one explanation for SUA. **(Right)** Thrombi in the placental circulation may embolize to the fetus. The calcified thrombus ➡ in this section of kidney is from a fetus with large fetal vessel occlusion in the placenta.*

Fetal Renal Vein Thrombosis

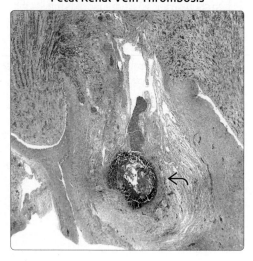

Chorionic Vessel Thrombus

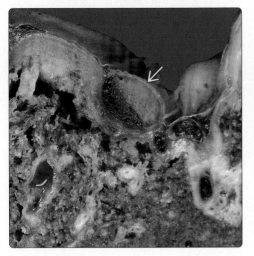

Chorionic Plate Occlusive Thrombus

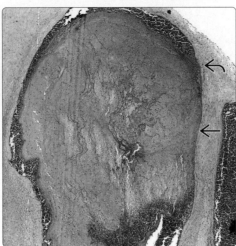

(Left) This chorionic plate vessel ➡ is distension by a partly red and partly gray-tan material that is highly suspicious for thrombus, but histologic examination is necessary for confirmation. (Right) This distended chorionic plate vessel has a nearly occlusive thrombus composed mostly of fibrin. Subacute thrombi such as this contain more fibrin than red blood cells. There is early calcification ➡ where the thrombus is attached to the vessel wall ➡.

Acute Fetal Vessel Thrombosis

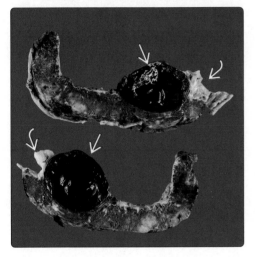

Marked Chorionic Plate Vascular Ectasia

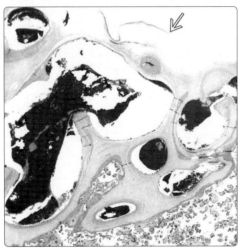

(Left) This placenta is from a 36-week intrauterine fetal demise (IUFD) with a well-circumscribed mass ➡ on the placental surface near the cord insertion ➡. Histologically, this is a markedly ectatic chorionic vessel with thrombosis. This appearance could also be a large subchorionic hematoma (Breu mole). Histology is necessary to show its origin. (Right) There is marked dilation of the chorionic plate vessels, as shown here. This is suggestive of an umbilical cord obstruction. Amnion is seen at the top of the section ➡.

Intramural Fibrin Deposition

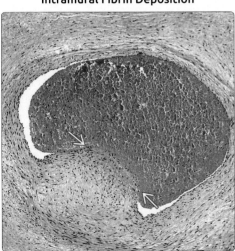

Intramural Fibrin Deposition

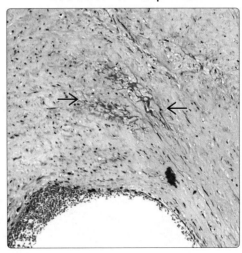

(Left) This chorionic plate vessel shows a myxoid-appearing intimal proliferation that has a fibrin thrombus cap ➡ beneath the endothelium. (Right) This stem villous vessel has no luminal abnormality, but the eosinophilic fibrin strands ➡ incorporated into the wall suggest a probable organized thrombus. Additional level sections can be useful to identify further features of thrombosis.

(Left) *Dense pink fibrin ⇥ in the wall of this stem vessel is present. Global fetal vascular malperfusion may show multiple similar lesions.* **(Right)** *Both a large ⇥ and small ⇥ stem villous vessel are occluded by a fibrointimal proliferation with red cell fragmentation. Cessation of proximal fetal blood flow due to either fetal death or upstream antemortem vascular occlusion shows similar vasoobliterative changes.*

Non-Occlusive Thrombus/Intramural Fibrin Deposition

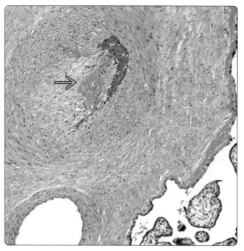

Stem Vessel Obliteration

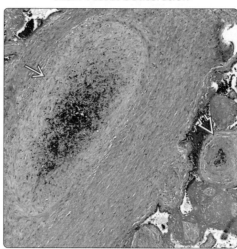

(Left) *Later in the course of stem villous obliteration, only rare fibrous strands or red cell fragments are seen. The lumen is septated into multiple small channels, often forming a ring where the endothelium once lay.* **(Right)** *Chronic fetal vascular obstruction ultimately produces this pattern where the stem vessel lumen ⇥ is completely replaced by fibrous tissue. There are abundant avascular villi surrounding the stem villus.*

Stem Vessel Obliteration

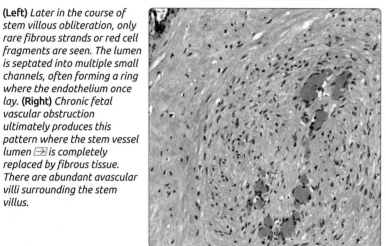

Complete Stem Vessel Obliteration

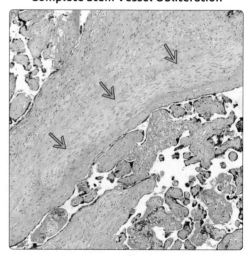

(Left) *This stem vessel lumen is almost completely filled with a bulging mass of fibrous tissue, leaving only a slit-like lumen ⇥. This finding is not diagnostic of fetal vascular malperfusion.* **(Right)** *Isolated luminal aggregates of fibrin alone are common and should not be diagnosed as a thrombus.*

Stem Vessel With Fibrointimal Proliferation

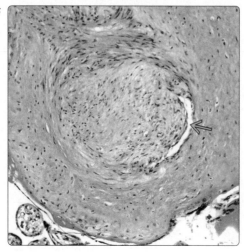

Normal Stem Vessel

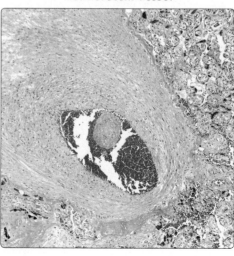

Refrigeration Artifact

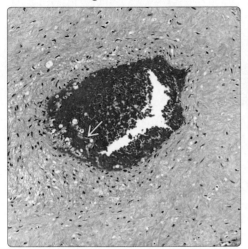

Necrotizing Funisitis With Thrombosis

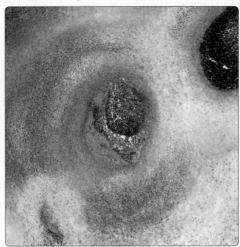

(Left) *Detachment of the endothelium* ➡️ *due to a refrigeration artifact, as seen in this chorionic plate vessel, should be distinguished from loss of endothelial integrity or fibrin strands of a vasoocclusive process.* (Right) *These umbilical vessels show severe funisitis with a dense layer of necrotic debris around the vessel. The lumen is thrombosed. This was from a stillborn infant with congenital syphilis.*

Amnion Band With Cord Constriction

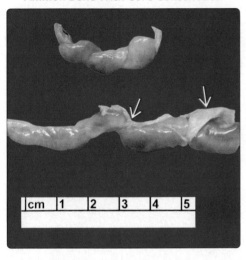

Chronic Villitis With Stem Vessel Obliteration

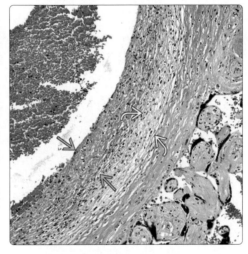

(Left) *This gross photograph shows membranous strands of tissue* ➡️ *wrapped around the umbilical cord in the case of an IUFD due to amniotic band sequence. There was increased coiling and umbilical vessel thrombosis.* (Right) *This high-power image of a stem villous vessel demonstrates how the chronic inflammatory infiltrates of villitis lead to vessel wall inflammation* ➡️, *endothelial cell effacement/injury, and then intramural fibrin deposition/thrombus* ➡️.

Acute Chorionic Vasculitis With Thrombosis

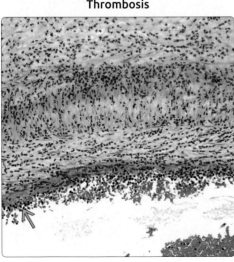

Eosinophilic/T-Cell Chorionic Vasculitis

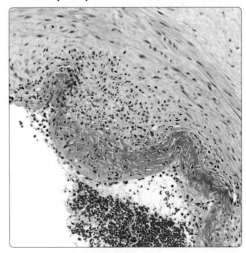

(Left) *In this case of amniotic fluid infection sequence, a large fetal vessel shows numerous neutrophils migrating from the vessel lumen to the amniotic cavity (top). The acute inflammation has resulted in endothelial injury and fibrin deposition* ➡️. (Right) *This form of chorionic plate vasculitis is not associated with infection, but is frequently seen with thrombosis. It is unclear if the inflammation causes the thrombus or if the thrombus attracts the inflammatory cells.*

TERMINOLOGY

- Fetal vascular malperfusion (FVM) is now preferred term for entities previously known as fetal thrombotic vasculopathy and hemorrhagic endovasculitis

ETIOLOGY/PATHOGENESIS

- Any condition that obstructs or impairs blood flow upstream of distal villi can cause VSVK and avascular villi

CLINICAL ISSUES

- FVM is associated with numerous fetal/neonatal morbidities and mortality
- ~ 5% of placentas from live births submitted for pathologic examination show VSVK or avascular villi
- 1% of placentas from all term births show high-grade FVM
- 9x increase in stillbirth

MACROSCOPIC

- Larger foci consist of well-demarcated area of villous pallor on cut surface of placenta

- Always look for thrombi in large chorionic plate or stem vessels
- Always take note of any umbilical cord abnormalities

MICROSCOPIC

- Avascular villi, VSVK
- Large vessel occlusion may or may not also be present

TOP DIFFERENTIAL DIAGNOSES

- FVM must be distinguished from changes occurring after fetal demise
  - Very difficult with prolonged retention of fetus after demise

REPORTING

- Diagnosis of FVM should include type and extent of VSVK &/or avascular villi
  - Grade: Low or high
  - Pattern: Segmental or global

(Left) This placenta from a term stillbirth was associated with a tight nuchal cord. Note the dilated, firm, white, thrombosed chorionic plate vessel ➡. The thrombosed vessel crosses over another vessel ➡, consistent with an arterial thrombus. (Right) Cut surface of the placenta shows large pale areas that appear more granular than typical infarcts. These represent large areas of avascular villi and villous stromal-vascular karyorrhexis (VSVK). Extravasation of blood products from a chorionic vessel thrombus is seen ➡.

Thrombosed Chorionic Plate Vessel

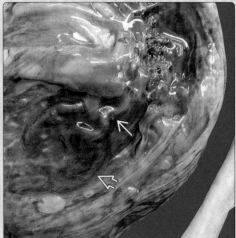

Large Areas of Avascular Villi

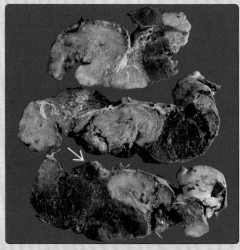

(Left) The chorionic plate vessels appear ectatic but not thrombosed ➡. A large area of pale, avascular villi occupies an area consistent with an obliterated stem vessel ➡, which is not seen in this section. (Right) Fetal vascular malperfusion (FVM) is segmental in this placenta, with the pallor of avascular villi restricted to a region ➡. The lesion would be high grade, as far more than 45 villi would be involved.

FVM

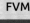
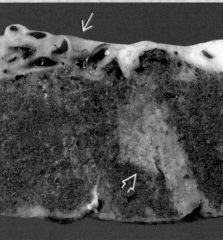

Gross Appearance of FVM

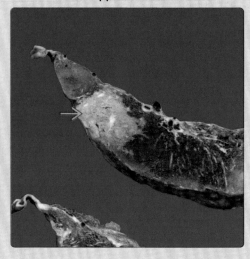

TERMINOLOGY

Synonyms

- Pathologic changes of fetal vascular occlusion are now referred to as fetal vascular malperfusion (FVM)
- Many terms have been used to describe histologically similar changes that are no longer preferred
  - Hemorrhagic endovasculitis or endovasculosis
  - Fetal thrombotic vasculopathy

Definitions

- Distal lesions of FVM
  - Avascular villi
    - Small focus; 3 or more foci of 2-4 villi
    - Intermediate focus; 5-10 villi
    - Large focus; > 10 villi
  - Villous stromal-vascular karyorrhexis (VSVK)
    - 3 or more foci of 2-4 terminal villi showing karyorrhexis of fetal cells
    - Also involves intermediate and large foci as avascular villi
- Grading of distal villous lesions of FVM
  - Low grade
    - Avascular villi or VSVK, involving < 45 villi
  - High grade
    - Avascular villi or VSVK, 2 or more foci, totaling ≥ 45 over 3 sections or average of > 15 villi per section
- Pattern of distal villous lesions of FVM
  - Segmental: Due to complete occlusion of branch of fetal vasculature
    - Large (possibly grossly visible) segmental focus of avascular villi or VSVK
    - Usually associated with occlusive thrombi in large fetal vessels
  - Global: Due to partial or intermittent obstruction at level of umbilical cord
    - Numerous small (< 5 villi per foci) of avascular villi or VSVK, usually basal
    - Often associated with multiple foci of intramural fibrin deposition, abnormalities of cord or cord insertion

ETIOLOGY/PATHOGENESIS

Loss of Perfusion From Proximal Fetal Vasculature

- Any condition that results in obstruction of upstream vasculature, loss of perfusion pressure or marked anemia can cause avascular villi or VSVK
  - Umbilical cord compromise, arterial thrombi, fetal heart failure, fetal demise
  - Villous capillaries degenerate secondary to lack of fetal perfusion
- VSVK is considered early stage and avascular villi later stage
  - Supported by progression of capillary changes that occur between fetal demise and delivery
  - Estimated to take 7 days to result in avascular villi
- VSVK with villous stromal hemorrhage may occur secondary to venous obstruction

CLINICAL ISSUES

Epidemiology

- Incidence
  - ~ 5% of placentas from live births submitted for pathologic examination show VSVK or avascular villi
  - 1% of placentas from all term births show high-grade FVM
  - Many more placentas from stillbirths have VSVK or avascular villi as part of normal involution of fetal vasculature after fetal death

Prognosis

- FVM is associated with numerous fetal/neonatal morbidities and mortality
  - FVM has 9x rate of stillbirth when compared with control placentas without FVM
  - Most infants born with these lesions in placenta will be healthy, especially with small lesions

Obstetrical Complications Associated With Fetal Vascular Malperfusion

- Preeclampsia
- Pregnancy-associated recurrent hemolytic-uremic syndrome
- Intrauterine growth restriction
- Oligohydramnios
- Abnormal umbilical artery Doppler velocimetry
- Decreased umbilical cord blood arterial and venous pH
- Stillbirth

Associated Placental Pathologies

- Umbilical cord abnormalities
  - Single umbilical artery, thrombi
  - Abnormal cord insertion, coiling, knots or strictures
- Changes of severe maternal vascular malperfusion
- Chronic villitis of unknown etiology with obstructive fetal vasculopathy
- Severe fetal anemia

Neonatal Morbidity Associated With Fetal Vascular Malperfusion

- Central nervous system injury; infarcts (stroke), neonatal encephalopathy, developmental delay, and cerebral palsy
- Visceral ischemic disease; perinatal liver disease, Budd-Chiari syndrome, renal vein thrombosis, small bowel atresia, myocardial infarction
- Transverse ischemic limb reduction defects
- Fetal cardiac abnormalities
- Thrombocytopenia
- Increased nucleated erythrocytes
- Thrombophilia
  - Few cases with FVM have confirmed mutations

MACROSCOPIC

General Features

- Avascular villi
  - Small foci are not detectable grossly
  - Larger foci consist of well-demarcated area of villous pallor on cut surface of placenta
    - Normal dark red parenchymal color is derived predominantly from fetal red blood cells
    - Avascular villi have no fetal capillaries or blood, so they appear pale

- – Pale foci retain fine granularity of villous parenchyma but will be soft
  - ○ Classically, arterial occlusion is characterized by wedge-shaped area of pallor with apex of wedge pointing to occluded vessel (toward chorionic plate)
  - ○ Gross lesions may be easier to appreciate after fixation
- VSVK
  - ○ Small foci are not detectable grossly
  - ○ Larger foci may show villous pallor
  - ○ Foci with villous stromal hemorrhage may appear more hemorrhagic
- Gross abnormalities of umbilical cord or chorionic plate vessels should not be overlooked

MICROSCOPIC

Histologic Features

- Avascular villi
  - ○ Terminal villi with total loss of villous capillaries and bland hyaline fibrosis of villous stroma
  - ○ Distribution consistent with obstructed flow in large supplying or draining fetal vessel
    - – Linear or finger-like pattern, like withered branch(es) of tree
    - – Often clustered together
  - ○ Small amount of residual karyorrhectic debris is allowable
  - ○ Hemosiderin-laden Hofbauer cells may be present
  - ○ Surrounding villous syncytiotrophoblast and intervillous space are preserved
- VSVK
  - ○ Terminal villi with karyorrhexis of fetal cells, including intravascular nucleated red blood cells, leukocytes, endothelial cells, &/or villous stromal cells
  - ○ Villi can be hypovascular or show only capillary degenerative changes
  - ○ Extravasated fetal red blood cells and red blood cell fragments are often seen
  - ○ Hemosiderin-laden macrophages may be present
  - ○ Surrounding villous syncytiotrophoblast and intervillous space are preserved
- Large vessel occlusion may or may not also be present

Overlap With Histologic Changes in Stillbirth

- Stasis of fetal blood flow after fetal death leads to involutional changes in fetal vasculature that mimic antemortem changes of FVM
  - ○ Large chorionic plate and stem vessels can show fibroblast proliferation, septation with appearance of recanalized thrombus, and even total fibrous obliteration
  - ○ Distal villi show intravascular karyorrhexis, stromal debris, and, ultimately, avascular villi
- True fibrin or layered thrombus and vascular ectasia of fetal vessels are not part of fetal vascular involutional changes after fetal death
- Regionally (as opposed to diffusely) distributed avascular villi also signify premortem fetal vascular occlusion
- Variability from area to area of hemosiderin-laden Hofbauer cells may help identify progressive villous injury as premortem event
- Prolonged retention after demise will make differentiation of pre- vs. postmortem changes very difficult

DIFFERENTIAL DIAGNOSIS

Infarcts

- Grossly visible foci of avascular villi can be mistaken for infarcts
  - ○ Infarcts are firmer, more homogeneous, less granular, and are usually marginal
  - ○ Avascular villi follow pattern of villous tree and are softer than infarcts
  - ○ Either can be wedge-shaped with base towards maternal surface

Villous Stromal Hemorrhage Associated With Abruption

- Acute intravillous hemorrhage may mimic VSVK but usually lacks karyorrhexis

Chronic Villitis of Unknown Etiology

- VSVK and avascular villi may be found with chronic villitis when stem villi are inflamed

Massive Perivillous Fibrin Deposition

- Avascular villi may be associated with massive perivillous fibrin deposition
- Presence of large vessel occlusive lesions and villi not enveloped by fibrin, distinguish FVM

REPORTING

Key Elements to Report

- As part of constellation of findings in FVM, type and extent of distal villous lesions (avascular villi and VSVK) should be reported
- Grade: Low or high
- Pattern: Segmental or global

SELECTED REFERENCES

1. Bernson-Leung ME et al: Placental pathology in neonatal stroke: a retrospective case-control study. J Pediatr. 195:39-47.e5, 2018
2. Stanek J: Fetal vascular malperfusion. Arch Pathol Lab Med. 142(6):679-681, 2018
3. Battarbee AN et al: Placental abnormalities associated with isolated single umbilical artery in small-for-gestational-age births. Placenta. 59:9-12, 2017
4. Heider A: Fetal vascular malperfusion. Arch Pathol Lab Med. 141(11):1484-1489, 2017
5. Khong TY et al: Sampling and definitions of placental lesions: Amsterdam Placental Workshop Group consensus statement. Arch Pathol Lab Med. 140(7):698-713, 2016
6. Chisholm KM et al: Fetal thrombotic vasculopathy: significance in liveborn children using proposed society for pediatric pathology diagnostic criteria. Am J Surg Pathol. 39(2):274-80, 2015
7. Ernst LM et al: Gross patterns of umbilical cord coiling: correlations with placental histology and stillbirth. Placenta. 34(7):583-8, 2013
8. Ryan WD et al: Placental histologic criteria for diagnosis of cord accident: sensitivity and specificity. Pediatr Dev Pathol. 15(4):275-80, 2012
9. Saleemuddin A et al: Obstetric and perinatal complications in placentas with fetal thrombotic vasculopathy. Pediatr Dev Pathol. 13(6):459-64, 2010
10. Parast MM et al: Placental histologic criteria for umbilical blood flow restriction in unexplained stillbirth. Hum Pathol. 39(6):948-53, 2008
11. Ariel I et al: Placental pathology in fetal thrombophilia. Hum Pathol. 35(6):729-33, 2004
12. Redline RW et al: Fetal vascular obstructive lesions: nosology and reproducibility of placental reaction patterns. Pediatr Dev Pathol. 7(5):443-52, 2004
13. Vik R et al: The placenta in neonatal encephalopathy: a case-control study. J Ped 2018.06.005

Avascular Villi

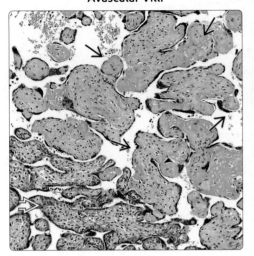

VSVK and Avascular Villi

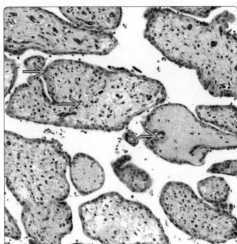

(Left) *Avascular villi* ⇨ *show eosinophilic, paucicellular stroma without capillaries. The trophoblast layer is intact. In comparison, the unaffected villi have cellular stroma* ⇨. *The villous capillaries are collapsed and indistinct.* (Right) *Karyorrhexis of villous vessels* ⇨ *and stromal cells yields sclerotic-appearing avascular villi* ⇨. *The processes result from poor perfusion by fetal vessels.*

Avascular and Hypovascular Villi

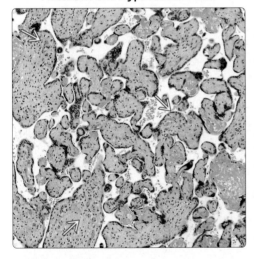

VSVK

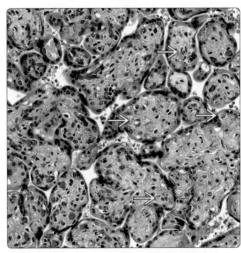

(Left) *Avascular villi show eosinophilic, paucicellular stroma with only a few residual capillaries* ⇨. *On low-power examination, these foci stand out because of their lack of blood within the capillaries.* (Right) *VSVK may be more subtle on low power because capillaries may not be completely lost. The eye is directed to paler foci, and high-power examination confirms the presence of karyorrhexis* ⇨.

Chronic Villitis With Fetal Obstructive Vasculopathy

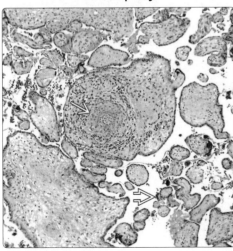

Villous Stromal Hemorrhage and VSVK

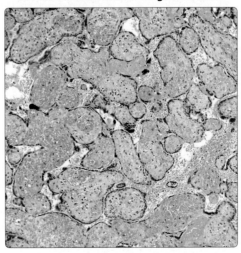

(Left) *This placenta had high-grade chronic villitis with stem villous involvement* ⇨, *which has led to obliteration of the stem vessel and avascular villi* ⇨. *The preferred terminology is "chronic villitis with fetal obstructive vasculopathy."* (Right) *In this case, the villi show stromal and vascular karyorrhexis in addition to villous stromal hemorrhage. The combination of these features suggests obstruction of fetal venous flow in the proximal vasculature. Iron stains may show extensive hemosiderin deposition.*

KEY FACTS

TERMINOLOGY

- Abruption and retroplacental hematoma are not synonymous
- Abruption is clinical diagnosis of premature placental separation
  - Vaginal bleeding or concealed retroplacental clot
  - Painful contractions or failure of uterine relaxation between contractions
  - Nonreassuring fetal status or fetal demise

ETIOLOGY/PATHOGENESIS

- Multifactorial but poorly understood
- Separation occurs from disruption of abnormal maternal vessels
- Traumatic separation of placenta secondary to severe maternal trauma
- Decidual necrosis with acute necrotizing chorioamnionitis

CLINICAL ISSUES

- Abruption has potentially devastating maternal and fetal consequences

MACROSCOPIC

- Retroplacental hematoma consisting of fresh to organizing blood clot adherent to basal plate
- Complete, acute abruption may have no pathologic placental abnormalities

MICROSCOPIC

- Fresh hematomas may be associated with villous edema, congestion, and stromal hemorrhage
- Established hematomas result in villous infarction and decidual devitalization
- Features of maternal malperfusion may be present; decidual arteriopathy
- Severe acute or subacute necrotizing chorioamnionitis, common in midgestation

Large Retroplacental Hematoma

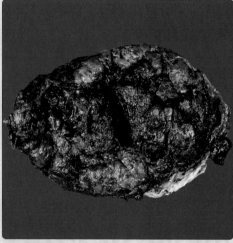

Retroplacental Hematoma Compressing Disc

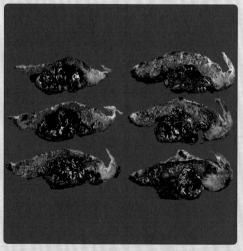

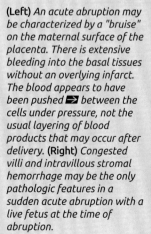

(Left) *Massive abruption caused intrauterine fetal demise at 33-weeks gestation in a mother with severe preeclampsia and chronic hypertension. The large blood clot obscures > 50% of the maternal surface.* (Right) *Cross sections of the same placenta demonstrate the adherent, dark red clot with compression of the adjacent villous parenchyma.*

Blood Dissecting Into Basal Plate

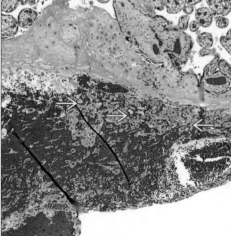

Villous Congestion and Stromal Hemorrhage

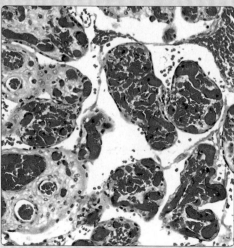

(Left) *An acute abruption may be characterized by a "bruise" on the maternal surface of the placenta. There is extensive bleeding into the basal tissues without an overlying infarct. The blood appears to have been pushed ➡ between the cells under pressure, not the usual layering of blood products that may occur after delivery.* (Right) *Congested villi and intravillous stromal hemorrhage may be the only pathologic features in a sudden acute abruption with a live fetus at the time of abruption.*

TERMINOLOGY

Synonyms

- Placental abruption: Abruptio placentae, premature placental separation, placental detachment

Definitions

- Abruption: Clinical diagnosis of complete or partial detachment of placenta prior to delivery
- Retroplacental hematoma: Hemorrhage or blood clot between basal plate and uterine wall

ETIOLOGY/PATHOGENESIS

Proposed Etiology and Pathogenesis

- Rupture of decidual artery, impaired placentation, chronic inflammation
- Acute inflammation and necrosis of implantation site

CLINICAL ISSUES

Epidemiology

- Incidence
  - Clinical abruption affects 1-2% of pregnancies
  - Increases to 2-4% when including partial/small retroplacental hematomas based on pathological exam
  - Over 50% are preterm, most are late preterm

Presentation

- Clinical syndrome based on maternal &/or fetal signs and symptoms
  - Sudden-onset, painful vaginal bleeding
    - Blood is usually dark
    - Bright red blood may be associated with placenta previa or bleeding of fetal origin
  - Retroplacental hematoma
    - Concealed retroplacental hematoma will not be associated with vaginal bleeding
    - US diagnosis is made in only 15% of cases
  - Abdominal pain, often described as tearing or uterine tenderness
  - Tetanic uterine contractions or uterine hypertonicity
  - Nonreassuring fetal status, including fetal demise
- May be asymptomatic and only identified at time of delivery

Treatment

- Emergent cesarean delivery may be necessary for fetal distress
- Transfusion as necessary for maternal &/or fetal hemorrhage
  - Abruption usually does not result in significant fetal anemia
  - Increased fetal hemorrhage more common in trauma-induced abruption; generally fetal maternal transfusion
    - Kleihauer-Betke on maternal blood to determine amount of fetal hemorrhage
  - Increased risk for postpartum hemorrhage and hysterectomy
- Recognition and management of maternal disseminated intravascular coagulopathy
  - Presence of retroplacental hematoma associated with hypofibrinogemia

Prognosis

- Fetal morbidity dependent on extent of abruption and gestational age
  - Risk of stillbirth or neonatal death with massive abruption at or near term, > 50% of placental surface

Risk Factors

- Preeclampsia/eclampsia, chronic hypertension
- History of prior abruption
- Smoking often associated with placenta previa
- Opioid use
- Abdominal trauma, usually severe, associated with maternal pelvic fracture
- Thrombophilia
- Preterm premature rupture of membranes
- Polyhydramnios with sudden decompression
- Multifetal gestations, particularly twin B
- Chorioamnionitis, usually associated with extreme prematurity
- Diffuse decidual leukocytoclastic necrosis and laminar necrosis preterm

Recurrence Risk

- Abruption secondary to decidual arteriopathy has ~ 23% recurrence risk
- Abruption secondary to acute chorioamnionitis & decidual necrosis has ~ 3% recurrence risk

IMAGING

General Features

- Ultrasound will identify retroplacental hematoma in 15% of cases
- Fresh retroplacental hematoma appears very similar to placental parenchyma

MACROSCOPIC

General Features

- Normal gross placental exam possible even with complete acute abruption
- Congealed, nonadherent blood clot submitted with placenta
  - Weigh loose clot
  - Liquid blood in excess of 100 ml in specimen container may be indicative of acute abruption
  - Blood clots are frequently described at time of delivery, but they may not be submitted in pathology specimen container
- Placenta with fresh (intrapartum) hematoma
  - Soft, red clot loosely adherent to basal plate or retromembranous tissues
  - Indentation of maternal surface may occur within minutes of clot formation
  - Overlying parenchyma may appear more congested, secondary to villous stromal hemorrhage
- Placenta with older hematoma
  - Firm, brown clot adherent to basal plate
  - Concavity or compression of overlying disc
  - Pale, firm infarct of overlying parenchyma

Sections to Be Submitted

- Routine sections to include assessment of maternal decidual vessels
- Basal plate with hematoma and adjacent parenchyma

MICROSCOPIC

Histologic Features

- No alterations in cases of sudden, complete placental separation
- Nonadherent blood clot
  - ○ Congealed with layered aggregate of red blood cells (RBCs) and fibrin
  - ○ May contain portions of decidua
- Placenta with fresh hematoma
  - ○ Hematoma with predominance of RBCs and few fibrin strands
  - ○ Hemorrhage dissecting into basal plate, which may extend into intervillous space
  - ○ Villous congestion with intravillous stromal hemorrhage with live fetus at time of abruption
    - – Loss of maternal blood pressure in intervillous space
    - – Fetal reaction to hypoxia
    - – Rupture of villous capillaries
  - ○ Acute villous infarction
  - ○ Villous edema
  - ○ Inflammation in decidua basalis or admixed with hematoma
- Placenta with older hematoma
  - ○ Hematoma with degenerating RBCs and thick bands of fibrin
  - ○ Basal plate necrosis with acute inflammation as secondary response to tissue injury
  - ○ Hemosiderin-laden macrophages after 48-72 hours
  - ○ Complete villous infarction with avascular and sclerotic stroma
- Abruption secondary to decidual arteriopathy
  - ○ Decidual arteriopathy in basal plate or decidua parietalis
    - – Persistent vascular mural smooth muscle in basal plate
    - – Mural hypertrophy
    - – Fibrinoid necrosis, foamy macrophages (atherosis)
    - – Maternal vessel thrombi
      - □ May be associated with laminar decidual necrosis
    - – Perivascular or subendothelial lymphocytes
  - ○ Chronic inflammation
    - – Chronic deciduitis, lymphocytes, &/or plasma cells in decidua parietalis or basal plate
    - – Chronic inflammation in chorionic plate
    - – Chronic villitis
  - ○ Accelerated villous maturation
- Abruption secondary to acute chorioamnionitis
  - ○ Severe acute or subacute necrotizing chorioamnionitis
  - ○ Extensive necrosis of decidua precedes abruption
  - ○ Villous edema

DIFFERENTIAL DIAGNOSIS

Intervillous Hematoma

- Common finding in 30% of term placentas; may be basally oriented but usually not associated with significant villous injury

Villous Stromal Hemorrhage Associated With Fetal Thrombotic Vasculopathy

- Generally small areas of villous tissue in pattern of villous tree
- Obliterated stem vessels usually present
- More karyorrhexis of stromal and intravascular cells

Vaginal Bleeding May Be of Fetal Origin

- Disruption of fetal blood vessels can also be associated with nonreassuring fetal status
  - ○ Careful gross examination of vessels in all abnormal cord insertions

DIAGNOSTIC CHECKLIST

Clinically Relevant Pathologic Features

- Describe extent of placental surface involvement
- Describe quality of clot
- Describe whether overlying placenta is compressed or infarcted, which helps determine relative age
- Microscopic assessment of maternal vessels
- Evaluate for features of maternal malperfusion

Pathologic Interpretation Pearls

- Distinguish fresh retroplacental hematoma from physiologic postpartum layering of blood
- Normal placental exam does not exclude clinical abruption

SELECTED REFERENCES

1. Chisholm KM et al: Classification of preterm birth with placental correlates. Pediatr Dev Pathol. 1093526618775958, 2018
2. Chen AL et al: The histologic evolution of revealed, acute abruptions. Hum Pathol. 67:187-197, 2017
3. Downes KL et al: Maternal, labor, delivery, and perinatal outcomes associated with placental abruption: a systematic review. Am J Perinatol. 34(10):935-957, 2017
4. Ananth CV et al: Severe placental abruption: clinical definition and associations with maternal complications. Am J Obstet Gynecol. 214(2):272.e1-272.e9, 2016
5. Kuo K et al: Contemporary outcomes of sickle cell disease in pregnancy. Am J Obstet Gynecol. 215(4):505.e1-5, 2016
6. Ananth CV et al: An international contrast of rates of placental abruption: an age-period-cohort analysis. PLoS One. 10(5):e0125246, 2015
7. Kitsantas P et al: Smoking and respiratory conditions in pregnancy: associations with adverse pregnancy outcomes. South Med J. 106(5):310-5, 2013
8. Han CS et al: Abruption-associated prematurity. Clin Perinatol. 38(3):407-21, 2011
9. Elsasser DA et al: Diagnosis of placental abruption: relationship between clinical and histopathological findings. Eur J Obstet Gynecol Reprod Biol. 148(2):125-30, 2010
10. Tikkanen M: Etiology, clinical manifestations, and prediction of placental abruption. Acta Obstet Gynecol Scand. 89(6):732-40, 2010
11. Hall DR: Abruptio placentae and disseminated intravascular coagulopathy. Semin Perinatol. 33(3):189-95, 2009
12. Goldenberg RL et al: The Alabama Preterm Birth Study: diffuse decidual leukocytoclastic necrosis of the decidua basalis, a placental lesion associated with preeclampsia, indicated preterm birth and decreased fetal growth. J Matern Fetal Neonatal Med. 20(5):391-5, 2007
13. Oyelese Y et al: Placental abruption. Obstet Gynecol. 108(4):1005-16, 2006

Partial Acute Abruption

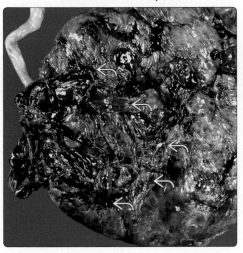

Acute Retroplacental Hematoma

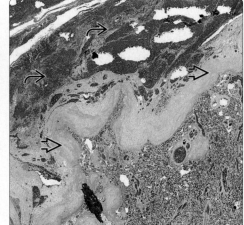

(Left) *A partial acute abruption* ➡ *obscuring 25% of the maternal surface is shown; emergent cesarean delivery was required due to intrapartum fetal distress. The placenta was described as partially detached upon entry into the uterine cavity per the operative note.* (Right) *H&E stain from the placenta with the partial abruption demonstrates the region of the maternal surface* ➡ *with an adherent fresh blood clot* ➡ *showing red blood cells layered with few fibrin strands.*

Postdelivery Pooling of Blood on Basal Plate

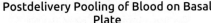
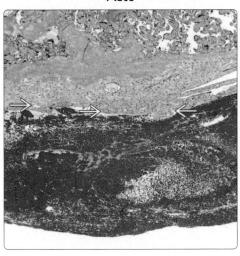

Extension of Retroplacental Hemorrhage

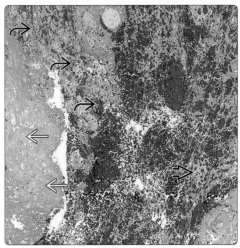

(Left) *Blood from the maternal intervillous space will pool at the basal plate* ➡ *during storage of the placenta after delivery. There is minimal fibrin, no extension of blood into the basal tissue or intervillous space, and no changes in the overlying villi. This could, however, be a finding of very acute abruption.* (Right) *Hemorrhage extends through the basal plate* ➡ *into the intervillous space with direct continuity with villi* ➡. *The decidua basalis shows bland necrosis* ➡.

Early Acute Villous Infarct

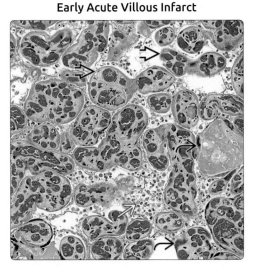

Small Vessel Fetal Thrombotic Vasculopathy

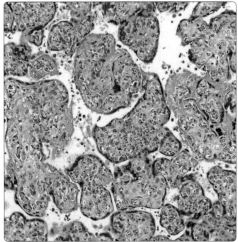

(Left) *Acute abruption resulted in acute infarction of the overlying villi. The syncytiotrophoblasts have lost the majority of the nuclear basophilia* ➡ *with only focal smudging of nuclei* ➡. *An acute maternal inflammatory response is present in the intervillous space* ➡. (Right) *Villous stromal hemorrhage may also be seen in fetal thrombotic vasculopathy. There is generally more stromal karyorrhexis and fragmentation of red blood cells than is seen in abruption.*

Marginal Retroplacental Hematoma

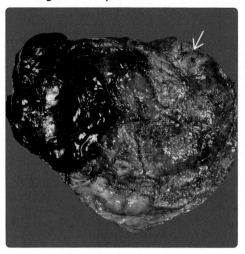

Infarction Hematomas

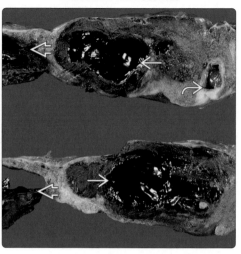

(Left) A marginal hematoma is present on the maternal surface of a placenta delivered at 31-weeks gestation following intrauterine fetal demise in the setting of maternal preeclampsia. Maternal vessels ⊟ on the surface may be thrombosed. (Right) Cut sections of this placenta demonstrate multiple infarcts of varying age. An acute marginal hematoma ⊟ compresses the underlying parenchyma. There is a recent large central infarction hematoma ⊟ and a smaller, remote one ⊟.

Acute Infarction Hematoma

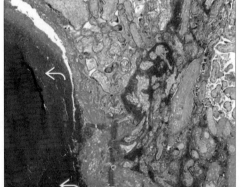

Remote Infarction Hematoma

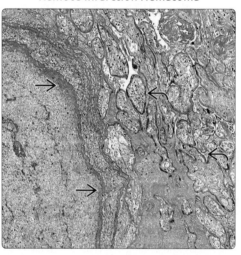

(Left) The hemorrhage ⊟ within an infarct usually does not form the layering of fibrin (lines of Zahn) as is present in the majority of usual intervillous hematomas. (Right) An older infarction hematoma consists of a central laminated fibrin clot with dissolution of red blood cells ⊟ and an adjacent rim of infarcted villi ⊟.

Basal Hemosiderin Deposition

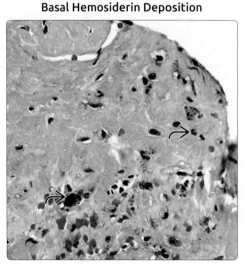

Thrombosis of Maternal Spiral Arteries

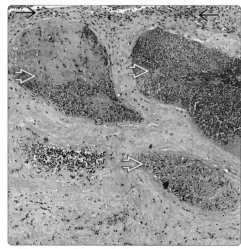

(Left) This section of the maternal surface contains abundant hemosiderin pigment ⊟ and macrophages, consistent with remote episodes of retroplacental hemorrhage. (Right) The maternal vessels in the placenta with the marginal hematoma demonstrate focal acute thrombosis ⊟ and lymphocytic inflammation ⊟.

Acute Abruption and Retroplacental Hematoma

Acute Abruption in Sickle Cell Disease

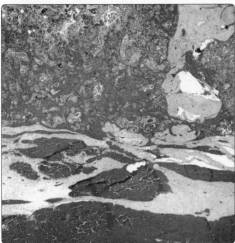

Sickle Cell Disease Placental Sequestration

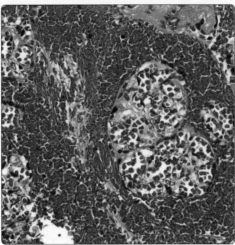

(Left) *Sickle cell disease has an increased risk for abruption. There can be sequestration of the sickled cells within the intervillous space.* **(Right)** *The maternal intervillous space is distended by sickled red blood cells in a manner similar to sickle crises elsewhere in a patient with sickle cell disease.*

Acute Abruption With Acute Chorioamnionitis

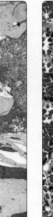

Acute Retroplacental Hematoma at 16 Weeks

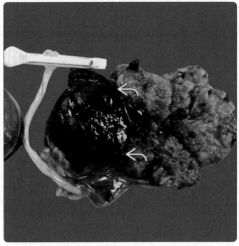

(Left) *This 20-week placenta has markedly discolored membranes with severe necrotizing chorioamnionitis and an acute retroplacental hematoma ⟹.* **(Right)** *This patient presented at 16-weeks gestation with advanced cervical dilation. The placenta shows a partial abruption ⟹. There was no acute inflammation or clinical features of preeclampsia.*

Acute Abruption Due to Acute Chorioamnionitis

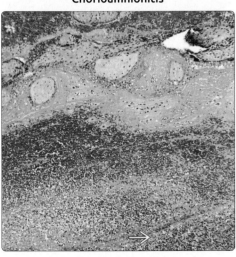

Acute Deciduitis and Necrosis

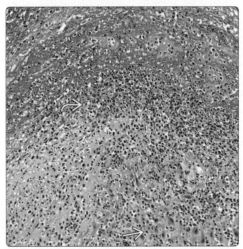

(Left) *Midgestation abruptions are most commonly secondary to acute chorioamnionitis with acute inflammation and necrosis of the implantation decidua ⟹.* **(Right)** *Placental abruption associated with acute chorioamnionitis is seen with extreme prematurity. The separation is usually marginal and associated with severe inflammation ⟹ and necrosis of the basal decidua ⟹. Diffuse decidual leukocytoclastic necrosis has a similar appearance but is not associated with other changes of amniotic fluid infection.*

ETIOLOGY/PATHOGENESIS

- Retromembranous or retroplacental hemorrhage with delayed interval from bleed to delivery
  - Usually repetitive or persistent vaginal bleeding with progression of sonographic lesion
  - Peripheral in location
  - Most likely of venous origin

CLINICAL ISSUES

- Recurrent or prolonged vaginal bleeding
- Obstetric management based on volume of hematoma and gestational age, and fetal well being, including surveillance of amniotic fluid level
- May precipitate preterm labor
- ~ 60% develop chronic abruption-oligohydramnios sequence
  - Defined entity associated with higher incidence of low birthweight, chronic lung disease, and neonatal mortality
- Subchorionic hematoma in 1st trimester
- Bleeding behind the membranes
- Increased risk for abortion, stillbirth, abruption, prematurity, and preterm premature rupture of membranes

MACROSCOPIC

- Hematomas located at disc margin with extension into subchorionic region
- Circumvallate membrane insertion with associated marginal blood clot
- Hemosiderotic discoloration of membranes
- Subchorionic hematoma: Focal green-brown discoloration on maternal surface of free membranes

MICROSCOPIC

- Blood clots of variable age
- Hemosiderin pigment deposition
- Potential infarction of adjacent villous parenchyma
- Inflammation associated with hematoma or frank chorioamnionitis

(Left) *Marginal hematoma results in displacement of membranes off the disc surface, creating a palpable rim or lip* ⇨ *at the membrane insertion. Fresh hematoma is present at the edge of the disc* ⇨ *and may extend into the subchorionic region.* (Right) *A remote marginal hematoma is variable in color, composed of brown to rust-colored remote clot* ⇨ *and a red portion* ⇨*, suggesting more recent clot formation. The clot may show laminations on a further cut section.*

Circumvallation With Marginal Hematoma

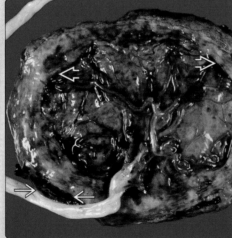

Remote Marginal Hematoma

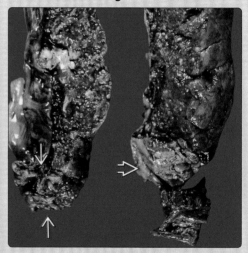

(Left) *Remote retromembranous hemorrhage resulting in red-brown to rusty discoloration of the membranes with relative preservation of the color of the umbilical cord* ⇨ *is shown. Adherent blood clot or necrotic tissue may be present opposite the fetal surface.* (Right) *Hemosiderin-laden macrophages are usually slightly granular and refractile. An iron stain will confirm the presence of iron. Meconium will not stain but may accompany hemosiderin.*

Hemosiderotic Membrane Discoloration

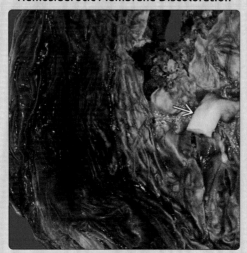

Hemosiderosis Iron Stain

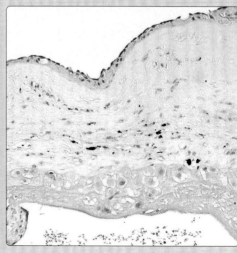

TERMINOLOGY

Synonyms

- Variable usage of language
  - Chronic peripheral separation/marginal abruption
  - Retroplacental hemorrhage with delay in delivery > 7 days
  - Marginal placental bleeding
  - Marginal sinus thrombosis or rupture
  - Venous hemorrhage/abruption

Definitions

- Chronic abruption: Repetitive or persistent hemorrhage with associated placental separation usually involving peripheral plate or membranes not associated with imminent delivery
- Chronic abruption-oligohydramnios sequence (CAOS): Clinical condition with persistent vaginal bleeding without placenta previa and oligohydramnios with amniotic fluid index ≤ 5, without ruptured membranes

CLINICAL ISSUES

Epidemiology

- There are no identified risk factors for chronic abruption or subchorionic hematoma in 1st trimester
- Incidence of chronic abruption is unknown; up to 4.5% in some studies
  - More common than acute abruption, which occurs in 1%
- Chronic abruption commonly manifests as decreased uteroplacental blood flow
- ~ 60% of patients with chronic abruption will develop CAOS
- Subchorionic hematoma in 1st trimester
  - Increased risk for spontaneous abortion, stillbirth, abruption, and preterm premature rupture of membranes

Presentation

- May be asymptomatic
- Vaginal bleeding may begin in 1st trimester and continues into 2nd trimester
- Placenta previa
- Abdominal pain
- Premature delivery
  - False/threatened or preterm labor
  - Preterm premature rupture of membranes
  - Mean gestational age at delivery with CAOS is 28 weeks
- Persistent amniorrhea, loss of fluid per vagina
- Evolving oligohydramnios
- Intrauterine fetal growth restriction
- Intrauterine fetal death
- Subchorionic hematoma in 1st trimester
  - Subchorionic hematoma is clinical term to imply blood found around gestational sac
  - Pathologically found behind membranes, not beneath chorionic plate

Treatment

- Subchorionic hematoma, expectant management with risk awareness
  - Possible precursor to spontaneous abortion

- Increased incidence of true abruption and preterm delivery
- Increased fetal monitoring with elective delivery for poor fetal growth or fetal distress
- Surveillance of amniotic fluid levels
  - Some have advocated serial amnioinfusions for CAOS
    - Decreases toxic substances in amniotic fluid
    - May improve fetal lung volume
- Serial imaging for detection of resolution vs. extension of lesion
- Tocolytics and corticosteroids as appropriate for gestational age and clinical parameters

Prognosis

- Less favorable outcomes with larger volume of hematoma and longer duration of bleeding
- Less favorable neonatal outcomes related to earlier gestational age
  - Low birthweight
  - Complications of prematurity, including chronic lung disease
  - Risk of adverse neurodevelopmental outcome
- CAOS has increased incidence of chronic lung disease and neonatal mortality
  - Lung disease may be due to toxic effects of inhaled blood products

IMAGING

Ultrasonographic Findings

- Sonolucency at site of marginal hematoma/clot
  - Circumvallate placenta is difficult to diagnose on US
    - Irregular, uplifted placental edge
    - Marginal shelf or rim, thick peripheral ring, "valley" is present in folded membranes
    - Thickened placenta ≥ 3.0 cm
  - As hematoma organizes, it progresses then resolves
    - Acute hematoma may be hyperechoic to isoechoic when compared to placenta and difficult to visualize
    - Within 1 week, hematoma appears hypoechoic
    - Within 2 weeks, hematoma may be anechoic
- Decreased amniotic fluid/oligohydramnios in CAOS
- Subchorionic hematoma; US shows low-echoic area around gestational sac during 1st trimester

MR Findings

- Increased T1-weighted images of amniotic fluid suggest presence of blood products in CAOS

MACROSCOPIC

General Features

- Degenerating blood clot ± more recent hemorrhage
- Circumvallate membrane insertion with associated degenerating marginal blood clot
- Extension of clot into subchorionic space from marginal hematoma
- Depression of maternal surface
  - Often associated with scant fibrin deposition
- Infarction of overlying villi
- Subchorionic hematoma in 1st trimester

o Focal retromembranous hemorrhage, green-tan thickened areas

Less Common Features

- Diffuse brown-green to rusty discoloration of fetal surfaces
- Associated parenchymal lesions, including infarcts overlying retroplacental hematomas

MICROSCOPIC

Histologic Features

- Marginal or peripheral subchorionic hematomas
  o Expansion of margin of placental disc with displacement of chorionic plate, peripheral membranes, or basal decidua by hematoma
    - Intermediate hematomas consist of laminated fibrin
    - Remote hematomas may be dissolved, appearing as lightly eosinophilic granular or fibrillary material
  o Adjacent parenchyma is variably affected by increased perivillous fibrin or villous infarction
- Subchorionic hematoma in 1st trimester
  o Homogeneous eosinophilic to granular debris in retromembranous tissues
  o May or may not have hemosiderin-laden macrophages
- Diffuse chorioamniotic hemosiderosis
  o Increased chorionic macrophages
  o Accumulation of hemosiderin pigment in chorionic plate, extraplacental membranes, or basal decidua
- Associated lesions
  o Regions of decidual necrosis
  o Inflammatory infiltrate associated with hematoma usually secondary to necrosis of decidua
  o Necrotizing chorioamnionitis, more often associated with acute abruption

DIFFERENTIAL DIAGNOSIS

Perivillous Fibrin Deposition

- Perivillous fibrin deposition (PVF) can be seen at periphery of infarcts
- PVF fills intervillous space, while infarcts will have collapsed intervillous space
- Extensive or massive PVF may appear as more diffuse marbling of parenchyma

Intervillous Hematoma

- Common finding in term placenta
- Lamination of hematoma occurs over time with development of lines of Zahn
- Blood pushes villi to periphery of hematoma without significant ischemic effects

DIAGNOSTIC CHECKLIST

Clinically Relevant Pathologic Features

- Volume of hematoma or percentage of affected parenchyma relative to total should be estimated and reported
- Conflicting evidence of significance of hemosiderosis in literature

Pathologic Interpretation Pearls

- Chronic abruption is variably defined and accepted as clinicopathologic entity
- CAOS is specific, clinically defined entity
  o Clinical hemorrhage with delay of delivery > 7 days
  o Lack of predisposing factor, such as placenta previa
  o Evolving oligohydramnios without rupture of membranes
  o Increased preterm delivery
  o Increased incidence of chorioamnionitis
  o Increased neonatal morbidity and mortality, especially chronic lung disease

SELECTED REFERENCES

1. Kurata Y et al: MRI findings of chronic abruption-oligohydramnios sequence (CAOS): report of three cases. Abdom Radiol (NY). 42(7):1839-1844, 2017
2. Kobayashi A et al: Adverse perinatal and neonatal outcomes in patients with chronic abruption-oligohydramnios sequence. J Obstet Gynaecol Res. 40(6):1618-24, 2014
3. Morita A et al: Therapeutic amnioinfusion for chronic abruption-oligohydramnios sequence: a possible prevention of the infant respiratory disease. J Obstet Gynaecol Res. 40(4):1118-23, 2014
4. Taniguchi H et al: Circumvallate placenta: associated clinical manifestations and complications-a retrospective study. Obstet Gynecol Int. 2014:986230, 2014
5. Han CS et al: Abruption-associated prematurity. Clin Perinatol. 38(3):407-21, 2011
6. Elsasser DA et al: Diagnosis of placental abruption: relationship between clinical and histopathological findings. Eur J Obstet Gynecol Reprod Biol. 148(2):125-30, 2010
7. Khong TY et al: Haemosiderosis in the placenta does not appear to be related to chronic placental separation or adverse neonatal outcome. Pathology. 42(2):119-24, 2010
8. Norman SM et al: Ultrasound-detected subchorionic hemorrhage and the obstetric implications. Obstet Gynecol. 116(2 Pt 1):311-5, 2010
9. Walker M et al: Sonographic diagnosis of chronic abruption. J Obstet Gynaecol Can. 32(11):1056-8, 2010
10. Ohyama M et al: Maternal, neonatal, and placental features associated with diffuse chorioamniotic hemosiderosis, with special reference to neonatal morbidity and mortality. Pediatrics. 113(4):800-5, 2004
11. Redline RW et al: Chronic peripheral separation of placenta. The significance of diffuse chorioamnionic hemosiderosis. Am J Clin Pathol. 111(6):804-10, 1999
12. Elliott JP et al: Chronic abruption-oligohydramnios sequence. J Reprod Med. 43(5):418-22, 1998
13. Harris BA Jr: Peripheral placental separation: a review. Obstet Gynecol Surv. 43(10):577-81, 1988
14. Sauerbrei EE et al: Placental abruption and subchorionic hemorrhage in the first half of pregnancy: US appearance and clinical outcome. Radiology. 160(1):109-12, 1986
15. Naftolin F et al: The syndrome of chronic abruptio placentae, hydrorrhea, and circumvallate placenta. Am J Obstet Gynecol. 116(3):347-50, 1973

Placental Marginal Sinus

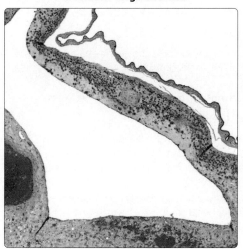

Thrombosis of Placental Marginal Sinus

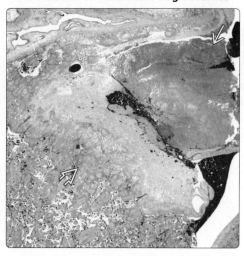

(Left) *The marginal sinus is at the junction of the free membranes with the margin of the placenta. There is some debate whether this is an actual vascular structure, but there does appear to be an endothelial lining.* (Right) *The marginal sinus is obliterated by a remote hematoma ➡. The adjacent villi ➡ are infarcted and ghost-like.*

Remote Retroplacental Hematoma With Hemosiderin

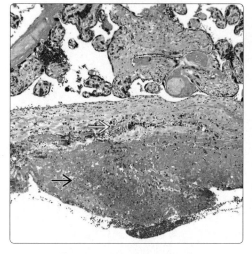

Remote Retroplacental Hematoma With Infarction

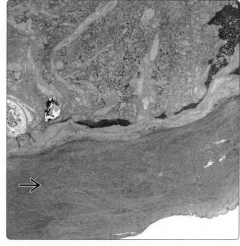

(Left) *The hematoma ➡ is remote with abundant hemosiderin extending into the basal plate ➡. The overlying villi are not infarcted, which implies good collateral circulation within the intervillous space.* (Right) *This large remote retroplacental hematoma ➡ has resulted in infarction of the overlying villi. This implies that there is a large area of maternal surface involvement.*

Remote Retromembranous Hemorrhage

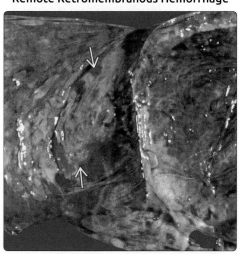

Remote Retromembranous Hematoma

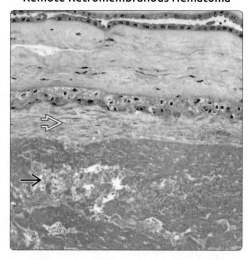

(Left) *The free membranes have a large area of green-tan discoloration ➡ from hemorrhage into the maternal tissues of the decidua parietalis. This usually correlates with a history of a subchorionic hematoma in the 1st trimester.* (Right) *There is a large amount of homogeneous eosinophilic debris within the decidua parietalis ➡ resulting from resolution of a remote retromembranous (subchorionic) hemorrhage. The decidua overlying the hemorrhage is devitalized ➡.*

TERMINOLOGY

- Villous hypercapillarization

ETIOLOGY/PATHOGENESIS

- Likely adaptive response to chronic placental underperfusion/hypoxia
- More frequent in setting of diabetes, preeclampsia, and hypertension
- May be seen in association with multiple cord lesions (true knots, abnormal insertion, and increased length or twist)

CLINICAL ISSUES

- Has been variably associated with poor fetal outcome, including nonreassuring fetal heart tones, increased rate of cesarean delivery, intrauterine growth restriction, and stillbirth

MACROSCOPIC

- Placentas with chorangiosis can be large for gestational age

- May see concurrent umbilical cord abnormalities or hypoxic lesions (infarcts or hematomas)

MICROSCOPIC

- ≥ 10 medium-powered fields of placental parenchyma with ≥ 10 terminal villi, each containing ≥ 10 capillaries, in at least 3 areas
- Capillaries are **not** surrounded by layer of pericytes

DIAGNOSTIC CHECKLIST

- Diagnosis reserved for mature placenta (> 37-weeks gestation)
- Hypervascular villi found in at least 3 different areas on H&E-stained slides
- Do not use immunohistochemistry for vascular markers (CD31 or CD34) because of risk of overdiagnosis
- Do not evaluate areas adjacent to infarction (can have focal chorangiosis-like reaction)
- Can be mimicked by vascular congestion

Hypervascular Terminal Villi

Diffuse Hypervascularity

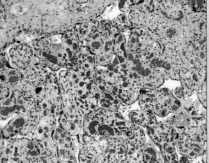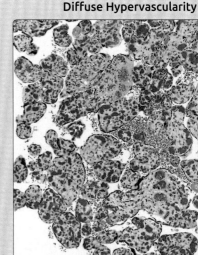

(Left) Even under low power, the impression of hypervascularity raises suspicion for chorangiosis. (Right) At least 3 separate areas should be involved to make a diagnosis of chorangiosis.

Increased Capillarization

Capillaries Without Pericytes

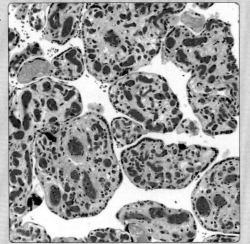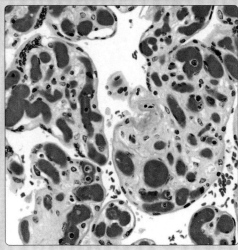

(Left) At least 10 villi in each of the 3 areas should contain ≥ 10 capillaries in order to meet the recommended diagnostic criteria. (Right) High-power view helps confirm the absence of a continuous pericyte layer around the capillaries.

TERMINOLOGY

Synonyms

- Villous hypercapillarization
- Villous hypervascularity

Definitions

- ≥ 10 fields of placental parenchyma with ≥ 10 terminal villi, each containing ≥ 10 capillaries, in at least 3 different areas

ETIOLOGY/PATHOGENESIS

Environmental Exposure

- Likely adaptive response to chronic placental underperfusion/hypoxia
- Cytotrophoblast proliferates more rapidly under hypoxic conditions and induces capillary endothelial proliferation; capillaries are excessively coiled in distal villi
- Vascular proliferation exceeds stromal growth resulting in increased capillary:villus area ratio
- Stimulated by cytokines, growth factors (VEGF and FGF), &/or increased vascular pressure

Incidence

- 5-10% of all placentas
- Typically only diagnosed in placentas after 37-weeks gestation

Associations

- More frequent in diabetic pregnancies
- More frequent in severely anemic mothers
- More frequent in setting of preeclampsia and hypertension
- More frequent at higher elevations
- More frequent with exposure to smoking and air pollution
- Associated with Beckwith-Wiedemann syndrome and congenital heart disease
- May be seen in association with multiple cord lesions (true knots, abnormal insertion, and increased length or twist)

CLINICAL ISSUES

Prognosis

- Chorangiosis itself may not confer worse prognosis, but underlying chronic hypoxia and associated conditions do
- Has been variably associated with poor fetal outcome, including nonreassuring fetal heart tones, increased rate of cesarean delivery, intrauterine growth restriction, and stillbirth

IMAGING

Ultrasonographic Findings

- Chorangiosis usually occurs in setting of normal umbilical artery Doppler ultrasound examinations

MACROSCOPIC

General Features

- Lesion(s) are not usually visible grossly
- Placentas can be large for gestational age
- May see concurrent umbilical cord abnormalities

MICROSCOPIC

Histologic Features

- ≥ 10 medium-powered fields of placental parenchyma with ≥ 10 terminal villi, each containing ≥ 10 capillaries
  - Normal: 2-6 capillaries/villus
- Capillaries are **not** surrounded by layer of pericytes
- May see concurrent villous infarcts, intervillous hematomas, and persistent nucleated fetal red blood cells

ANCILLARY TESTS

Immunohistochemistry

- Muscle-specific actin marks pericytes in chorangioma and chorangiomatosis, which are absent in chorangiosis
- Endothelial markers, such as CD31 and CD34, should **not** be used
  - Not part of accepted diagnostic criteria; will lead to overdiagnosis

DIFFERENTIAL DIAGNOSIS

Congestion of Normal Terminal Villi

- Fetal capillary bed is normally only ~ 50% filled
  - Congestion will appear hypervascular
- True chorangiosis may have nearly 20 capillaries per villus, many more than would be apparent with vascular congestion

Chorangioma

- Single expansile nodule
- Capillaries have continuous layer of pericytes

Chorangiomatosis

- Involves intermediate villi, stem villi
- Capillaries have continuous layer of pericytes

DIAGNOSTIC CHECKLIST

Pathologic Interpretation Pearls

- Diagnosis should be made on H&E-stained slides, not by immunohistochemistry
- Present in ≥ 10 fields in ≥ 3 areas of sampled parenchyma
- Do not evaluate areas adjacent to infarction (can have focal, chorangiosis-like reaction)
- Can be mimicked by vascular congestion

SELECTED REFERENCES

1. Bhattacharjee D et al: Histopathological study with immunohistochemical expression of vascular endothelial growth factor in placentas of hyperglycemic and diabetic women. J Lab Physicians. 9(4):227-233, 2017
2. Stanek J: Chorangiosis of chorionic villi: what does it really mean? Arch Pathol Lab Med. 140(6):588-93, 2016
3. Barut A et al: Placental chorangiosis: the association with oxidative stress and angiogenesis. Gynecol Obstet Invest. 73(2):141-51, 2012
4. Chan JS et al: Gross umbilical cord complications are associated with placental lesions of circulatory stasis and fetal hypoxia. Pediatr Dev Pathol. 15(6):487-94, 2012
5. Akbulut M et al: Chorangiosis: the potential role of smoking and air pollution. Pathol Res Pract. 205(2):75-81, 2009
6. Ogino S et al: Villous capillary lesions of the placenta: distinctions between chorangioma, chorangiomatosis, and chorangiosis. Hum Pathol. 31(8):945-54, 2000
7. Altshuler G: Chorangiosis. An important placental sign of neonatal morbidity and mortality. Arch Pathol Lab Med. 108(1):71-4, 1984

TERMINOLOGY

- Localized chorangiomatosis
  - Hypervascularization of multiple adjacent stem villi in single focus
- Multifocal chorangiomatosis
  - Hypervascularization of multiple adjacent stem villi in multiple foci
  - Multiple chorangioma-like lesions scattered throughout placenta

CLINICAL ISSUES

- < 1% of all placentas
- Localized chorangiomatosis is associated with maternal preeclampsia and multiple gestation pregnancies
- Multifocal chorangiomatosis is associated with placentomegaly, advanced maternal age, avascular villi, preterm delivery, intrauterine growth restriction, and congenital malformations

MICROSCOPIC

- Localized chorangiomatosis
  - Similar to chorangioma, but rather than forming single nodule, it involves multiple adjacent stem villi
  - Capillary vessel proliferation throughout involved stem villi
  - Lesional vessels are surrounded by pericytes and lattice-like reticulin fibers
  - Increased stromal collagenization, sometimes with central dense fibrotic core (similar to stem villi)
- Multifocal chorangiomatosis
  - Involves multiple foci of multiple stem villi or intermediate villi
  - Small anastomosing capillaries at periphery of stem villi surrounding central vessel
  - Lesional vessels surrounded by pericytes and increased stromal collagen

Villous Hypervascularity

Capillaries With Pericytes

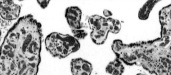

(Left) *Localized chorangiomatosis shows expansion of multiple adjacent intermediate villi by proliferating capillaries that are similar to those seen in chorangioma.* (Right) *The lesional capillaries are surrounded by pericytes, unlike those in chorangiosis.*

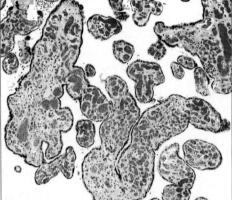

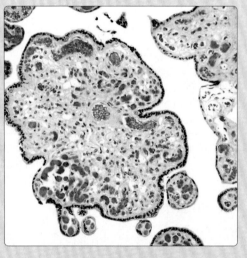

Villous Stromal Alterations

Placental Mesenchymal Dysplasia

(Left) *The villi have increased stromal cellularity and matrix with areas of collagenization ➡ and a lattice-like pattern on reticulin stain.* (Right) *Chorangiomatosis can also be seen in the setting of placental mesenchymal dysplasia, as seen here with large, edematous, irregularly shaped villi and occasional cisterns.*

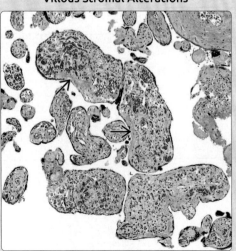

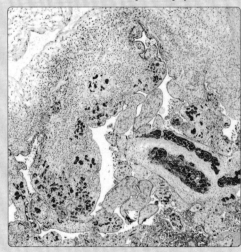

TERMINOLOGY

Synonyms

- Localized chorangiomatosis
  - Focal chorangiomatosis
  - Segmental chorangiomatosis
- Multifocal chorangiomatosis
  - Diffuse chorangiomatosis
  - Diffuse multifocal chorangiomatosis
  - Multiple chorangiomas

Definitions

- Localized chorangiomatosis
  - Hypervascularization of multiple adjacent stem villi in single focus
- Multifocal chorangiomatosis
  - Hypervascularization of multiple adjacent stem villi in multiple foci
  - Multiple chorangioma-like lesions scattered throughout placenta

ETIOLOGY/PATHOGENESIS

Developmental Anomaly

- May arise from aberrant overgrowth of peripheral capillary net seen in immature intermediate villi maturing to early stem villi
- Typically manifest after 32-weeks gestation

CLINICAL ISSUES

Epidemiology

- Incidence
  - < 1% of all placentas

Presentation

- Localized chorangiomatosis is associated with maternal preeclampsia and multiple gestation pregnancies
- Multifocal chorangiomatosis is associated with placentomegaly, advanced maternal age, avascular villi, preterm delivery, intrauterine growth restriction, and congenital malformations
- Both forms are associated with other vascular abnormalities, including chorangiosis and chorangiomas
- Can be seen in setting of placental mesenchymal dysplasia
- Platelet sequestration in lesional vessels can lead to thrombocytopenia or disseminated intravascular coagulation in neonates

MACROSCOPIC

General Features

- Localized and multifocal chorangiomatosis are not usually grossly identifiable
- Multiple chorangiomas may be evident as scattered small, tan or red nodules

MICROSCOPIC

Histologic Features

- Localized chorangiomatosis
  - Similar to chorangioma, but rather than forming single nodule, it involves multiple adjacent stem villi
  - Capillary vessel proliferation throughout involved stem villi
  - Lesional vessels are surrounded by pericytes and lattice-like reticulin fibers
  - Increased stromal collagenization, sometimes with central dense fibrotic core (similar to stem villi)
- Multifocal chorangiomatosis
  - Involves multiple foci of multiple stem villi or intermediate villi
  - Small anastomosing capillaries at periphery of stem villi surrounding central vessel
  - Lesional vessels surrounded by pericytes and increased stromal collagen

ANCILLARY TESTS

Histochemistry

- Reticulin highlights stromal matrix surrounding capillaries

Immunohistochemistry

- Pericytes surrounding capillaries are positive for muscle-specific actin

DIFFERENTIAL DIAGNOSIS

Congestion of Normal Terminal Villi

- Capillaries should be counted to avoid overcalling prominent, distended vessels

Chorangioma

- Capillary expansion of single stem villus
- Similar appearance of capillaries invested by pericytes

Chorangiosis

- > 10 terminal villi, each with > 10 capillaries, in at least 10 fields in 3 different areas
- Hypervascularity confined to terminal villi
- Lesional vessels lack surrounding pericytes

REPORTING

Categorization

- Localized (1 area of involved villi) vs. multifocal (multiple areas)
- Focal (1-5 involved villi) vs. segmental (more than 5 involved villi) vs. diffuse multifocal

SELECTED REFERENCES

1. Rosefort A et al: Co-occurrence of multifocal chorioangiomatosis and mesenchymal dysplasia in preeclampsia. Pediatr Dev Pathol. 16(3):206-9, 2013
2. Bagby C et al: Multifocal chorangiomatosis. Pediatr Dev Pathol. 14(1):38-44, 2011
3. Amer HZ et al: Chorangioma and related vascular lesions of the placenta--a review. Fetal Pediatr Pathol. 29(4):199-206, 2010
4. Chopra A et al: Diffuse multifocal chorangiomatosis of the placenta with multiple intestinal stenosis of the fetus: combination of rare causes for nonimmune hydrops fetalis. Indian J Pathol Microbiol. 49(4):600-2, 2006
5. Caldarella A et al: Chorangiosis: report of three cases and review of the literature. Pathol Res Pract. 199(12):847-50, 2003
6. Ogino S et al: Villous capillary lesions of the placenta: distinctions between chorangioma, chorangiomatosis, and chorangiosis. Hum Pathol. 31(8):945-54, 2000

KEY FACTS

TERMINOLOGY

- Intraparenchymal nodule composed of capillaries, stromal cells, and surrounding trophoblast layers

ETIOLOGY/PATHOGENESIS

- Placental hypoxia → angiogenesis with excessive capillary proliferation
- May occur concurrently with infantile hemangiomas (as high as 50% in some studies)

CLINICAL ISSUES

- Most common placental tumor (~ 0.5-1.0% of all placentas)
- Small chorangiomas (< 1 cm) are usually asymptomatic
- Medium-sized chorangiomas (1-4 cm) can be associated with fetal growth restriction, preterm delivery, and stillbirth
- Large chorangiomas (> 4 cm) can cause preterm delivery, polyhydramnios, intrauterine growth restriction, fetal thrombocytopenia, arteriovenous shunting with high-output heart failure, and stillbirth

- Fetoscopic intervention is high risk but can be performed to ligate, cauterize, or ablate lesion and its feeding vessel

MACROSCOPIC

- Single or multiple nodules, 1 mm to > 10 cm
- Usually subchorionic or marginal

MICROSCOPIC

- Vascular proliferation expanding mature stem villus
- Capillary vessels set within variably cellular (fibroblasts and macrophages) and collagenous stroma
- Surrounding trophoblastic layer may have hyperplasia

ANCILLARY TESTS

- GLUT1(+) (like infantile hemangioma)

TOP DIFFERENTIAL DIAGNOSES

- Localized/"focal" chorangiosis
- Multifocal chorangiomatosis
- Chorangiocarcinoma

Chorangioma

Cellular Appearance of Chorangioma

(Left) Chorangioma is always well circumscribed. It consists of a stem villus expanded by a proliferation of capillaries and stroma. (Right) Chorangioma can appear cellular with a lobular architecture reminiscent of infantile hemangioma.

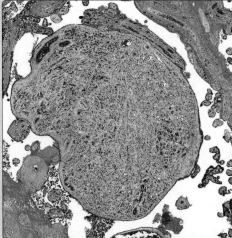
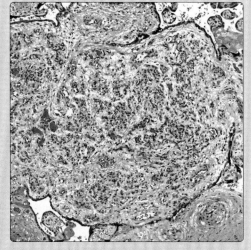

Mitotic Activity

Pericytes in Mature-Appearing Chorangioma

(Left) Chorangioma may show a proliferative phase of growth. Stromal mitoses ➡ are a common finding and do not indicate malignant potential. (Right) The small capillaries of a chorangioma are surrounded by pericytes ➡.

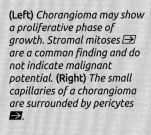
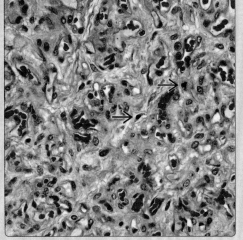
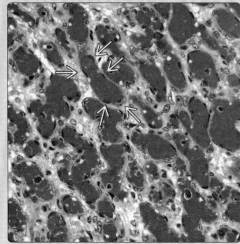

TERMINOLOGY

Synonyms

- Placental hemangioma
- Fibroangiomyxoma

Definitions

- Intraparenchymal nodule composed of capillaries, stromal cells, and trophoblast

ETIOLOGY/PATHOGENESIS

Environmental Exposure

- Reactive proliferation, not neoplasm
- Placental hypoxia may induce angiogenesis and excessive capillary proliferation

Associations

- Preeclampsia
- Multiple gestation
- High altitude
- May recur in subsequent pregnancies
- Often occurs concurrently with infantile hemangiomas (as high as 50% in some studies)

CLINICAL ISSUES

Epidemiology

- Incidence
  - Most common placental tumor
  - ~ 0.5-1.0% of all placentas

Presentation

- Usually develops between 32- to 37-weeks gestation
- Small chorangiomas (< 1 cm) are usually asymptomatic
- Medium-sized chorangiomas (1-4 cm) can be associated with fetal growth restriction, preterm delivery, and stillbirth
- Large chorangiomas (> 4 cm) can cause
  - Preterm delivery
  - Polyhydramnios
  - Intrauterine growth restriction
  - Platelet trapping in small tortuous vessels (with fetal thrombocytopenia, hemorrhage, &/or disseminated intravascular coagulation)
  - Arteriovenous shunting (with fetal hydrops, anemia, high-output heart failure, polyhydramnios, &/or death)
  - Maternal "mirror" syndrome (with maternal edema or preeclampsia in association with fetal hydrops)
  - Stillbirth
- May increase risk of fetal-maternal hemorrhage

Natural History

- Hamartomatous mesenchymal lesion
- Chorangiomas and infantile hemangiomas appear to be related
  - Often occur together
  - Have similar gene and protein expression patterns
  - Some propose that infantile hemangiomas develop from placental endothelial cells that enter fetal circulation, or that growth of infantile hemangioma may be mediated by growth factors and signaling molecules shed from chorangioma
- Can undergo infarction or spontaneous regression

Treatment

- Options, risks, complications
  - Often just carefully monitored; if fetal distress occurs, delivery can be induced
  - Symptomatic fetal therapy
    - Amnioreduction
    - Blood transfusion
- Surgical approaches
  - Fetoscopic intervention
    - Surgical ligation of feeding placental vessels
    - Alcohol injection to induce vascular sclerosis
    - Microcoil embolization
    - Bipolar coagulation
    - Laser ablation
    - These approaches have significant risk of rupture of chorangioma or its feeding vessel with subsequent hemorrhage and fetal exsanguination (as high as 50% in some series)

Prognosis

- Spontaneous involution/regression or treatment of large chorangiomas is associated with improvement of clinical symptoms
- Altered blood flow secondary to chorangioma or other fetoplacental vascular tumors may be associated with poorer neurodevelopmental outcomes

IMAGING

Ultrasonographic Findings

- Well-circumscribed, heteroechogenic mass by ultrasound
- Decreased blood flow on Doppler imaging is associated with fewer complications and better prognosis
- Associated polyhydramnios and fetal growth restriction

MACROSCOPIC

General Features

- Single or multiple nodules
- Usually subchorionic or marginal (sites of lower oxygen levels)
- Can be dark and soft (vascular) or firm and tan (fibrotic)
- Often occur in isolation but may see concurrent hypoxic lesions (infarcts, thrombi, cord lesions)
- Chorangiomas can separate and deliver separately from placenta
  - May occur after in utero infarction
  - May occur by shearing of feeding vessel during delivery/handling of placenta
  - Clinical differential diagnosis may include leiomyoma, acardiac twin, or other entity

Size

- Range: 1 mm to > 10 cm

MICROSCOPIC

Histologic Features

- Vascular proliferation expanding mature stem villus
  - Capillary vessels set within variably cellular and collagenous stroma, surrounded by trophoblast layers
  - Stroma contains fibroblasts, macrophages, and collagen

- May have associated trophoblastic hyperplasia
- Older lesions may have degenerative changes: Calcifications, infarcts, hemosiderin-laden macrophages
- Different subtypes (capillary, cavernous, endotheliomatous, fibrosing, fibromatous) have been described, but all have identical clinical behavior
- Never malignant despite variable mitotic activity, variable cellularity, and occasional atypical cytology
- Microscopic appearance mimics stages of infantile hemangioma growth and regression

ANCILLARY TESTS

Immunohistochemistry

- Not required, but CD31 and CD34 stain endothelial lining, and muscle-specific actin stains pericytes
- GLUT1(+) (like infantile hemangioma)

Genetic Testing

- Not required but shows normal karyotype
- Clonality has not been demonstrated in these lesions

DIFFERENTIAL DIAGNOSIS

Gross Mimics

- Villous infarct
- Laminated intervillous hematoma

Histologic Mimics

- Localized/"focal" chorangiosis
  - Capillary proliferation limited to distal chorionic villi
  - Lesional vessels lack surrounding pericytes
- Multifocal chorangiomatosis
  - Similar capillary proliferation expanding stem villi
    - Involves multiple stem or intermediate villi, in 1 or multiple areas

Chorangiocarcinoma

- Very rare lesion of intraplacental choriocarcinoma with hypervascular villous stroma
  - Trophoblastic proliferation is striking with extensive necrosis

- Differs from syncytiotrophoblast sprouting that may appear hyperplastic on surface of benign chorangioma

SELECTED REFERENCES

1. Sirotkina M et al: Clinical outcome in singleton and multiple pregnancies with placental chorangioma. PLoS One. 11(11):e0166562, 2016
2. Sirotkina M et al: Association of chorangiomas to hypoxia-related placental changes in singleton and multiple pregnancy placentas. Placenta. 39:154-9, 2016
3. Lim FY et al: Giant chorioangiomas: perinatal outcomes and techniques in fetoscopic devascularization. Fetal Diagn Ther. 37(1):18-23, 2015
4. Fan M et al: Placental chorioangioma: literature review. J Perinat Med. 42(3):273-9, 2014
5. Iacovella C et al: Fetal and placental vascular tumors: persistent fetal hyperdynamic status predisposes to poorer long-term neurodevelopmental outcome. Ultrasound Obstet Gynecol. 43(6):658-61, 2014
6. Selmin A et al: An epidemiological study investigating the relationship between chorangioma and infantile hemangioma. Pathol Res Pract. 210(9):548-53, 2014
7. Saksiriwuttho P et al: Prenatal three dimensional ultrasonography and expectant management of placental chorioangioma: a case report. J Med Assoc Thai. 96(4):496-500, 2013
8. Faes T et al: Chorangiocarcinoma of the placenta: a case report and clinical review. Placenta. 33(8):658-61, 2012
9. García-Díaz L et al: Prenatal management and perinatal outcome in giant placental chorioangioma complicated with hydrops fetalis, fetal anemia and maternal mirror syndrome. BMC Pregnancy Childbirth. 12:72, 2012
10. Amer HZ et al: Chorangioma and related vascular lesions of the placenta--a review. Fetal Pediatr Pathol. 29(4):199-206, 2010
11. Sepulveda W et al: Endoscopic laser coagulation of feeding vessels in large placental chorioangiomas: report of three cases and review of invasive treatment options. Prenat Diagn. 29(3):201-6, 2009
12. Taori K et al: Chorioangioma of placenta: sonographic features. J Clin Ultrasound. 36(2):113-5, 2008

Gross Appearance of Chorangioma

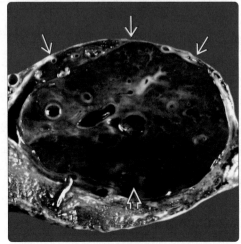

(Left) A medium-sized chorangioma ➡ bulges from the underside of the chorionic plate ➡. The circumscribed, red, firm appearance is characteristic of these highly vascular lesions. (Right) Histologically, the lesion is a well-circumscribed stem villus expanded by a capillary proliferation.

Chorangioma

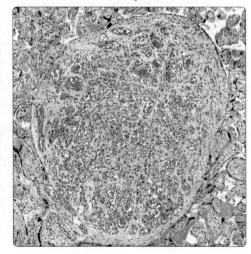

Infarcted Chorangioma

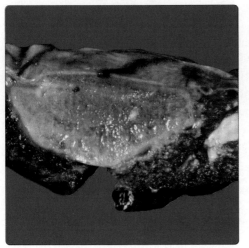

Infarcted Chorangioma

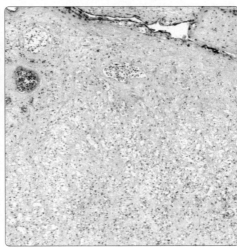

(Left) *Grossly, an infarcted chorangioma has a firm, tan appearance distinct from the usual soft red character of a viable lesion and may easily be mistaken for a more common villous infarct. It retains a glassy texture.* (Right) *Microscopically, an infarcted chorangioma has ghosted capillaries and stromal cells. Variable preservation of the overlying trophoblast and central areas may be seen.*

Trophoblast in Chorangioma

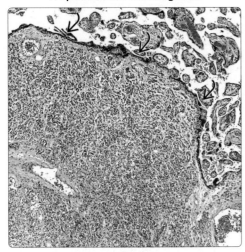

GLUT1 Staining of Chorangioma

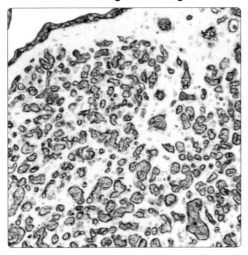

(Left) *Chorangiomas are composed of capillary proliferations expanding stem villi. The capillaries are surrounded by stromal cells, and the nodule is lined by villous cytotrophoblast and syncytiotrophoblast* ⊞. (Right) *Immunohistochemistry for glucose transporter GLUT1 strongly highlights the capillaries of chorangiomas (and stains the overlying trophoblast), similar to the vessels in infantile hemangiomas.*

Benign Syncytiotrophoblast Hyperplasia in Chorangioma

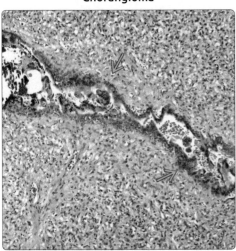

Chorangiocarcinoma

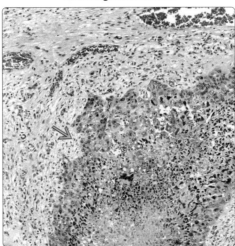

(Left) *The syncytiotrophoblast may show hyperplastic changes* ⊟ *such as elongated sprouts and occasionally lace-like proliferation. These findings are not diagnostic of chorangiocarcinoma.* (Right) *In chorangiocarcinoma, the trophoblastic proliferation* ⊟ *is malignant (intraplacental choriocarcinoma). It is unclear if the villous capillary proliferation is a reactive change, or if it truly represents intraplacental choriocarcinoma arising in a chorangioma. The former seems more likely.*

Hydropic Degeneration

TERMINOLOGY

- Hydropic degeneration (HD) or hydropic abortion: Pathologic term referring to edematous microscopic appearance of nonmolar villi

CLINICAL ISSUES

- HD
  - Most present as missed abortion
  - Uterus small for dates
  - β-hCG low (mean 19,000 mIU/mL) or decreasing
  - In normal pregnancy, β-hCG increased 66% every 48 hours

IMAGING

- Gestational sac smaller than expected for gestational age or empty gestational sac with no fetal pole
- Embryo/fetus smaller than expected for gestation
- No cardiac activity
- Absent or abnormal yolk sac

MACROSCOPIC

- Varying amount of villous tissue, dependent on gestational age, but generally not increased
- Rarely identify embryonic or fetal tissues
- Hydropic villi up to 2.2 mm
- Rare cisterns < 3 mm

MICROSCOPIC

- Direct or indirect evidence of embryo/fetus
- Villi relatively uniform, round to oval
- Villous stroma edematous, frequently amphophilic, or fibrotic
- Residual vessels, rarely containing nucleated red blood cells
- Syncytiotrophoblast atrophy, corresponds to decreasing hCG
- Normal implantation site

Missed Abortion Photographed Under Dissecting Scope

HD With Atrophic Syncytiotrophoblasts

(Left) The villi have been rinsed and rehydrated in water. The villi are relatively uniform in diameter, with some distal tapering, like the branches of a tree. (Right) Hydropic degeneration (HD) shows amphophilic, hypocellular, avascular stroma. There is atrophy of surrounding syncytiotrophoblasts, consistent with low or decreasing hCG. The findings usually indicate embryo loss significantly before evacuation of the uterine contents.

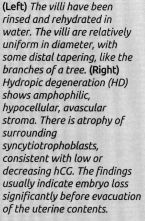
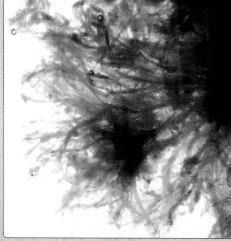
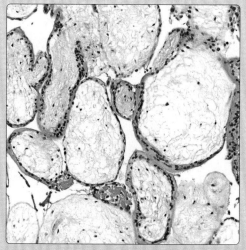

HD With Embryonic Tissue

Normally Adapted Maternal Spiral Artery

(Left) Embryonic/fetal tissues are rarely noted grossly after a suction D&C, but bone and cartilage may be firm to palpation and will remain intact. (Right) The implantation site associated with HD is normal. The invasive trophoblasts will invade and destroy the vascular smooth muscle. Early in gestation, these maternal vessels will be contained or plugged ➡ by trophoblasts.

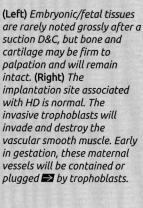
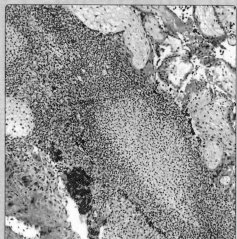
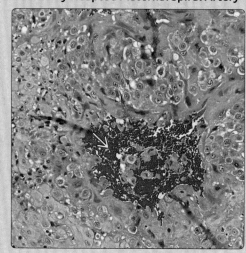

TERMINOLOGY

Abbreviations

- Hydropic degeneration (HD), nonmolar abortion (NMA), hydropic abortion (HA)
- Partial hydatidiform mole (PHM)
- Complete hydatidiform mole (CHM)
- Very early complete hydatidiform mole (VECHM)
- Human chorionic gonadotropin (hCG) (generally refers to β subunit)
- Gestational trophoblastic disease (GTD); CHM, PHM, placental site nodule (PSN), exaggerated placental site (EPS)
- Gestational trophoblastic neoplasm (GTN); choriocarcinoma, placental site trophoblastic tumor (PSTT), epithelioid trophoblastic tumor (ETT)

Definitions

- HD
  - Pathologic term referring to edematous microscopic appearance of nonmolar villi
- Blighted ovum, anembryonic pregnancy
  - Empty gestational sac
- Missed abortion
  - Presentation at routine visit and found to have nonviable pregnancy
- Incomplete abortion
  - Presentation with open cervix and vaginal bleeding, possibly with passage of clots and tissue

ETIOLOGY/PATHOGENESIS

HD

- 50-75% secondary to chromosomal abnormalities
  - 80% autosomal chromosome aberrations, 15% sex chromosome aneuploid, 5% polypoid
- Majority diploid, but can be triploid or tetraploid HD

CLINICAL ISSUES

Epidemiology

- Incidence
  - Vast majority of fertilized ova do not develop into viable pregnancy
  - 60% of pregnancies lost prior to 1st missed period

Presentation

- HD
  - Most present as missed abortion
  - Uterus small for dates
  - Decreasing or low β-hCG, mean < 19,000 mIU/mL
    - In normal early gestation, serum hCG increases 66% every 48 hours

Treatment

- Options, risks, complications
  - Expectant management
    - 71% will spontaneously pass products of conception; increased incidence of bleeding
  - Medical therapy
    - Misoprostol in 1st trimester (sublingual or vaginal) will be successful in 66% of cases within 18 hours; increased incidence of pain
    - Pregnancy with higher hCG levels less likely to successfully respond to misoprostol
  - Surgical treatment
    - Dilation and suction curettage may be primary choice or become necessary if expectant management or medical therapy does not result in complete evacuation of uterine contents; increased risk for uterine perforation
    - Dilation and evacuation treatment of choice in 2nd trimester
  - Follow-up
    - Transvaginal US to assure complete evacuation after any of above therapies
    - β-hCG should return to normal 6-8 weeks after evacuation

Prognosis

- Rare incidence of GTD
  - 25% of choriocarcinomas believed to occur after spontaneous abortion
- Persistent positive hCG may indicate retained placental tissue

IMAGING

Ultrasonographic Findings

- HD
  - Gestational sac smaller than expected for gestational age or empty gestational sac with no fetal pole
  - Embryo/fetus smaller than expected for gestation
  - No cardiac activity
  - Absent, small, or abnormally shaped or cystic yolk sac

MACROSCOPIC

General Features

- HD
  - Varying amount of villous tissue, dependent on gestational age, but generally not increased
  - Gestational sac, chorionic plate usually present; rarely umbilical cord
  - Rarely identify embryonic or fetal tissues
    - Cartilage and bone will be firm to palpation and remain intact during D&C process
  - Hydropic villi, < 2 mm
  - Rare small cisterns, < 2 mm
    - Do not mistake primary chorionic plate of gestational sac for large cistern
- Dysmorphic villi, may be associated with chromosomal abnormalities or congenital malformations
  - Scant tissue
  - Slightly larger villi, 2-3 mm

Sections to Be Submitted

- Careful examination of gross tissue will usually yield villi
  - Rinse tissue through fine mesh strainer and resuspend in water
    - Removing blood will aid in visualization of placental tissue

- Placing tissue in hypotonic water for a few minutes will rehydrate villi
  - □ This technique will work even after formalin fixation
  - o Majority of tissue will be sheets of lush decidua
    - Decidua vera will be present in intrauterine and ectopic pregnancy
- Implantation site should be submitted
  - o Implantation site slightly firm with yellow hyalinized appearance due to presence of fibrinoid
  - o Implantation site confirms intrauterine pregnancy, even in absence of villi
  - o Implantation site may identify abnormalities responsible for pregnancy loss
  - o CHM has atypical implantation site that is especially useful in identification of VECHM

MICROSCOPIC

Histologic Features

- HD
  - o Direct evidence of fetus
    - Embryonic or fetal tissues
  - o Indirect evidence of fetus
    - Chorionic plate, amnion, umbilical cord, nucleated red blood cells, yolk sac
  - o Villi relatively uniform in size and are round to oval
    - Villous stroma edematous, paucicellular, or fibrotic
    - Residual vessels may be present, sometimes containing nucleated red blood cells or karyorrhectic debris
    - Variable number of Hofbauer cells; some may contain eosinophilic granules
  - o Trophoblasts
    - Syncytiotrophoblast atrophy, corresponds to decreasing hCG
    - Anchoring villi with polar orientation of cytotrophoblast columns
    - Normal invasive trophoblasts at implantation site
- Abnormal villous morphology (dysmorphic villi)
  - o Dysmorphic changes frequently raise concern for molar pregnancy, especially partial mole
    - May be associated with chromosomal abnormalities or malformation syndromes
  - o May see dimorphic villous populations, small fibrotic and larger edematous villi
  - o Variation in villous size and shape, irregular contours with infrequent trophoblast pseudoinclusions
  - o Calcification of trophoblast basement membrane, stromal/vascular karyorrhexis in older gestations
  - o Rare atypical intrastromal trophoblasts
  - o May see abnormal maze-like vasculature
  - o No abnormal trophoblast proliferation
  - o Rare cisterns, < 3 mm in size

ANCILLARY TESTS

Immunohistochemistry

- p57, cyclin-dependent kinase inhibitor 1C (CDKN1C, p57, KIP2)

- o Extravillous trophoblast at tips of anchoring villi, invasive trophoblasts and decidual cells are positive in all gestations
- o Positive nuclear staining in > 10% of villous cytotrophoblasts and stromal cells in HD and PHM
- o < 10% nuclear staining of villous cytotrophoblast and stromal cells in CHM
- Ki-67
  - o Minimal staining of cytotrophoblasts in HD

Flow Cytometry

- Useful to determine ploidy
  - o HD and CHM are diploid
  - o PHM is triploid
    - Diandric triploids are PHM, digynic triploids are nonmolar
  - o Flow can only identify aneuploidy when > 10% abnormal population, ≥ 2 chromosomes

Genetic Testing

- Considered gold standard in diagnosis, but cost may limit practical utility
- Routine karyotype has high rate of failure in cases with HD
- Chromosomal microarray recommended in cases of repeated pregnancy loss
  - o Microarray does not always identify triploidy
- Short tandem repeat (STR) loci genotyping identifies maternal and paternal genomic contributions, most useful genetic test for diagnosing molar disease
  - o Androgenetic diploid (2 copies of paternal genes only, no maternal) = CHM
  - o Diandric triploid (2 copies of paternal genes and 1 set of maternal) = PHM
  - o Digynic triploid (2 copies of maternal genes and 1 set of paternal) = nonmolar

Algorithm for Use in HD Diagnosis

- Morphologic assessment to see if molar features present or absent; in most cases of HD, diagnosis straightforward; in cases with abnormal villous morphology, may need ancillary studies
- Supplementation with p57 immunostain to exclude CHM if concern for mole
  - o p57 will not distinguish HD from PHM
- For p57(-) cases with concern for PHM, molecular STR genotyping can identify PHM
- Chromosomal microarray has higher yield than cytogenetics for identifying chromosomal abnormalities as well as smaller gene deletions or duplications
  - o Comparison with maternal and paternal blood samples best for interpretation of gene results
- Always check hCG and compare to expected normal levels for gestational age

DIFFERENTIAL DIAGNOSIS

VECHM

- Atypical implantation site, bulbous cauliflower-like villi, myxoid stroma, abundant karyorrhexis and mixed trophoblast proliferation

Serum β-hCG Levels During Normal Pregnancy

Weeks	5th Percentile	Mean	95th Percentile
4	318	719	1,065
6	16,451	41,642	81,650
8	81,313	133,885	232,315
10	50,155	95,670	151,440
12	37,990	79,236	129,005
14	30,500	67,630	136,900
16	15,942	32,889	87,115
18	7,400	26,560	50,000
20	8,963	19,920	37,217
22	12,600	23,855	40,800
24	9,328	19,560	33,130
26	6,800	24,707	57,200
28	13,030	31,584	72,970
30	12,071	21,690	46,650
32	9,160	28,860	77,100
34	5,198	26,374	93,405
36	8,120	30,290	96,700
38	10,360	34,763	10,360
40	5,943	23,138	71,556

β-hCG Values in Pregnancy, Clinical Assays, 1982.

PHM

- 2 villous populations, prominent villous irregularity, trophoblastic pseudoinclusions, central cisterns and syncytiotrophoblast proliferation

DIAGNOSTIC CHECKLIST

Pathologic Interpretation Pearls

- Most important part of grossing specimen is to rinse out blood and float/rehydrate villi in water
- Implantation site decidua basalis will confirm intrauterine pregnancy in absence of villi

SELECTED REFERENCES

1. Mählck CG et al: Follow-up after early medical abortion: comparing clinical assessment with self-assessment in a rural hospital in northern Norway. Eur J Obstet Gynecol Reprod Biol. 213:1-3, 2017
2. Petersen SG et al: Utility of βhCG monitoring in the follow-up of medical management of miscarriage. Aust N Z J Obstet Gynaecol. 57(3):358-365, 2017
3. Rosenfeld JA et al: Diagnostic utility of microarray testing in pregnancy loss. Ultrasound Obstet Gynecol. 46(4):478-86, 2015
4. Stomornjak-Vukadin M et al: Combined use of cytogenetic and molecular methods in prenatal diagnostics of chromosomal abnormalities. Acta Inform Med. 23(2):68-72, 2015
5. Banet N et al: Characteristics of hydatidiform moles: analysis of a prospective series with p57 immunohistochemistry and molecular genotyping. Mod Pathol. 27(2):238-54, 2014
6. Levy B et al: Genomic imbalance in products of conception: single-nucleotide polymorphism chromosomal microarray analysis. Obstet Gynecol. 124(2 Pt 1):202-9, 2014
7. Gupta M et al: Diagnostic reproducibility of hydatidiform moles: ancillary techniques (p57 immunohistochemistry and molecular genotyping) improve morphologic diagnosis for both recently trained and experienced gynecologic pathologists. Am J Surg Pathol. 36(12):1747-60, 2012
8. Wapner RJ et al: Chromosomal microarray versus karyotyping for prenatal diagnosis. N Engl J Med. 367(23):2175-84, 2012
9. Sotiriadis A et al: Expectant, medical, or surgical management of first-trimester miscarriage: a meta-analysis. Obstet Gynecol. 105(5 Pt 1):1104-13, 2005

Fresh D&C

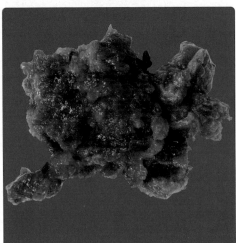

Fresh D&C Floated in Water

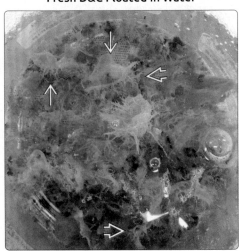

(Left) *Fresh tissue removed from a suction evacuation device without any additional manipulation does not show distinct villous tissue.* (Right) *This is the same specimen after rinsing through a fine mesh strainer and floating the tissue in water. The placental membranes ➡ and villous tissue ➡ are easily identified.*

HD Anchoring Villi

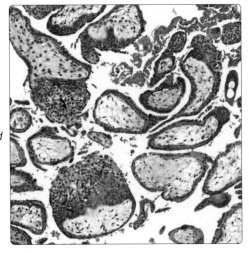

HD

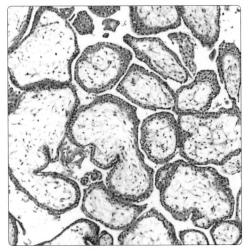

(Left) *The polar-oriented cytotrophoblast columns of the anchoring villi are very prominent in this case.* (Right) *The villi in HD are relatively uniform in size and round to oval. The stroma is myxoid with mild edema, and residual vessels are empty and collapsed. The villi are 1st trimester with a dual cyto- and syncytiotrophoblast covering. The plump syncytiotrophoblasts may be associated with a higher than expected hCG.*

HD, p57

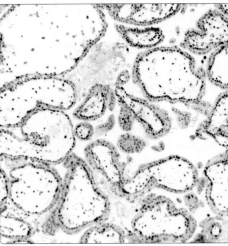

HD, Ki-67

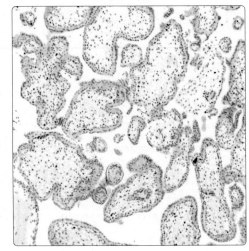

(Left) *Diffuse positive cytotrophoblast and stromal staining with p57 is noted in this relatively well preserved 1st-trimester HD. Staining may be less prominent when there is significant degeneration of the tissue.* (Right) *The HD has very limited Ki-67 cytotrophoblast staining. There is a progressive increase in staining from HD to partial hydatidiform mole (PHM) to complete hydatidiform mole (CHM).*

Implantational Decidua, Gross

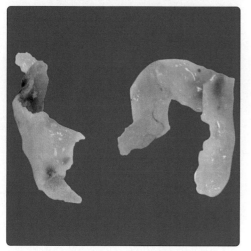

Implantational Decidua

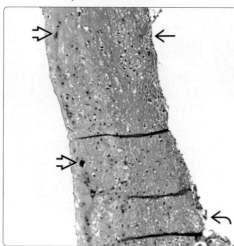

(Left) *Implantation decidua grossly has a yellow hyalinized appearance due to fibrinoid deposition. It is thinner and also has increased resistance compared to the more abundant nonimplantational decidua.* (Right) *Implantational decidua shows the thick layer of fibrinoid ⟹ with extravillous trophoblasts ⟹ in the decidua vera. On the surface of the fibrinoid, there are a few multinucleated syncytiotrophoblasts ⟹. If necessary, a cytokeratin can be performed to confirm the presence of invasive trophoblasts.*

Normal Basal Implantation

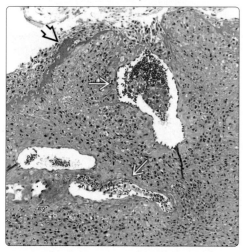

Chorion Laeve of Free Membranes

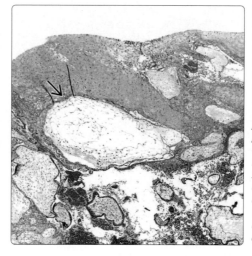

(Left) *The basal implantation site should also have maternal vessels that are undergoing adaptation to pregnancy. The vessel lumens normally contain, and may be completely plugged by, invasive trophoblasts ⟹ in the 1st trimester. Nitabuch fibrinoid ⟹ is also noted focally.* (Right) *Villi within the chorion laeve of the free membrane frequently have significant hydropic degeneration ⟹ and may even show central cisterns. This is due to devitalization of the villi as the free membranes are forming.*

Nonimplantional Decidua, Decidua Vera, Gross

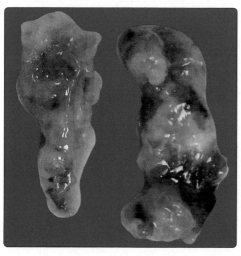

Nonimplantational Decidua, Decidua Vera

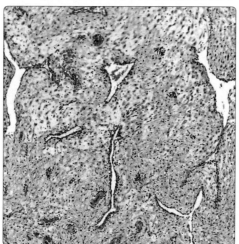

(Left) *The nonimplantation site decidua (decidua vera) may represent the majority of tissue in early gestation. It is tan-pink, spongy, and usually present in sheets. There may be focal acute hemorrhage.* (Right) *Nonimplantation decidua shows changes of pregnancy hormones on the endometrium, but these changes are not diagnostic of an intrauterine pregnancy. Ectopic pregnancy would show the same decidualization. There is usually only a minimal amount of acute decidual inflammation in a spontaneous abortion.*

(Left) In the 1st trimester, trophoblastic islands are a normal component. They are composed of villi with extravillous trophoblasts and fibrinoid deposition. They become inconspicuous later in pregnancy and may become calcified. **(Right)** HD may be associated with increased numbers of Hofbauer cells ⊟. The cytoplasm may be vacuolated and sometimes will contain eosinophilic globules.

Trophoblastic Island

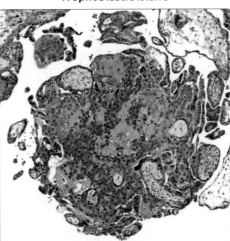

HD, Hofbauer Cell Hyperplasia

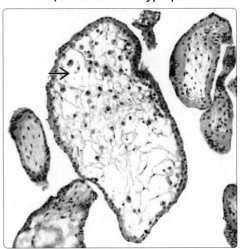

(Left) The yolk sac will involute ~ 9-weeks gestation and may calcify (as seen here) or become fibrotic. The presence of amnion ⊟ and yolk sac ⊟ are indirect features of a fetus. **(Right)** The majority of the red cells in the fetal capillaries are nucleated, a feature of early gestation (6-8 weeks).

Calcified Yolk Sac

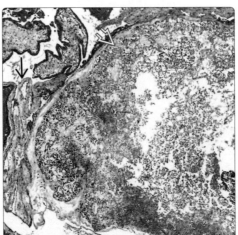

Nucleated Red Blood Cells

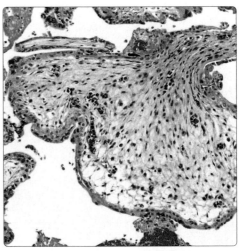

(Left) These large vessels containing large numbers of nucleated cells may represent an umbilical cord, indirect evidence of a fetus. **(Right)** This late 1st-trimester pregnancy has significant chronic inflammation in the chorionic plate and villi. This could be due to an infectious etiology or a heightened maternal response against the placental tissues.

Possible Umbilical Cord

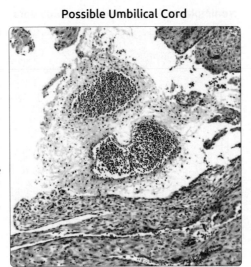

HD With Chronic Inflammation

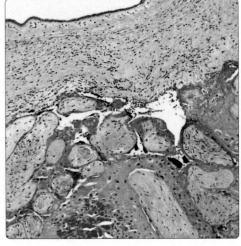

Dysmorphic Villi, 2 Villous Populations

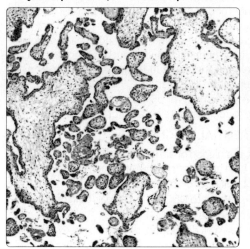

Dysmorphic Villi, Trisomy 13

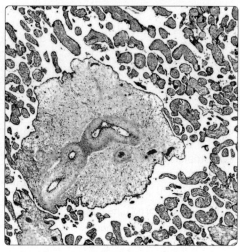

(Left) There is a significant difference in villous size with 2 villous populations. This is a feature often associated with chromosomal abnormality or congenital malformations. The features are also seen in PHM. (Right) Trisomy 13 may show dysmorphic villous features. Rare vesicles may be present, even visible grossly. There is no abnormal trophoblast proliferation.

Trophoblast Pseudoinclusion Dysmorphic Villi

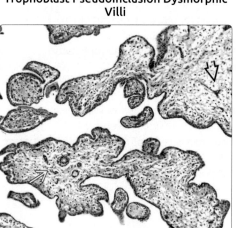

Dysmorphic Villi, Pseudoinclusions, and Calcifications

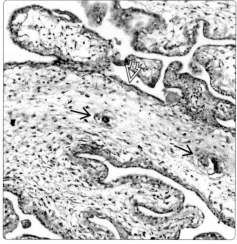

(Left) Villous irregularity is pronounced in this case with several trophoblast pseudoinclusions ➡. There are residual blood vessels ⊡ containing red blood cells. (Right) The irregular shape may be associated with trophoblast pseudoinclusions ➡. Abnormal stromal calcification, and especially calcification of the trophoblast basement membrane ⇒, is also a dysmorphic feature.

Calcified Trophoblast Basement Membrane, 45,X

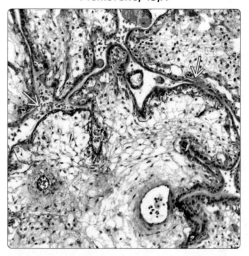

Atypical Stromal Trophoblast

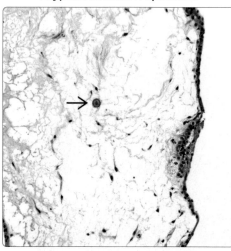

(Left) Mineralization of the trophoblastic basement membrane ➡ may be seen in dysmorphic villi. The etiology is unknown. (Right) A dysmorphic, hydropic villus with an isolated atypical cell ⊡ is shown. Staining shows that these are consistent with extravillous trophoblasts. There is no stromal karyorrhexis and no trophoblast proliferation. Similar atypical cells may be seen in PHM and CHM.

Partial Hydatidiform Mole

TERMINOLOGY

- Partial hydatidiform mole (PHM)
- Diandric triploidy: 3 sets of chromosomes (2 paternal, 1 maternal)
- Digynic triploidy: 3 sets of chromosomes (1 paternal, 2 maternal)

ETIOLOGY/PATHOGENESIS

- PHM is triploid gestation with 2 paternal genomes and 1 maternal genome (diandric triploidy)
  - Triploidy can also be composed of 2 maternal genomes and 1 paternal genome (digynic triploidy): These are not associated with PHM

MICROSCOPIC

- Morphology alone is generally diagnostic for PHM when at least 3 of 4 following features of PHM are well developed
  - 2 populations of villi (large hydropic and smaller fibrotic)
  - Enlarged, irregular, dysmorphic villi with trophoblast inclusions
  - Enlarged villi with cisterns (at least 3 mm in size)
  - Syncytiotrophoblast hyperplasia/atypia
- Nonmolar triploidy (digynic triploidy) may show some of these features but not significant syncytiotrophoblast hyperplasia

ANCILLARY TESTS

- If at least 3 of 4 histologic features are not well developed (as is often case in very early PHM), consider following next steps
  - Short tandem repeat (STR) genotyping to identify diandric triploidy, confirming diagnosis of PHM
  - Flow cytometry or FISH for ploidy
    - Can be performed on fresh, formalin-fixed or formalin-fixed paraffin embedded tissue
    - Useful for diagnosing triploidy vs. other chromosomal abnormalities common in HD and cases with abnormal villous morphology

- Will not tell digynic triploidy from PHM; histologic features of diandric and digynic triploidy can overlap in 1st trimester
  - If resources do not accommodate additional molecular testing, issue general diagnosis, such as "abnormal villous morphology, cannot exclude PHM," and recommend follow-up serum HCG testing
- Immunohistochemistry for p57 immunohistochemistry is useful to exclude complete hydatidiform mole (CHM)

TOP DIFFERENTIAL DIAGNOSES

- Dimorphic population of abnormal and normal villi can be seen with twin gestation of CHM and nonmolar twin
  - Nonmolar villi lack dysmorphic changes
  - Ultrasound prior to D&C usually reveals twin gestation
- Very early complete mole (CM)
  - Cisterns less well developed, can be mistaken for partial mole
  - Cytotrophoblast and syncytiotrophoblast proliferation around villi and at implantation site in CM
  - Immunostaining for p57 distinguishes CM from PHM
- Placental mesenchymal dysplasia
  - Can have cystic villi but no syncytiotrophoblast proliferation
- Androgenetic/biparental mosaic/chimeric conceptions with CM component
  - Can be confusing, as only subset of villi appear molar
  - Can be associated with embryo/fetus
  - Immunohistochemistry for p57 shows characteristic lack of reactivity in molar villi
    - Risk of gestational trophoblastic disease after these conceptions in cases with CM component

PHM

PHM Floated in Water

(Left) A formalin-fixed partial hydatidiform mole (PHM) without rehydration in water is difficult to evaluate. (Right) The curettage was rinsed and floated in water. Membranes ⊅ are visible in addition to small vesicles ⊳.

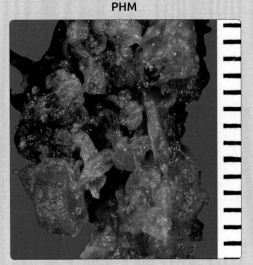
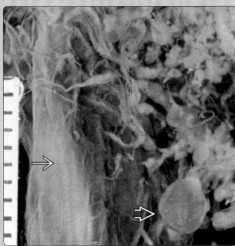

TERMINOLOGY

Abbreviations
- Partial hydatidiform mole (PHM)
- Complete hydatidiform mole (CHM)
- Human chorionic gonadotropin (hCG)

Definitions
- Diandric triploidy: 3 sets of chromosomes (2 paternal, 1 maternal)
- Digynic triploidy: 3 sets of chromosomes (2 maternal, 1 paternal)
- Androgenetic conception: Chromosomes from paternal origin only
- Androgenetic/biparental mosaic conception: Mixed population where some cell lineages have only paternal chromosomes, other cell lineages have both maternal and paternal chromosomes
- Gestational trophoblastic disease (GTD): PHM, CHM, invasive mole, choriocarcinoma, epithelioid trophoblastic tumor, placenta site trophoblastic tumor

ETIOLOGY/PATHOGENESIS

Triploidy
- May be due to extra maternal (digynic triploidy) or paternal (diandric triploidy) genome
- Accounts for 1-3% of conceptions
  o Associated with early pregnancy loss
  o Rarely associated with live birth (1/10,000 to 1/250,000)
    - Neonatal death due to malformations
    - Males account for 50-70% of live births
  o Malformations include cleft lip, cardiac malformations, neural tube defects, holoprosencephaly, microcephaly, cystic kidneys, single umbilical artery, and syndactyly of 3rd and 4th fingers and toes
  o 64% diandric dispermy, 24% diandric monospermy, and 10% digynic in origin
- Nearly all partial moles are triploid, but not all triploid conceptions are partial mole
- PHM
  o Diandric triploidy: 2 paternal genomes and 1 maternal genome
    - Rarely tetraploid with 3 paternal components
    - Excess paternal genome drives placental overgrowth
  o Normal ovum fertilized by 1 sperm that replicates (monospermy) or by 2 sperm (dispermy)
  o 69,XXY > 69,XXX > > 69,XYY karyotypes
- Nonmolar triploid
  o Digynic triploidy: 2 maternal genomes and 1 paternal genome
  o Attributed to errors in 2nd meiotic division
  o Usually 1st-trimester embryonic loss
  o 69, XXX karyotype more common in cases with fetus
    - Growth restriction may be due to placental insufficiency

CLINICAL ISSUES

Presentation
- PHM
  o Usually present as missed abortion
    - Rarely associated with liveborn fetus, appropriate for gestational age growth, or with symmetric growth restriction with multiple congenital anomalies associated with triploidy
  o Uterus typically small for dates
  o Rarely has mildly increased hCG, mean: < 80,000 mIU/mL
  o Rarely diagnosed in ectopic pregnancy
- Nonmolar triploid
  o Most present as missed abortion or embryonic loss
    - Prevalence of triploidy in second trimester estimated at 1/5,000 pregnancies
  o Rarely associated with with liveborn fetus with asymmetric growth restriction with multiple congenital anomalies associated with triploidy

Treatment
- Options, risks, complications
  o Follow-up for PHM
    - Complete evacuation either medically or surgically is usually sufficient treatment
    - Serum hCG monthly until negative and then 1 more measurement 1 month after 1st negative

Prognosis
- Persistent GTD after PHM in < 1%
- Most persistent GTD after PHM is due to retained molar tissue or invasive mole
  o More aggressive forms of GTD after diagnosis of PHM are very rare

IMAGING

Ultrasonographic Findings
- Only 15% of PHM are diagnosed prior to pathologic examination
- Empty gestational sac or may have embryo/fetus, usually with significant growth restriction
- Rare vesicles, best seen on transvaginal ultrasound

MACROSCOPIC

General Features
- PHM
  o Volume of villous parenchyma normal or increased, especially compared to hydropic degeneration (HD)
  o Gestational sac and chorionic plate are usually present
  o Gross vesicles measuring 3-5 mm present in subset of villi (usually ~ 20% of villi)
  o Diandric triploidy fetus shows severe symmetric growth restriction, may be normally grown in subset of cases
    - Syndactyly of 3rd and 4th fingers &/or toes
    - Cleft lip and palate, holoprosencephaly, microcephaly
    - Similar malformations seen in digynic triploidy with exception of asymmetric growth restriction
- Nonmolar digynic triploidy, small placenta
  o Very small placenta, no molar features
  o Embryo/fetus, asymmetric growth restriction with preservation of head growth
    - Syndactyly of 3rd and 4th fingers &/or toes
    - Cleft lip and palate, holoprosencephaly

Sections to Be Submitted

- If there is clinical diagnosis of mole or grossly identified vesicles, submit all of villous tissue or 10 cassettes
  - Include implantation site decidua

MICROSCOPIC

Histologic Features

- PHM
  - Direct or indirect evidence of embryo/fetus
    - Direct = embryonic/fetal tissues
    - Indirect = chorionic plate, amnion, umbilical cord, yolk sac, nucleated red blood cells
  - Abnormal villi
    - 2 villous populations: Larger edematous villi and smaller fibrotic villi
    - Hydropic villi, 3-5 mm, involving < 20% of villi
    - Irregular villous shape (scalloped or dentate) resulting in formation of rare to many round or oval trophoblast pseudoinclusions
    - Central cisterns without karyorrhectic stromal cells
    - After 16 weeks, villi may have maze-like spaces that are actually dilated vascular structures
    - Syncytiotrophoblast proliferation only; may be inconspicuous, rarely circumferential, discontinuous, or with lacy appearance
  - Normal anchoring villi with polar orientation of cytotrophoblast columns
  - Normal invasive trophoblast at implantation site
    - Mild nuclear atypia with enlargement at implantation site noted in some cases
- Very early PHM (1st trimester)
  - Direct or indirect evidence of embryo/fetus
  - Abnormal villi
    - Spectrum of villus sizes (dimorphic population not well developed)
    - Scattered hydropic villi with rare cisterns
    - Some irregularly shaped villi with trophoblast pseudoinclusion
      - "Dentate" outline described, often with right angles
    - Focal syncytiotrophoblastic proliferation, nonpolar
    - Persistence of nucleated red blood cells beyond expected gestational age
  - Normal anchoring villi with polar orientation of cytotrophoblast columns
  - Normal invasive trophoblast at implantation site
- Nonmolar digynic triploidy
  - Dysmorphic villi
    - Irregular size and shape with rare cisterns and rare trophoblastic pseudoinclusions
    - Occasional polypoid projections of syncytiotrophoblast but no striking proliferation
  - Normal anchoring villi and implantation site

ANCILLARY TESTS

Immunohistochemistry

- p57: Cyclin-dependent kinase inhibitor 1C (CDK1C, p57, KIP2)
  - Extravillous trophoblast at tips of columns and some decidual cells are positive in HD, PHM, and CHM

- Positive nuclear staining in > 10% of villous cytotrophoblast cells and stromal cells in PHM or HD
- Lack of villous cytotrophoblast cell and villous stromal cell staining in CHM
- Ki-67 of PHM
  - Intermediate staining between near absence in HD and diffuse positivity in CHM
  - Interpretation of this stain requires significant experience, less straightforward than p57

Flow Cytometry

- Useful to determine ploidy
  - PHM are predominantly triploid, although aneuploid and tetraploid PHM have been identified
  - Triploid conceptions may also be nonmolar (digynic triploidy)
  - Placental mesenchymal dysplasia (PMD), diploid

Genetic Testing

- Considered gold standard in diagnosis, but cost may limit practical utility
  - Molecular short tandem repeat genotyping identifies maternal and paternal genomic contributions
    - Best test for diagnosis of very early PHM, identifying diandric triploidy
  - Karyotype or FISH will identify triploidy
    - Does not distinguish diandric from digynic triploidy
  - Chromosome microarray may not identify triploidy with some methodologies

Algorithm for Use in Partial Hydatidiform Mole Diagnosis

- Morphology alone is generally diagnostic for cases with at least 3 of 4 following features of PHM
  - 2 populations of villi: Large hydropic and smaller fibrotic
  - Enlarged, irregular dysmorphic villi with trophoblast inclusions
  - Enlarged villi with cisterns (at least 3 mm in size)
  - Syncytiotrophoblast hyperplasia/atypia
- If at least 3 features are not well developed (as is often case in very early PHM), consider following next steps
  - Short tandem repeat (STR) genotyping to identify diandric triploidy, confirming diagnosis of PHM
  - Issue general diagnosis, such as "abnormal villous morphology, cannot exclude PHM," and recommend follow-up serum HCG testing
    - Reasonable approach in resource-limited setting
    - May be clinically unacceptable when mother is having difficulty getting pregnant and does not want to delay getting pregnant again
- Immunohistochemistry for p57 immunohistochemistry is useful to exclude CHM
  - Will not distinguish PHM from HD
- Flow cytometry or FISH for ploidy is useful for diagnosing triploidy
  - Can be performed on fresh, formalin-fixed or formalin-fixed paraffin embedded tissue
  - Will not tell digynic triploidy from partial mole, histologic features of diandric and digynic triploidy can overlap in 1st trimester

DIFFERENTIAL DIAGNOSIS

Very Early Complete Mole

- CHM is easier histologic diagnosis in 1st trimester
  - No direct evidence of embryo/fetus (except for mosaic cases with complete mole component)
  - Villi are more bulbous with rounded, cauliflower-like contours
  - Amphophilic cytoplasm with karyorrhectic stromal cells precedes cavitation
  - Proliferation of cytotrophoblast and syncytiotrophoblast surrounding abnormal villi
  - Proliferation of pleomorphic and hyperchromatic extravillous trophoblast in implantation site

Placental Mesenchymal Dysplasia

- Formerly known as "pseudopartial mole"
- PMD incidence: 0.02%
- Androgenetic/biparental mosaicism with androgenetic component confined to placental mesenchyme
- Associated with intrauterine growth restriction and Beckwith-Wiedemann syndrome (BWS) in subset of cases
- Morphology
  - Characterized by large, cystically dilated stem villi with central cistern formation and very cellular stroma, often hypervascular
    - Resembles hydropic villi of PHM on gross exam
  - Aneurysmally dilated, often thrombosed chorionic plate vessels
  - ± chorangiosis and changes of fetal vascular malperfusion
- Lacks trophoblastic proliferation of PHM
- 1st-trimester specimens of likely PMD show enlarged villi with cisterns but no trophoblastic proliferation
  - p57 immunostaining shows loss of staining in villous mesenchyme with preservation in cytotrophoblast
  - Genotyping shows androgenetic/bipaternal mosaic conception with androgenetic stroma and bipaternal cytotrophoblast

Androgenetic/Biparental Mosaic/Chimeric Conceptions With Complete Mole Component

- Subset of villi appear molar with large cisterns and trophoblastic proliferation
- Rarely may have embryo/fetal tissues suggesting diagnosis of partial mole
- CHM component demonstrates trophoblastic proliferation on hydropic villi
  - Implantation site may have atypical extravillous trophoblast proliferation of complete mole
  - p57 staining will be compatible with complete mole in subset of villi that have trophoblast proliferation
  - Short tandem repeat (STR) genotyping confirms androgenetic component

DIAGNOSTIC CHECKLIST

Pathologic Interpretation Pearls

- Villous trophoblast proliferation in PHM consists of syncytiotrophoblast only

SELECTED REFERENCES

1. Kaur B et al: p57KIP2 immunostaining for diagnosis of hydatidiform mole. BJOG. ePub, 2018
2. Kolarski M et al: Genetic counseling and prenatal diagnosis of triploidy during the second trimester of pregnancy. Med Arch. 71(2):144-147, 2017
3. Toufaily MH et al: Triploidy: variation of phenotype. Am J Clin Pathol. 145(1):86-95, 2016
4. Banet N et al: Characteristics of hydatidiform moles: analysis of a prospective series with p57 immunohistochemistry and molecular genotyping. Mod Pathol. 27(2):238-54, 2014
5. Buza N et al: Partial hydatidiform mole: histologic parameters in correlation with DNA genotyping. Int J Gynecol Pathol. 32(3):307-15, 2013
6. Lewis GH et al: Characterization of androgenetic/biparental mosaic/chimeric conceptions, including those with a molar component: morphology, p57 immnohistochemistry, molecular genotyping, and risk of persistent gestational trophoblastic disease. Int J Gynecol Pathol. 32(2):199-214, 2013
7. Sundvall L et al: Tetraploidy in hydatidiform moles. Hum Reprod. 28(7):2010-20, 2013
8. Armes JE et al: The placenta in Beckwith-Wiedemann syndrome: genotype-phenotype associations, excessive extravillous trophoblast and placental mesenchymal dysplasia. Pathology. 44(6):519-27, 2012
9. Gupta M et al: Diagnostic reproducibility of hydatidiform moles: ancillary techniques (p57 immunohistochemistry and molecular genotyping) improve morphologic diagnosis for both recently trained and experienced gynecologic pathologists. Am J Surg Pathol. 36(12):1747-60, 2012
10. Baasanjav B et al: The risk of post-molar gestational trophoblastic neoplasia is higher in heterozygous than in homozygous complete hydatidiform moles. Hum Reprod. 25(5):1183-91, 2010
11. Kim KR et al: The villous stromal constituents of complete hydatidiform mole differ histologically in very early pregnancy from the normally developing placenta. Am J Surg Pathol. 33(2):176-85, 2009
12. McFadden DE et al: Phenotype of triploid embryos. J Med Genet. 43(7):609-12, 2006
13. Vaisbuch E et al: Twin pregnancy consisting of a complete hydatidiform mole and co-existent fetus: report of two cases and review of literature. Gynecol Oncol. 98(1):19-23, 2005
14. Sebire NJ et al: Histopathological diagnosis of partial and complete hydatidiform mole in the first trimester of pregnancy. Pediatr Dev Pathol. 6(1):69-77, 2003
15. Genest DR: Partial hydatidiform mole: clinicopathological features, differential diagnosis, ploidy and molecular studies, and gold standards for diagnosis. Int J Gynecol Pathol 20(4):315-322, 2001

PHM After Prolonged Formalin Fixation Floated in Water

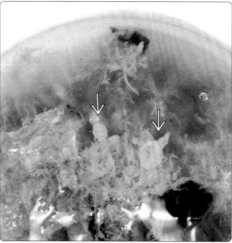

Direct and Indirect Evidence of Fetus in PHM

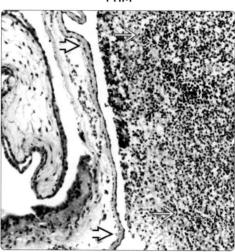

(Left) *This is a PHM that has been rinsed and immersed in water. Most villi are normal in appearance with only a few grossly evident vesicles ➡. This method is successful in rehydrating villi even after prolonged formalin fixation.* (Right) *Embryonic tissue in this section of a PHM shows direct evidence of an embryo/fetus ➡. Placental membranes ➡ provide indirect evidence of an embryo/fetus.*

Dimorphic Villous Populations

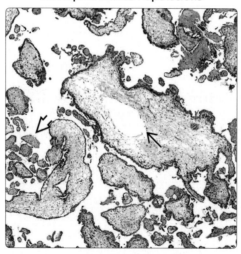

PHM With Trophoblast Pseudoinclusions

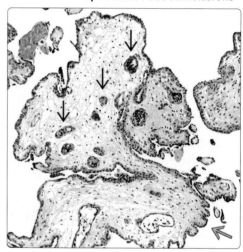

(Left) *Section of PHM shows 2 villous populations. There are a few, large hydropic villi, including one with a central cistern ➡, and more abundant smaller, fibrotic villi ➡. The villi are irregular in shape, resulting in a jigsaw puzzle piece or dentate appearance.* (Right) *Exuberant trophoblast pseudoinclusions ➡ are seen in this PHM. They result from sectioning of irregular villous contours. Note the angular, tooth-like contour (dentate) ➡.*

2 Villous Populations and Large Cistern in PHM

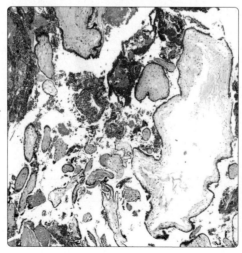

Syncytiotrophoblast Proliferation and Inclusions in PHM

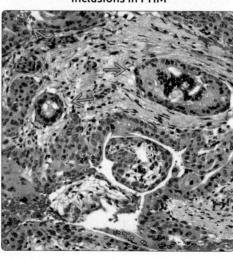

(Left) *Two of the 4 major histologic features of PHM are seen here: Dimorphic population with small fibrotic and enlarged abnormal villi and the presence of a large cistern (> 3 mm).* (Right) *The other 2 major findings are seen here: Syncytiotrophoblast proliferation ➡ and irregular contours with multiple trophoblast inclusions ➡. When all 4 features are well developed, a histologic diagnosis is straightforward. When < 3 are present, ancillary studies are needed to be definitive.*

PHM Chorionic Plate

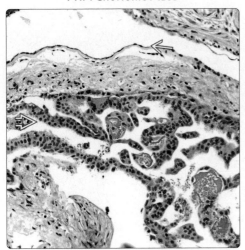

PHM Cisterns

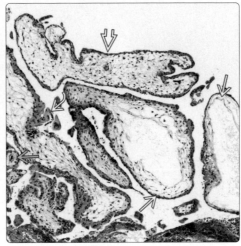

(Left) *An intact gestational sac was present in this PHM. The amnion ➡ and chorion are present. There is prominent syncytiotrophoblast proliferation ➡ beneath the primary chorionic plate, similar to what is seen on the villi.* **(Right)** *Two of the larger villi have central cisterns ➡ without stromal karyorrhexis. Villous irregularity is noted with rare trophoblastic pseudoinclusion ➡. There are a few vessels with red blood cells ➡. The syncytiotrophoblast proliferation ➡ is inconspicuous.*

PHM With Syncytiotrophoblast Proliferation

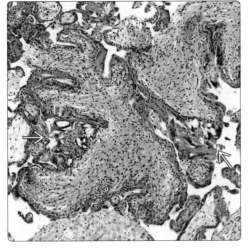

PHM With Maze-Like Cisterns

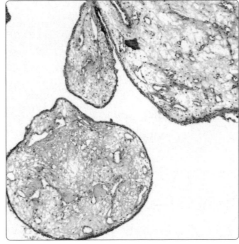

(Left) *The syncytiotrophoblast proliferation ➡ is much more prominent in this PHM. The proliferation has a lace-like appearance.* **(Right)** *PHM after 16-weeks gestation may show prominent stromal vascularity, which has been termed maze-like cisterns.*

p57 Staining of PHM

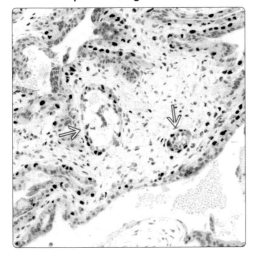

Discordant Cytotrophoblast and Stromal p57 Staining

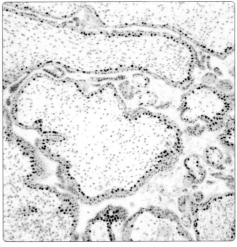

(Left) *Both the cytotrophoblast and villous stromal cell populations retain p57 staining because a maternal copy of the allele of this imprinted gene is present. Cytotrophoblast cells of the inclusions ➡ are also staining. Syncytiotrophoblast often lose expression; this does not affect interpretation of the stain.* **(Right)** *Staining of the cytotrophoblast, but not villous stromal cells, can be seen in PMD as well as androgenetic/biparental mosaic conceptions, both of which are in the differential diagnosis of PMD.*

(Left) *The placenta is small and fibrotic without molar features. The fetus has asymmetric growth restriction with preservation of brain growth. There is syndactyly ➡ of the 3rd and 4th fingers on both hands.* **(Right)** *Digynic triploidy may show some features associated with a partial mole, such as the irregular villous shapes and inclusions seen here with some early cavitation ⇥. There is no syncytiotrophoblast proliferation. Flow confirmed triploidy.*

Digynic Triploidy Placenta and Fetus

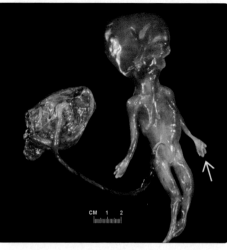

Nonmolar Triploid Placenta

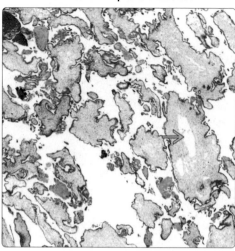

(Left) *Syndactyly of the 3rd and 4th fingers is characteristic of triploid fetus, regardless of diandric or digynic origin.* **(Right)** *A relatively consistent finding in triploidy is cystic renal dysplasia.*

Triploid Fetus With Syndactyly of 3rd and 4th Fingers

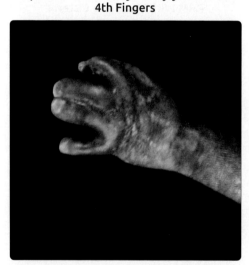

Cystic Dysplastic Kidney Triploidy

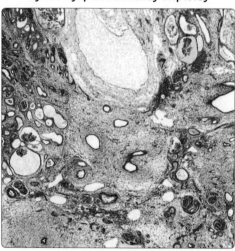

(Left) *The fetus with diandric triploidy (PHM) is often severely growth restricted. This fetus had hypotelorism, absent nose, and cleft lip/palate, consistent with holoprosencephaly.* **(Right)** *The syncytiotrophoblast proliferation of PHM may be lacy ➡ or associated with fibrin deposition ⇥. The small, fibrotic villi ➤ are often inconspicuous, especially in early PHM.*

Fetus With Holoprosencephaly and PHM

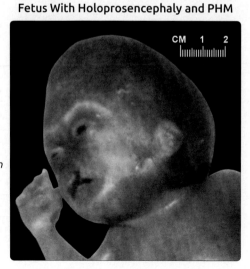

Syncytiotrophoblast of PHM

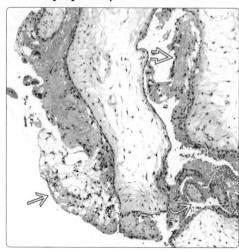

PHM Implantation Site

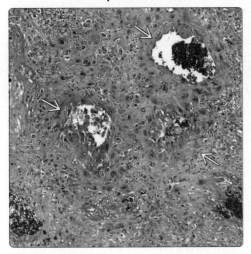

PHM Abnormal Implantation Site

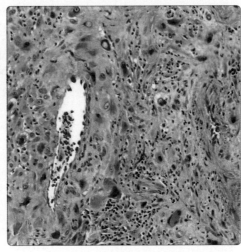

(Left) *The implantation site of this PHM shows normal trophoblast invasion of the maternal spiral arteries* ➡. *The invasive trophoblasts have no significant atypia.* **(Right)** *The invasive trophoblast cells of the implantation site in this case show mild atypia with nuclear enlargement and hyperchromasia. Careful exclusion of a diagnosis of complete mole or a mosaic conception with a component of complete mole (by p57 staining of villi) should be made in such cases.*

Placental Mesenchymal Dysplasia Gross

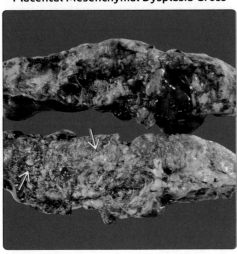

Placental Mesenchymal Dysplasia Stem Villus

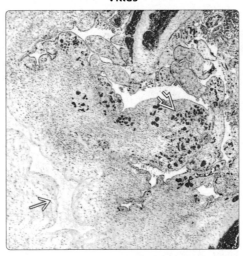

(Left) *PMD has been termed "pseudopartial mole" in the literature. The cut surface of the placenta shows cystic structures* ➡ *within the parenchyma, which are the abnormal stem villi.* **(Right)** *The cysts* ➡ *in PMD are within the stem villi, not the terminal villi as with PHM and complete hydatidiform mole. The stroma is very cellular. Marked vascular proliferation* ➡ *of the stem villus and terminal villi is also present in some cases.*

Placental Mesenchymal Dysplasia

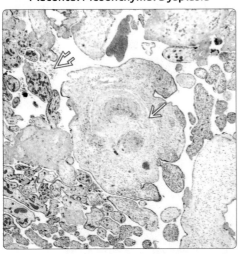

Placental Mesenchymal Dysplasia With Discordant p57 Staining

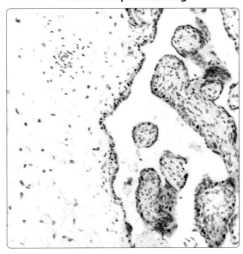

(Left) *The abnormal villi in PMD are stem villi, identified by the muscular vessels* ➡. *The terminal villi are not vesicular but may be hypervascular* ➡. **(Right)** *There is p57 staining of the cytotrophoblasts in both the enlarged cystic stem villous and the smaller normal villi. The stromal cells are uniformly negative in both; positive stromal staining in a subpopulation of villi suggests mosaicism.*

Complete Hydatidiform Mole

KEY FACTS

MACROSCOPIC

- Complete hydatidiform mole (CHM)
  - Increased amount of tissue for gestational age
  - Majority of villi are vesicular, 1-2 cm in diameter, attached to one another by thin fibrous strands
- Very early CHM, < 10-weeks gestation
  - Usually scant tissue
  - Villi may have bulbous appearance but are usually not vesicular; may measure up to 0.7 cm

MICROSCOPIC

- CHM
  - No direct or indirect evidence of fetus
  - All villi are enlarged with central cisterns
  - Mixed trophoblast proliferation is circumferential but may be discontinuous
  - Implantation site with markedly abnormal invasive trophoblasts
- Very early CHM
  - Variation in villous size
  - Subtle scalloping with bulbous projections
  - Marked stromal cellularity, amphophilic appearing, karyorrhexis and rare cisterns
  - Implantation site with markedly abnormal invasive trophoblasts

ANCILLARY TESTS

- p57 is very useful in diagnosis of CHM
  - Negative in villous cytotrophoblasts and villous stroma in CHM
    - Always positive in extravillous trophoblast, serves as internal positive control
  - Positive in cytotrophoblasts and villous stroma in hydropic degeneration and partial hydatidiform mole
  - Discordant staining seen in androgenetic/biparental mosaic/chimeric conceptions
  - Divergent p57 staining CHM and twin

Classic CHM Gross

Classic CHM

(Left) This D&C is from a 2nd-trimester, classic complete hydatidiform mole (CHM) that has been rinsed to remove blood, then rehydrated in water. All villi are vesicular and connected by thin fibrous strands ➡. It is rare to see this form of CHM, as most are now being diagnosed in the 1st trimester. (Right) Microscopically, a classic CHM shows well-developed central cisterns ➡, mixed circumferential trophoblast hyperplasia ➡, and focal remote hemorrhage ➡.

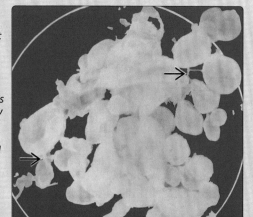

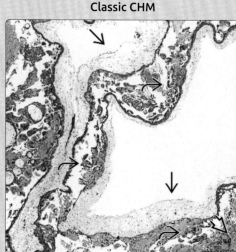

VECHM Gross

VECHM

(Left) This 1st-trimester, very early complete hydatidiform mole (VECHM) is visualized under a dissecting scope after it has been rinsed and floated in water. Note the uniformly dilated and bulbous appearance of the villi ➡. (Right) The grossly bulbous villi of VECHM have a gently scalloped, cauliflower-like appearance ➡. There is marked mixed trophoblast proliferation, which may not be circumferential but multifocal and discontinuous. The stroma is cellular without central cistern formation.

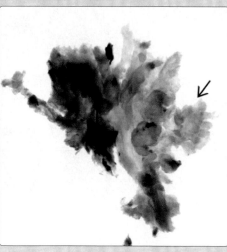

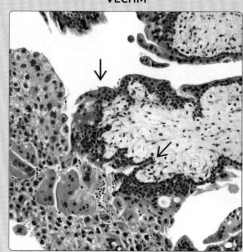

TERMINOLOGY

Abbreviations

- Complete hydatidiform mole (CHM)

Definitions

- Gestational trophoblastic disease (GTD): CHM, partial hydatidiform mole (PHM)
- Gestational trophoblastic neoplasm (GTN): Invasive mole, choriocarcinoma, placental site trophoblastic tumor, epithelioid trophoblastic tumor
- Hydropic change: Edematous microscopic appearance of villi due to stromal pallor and hypocellularity

ETIOLOGY/PATHOGENESIS

CHM

- Diandrogenetic
  - 80% anucleate ovum
    - Fertilized by 1 sperm that replicates (monospermy)
    - Fertilized by diploid sperm resulting from failure of 2nd meiotic division
  - 20% anucleate ovum fertilized by 2 sperm (dispermy, heterozygous)
  - Because it is an abnormal ovum, CHM occurs more commonly at early and late reproductive ages, < 20 and > 35 years of age
  - What happens to maternal chromosomes is unknown; error during meiosis would result in anucleate ovum
- Most are diploid
  - 93% are 46,XX and 4-12% are 46,XY; 46,YY is nonviable
  - 2% of 46,XX are dispermic, almost all 46,XY are dispermic
  - So-called diploid PHM most likely represents misdiagnosed very early complete hydatidiform mole (VECHM)
- Rare cases are tetraploid; majority are 92,XXXX
- Biparental familial recurrent CHM
  - Accounts for 0.6-2.6% of all moles
  - Autosomal recessive due to mutations in maternal genes that repress expression of imprinted genes from maternal chromosomes
  - 50-80% due to mutations of *NLRP7* on 19q13.4, more than 60 mutations identified
    - Severity of mutation affects morphology, varying p57 expression
      □ Some have features more closely resembling PHM
    - *NLRP7* mutations are associated with early embryonic developmental arrest, before blastocyst stage
  - 5-10% due to mutations of *KHDC3L* on 6q13, 4 mutations identified
  - Patients with either mutation have history of recurrent pregnancy loss, may account for 0.3% of spontaneous abortions

Invasive Mole

- Complicates 2-8% of CHM
- Molar villi invade into myometrium and venous channels
- Molar villi can metastasize, primarily to lung

Complete Mole and Twin

- CHM and twin occurs in 1/20,000-100,000 pregnancies
- Fertilization of 2 ova, 1 normal and 1 anucleate

- Increased incidence with induced ovulation

Androgenetic/Biparental Mosaic/Chimeric-Molar and Nonmolar Conceptions

- Has morphologic features that may overlap with CHM, PHM, but are genetically distinct as evidenced by molecular genotyping
  - Mosaic forms due to mitotic error in single zygote
  - Chimeric forms due to fusion of 2 different zygotes
- Molar forms associated with androgenetic trophoblast cells, demonstrating CHM morphology in subset of villi
- Often have discordant p57 staining in villous cytotrophoblast (CT) and stromal cells
  - Includes some cases of placental mesenchymal dysplasia

CLINICAL ISSUES

Epidemiology

- ~ 1-3/1,000 pregnancies are CHM
- Account for approximately 2% of spontaneous abortions
- Higher incidence associated with certain nationalities, 10x greater in Southeast Asia, Japan, Brazil, Africa
  - Increased incidence of biparental familial recurrent CHM with consanguinity and East African ancestry
- Higher incidence associated with certain nutritional deficiencies (vitamin A and folate)

Presentation

- CHM
  - Usually present as 1st-trimester spontaneous abortion with dark brown vaginal bleeding
  - Uterus usually large for dates
  - Human chorionic gonadotrophin (hCG) often elevated, mean 160,000 IU/L
    - High hCG associated with hyperemesis, theca lutein ovarian cysts, hyperthyroidism, early-onset preeclampsia
    - Tetraploid CHM may have higher hCG
    - May present with falsely low hCG due to biochemical phenomenon when hCG is > 1,000,000 IU/L (Hook effect)
  - May be associated with significant bleeding at time of uterine curettage
  - CHM has been diagnosed in ectopic pregnancy
- Invasive mole
  - Persistent elevation of hCG after CHM
  - Uterine bleeding after evacuation of CHM
  - May have mass in endometrial cavity or in myometrium
  - 15% of cases present with lung or vaginal metastases
- CHM and twin
  - May be misdiagnosed as partial mole because of presence of placental vesicles and fetus

Treatment

- Options, risks, complications
  - Follow-up for CHM is serial serum hCG levels, weekly until 3 consecutive negatives, then monthly for 6 months
    - Half-life of hCG is 24 hours
    - hCG should return to negative within 6-8 weeks post evacuation
    - Patients with CHM are advised not to get pregnant for 6 months to allow for adequate follow-up

- ○ GTN is diagnosed after evacuation of CHM when one of following occurs
  - – HCG plateaued for 3 weeks or longer, or rising over 3 weeks, or remains elevated 6 months or more
  - – Histologic evidence of choriocarcinoma or metastases
  - – Heavy vaginal bleeding or intraperitoneal or gastrointestinal hemorrhage
- Surgical approaches
  - ○ Uterine evacuation by D&C is usually sufficient in CHM
  - ○ Primary hysterectomy may be performed for CHM
    - – Women > 40 years due to increased risk for choriocarcinoma
    - – May reduce number of cycles of chemotherapy
  - ○ Hysterectomy may be performed for invasive CHM
  - ○ Increased risk for pulmonary embolization of molar tissue with D&C when pregnancy > 16-weeks gestation
- Adjuvant therapy
  - ○ Some have advocated use of prophylactic chemotherapy in CHM with high risk factors for GTN; currently not recommended
- CHM and twin
  - ○ Early in gestation, termination of pregnancy is generally recommended
  - ○ Close follow-up for those who wish to continue pregnancy
- Patient with gene mutations of familial biparental CHM achieve successful pregnancy with donor oocytes

Prognosis

- Recurrence risk for developing subsequent molar pregnancy after first CHM is 1-2%, 10-20x normal risk
  - ○ Recurrence risk after 2 consecutive CHM is 25%
- Low-risk GTD, accounts for 95% of cases with nearly 100% survival
  - ○ Serum hCG < 20,000 IU/L 4 weeks after evacuation; negative hCG ≤ 56 days after evacuation of molar pregnancy, ectopic pregnancy, or spontaneous abortion
  - ○ < 40 years old, no metastases, no prior chemotherapy, lesion < 3 cm, confined to uterus
- High risk GTD
  - ○ Serum hCG ≥ 20,000 IU/L 4 weeks after evacuation; persistent hCG > 56 days after evacuation
    - – Higher hCG associated with tetraploid mole does not increase risk
  - ○ ≥ 40 years old
  - ○ Metastases, location and number, worse with liver or brain mets
  - ○ Following term pregnancy
  - ○ Failed previous chemotherapy
  - ○ Heavy vaginal bleeding or any intraperitoneal or gastrointestinal hemorrhage
- CHM and twin
  - ○ 55% incidence of GTN, 22% metastatic disease
    - – 38% result in live birth
      - □ Better outcome for fetus when hCG is < 400,000 IU/L
      - □ Worse outcome for fetus with maternal symptoms < 20 weeks
    - – Diagnosed later in gestation; may increase incidence of GTN
- Biparental familial recurrent CHM

- ○ Autosomal recessive, 25% recurrence risk for CHM in subsequent pregnancy
- ○ Similar risk for GTN as seen in diandrogenetic CHM
- Androgenetic/biparental mosaic/chimeric conception with molar component
  - ○ Those cases with trophoblastic proliferation have risk for GTN and should be followed as diandrogenetic CHM

IMAGING

Ultrasonographic Findings

- CHM
  - ○ Classic appearance is snow storm due to multiple echogenic interfaces of diffuse 1-2 cm cysts
    - – In contrast to Swiss cheese appearance of PHM
  - ○ May have normal gestational sac at 4 weeks, polypoid mass at approximately 6 weeks, and vesicular after 8 weeks
  - ○ No fetal pole or fetus
- Invasive mole
  - ○ May have mass in endometrium or myometrium
- CHM and twin
  - ○ Often misdiagnosed as partial mole; molar villi with fetus

MACROSCOPIC

General Features

- CHM
  - ○ Increased amount of tissue for gestational age
  - ○ Majority of villi are vesicular, 1-2 cm in diameter, attached to one another by thin fibrous strands
  - ○ Increased amount of old hemorrhage with well-formed clots almost always present
- VECHM, diagnosis before 10-weeks gestation
  - ○ Usually scant tissue
  - ○ Villi may have bulbous appearance but are usually not vesicular; may measure up to 0.7 cm
    - – Best seen after rehydration in water
- Invasive CHM
  - ○ Hemorrhagic mass invades into myometrium
- Mole and twin
  - ○ Both complete and partial moles may be associated with normal cotwin
  - ○ Molar and nonmolar tissues may be intermixed in curettage specimens

Sections to Be Submitted

- D&C specimen; if there is clinical diagnosis of mole or grossly identified vesicles, submit all of villous tissue or 10 cassettes
- Implantation site is characterized by increased firmness and yellow color due to fibrinoid deposition
  - ○ CHM has an atypical implantation site that is especially useful in identification of VECHM

MICROSCOPIC

Histologic Features

- CHM
  - ○ All villi are enlarged and rounded
    - – Vessels may persist until 10 weeks (vasculogenesis); nucleated red blood cells (NRBCs) are scant or absent

- Central cisterns with abundant karyorrhectic villous stromal cells, decreased Hofbauer cells
- Trophoblast proliferation is mixed, syncytiotrophoblast, CT, and intermediate trophoblasts
- Trophoblastic proliferation is circumferential but may be discontinuous
- Syncytiotrophoblast proliferation may have lacy appearance; often hypereosinophilic due to fibrinoid necrosis
  ○ Anchoring villi with normal polar proliferations of trophoblast are usually not found
  ○ Implantation site trophoblast atypia, moderate to severe, usually diffuse
    - Invasive trophoblasts are enlarged with nucleomegaly, nuclear pleomorphism, with hyperchromasia and increased mitotic activity
    - May have multiple nucleoli or intranuclear pseudoinclusions
    - Trophoblast invasion of maternal spiral arteries for remodeling is diminished
  ○ Excessive remote hemorrhage
  ○ Degree of cytologic atypia does not predict which patients will develop persistent GTN
  ○ Tetraploid CHM associated with larger villi and persistence of villous vessels
- VECHM (CHM in 1st trimester)
  ○ Variation in villous size
  ○ Villi have bulbous, cauliflower-like projections
    - Stroma appears amphophilic due to stromal mucin
    - Cellular stroma with karyorrhexis of stromal cells
    - Few residual villous linear interconnective vessels (vasculogenesis), rare or absent NRBCs
    - Mixed trophoblast proliferation, circumferential but frequently syncytiotrophoblasts predominate
  ○ Implantation site with atypical features same as classic CHM
- Mole and twin
  ○ May have totally separate populations of normal and molar villi
  ○ Curetted samples are usually extensively intermixed, which can be confusing
- Invasive mole
  ○ Villi that are invasive into myometrium generally lose their molar characteristics
    - May be smaller than intracavitary villi
    - Rarely have central cisterns
    - May need multiple sections to confirm presence of villi and not overcall choriocarcinoma
  ○ Trophoblastic proliferation is more pronounced and may invade deeply into myometrium
- Biparental familial recurrent CHM
  ○ Indistinguishable from androgenetic CHM, but possibly less pronounced molar features have been reported
- Androgenetic/biparental mosaic/chimeric conceptions
  ○ Enlarged, hydropic villi, hypercellular villous stroma
  ○ Variable shape with trophoblastic pseudoinclusions and cisterns
  ○ Trophoblast proliferation may be absent or present
  ○ May be 2 distinct villous populations, 1 with and 1 without trophoblast proliferation

- Need evaluation with p57 to confirm component of complete mole

ANCILLARY TESTS

Immunohistochemistry

- Cyclin-dependent kinase inhibitor 1C (CDKN1C, p57, KIP2)
  ○ p57 is strongly paternally imprinted and expressed on maternal allele of chromosome 11p15
    - Positive staining in all intermediate/invasive trophoblasts and some maternal decidual cells regardless of diagnosis, serves as internal positive control
  ○ Positive nuclei (> 10%) of villous CT and stromal cells in hydropic degeneration and PHM characteristic of maternal and paternal genetic components
    - Syncytiotrophoblast nuclei may show weak or absent staining
  ○ Negative or limited (< 10%) nuclear staining in CT and stromal cells is characteristic of diandrogenetic paternally derived CHM
    - Tetraploid CHM may have absent or low p57 staining of CT and stromal cells
    - Biparental familial recurrent CHM usually has negative p57 despite maternal component due to shutdown of maternally imprinted gene expression
  ○ Discordant p57 expression (usually in androgenetic/biparental mosaic/chimeric conception)
    - Negative and positive results for villous stromal cells and CT within individual villi
      □ Positive CT and negative stromal cells, lack trophoblastic proliferation
      □ Villi with trophoblastic proliferation are negative in both CT and stroma; indicates component of CHM
  ○ Divergent p57 expression (usually in CHM and twin)
    - 2 different villous populations with different staining patterns (some villi negative for p57, others with normal positive expression)
  ○ Cases with significant autolysis/necrosis may be nonreactive; should be considered unsatisfactory for interpretation
    - Positive staining of intermediate/invasive trophoblasts and decidual cells are internal control

Genetic Testing

- Molecular genotyping considered "gold standard" in diagnosis, but cost may limit practical utility in some settings; morphology with p57 staining is usually sufficient for diagnosis of CHM
  ○ PCR for short tandem repeats identifies maternal and paternal contributions in specimen
    - Only method to tell if diploid chromosomes are biparental or diandric
    - Complex results in androgenetic/biparental mosaic/chimeric conceptions
- Consider analysis for genes mutated in familial biparental recurrent CHM in patients with > 2 pregnancies with CHM or when molecular results show biparental genotype in CHM

Comparison of Early Complete Hydatidiform Mole, Partial Hydatidiform Mole, and Hydropic Abortus

Feature	Complete Hydatidiform Mole	Partial Hydatidiform Mole	Hydropic Abortus
Villous size	Varied	Varied	Uniform
Villous contour	Budding	Irregular	Smooth
Villous stroma	Mucoid/myxoid, amphophilic	Fibrotic in subpopulation	Hydropic
Villous hydrops	Varied	Varied	Present
Cistern formation	Varied	Varied	None
Stromal karyorrhectic debris	Present	Absent	Absent
Villous vessels	Absent/collapsed	Present	Absent/collapsed
Nucleated RBC	Very rare	Present	Present
Trophoblast pseudoinclusion	Present	Present	Rare
Trophoblast hyperplasia (> 2 cell layers)	Present, circumferential, cytotrophoblast, and syncytiotrophoblast	Present, may be focal, lace-like, syncytiotrophoblast only	Polar, normal cell columns
Implantation site	Florid trophoblast proliferation with hyperchromasia, pleomorphism	Normal	Normal
Fetal parts/amnion	Absent*	Present	Present
p57 immunohistochemistry	Negative staining in villous cytotrophoblast and stromal cells	Positive	Positive

Excepting cases of CHM and twin, or rare cases of androgenetic/biparental mosaic/chimeric conceptions with molar component

Modified from: Sebire NJ, Fisher R and Rees H: Histopathologic diagnosis of partial and complete hydatidiform mole in the first trimester of pregnancy. Pediatric and Developmental Pathology. 6:69-77, 2002.

DIAGNOSTIC CHECKLIST

Pathologic Interpretation Pearls

- Most important part of grossing specimen is to rinse out blood and float/rehydrate villi in water
  - This technique can be used even after formalin fixation
- Implantation site shows invasive trophoblasts with marked atypia, helpful in morphologic diagnosis of VECHM
- Villous trophoblast proliferation in CHM is mixed (syncytiotrophoblast, CT, extravillous trophoblast) and is circumferential
- Villous trophoblast proliferation in PHM consists of syncytiotrophoblasts only
- When morphology is classic for complete mole, but genotyping shows biparental diploid conception, consider biparental familial recurrent CHM
- When morphology is classic for complete mole, but p57 staining is retained, additional molecular characterization is warranted; can have retention of maternal chromosome 11 in otherwise androgenetic conception

SELECTED REFERENCES

1. Jauniaux E et al: New insights in the pathophysiology of complete hydatidiform mole. Placenta. 62:28-33, 2018
2. Hui P et al: Hydatidiform moles: genetic basis and precision diagnosis. Annu Rev Pathol. 12:449-485, 2017
3. Eagles N et al: Risk of recurrent molar pregnancies following complete and partial hydatidiform moles. Hum Reprod. 30(9):2055-63, 2015
4. Niemann I et al: Gestational trophoblastic diseases - clinical guidelines for diagnosis, treatment, follow-up, and counselling. Dan Med J. 62(11):A5082, 2015
5. Sanchez-Delgado M et al: Absence of maternal methylation in biparental hydatidiform moles from women with NLRP7 maternal-effect mutations reveals widespread placenta-specific imprinting. PLoS Genet. 11(11):e1005644, 2015
6. Banet N et al: Characteristics of hydatidiform moles: analysis of a prospective series with p57 immunohistochemistry and molecular genotyping. Mod Pathol. 27(2):238-54, 2014
7. Lewis GH et al: Characterization of androgenetic/biparental mosaic/chimeric conceptions, including those with a molar component: morphology, p57 immunohistochemistry, molecular genotyping, and risk of persistent gestational trophoblastic disease. Int J Gynecol Pathol. 32(2):199-214, 2013
8. Sebire NJ et al: Histopathological features of biparental complete hydatidiform moles in women with NLRP7 mutations. Placenta. 34(1):50-6, 2013
9. Gupta M et al: Diagnostic reproducibility of hydatidiform moles: ancillary techniques (p57 immunohistochemistry and molecular genotyping) improve morphologic diagnosis for both recently trained and experienced gynecologic pathologists. Am J Surg Pathol. 36(12):1747-60, 2012
10. Ronnett BM et al: Hydatidiform moles: ancillary techniques to refine diagnosis. Int J Gynecol Pathol. 30(2):101-16, 2011
11. Kim KR et al: The villous stromal constituents of complete hydatidiform mole differ histologically in very early pregnancy from the normally developing placenta. Am J Surg Pathol. 33(2):176-85, 2009

US of Classic CHM

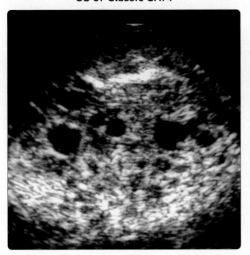

Classic CHM Gross

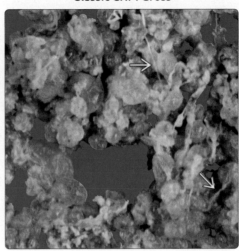

(Left) *This transvaginal US shows the classic snowstorm appearance of a CHM in the 2nd trimester.* (Right) *This CHM has previously been formalin fixed. Immersion in water will rehydrate the vesicles. All of the tissue is vesicular with fibrous strands ⇒ connecting the vesicles together. There is usually a moderate amount of remote hemorrhage, which was removed for this photograph.*

Central Cistern in Classic CHM

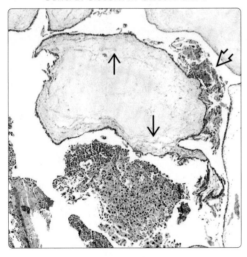

CHM With Mixed Trophoblast Proliferation

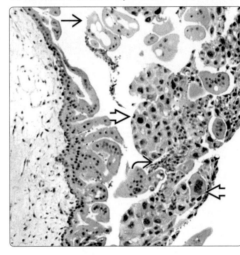

(Left) *A classic CHM typically shows huge villi with central cisterns ⇒ and mixed trophoblast proliferation that may be focally necrotic ⇒.* (Right) *CHM has mixed trophoblast proliferation that is not as well organized as the normal anchoring villus. Syncytiotrophoblasts may have a lacy appearance ⇒. The intermediate trophoblast nuclei are atypical ⇒ and pleomorphic. The small, more regular cytotrophoblasts ⇒ are inconspicuous in this section.*

CHM Implantation Site

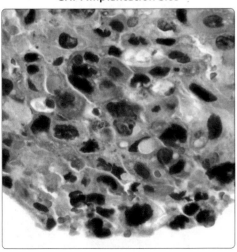

CHM With Negative p57 Staining

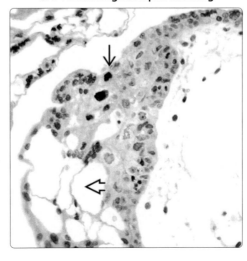

(Left) *This is a section from the implantation site of a CHM, showing the marked nuclear enlargement, pleomorphism, and hyperchromasia of the invasive trophoblasts.* (Right) *CHM stained with p57 shows only nuclear positivity of the extravillous trophoblast ⇒. There is negative or minimal staining of villous stromal cells or cytotrophoblasts by p57. Also note the lacy appearance of the syncytiotrophoblast ⇒ proliferation.*

Placental Diagnoses

VECHM

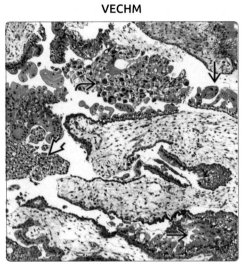

VECHM

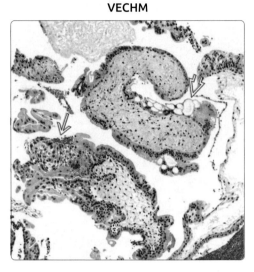

(Left) *This VECHM shows characteristic marked mixed syncytiotrophoblast* ➡, *cytotrophoblast* ⬄, *and intermediate trophoblast* ⬌ *proliferation. The villous stroma is highly cellular without central cisterns.* **(Right)** *The VECHM has myxoid stroma. There is inconspicuous mixed trophoblast proliferation* ➡ *and a lacy appearance* ⬄ *of the more prominent proliferating syncytiotrophoblasts.*

VECHM With Vessels

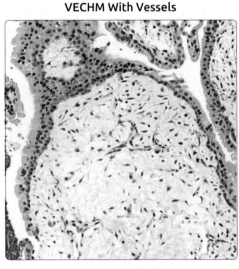

VECHM With Stromal Karyorrhexis

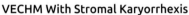
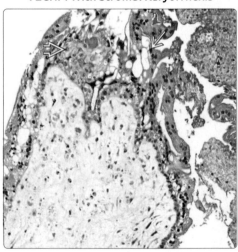

(Left) *Vasogenesis occurs during early villous development, arising from the villous stroma. No angiogenesis is present in CHM. The vessels are empty and do not contain nucleated red blood cells. The vessels often have a linear interconnected appearance.* **(Right)** *The stroma of the VECHM will show cellular karyorrhexis, which is the precursor of central cistern formation. Note the lacy syncytiotrophoblasts* ➡ *admixed with* ⬄ *cytotrophoblasts.*

VECHM With Atypical Invasive Trophoblasts

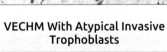
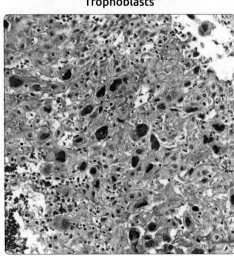

Atypical Extravillous Trophoblasts

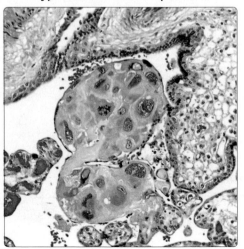

(Left) *The implantation site of the VECHM already exhibits the marked nuclear atypia of the invasive trophoblasts. This is extremely helpful in identifying VECHM when scant villous tissue is present.* **(Right)** *Occasionally there can be atypia within extravillous trophoblast proliferation in an otherwise normal placenta. This is usually associated with perivillous fibrin deposition. This may be due to ischemia of the cells and does not seem to be a precursor to gestational trophoblastic neoplasm.*

VECHM p57

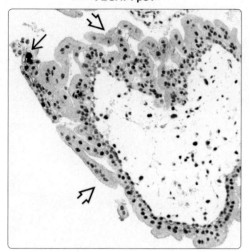

Divergent p57 Staining

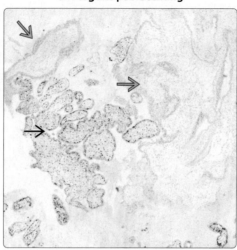

(Left) *p57 immunohistochemical staining in VECHM shows negative nuclear staining of villous cytotrophoblasts and stroma. There is nuclear staining of the intermediate trophoblast ➡️. There is circumferential syncytiotrophoblast ➡️ proliferation.* (Right) *This D&E specimen from a mole and twin pregnancy shows an admixture of smaller normal villi ➡️ with p57 staining the villous cytotrophoblast and stromal cells, and molar villi ➡️ negative in both populations.*

Tetraploid CHM

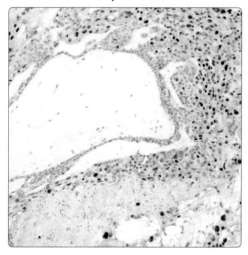

Abnormal Villous Morphology in Case With Discordant p57 Staining

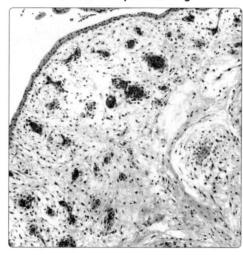

(Left) *p57 staining of tetraploid CHM is usually negative in the cytotrophoblast and stroma.* (Right) *This case had a population of molar villi admixed with these large villi with stromal overgrowth and no trophoblastic hyperplasia. An embryo was present. The component of molar villi with loss of p57 staining and trophoblastic hyperplasia warrants follow up as gestational trophoblastic disease.*

Discordant p57 in Nonmolar Villi

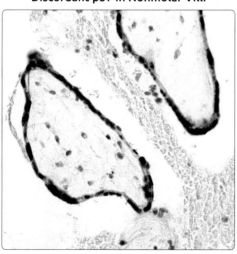

CHM Discordant p57 Staining

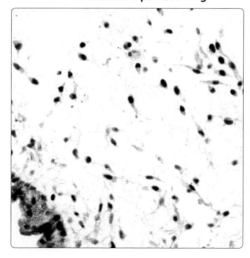

(Left) *These nonmolar villi show positive CT staining and negative stromal staining; the most common discordant p57 pattern. This most likely represents a nonmolar androgenetic/biparental mosaic/chimeric conception.* (Right) *This case showed all of the histologic features characteristic of a VECHM; however, the p57 staining is discordant with positive stromal cells and negative CT. This most likely represents an androgenetic/biparental mosaic/chimeric molar conception.*

Persistent Gestational Trophoblastic Disease Gross

Invasive CHM Gross

(Left) *A hemorrhagic intracavitary mass is grossly noted in this hysterectomy specimen. The patient had a previous diagnosis of CHM with persistent elevation of serum human chorionic gonadotrophin (hCG) and uterine bleeding.* **(Right)** *Cross section of this uterus shows a deeply invasive friable mass of an invasive mole.*

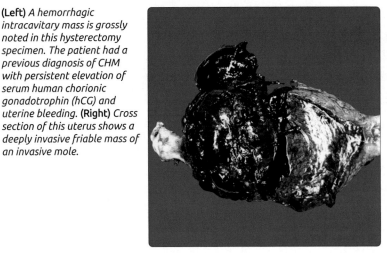

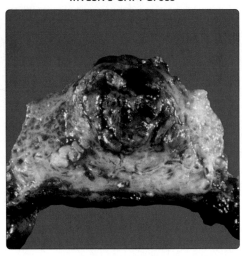

Invasive CHM

Invasive CHM

(Left) *The villi in an invasive mole are less molar in appearance. Similar to placenta accreta, they are found in the myometrium, often in venous channels. Atypical invasive trophoblasts ➡ are present.* **(Right)** *The trophoblastic proliferation in an invasive mole may be marked. Villi may be infrequent and a careful search should occur so as not to overdiagnose an invasive mole as choriocarcinoma. Some experts view similar lesions as "emerging choriocarcinoma," but this is controversial.*

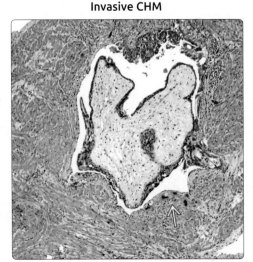

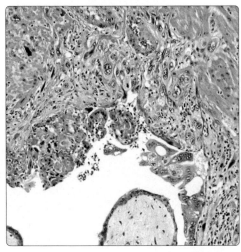

Invasive CHM

Syncytiotrophoblast of Invasive Mole

(Left) *This invasive CHM could easily be interpreted as a choriocarcinoma if the residual villus ➡ were not recognized. The trophoblastic proliferation shows prominent cytotrophoblast columns ➡, partially covered by syncytiotrophoblasts. The invasive trophoblasts ➡ are less conspicuous in this section.* **(Right)** *The syncytiotrophoblasts of invasive CHM are hCG positive. This high-power field is indistinguishable from choriocarcinoma.*

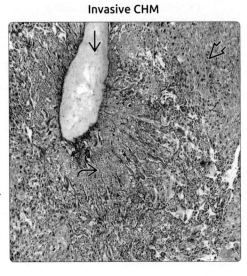

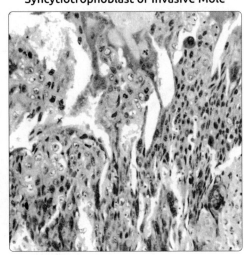

Ultrasound of Complete Mole and Twin

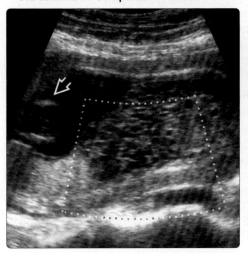

Complete Mole and Twin

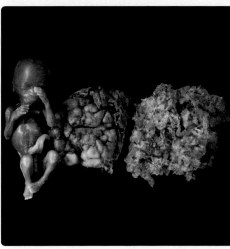

(Left) *This US shows a CHM and twin at 26-weeks gestation. Although the placenta has the characteristic snow storm appearance of CHM, the presence of the fetus ➡ resulted in misinterpretation as a partial mole.* (Right) *The twin and CHM have totally separate placental masses. This patient developed severe preterm preeclampsia that necessitated preterm delivery.*

Fused Disc of Complete Mole and Twin

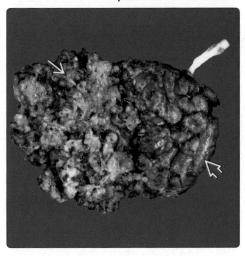

Fused Disc of Complete Mole and Twin

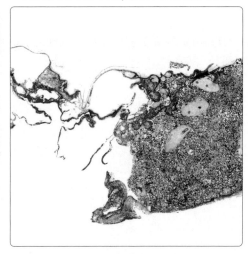

(Left) *This twin ➡ and CHM ➡ have molar and normal villous tissue.* (Right) *This section is taken from the interface between the CHM and the normal placenta, showing that they are separate.*

Divergent Histology in Complete Mole and Twin

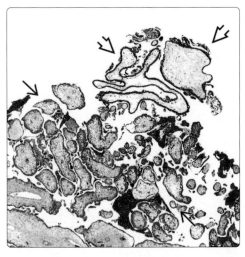

Divergent p57 Staining in Complete Mole and Twin

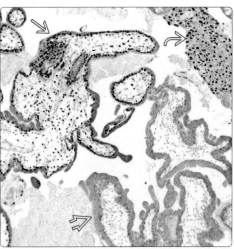

(Left) *This 12-week-gestation pregnancy was diagnosed as partial mole by imaging studies due to the presence of molar villi and a fetus. There are normal immature villi ➡ intermixed with molar villi characteristic of CHM ➡, indicative of a twin and CHM.* (Right) *D&C specimen with discordant p57 positive normal villi ➡ and negative molar villi ➡ is shown here. Extravillous trophoblasts ➡ are positive as an internal control. Only nuclear staining counts as "positive."*

Gestational Choriocarcinoma

ETIOLOGY/PATHOGENESIS

- Gestational choriocarcinoma includes paternal chromosomal complement; choriocarcinoma arising as germ cell tumor does not
- > 50% occur after complete hydatidiform mole, remainder after term deliveries (22%), preterm deliveries, spontaneous abortion (25%), or ectopic pregnancy (3%)

MACROSCOPIC

- Choriocarcinoma: Hemorrhagic, necrotic mass
- Intraplacental choriocarcinoma: Tan-white, granular parenchymal lesion, rarely multifocal

MICROSCOPIC

- Choriocarcinoma
  - No residual villi
  - Biphasic with central cytotrophoblast core and syncytiotrophoblast covering, rare intermediate trophoblasts

- Invasive and destructive growth pattern with necrosis, recent and remote hemorrhage
- Intraplacental choriocarcinoma
  - Extensive mixed trophoblast proliferation, usually limited to villous surface, rarely invades villous stroma, focal necrosis

TOP DIFFERENTIAL DIAGNOSES

- Choriocarcinoma vs. invasive mole
  - Choriocarcinoma has no residual villi
- Choriocarcinoma vs. epithelioid trophoblastic tumor (ETT)
  - Choriocarcinoma is invasive and hemorrhagic; ETT is well circumscribed with eosinophilic matrix
  - Choriocarcinoma is intimate mixture of syncytiotrophoblasts and cytotrophoblasts; ETT is tumor of intermediate trophoblast (extravillous cytotrophoblast) with rare syncytiotrophoblasts

Choriocarcinoma With Blood Lakes

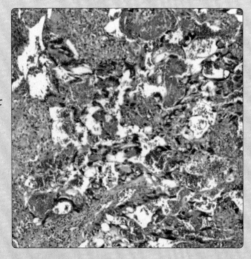

Choriocarcinoma Invading Myometrium

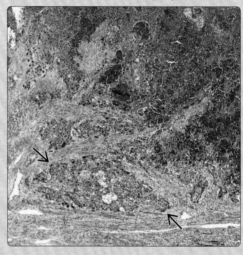

(Left) *H&E shows choriocarcinoma with blood-filled lakes, some of which contain fibrin thrombi. The syncytiotrophoblasts are seen lining the vascular spaces.* (Right) *Choriocarcinoma is a very hemorrhagic and necrotic lesion. Residual viable tumor cells may be hard to find. In this case, there are sheets of tumor cells ➡ invading the myometrium.*

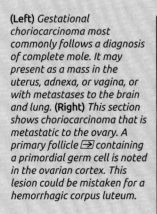

Gestational Choriocarcinoma, Gross

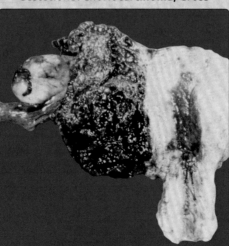

Choriocarcinoma Metastatic to Ovary

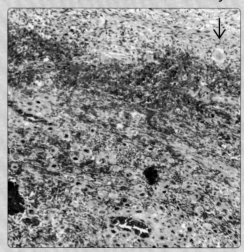

(Left) *Gestational choriocarcinoma most commonly follows a diagnosis of complete mole. It may present as a mass in the uterus, adnexa, or vagina, or with metastases to the brain and lung.* (Right) *This section shows choriocarcinoma that is metastatic to the ovary. A primary follicle ➡ containing a primordial germ cell is noted in the ovarian cortex. This lesion could be mistaken for a hemorrhagic corpus luteum.*

TERMINOLOGY

Definitions

- Gestational choriocarcinoma: Malignant tumor of syncytiotrophoblast and cytotrophoblast in absence of chorionic villi
- Intraplacental choriocarcinoma: Focal features of choriocarcinoma in nonmolar placenta

ETIOLOGY/PATHOGENESIS

Gestational Choriocarcinoma

- Gestational choriocarcinoma includes paternal chromosomal complement; choriocarcinoma arising as germ cell tumor does not
- > 50% occur after complete hydatidiform mole, remainder after term deliveries (22%), preterm deliveries, spontaneous abortion (25%), or ectopic pregnancy (3%)
  - Occurrence after partial hydatidiform mole is rare but documented
  - Genetic studies have shown immediately antecedent or concurrent pregnancy is not always causative pregnancy
  - Short tandem repeat (STR) genotyping demonstrates androgenetic genomes in cases without clinically recognized concurrent or antecedent molar pregnancy

CLINICAL ISSUES

Epidemiology

- Incidence
  - Choriocarcinoma: 1 in 25,000 to 40,000 pregnancies
  - Intraplacental choriocarcinoma: 1 in 160,000 placentas, probably underreported

Presentation

- Choriocarcinoma
  - May present with vaginal bleeding after pregnancy or concurrently with normal term pregnancy
  - Headache or cough due to metastasis, metastasis to vagina 50%, lung 80%, brain 10%
- Intraplacental choriocarcinoma
  - Usually incidental finding in placenta
  - May be source of fetal-maternal transfusion, newborn rarely presents with metastatic disease
  - May have maternal metastatic disease at time of delivery, usually to lungs

Prognosis

- Gestational choriocarcinoma is highly treatable
  - > 90% of patients are cured by chemotherapy
  - Nongestational choriocarcinoma has worse prognosis

MACROSCOPIC

Choriocarcinoma

- Hemorrhagic, necrotic mass

Intraplacental Choriocarcinoma

- Tan-white, granular parenchymal lesion, usually interpreted as infarct grossly

MICROSCOPIC

Histologic Features

- Choriocarcinoma
  - No residual villi, intimate admixture of cytotrophoblast and syncytiotrophoblast
  - Invasive and destructive growth pattern, invades maternal vessels, with recent and remote hemorrhage
  - No intrinsic blood supply; results in extensive ischemic necrosis
- Intraplacental choriocarcinoma
  - Striking proliferation of cytotrophoblast and syncytiotrophoblast on villous surface with extensive necrosis
    - Rarely invades villous stroma
  - Rare variant associated with villous hypervascularity, termed "chorangiocarcinoma"

ANCILLARY TESTS

Immunohistochemistry

- β-HCG: Strongly positive in syncytiotrophoblasts, weak and focal in cytotrophoblasts and intermediate trophoblasts
- HPL (human placental lactogen): Focal positivity
- Inhibin: Negative

Genetic Testing

- Molecular genetic studies (STR, DNA polymorphism analysis) may be used to distinguish gestational from nongestational choriocarcinoma
  - Gestational choriocarcinoma: Includes paternal chromosomal complement
    - Majority are androgenetic/homozygous XX, lacking maternal component, as in complete hydatidiform mole
    - Subset are biparental, including all cases of intraplacental choriocarcinoma
  - Nongestational choriocarcinoma: Homology with patient's DNA, no significant copy number alterations

DIFFERENTIAL DIAGNOSIS

Invasive Mole

- Choriocarcinoma has no residual villi

Epithelioid Trophoblastic Tumor

- Choriocarcinoma is invasive and hemorrhagic; epithelioid trophoblastic tumor (ETT) is well circumscribed with eosinophilic matrix
- Choriocarcinoma is admixture of syncytiotrophoblast and cytotrophoblast cells; ETT is tumor of intermediate trophoblast with rare syncytiotrophoblast

Atypical Extravillous Trophoblast Proliferation

- These foci lack primitive-appearing cytotrophoblast, syncytiotrophoblast proliferation, and necrosis

SELECTED REFERENCES

1. Mello JB et al: Genomic profile in gestational and non-gestational choriocarcinomas. Placenta. 50:8-15, 2017
2. Savage J et al: Choriocarcinoma in women: analysis of a case series with genotyping. Am J Surg Pathol. 41(12):1593-1606, 2017
3. Jiao L et al: Intraplacental choriocarcinoma: systematic review and management guidance. Gynecol Oncol. 141(3):624-631, 2016

(Left) *Choriocarcinoma is a neoplastic proliferation of cytotrophoblast cells and syncytiotrophoblast. Cytotrophoblast cells include a central core of primitive cells similar to cell columns of early villi, as well as occasional intermediate trophoblasts similar to EVT. Villi are absent.* **(Right)** *Syncytiotrophoblasts ⮕ are frequently lining blood-filled lakes. While described as "triphasic," recognition of intermediate trophoblasts can be difficult in regions like this. The more primitive cytotrophoblast component ⮕ is easier to recognize.*

Choriocarcinoma Cytotrophoblast Core

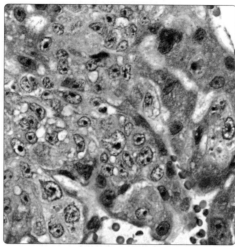

Choriocarcinoma

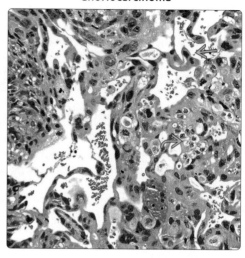

(Left) *The intimate association of cytotrophoblast ⮕ with syncytiotrophoblast ⮕ distinguishes choriocarcinoma from epithelioid trophoblastic tumor and placental-site trophoblastic tumor.* **(Right)** *Choriocarcinoma frequently spreads through the bloodstream to the lungs and brain. This image shows a pulmonary metastasis ⮕.*

Choriocarcinoma With Old Hemorrhage

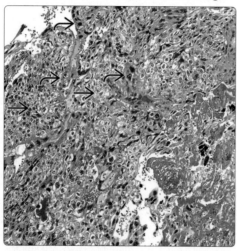

Metastatic Choriocarcinoma to Lung

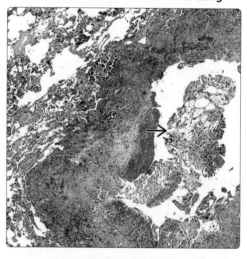

(Left) *Choriocarcinoma may present with headache in the postpartum period due to metastasis to the brain ⮕, as seen in this imaging study.* **(Right)** *At autopsy, metastatic choriocarcinoma to the brain shows characteristic hemorrhage.*

Choriocarcinoma Metastatic to Brain, Neuroimaging

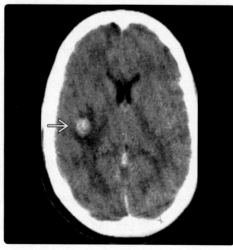

Choriocarcinoma Metastatic to Brain, Gross

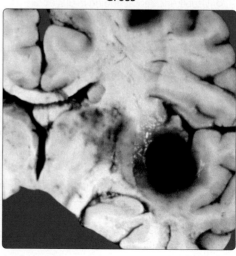

Intraplacental Choriocarcinoma, Gross

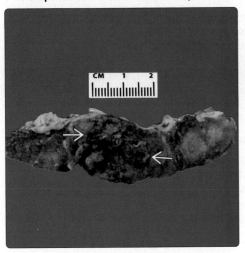

Intraplacental Choriocarcinoma

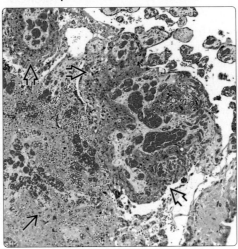

(Left) *Intraplacental choriocarcinoma was an incidental finding in this term placenta from an uncomplicated pregnancy. It was grossly thought to be an infarct, although not wedge-shaped. Close inspection reveals a more ➡ variegated and friable appearance than the usual infarct.* (Right) *Intraplacental choriocarcinoma shows malignant trophoblasts ➡, often with necrosis ➡. The tumor spreads along the surface of contiguous villi. The underlying stroma does not appear invaded.*

Intraplacental Choriocarcinoma Invading Villous Stroma

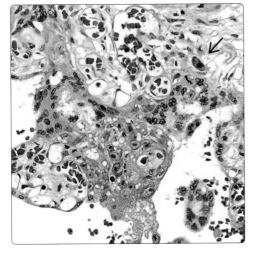

Intraplacental Choriocarcinoma

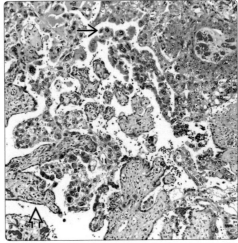

(Left) *Intraplacental choriocarcinoma usually involves only the surface of the villi, but invasion into the villous stroma may occur ➡. This does not necessarily imply greater risk of metastasis to the fetus, but all newborns associated with an intraplacental choriocarcinoma should be carefully evaluated to exclude metastatic disease.* (Right) *The trophoblast nuclei ➡ of intraplacental choriocarcinoma are markedly enlarged compared to neighboring normal trophoblast populations ➡.*

Chorangiocarcinoma

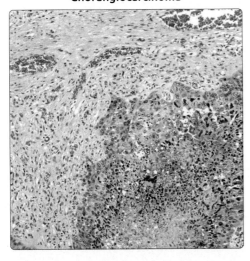

Reactive Extravillous Trophoblast Proliferation

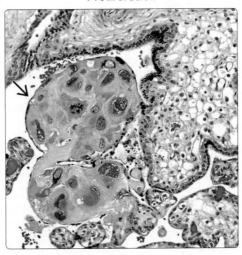

(Left) *Rarely, intraplacental choriocarcinoma has hypervascular villi associated with the neoplasm.* (Right) *Markedly pleomorphic extravillous trophoblast cells may be occasionally seen in otherwise unremarkable placentas. Some authors associate them with hypoxia. Nonneoplastic syncytiotrophoblasts ➡ appear to wall off the cells, much like they do to nodules of fibrin in the intervillous space.*

Placental Site Nodule and Exaggerated Placental Site

TERMINOLOGY

- Placental site nodule (PSN)
  - Foci of persistent intermediate trophoblasts (IT) and extracellular matrix remaining after pregnancy
- Atypical placental site nodule (APSN)
  - Intermediate lesion between PSN and epithelioid trophoblastic tumor (ETT)/placental site trophoblastic tumor (PSTT); more cellular, more mitoses
  - Subset of patients at risk for ETT/PSTT elsewhere
- Exaggerated placental site reaction (EPSR); term used for different entities
  - 1st trimester: Increased intermediate trophoblast numbers or mononuclear and multinucleated trophoblasts in myometrium
  - 2nd- or 3rd-trimester implantation with increased residual invasive trophoblasts
  - Implantation site of complete hydatidiform mole should not be diagnosed as EPSR

MICROSCOPIC

- PSN: Round to oval, lobulated borders with central hyalinized core, and scattered trophoblast arranged singly in clusters or in cords; and Ki-67 < 5-8%
- APSN: Similar to PSN but increased trophoblast cellularity, moderate pleomorphism, Ki-67 5-12%; size typically > 4 mm but < 50 mm
- EPSR: Variants of normal implantation site with increased numbers of IT, Ki-67 < 1%

DIAGNOSTIC CHECKLIST

- Clinical presentation key to distinguish these benign lesions of IT from malignant GTD
  - PSN is usually microscopic incidental finding
  - EPS is typically associated with products of conception or bed of recently delivered placenta

Placental Site Nodule in Endometrial Curettings

(Left) Discrete, pale pink nodules of modest cellularity are seen on low power. (Right) Placental site nodules are characteristically well circumscribed. This placental site nodule in the ➡ myometrium is paucicellular.

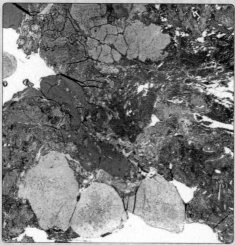

Placental Site Nodule

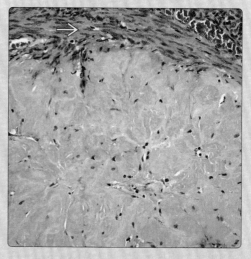

Exaggerated Placental Site Reaction

(Left) This curettage for missed abortion shows sheets of intermediate trophoblast cells in the implantation site decidua. The trophoblast cells have darker nuclei than decidual stromal cells and cover a low-power field. (Right) In this products of conception (POC) specimen, the implantation site decidua includes multiple low-power fields dense with trophoblast cells, including frequent multinucleate trophoblast cells ➡.

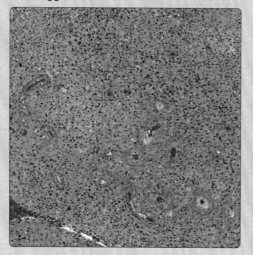

Exaggerated Placental Site Reaction

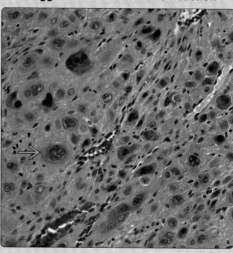

TERMINOLOGY

Synonyms

- Intermediate trophoblast (IT) and extravillous trophoblast (EVT)
- Older terms for exaggerated placental site reaction (EPSR) include "syncytial endometritis" and "benign chorionic invasion"

Definitions

- Placental site nodule (PSN)
  o Benign foci of persistent, chorionic-type IT and hyalinized extracellular matrix
  o Residual trophoblast population from prior pregnancy
- Atypical placental site nodule (APSN)
  o Intermediate lesion between PSN and epithelioid trophoblastic tumor (ETT)/placental site trophoblastic tumor (PSTT)
  o Larger focus of persistent, chorionic-type IT with increased cellularity, more cohesion of IT, mild nuclear atypia, and increased Ki-67 labeling compared to PSN
- EPSR
  o Term originated to distinguish histology from neoplasia
  o Normal variations of implantation site with numerous invasive-type IT
    - 1st-trimester implantation with increased number of IT in endometrium or myometrium
    - 2nd- or 3rd-trimester placenta with increased numbers of residual IT at basal plate, often associated with preeclampsia
  o Original descriptions included changes seen in implantation site of complete hydatidiform mole with increased numbers and pleomorphism of IT
    - Should not be diagnosed as EPSR, part of gestational trophoblastic disease of complete hydatidiform mole
- Chorionic-type IT
  o EVT of chorion laeve of free membranes, chorionic plate
- Invasive-type IT
  o Trophoblasts from cytotrophoblastic columns of anchoring villi that invade into endometrium and inner 1/3 of myometrium

ETIOLOGY/PATHOGENESIS

Placental Site Nodule

- Residual portion of otherwise normal population of chorionic-type IT
- Frequent history of cesarean delivery, or prior curettage
  o Decidua is usually shed spontaneously at delivery and with lochia
  o Cesarean delivery may bypass physiologic shedding
- Pathogenesis may be similar to placenta accreta, but no villi remain
  o Frequently seen in areas with minimal or no decidua (lower uterine segment, cervix, uterine cornua, or fallopian tube)
- Rarely reported in extrauterine sites including ovary, broad ligament, paratubal tissues, and rectovaginal septum peritoneum
  o Assumed to be remnant of previous ectopic pregnancy

Atypical Placental Site Nodule

- Also originate from chorionic-type IT, larger foci with more mitotic activity than PSN
- May represent 10% of PSN from literature, few case series reported
- Associated with 14% risk for gestational trophoblastic neoplasm (epithelioid trophoblastic tumor, placenta site trophoblastic tumor)

Exaggerated Placental Site Reaction

- Variants of normal implantation site
  o Incidence reported in 1.6% of 1st-trimester products of conception (POC)
  o Invasive trophoblasts normally extend through endometrium into inner 3rd of myometrium, invasion ends with transformation to multinucleation
  o "Superficial implantation" associated with preeclampsia, increased number of invasive trophoblasts at implantation site

CLINICAL ISSUES

Presentation

- PSN
  o Incidental finding on curettage, biopsy, or hysterectomy
    - Evaluation for uterine bleeding, infertility, or hysterectomy for other diagnoses
  o Serum HCG not elevated
  o 50% located in cervix, 50% in endometrium or superficial myometrium
- APSN
  o Same as for PSN
- EPSR
  o Diagnosed with POC in 1st trimester or on postpartum curettage or hysterectomy for bleeding
  o Unclear if causal association exists between EPS and uterine atony, postpartum hemorrhage or placenta increta in 2nd- and 3rd-trimester placental bed

Prognosis

- PSN
  o Benign, no treatment necessary
- APSN
  o Rare reports of development of ETT or PSTT months after initial diagnosis; 10-15% of patients
  o Patients should have imaging studies to exclude mass lesion, role of serum β-hCG monitoring unclear
- EPSR
  o No recurrence and no malignant potential reported with variants of normal implantation sites

MACROSCOPIC

Placental Site Nodule

- Described on hysteroscopy as small, white-red or yellow-white nodule with hemorrhage and necrosis, rarely as polypoid
- Rarely identified grossly as 1- to 14- mm tan, firm nodules or plaques, may be single or multiple

Exaggerated Placental Site Reaction

- No specific gross diagnostic features; resembles implantation site decidua in curettage specimen

MICROSCOPIC

Histologic Features

- PSN
  - Round to oval with lobulated margins, central hyalinized core
  - Rare decidualized stromal cells and chronic inflammation at periphery
  - Trophoblast cells dispersed as single cells, clusters, or cords with eosinophilic, hyalinized extracellular matrix
    - Minimal pleomorphism
    - Minimal mitotic activity, Ki-67 < 5%
  - Rarely associated with EVT cyst
- APSN
  - Features intermediate between PSN and ETT or PSTT; consider APSN when lesion resembles PSN but has increased
    - Size: Usually > 4 mm but < 50 mm
    - Cellularity with more cohesive nests and cords of cells; may have necrosis
    - Cytologic &/or nuclear atypia
    - Mitoses or Ki-67 staining
- EPSR
  - Variants of nonmolar implantation site
    - 1st trimester, increased numbers of mononuclear or multinucleated IT in decidua or superficial myometrium
      - □ Nuclei described as atypical in original reports (hyperchromatic, enlarged or multinucleate)
      - □ Uncommonly see superficial myometrium on curettage specimens for SAB
      - □ Unclear if presence of IT infiltrating myometrium on curettage is due to extent of curettage or relatively thin decidua
    - 2nd and 3rd trimester, increased IT remaining in basal plate
    - Ki-67 < 1%

ANCILLARY TESTS

Immunohistochemistry

- hPL: Focal staining in PSN, diffuse staining in EPSR
- PLAP: Diffuse staining in PSN, focal staining in EPSR
- Inhibin-α: Focal positive staining in trophoblast of PSN and EPSR
- Ki-67: Trophoblast nuclear staining < 5% in PSN, < 5-10% in APSN, < 1% in EPSR
- p-63: Positive nuclear staining in PSN, negative in EPSR (TA isoform expressed by EVT of membranous chorion)
- Melcam (CD146): Focal positive staining reported in both PSN and EPSR

DIFFERENTIAL DIAGNOSIS

APSN vs. PSTT/ETT

- Microscopic size, circumscription, abundant hyalin matrix, lower cellularity, and lack of necrosis favor APSN
- IHC of limited utility, Ki-67 8-10% in APSN, 5-20% in ETT/PSTT

PSN vs. Squamous Cell Carcinoma of Cervix

- Circumscription, abundant extracellular matrix, and lack of mitotic activity favor PSN
- Both are cytokeratin and p63(+)
- PSN is inhibin-α, cytokeratin 18, HLA-G +; squamous cell carcinoma (SCC) is not
- SCC is usually p16+; PSN is not

EPSR vs. PSTT

- PSTT forms tumor mass and is never associated with villi
- Ki-67 index is near 0 in EPSR but elevated in PSTT (7-21%)

EPSR vs. EVT of Complete Mole Implantation Site

- If changes of EPSR seen in curettage without villi, showing marked nuclear pleomorphism and hyperchromasia, consider diagnosis of complete mole; molar villi may have been passed with spontaneous abortion
- EVT of complete mole show increased ki-67 staining compared to near-absent staining in EPSR

DIAGNOSTIC CHECKLIST

Pathologic Interpretation Pearls

- Clinical presentation important in distinguishing these benign lesions of IT from malignant GTD; PSN is usually microscopic incidental finding, EPSR is typically associated with POC or bed of recently delivered placenta
- Only count trophoblast nuclei for Ki-67 index; lymphocytes may have high mitotic activity that is not relevant to differential
- APSN lacks straightforward diagnostic criteria, given 10-15% are associated with malignant ETT/PSTT; imaging studies to exclude mass lesion and close clinical follow-up are warranted

SELECTED REFERENCES

1. Cramer SF et al: Placenta increta presenting as exaggerated placental site reaction. Pediatr Dev Pathol. 20(2):152-157, 2017
2. McCarthy WA et al: Atypical placental site nodule arising in a postcesarean section scar: case report and review of the literature. Int J Gynecol Pathol. ePub, 2017
3. Pereira N et al: Sonographic, hysteroscopic, and histopathological findings of a placental site nodule. J Minim Invasive Gynecol. 24(6):891-892, 2017
4. Kaur B et al: Atypical placental site nodule (APSN) and association with malignant gestational trophoblastic disease; a clinicopathologic study of 21 cases. Int J Gynecol Pathol. 34(2):152-8, 2015
5. De Miguel JR et al: Exaggerated placental site/placental site trophoblastic tumor: an underestimated risk factor for emergency peripartum hysterectomy. Clin Exp Obstet Gynecol. 41(6):638-40, 2014
6. Kurman RJ et al: Discovery of a cell: reflections on the checkered history of intermediate trophoblast and update on its nature and pathologic manifestations. Int J Gynecol Pathol. 33(4):339-47, 2014
7. Pramanick A et al: Placental site nodule (PSN): an uncommon diagnosis with a common presentation. BMJ Case Rep. 2014, 2014
8. Dotto J et al: Lack of genetic association between exaggerated placental site reaction and placental site trophoblastic tumor. Int J Gynecol Pathol. 27(4):562-7, 2008
9. Shih IM et al: The pathology of intermediate trophoblastic tumors and tumor-like lesions. Int J Gynecol Pathol. 20(1):31-47, 2001
10. Shih IM et al: Placental site nodule and characterization of distinctive types of intermediate trophoblast. Hum Pathol. 30(6):687-94, 1999
11. Young RH et al: Proliferations and tumors of intermediate trophoblast of the placental site. Semin Diagn Pathol. 5(2):223-37, 1988

Placental Site Nodule

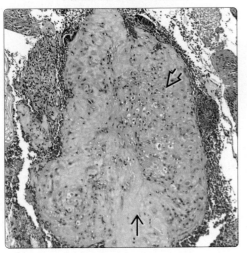

Placental Site Nodule PLAP

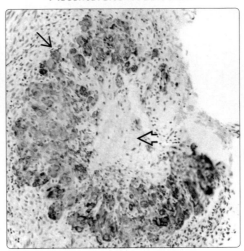

(Left) This curettage was obtained 6 weeks postpartum for abnormal abnormal uterine bleeding. A 1-mm placental site nodule shows central hyalinization ➡ surrounded by bland, intermediate trophoblast cells ➡. No residual placental tissue was present. (Right) Trophoblast cells of the placental site nodule are strongly positive with placental alkaline phosphatase (PLAP) ➡, which spares the area of central hyalinization ➡.

Placental Site Nodule

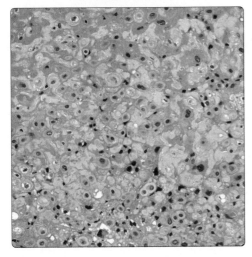

Ki-67 Staining in Placental Site Nodule

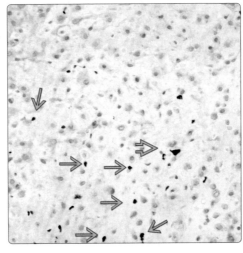

(Left) This patient had a C-section with bilateral salpingo-oophorectomy 3 years before endometrial curettage and ablation for menorrhagia. The PSN measured > 3 mm. High-power examination shows individual intermediate trophoblast cells and cords of cells with extracellular matrix. (Right) The Ki-67 stain in this case shows a proliferative index that is < 1% ➡. Ki-67 stains must be interpreted carefully to avoid counting lymphocyte nuclei ➡, which are frequently Ki-67 positive.

Placental Site Nodule in Hysterectomy Specimen

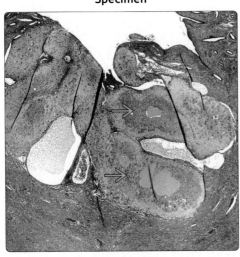

Hemosiderin Deposition in Placental Site Nodule

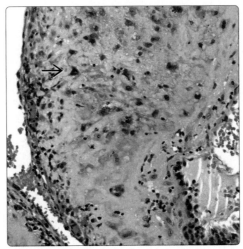

(Left) This hysterectomy specimen shows placental site nodule associated with cysts ➡, similar to microscopic extravillous trophoblast cysts of the extraplacental membranes. (Right) This small, polypoid focus from the same case shows focal hemosiderin laden macrophages ➡.

Atypical Placental Site Nodule

(Left) *This lesion was of small size (< 5 mm), but cellular areas displayed atypical mitoses ➡. (Right) The Ki-67 index is above 5%, warranting a diagnosis of atypical placental site nodule.*

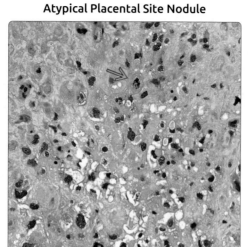

Atypical Placental Site Nodule

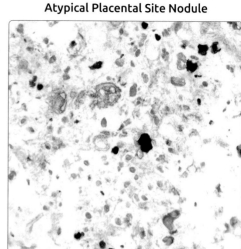

Atypical Placental Site Nodule

(Left) *This small focus lacks the typical abundant hyalin matrix of placental site nodule. Note the anastomosing cords of intermediate trophoblast cells ➡. (Right) Ki-67 staining is increased compared to that expected for placental site nodule for this same case, hence the diagnosis of atypical placental site nodule.*

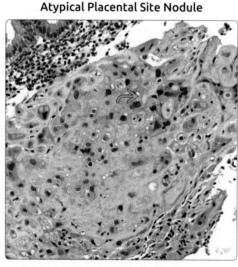

Atypical Placental Site Nodule

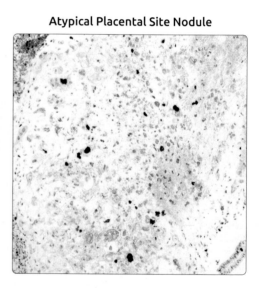

Regressed Villus

(Left) *The rounded contours of this regressed villus ➡ from retained POC might be confused with placental site nodule. Note the abundant fibrin surrounding the villus. Keratin staining may reveal numerous associated extravillous trophoblast cells ➡. (Right) The trophoblast cells associated with this regressed villus show more than minimal Ki-67 reactivity, leading to confusion with atypical placental site nodule.*

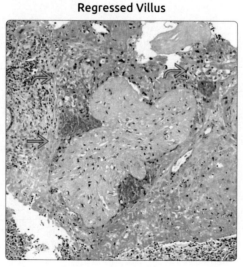

Retained POC

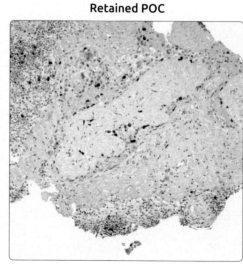

Exaggerated Placental Site Reaction

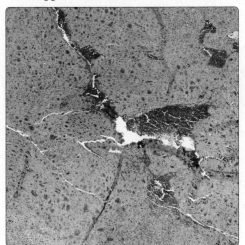

Exaggerated Placental Site Ki-67

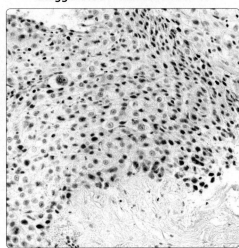

(Left) *Low-power examination of this 1st-trimester implantation site decidua shows numerous trophoblast cells at low power. The variation in cell size is due to numerous multinucleated trophoblast, not nuclear enlargement.* (Right) *The implantation site from this 1st-trimester missed abortion has a large number of invasive trophoblasts but shows low Ki-67 staining.*

Exaggerated Placental Site

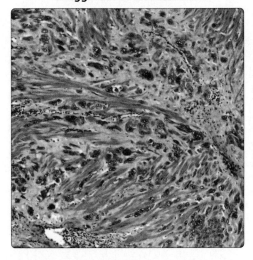

Exaggerated Placental Site Reaction

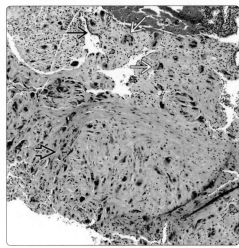

(Left) *Invasive trophoblasts normally invade into the inner 3rd of the myometrium. This D&C shows increased mononuclear and multinucleated trophoblasts between myometrial fibers.* (Right) *Increased numbers of ➡ multinucleated trophoblasts are present. Invasive trophoblasts become multinucleated when they stop invading, which may be associated with "superficial implantation" and pregnancy loss. Invasion into the endometrium ➡ and myometrium ➡ is normal.*

Implantation Site of Complete Mole

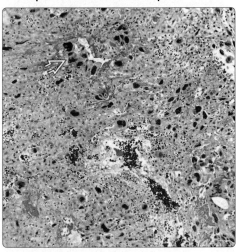

Implantation Site of Complete Mole

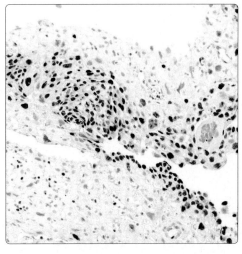

(Left) *The implantation site of complete hydatidiform shows marked hyperchromasia and nuclear pleomorphism of trophoblast cells. While these changes were part of the initial descriptions of exaggerated placental site reaction, they should be recognized as part of gestational trophoblastic disease. A maternal vessel ➡ has been invaded by the trophoblasts.* (Right) *In contrast to exaggerated placental site reaction, the implantation site of complete mole shows marked Ki-67 nuclear staining of EVT.*

KEY FACTS

TERMINOLOGY

- Placental site trophoblastic tumor (PSTT): Rare tumor of implantation site intermediate trophoblasts
  - Most occur after normal pregnancy or spontaneous abortion (SAB), 25% after molar gestation when studied by molecular genotyping
- Epithelioid trophoblastic tumor (ETT): very rare tumor of chorionic-type intermediate trophoblasts
  - Most occur after normal pregnancy or SAB, 25% after molar gestation when studied by molecular genotyping

MICROSCOPIC

- PSTT
  - Bland, polygonal cells forming sheets and cords of tumor cells
  - Cords of cells separate myometrial fibers with minimal necrosis
  - Eosinophilic extracellular matrix
  - Tumor cells remodel uterine blood vessels as in normal implantation site decidua
  - Ki-67 15-25%
- ETT
  - Well-circumscribed nests, cords, and masses of mildly to moderately atypical cells, often with central blood vessel
  - Nodular growth pattern with expansile border; may have decidualized cells adjacent to lesion
  - Eosinophilic extracellular matrix
  - Extensive geographic necrosis
  - Ki-67 10-25%
  - Lower uterine segment or cervix

TOP DIFFERENTIAL DIAGNOSES

- Squamous cell carcinoma vs. ETT
- Placental site nodule vs. ETT, PSTT
- Exaggerated placental site vs. PSTT
- Choriocarcinoma vs. ETT

PSTT

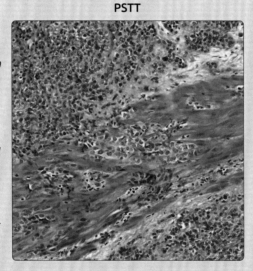

Exaggerated Placental Site

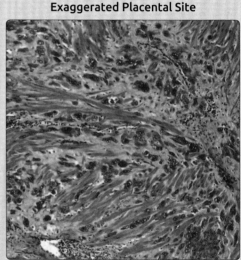

(Left) PSTT consists of sheets and cords of monomorphic polygonal trophoblasts that infiltrate between the smooth muscle of the uterus without significant hemorrhage or necrosis. (Right) This implantation site has prominent mononuclear and multinucleated trophoblasts invading between myometrial fibers, a variant of normal implantation that was previously termed "syncytial endometritis." Neoplastic PSTT was originally recognized from this group of lesions.

ETT

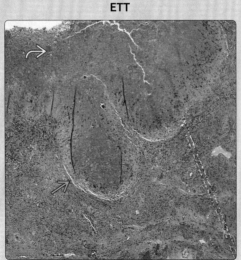

PSN

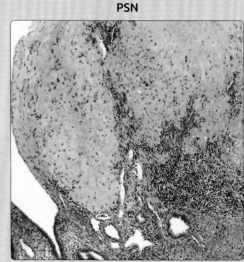

(Left) ETT is a well-circumscribed mass lesion with a characteristic pushing border ➡ and geographic necrosis ➤. (Right) Benign placental site nodule (PSN) has histologic overlap with ETT. Some atypical PSNs may be intermediate lesions. They are associated with development of ETT and PSTT. There are similarities with the nodular pattern, central hyalinization, and peripheral lymphocytes. A PSN is a microscopic diagnosis with low cellularity, minimal nuclear atypia, and virtually no mitotic activity.

TERMINOLOGY

Abbreviations

- Placental site trophoblastic tumor (PSTT)
- Epithelioid trophoblastic tumor (ETT)

Synonyms

- Intermediate trophoblast (IT), extravillous trophoblast, and X-cells are synonyms

Definitions

- PSTT: Rare malignant tumor of gestational trophoblastic neoplasia (GTN), 1-2% of trophoblastic tumors
  - Infiltrative tumor arising from placental implantation site trophoblast cells
  - Slower growth rate than choriocarcinoma; may present remote from last pregnancy
    - Treatment is primarily surgical, insensitive to chemotherapy
- ETT: Very rare malignant tumor of GTN, relatively recently described
  - Well-circumscribed tumor arising from chorionic-type trophoblast cells
  - Slower growth than choriocarcinoma
    - Treatment is primarily surgical, insensitive to chemotherapy
  - Some tumors have mixed features of PSTT and ETT

ETIOLOGY/PATHOGENESIS

Antecedent Pregnancy

- Most PSTT and ETT follow normal pregnancy with female neonate
- ~ 25% of cases follow molar pregnancy by genotyping, most of which were complete hydatidiform mole with one case of molecularly confirmed partial mole
- Genetic origin of tumor is not always immediately preceding pregnancy; rarely, it may be from prior conception

Genetics of PSTT/ETT

- Most diploid are 46,XX
- Subset (~ 25%) are diandrogenetic like complete mole

Cell of Origin

- PSTT and ETT are derived from intermediate trophoblast
  - IT morphology can be polygonal or decidual-like, spindle-shape resembling smooth muscle or endothelial like, lining vascular spaces
  - Universal markers positive for IT: Inhibin-α, HLA-G, cytokeratin, and EMA
- 3 types of IT: Villous, invasive, and chorionic type
  - Villous IT, proximal portion of anchoring villi, immature reserve cell population for invasive IT of implantation site
  - Invasive, implantation site IT, invade endometrium, inner 1/3 of myometrium, remodel spiral arteries
    - CD146 (MEL-CAM) (+)
      - Binds to surface of smooth muscle, limits invasion into superficial 3rd of myometrium
    - p63(-), PLAP(-), HPL(+), Ki-67(-), p57(+)
  - Chorionic IT from chorion laeve of extraplacental membranes
    - Secrete eosinophilic extracellular matrix

- p63(+), CD146 (MEL-CAM)(-), PLAP(+), HPL weak variable staining

CLINICAL ISSUES

Presentation

- PSTT
  - Most patients present with abnormal menstrual cycles (amenorrhea, menorrhagia, irregular bleeding)
  - Slight uterine enlargement in 25% of patients; may suggest missed abortion
  - Serum β-human chorionic gonadotrophin (hCG) only mildly elevated
  - May present with erythrocytosis, which resolves after removal of tumor
- ETT
  - Present with abnormal uterine bleeding, which may occur many years following last pregnancy
  - May be asymptomatic, even with metastatic disease
  - Usually low-level β-hCG (< 2,500 mIU/ml)
  - Often found in cervix or lower uterine segment

Treatment

- Surgical approaches
  - Hysterectomy is treatment of choice in PSTT and ETT
- Drugs
  - Chemotherapy is used only in metastatic disease; effectiveness is unclear

Prognosis

- PSTT
  - 10-23% metastasize to brain, lungs, liver, lower genital tract, and abdomen
  - Increased mitoses and antecedent pregnancy of > 2 years associated with recurrence
- ETT
  - 20-40% of patients have metastatic disease; 10% of cases may be fatal

MACROSCOPIC

General Features

- PSTT
  - Soft, tan-yellow, usually endophytic mass in uterine wall; may protrude into endometrial cavity
  - Often poorly circumscribed; variable size
  - May extend to serosa, perforate serosa, or extend into broad ligament or adnexa
  - Minimal necrosis or hemorrhage on cut section
- ETT
  - Expansile mass in endomyometrium of lower uterine segment or cervix, up to 5 cm in size, may protrude into endometrial cavity or invade myometrium
  - May be solid or cystic on cut section, ± hemorrhage and necrosis

MICROSCOPIC

Histologic Features

- PSTT
  - Sheets of bland round IT with eosinophilic to clear cytoplasm forming cords and nests at periphery; rare multinucleated cells

- o Cells separate myometrial fibers with minimal necrosis
- o Associated with eosinophilic extracellular matrix
- o Trophoblasts remodel uterine blood vessels as in normal implantation
- o Mitoses 2-5/10 HPF, Ki-67 15-25%
- o Rare tumors have mixed features of PSTT and choriocarcinoma (mixed choriocarcinoma PSTT), or mixed PSTT and ETT
- ● ETT
  - o Well-circumscribed nests, cords, and masses of IT with mild to marked nuclear atypia with prominent nucleoli, central small vessel
    - – Features resembling carcinoma, often mistaken for choriocarcinoma (Ki-67 > 50%)
  - o Extensive geographic necrosis surrounds foci of viable cells
  - o Eosinophilic extracellular matrix material may mimic keratin
  - o Cervical ETT can replace epithelium
  - o Mitoses 0-9/10 HPF, Ki-67 10-25%
  - o Increased lymphocytes
  - o Absence of vascular invasion

ANCILLARY TESTS

Immunohistochemistry

- ● Cytokeratin, EMA, inhibin-α, HLA-G, GATA-3
  - o Positive in all lesions of intermediate trophoblasts, PSTT and ETT
- ● Ki-67 proliferation marker
  - o Staining in 15-25% of nuclei in PSTT and 10-25% ETT but < 10% in placental site nodule (PSN)
- ● HPL
  - o Diffusely positive in PSTT, focal in ETT
- ● PLAP
  - o Diffuse staining in ETT, focal staining in PSTT
- ● MEL-CAM (CD146)
  - o Diffusely positive in PSTT, focal positive in ETT
- ● p63
  - o PSTT negative; ETT positive
- ● SALL4
  - o Positive in choriocarcinoma and negative in PSTT and ETT
- ● hCG
  - o Weak and focal staining in both PSTT, ETT

DIFFERENTIAL DIAGNOSIS

PSN vs. ETT, PSTT

- ● PSNs are incidental microscopic lesions, well-circumscribed and paucicellular with extensive hyalin-like extracellular matrix
- ● PSN that are more cellular, with mitotic activity may be termed "atypical PSN" - difficult diagnosis lacking clear criteria
  - o "Atypical PSN" associated with development of ETT and PSTT in some patients

Squamous Cell Carcinoma vs. ETT

- ● Eosinophilic extracellular matrix can mimic keratin; ETT growth pattern can mimic squamous cell carcinoma (SCC)
- ● Both ETT and SCC may express p16 and p63

- ● ETT expresses inhibin-α, HLA-G, and CK18, whereas SCC does not

Exaggerated Placental Site vs. PSTT

- ● Both consist of implantation site IT cells, similar immunophenotype
- ● PSTT shows confluent masses of IT with mitotic activity
- ● Exaggerated placental site is usually incidental finding with normal implantation site features including decidua; trophoblasts are not mitotically active

Choriocarcinoma vs. ETT

- ● Choriocarcinoma is biphasic tumor with cytotrophoblasts surrounded by syncytiotrophoblasts, may also have extensive necrosis, often hemorrhagic, Ki-67 > 50%
- ● Cases with mixed features of both tumors are reported

SELECTED REFERENCES

1. Sobecki-Rausch J et al: Surgery and platinum/etoposide-based chemotherapy for the treatment of epithelioid trophoblastic tumor. Int J Gynecol Cancer. 28(6):1117-1122, 2018
2. Horowitz NS et al: Placental site trophoblastic tumors and epithelioid trophoblastic tumors: biology, natural history, and treatment modalities. Gynecol Oncol. 144(1):208-214, 2017
3. Stichelbout M et al: SALL4 expression in gestational trophoblastic tumors: a useful tool to distinguish choriocarcinoma from placental site trophoblastic tumor and epithelioid trophoblastic tumor. Hum Pathol. 54:121-6, 2016
4. Stănculescu RV et al: Epithelioid trophoblastic tumor: a case report and literature review. Rom J Morphol Embryol. 57(4):1365-1370, 2016
5. Zhao S et al: Molecular genotyping of placental site and epithelioid trophoblastic tumours; female predominance. Gynecol Oncol. 142(3):501-7, 2016
6. Banet N et al: GATA-3 expression in trophoblastic tissues: an immunohistochemical study of 445 cases, including diagnostic utility. Am J Surg Pathol. 39(1):101-8, 2015
7. Davis MR et al: Epithelioid trophoblastic tumor: a single institution case series at the New England Trophoblastic Disease Center. Gynecol Oncol. 137(3):456-61, 2015
8. Kurman RJ et al: Discovery of a cell: reflections on the checkered history of intermediate trophoblast and update on its nature and pathologic manifestations. Int J Gynecol Pathol. 33(4):339-47, 2014
9. Luiza JW et al: Placental site trophoblastic tumor: immunohistochemistry algorithm key to diagnosis and review of literature. Gynecol Oncol Case Rep. 7:13-5, 2013
10. Chew I et al: p16 expression in squamous and trophoblastic lesions of the upper female genital tract. Int J Gynecol Pathol. 29(6):513-22, 2010
11. Ou-Yang RJ et al: Expression of glypican 3 in placental site trophoblastic tumor. Diagn Pathol. 5:64, 2010
12. Houghton O et al: The expression and diagnostic utility of p63 in the female genital tract. Adv Anat Pathol. 16(5):316-21, 2009
13. Kim SJ: Placental site trophoblastic tumour. Best Pract Res Clin Obstet Gynaecol. 17(6):969-84, 2003
14. Shih IM et al: The pathology of intermediate trophoblastic tumors and tumor-like lesions. Int J Gynecol Pathol. 20(1):31-47, 2001
15. Shih IM et al: Epithelioid trophoblastic tumor: a neoplasm distinct from choriocarcinoma and placental site trophoblastic tumor simulating carcinoma. Am J Surg Pathol. 22(11):1393-403, 1998

Ultrasound of PSTT

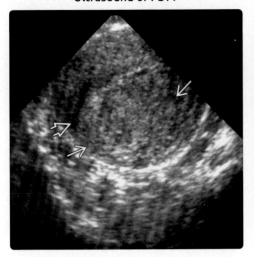

Gross Uterus With PSTT

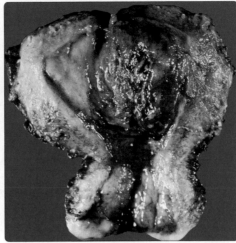

(Left) This ultrasound shows there is asymmetry to the uterus with a mass ➡ bulging into the ➡ endometrial cavity. (Right) The hysterectomy specimen shows the exophytic PSTT, bulging into the endometrial cavity.

Infiltrative Trophoblast of PSTT

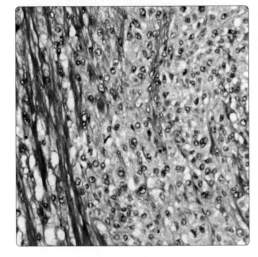

Nuclear Features of PSTT

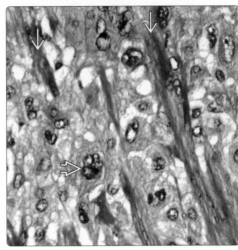

(Left) PSTT is characterized by regular polygonal trophoblasts that infiltrate between myometrial fibers with little or no necrosis. (Right) PSTT implantation site trophoblasts have minimal pleomorphism with rare ➡ multinucleated cells. They invade between myometrial fibers ➡ without necrosis.

PSTT With HPL

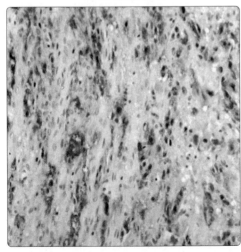

PSTT Metastatic to Salivary Gland

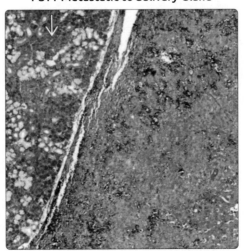

(Left) PSTT is strongly positive with HPL. (Right) Metastasis of PSTT occurs in 10-23% of cases but mostly to brain, lungs, liver, lower genital tract, and abdomen. This is an unusual metastasis to the ➡ salivary gland.

Geographic Necrosis in ETT

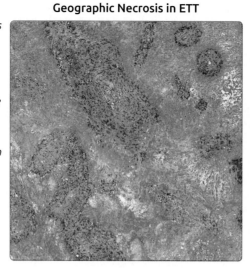

ETT Involving Cervical Mucosa

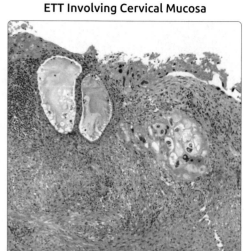

(Left) *Necrosis surrounds nests and islands of tumor cells, forming the characteristic geographic necrosis appearance of ETT.* (Right) *ETT is a mimic of squamous cell carcinoma (SCC). This case shows involvement of the cervical epithelium and endocervical glands. Both lesions express p63, a common pitfall.*

Perivascular Tumor Cells in ETT

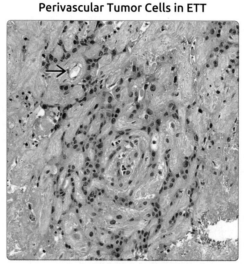

Nests and Cords of Tumor Cells in ETT

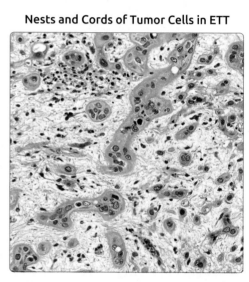

(Left) *The cords and nests of tumor cells in ETT may surround small blood vessels* ⮕. (Right) *ETT can strongly mimic invasive carcinoma. The tumor location within the lower uterine segment or cervix and cells with abundant eosinophilic cytoplasm, as seen here, can mimic SCC.*

ETT p63

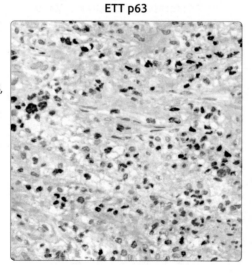

ETT Ki-67

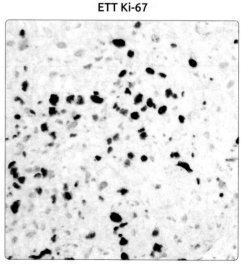

(Left) *ETT can be a difficult mimic of SCC, particularly in cervical lesions. Both may express p63, as seen here in this image of ETT.* (Right) *The Ki-67 index of ETT is ~ 10-25%, which may be helpful in differentiating ETT from PSN. This distinction is not always easy, as some cases of PSN, particularly atypical PSN, can have mitotic rates approaching 10%.*

ETT in Myometrium

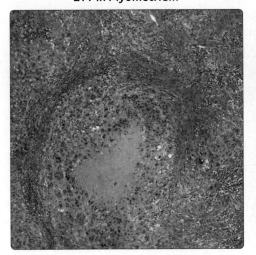

Lymphoid Infiltrates in ETT

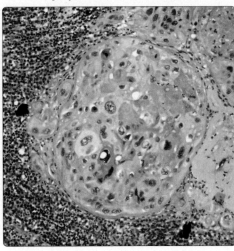

(Left) ETT usually has a pushing border into the myometrium. This tumor nodule has central necrosis. (Right) ETT usually has moderate nuclear atypia with varying amount of eosinophilic extracellular matrix. This nodule is surrounded by a large infiltrate of lymphocytes.

Abundant Matrix in ETT

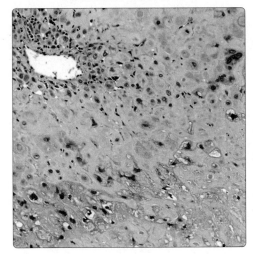

Extensive Necrosis in ETT

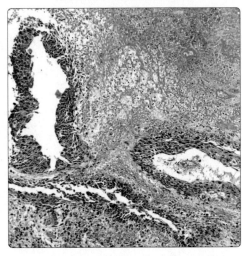

(Left) ETT will frequently show tumor cells surrounding a central vessel. This example has abundant eosinophilic matrix. The high-power appearance resembles the foci of PSN. (Right) Larger uterine vessels are surrounded by ETT with extensive tumor necrosis.

ETT, Ki-67

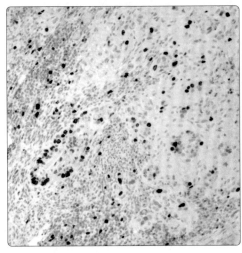

ETT Negative, or Only Weakly Positive, for hPL

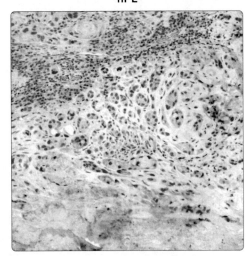

(Left) ETT has a Ki-67 index of ~ 10-25%, not significantly different from PSTT. (Right) ETT is negative or only weakly positive for hPL, in contrast to PSTT, which is strongly positive.

Metastatic Tumors

ETIOLOGY/PATHOGENESIS

- Malignant maternal tumor sheds cells into maternal bloodstream that are carried through decidual arteries into blood surrounding chorionic villi
- Malignant fetal tumor sheds cells into fetal bloodstream that are carried through umbilical artery into placental circulatory bed where they lodge in villous capillaries
- Ectopic fetal tissue thought to result from aberrant migration of tissue during development with implantation into umbilical cord, chorionic plate, or villi

CLINICAL ISSUES

- Most common malignant maternal tumors with placental metastasis: Melanoma and lymphoma/leukemia
- Most common malignant fetal tumors with placental metastasis: Neuroblastoma and lymphoma/leukemia
  - Massive amount of tumor cells in fetal vessels may result in fetal demise due to hypoxia
  - Often present with nonimmune hydrops

MACROSCOPIC

- Melanoma may form pigmented nodules
- Lymphoma and carcinoma may form white nodules

MICROSCOPIC

- Metastatic maternal tumors
  - Clusters of tumor cells within intervillous space, sometimes embedded within fibrinoid material
- Metastatic fetal tumors
  - Clusters of tumor cells within (often distended) fetal vessels and villous capillaries

TOP DIFFERENTIAL DIAGNOSES

- Metastatic maternal tumors: Chronic histiocytic intervillositis and inflammatory conditions
- Metastatic fetal tumors: Clusters of circulating immature hematopoietic cells (e.g., erythroblastosis fetalis)
- Heterotopic rests of fetal liver or nevus cells should not be confused with placental metastasis

Neuroblastoma Metastatic to Placenta

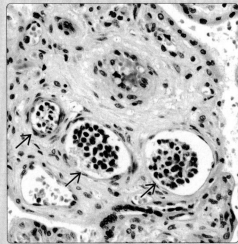

Villous Capillaries Filled With Neuroblastoma

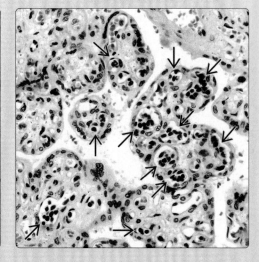

(Left) This placenta, from a 36-week gestation infant with a prenatally diagnosed abdominal mass, weighed 855 g (> 97th percentile). Large clusters of neuroblastoma cells ⮕ are present within the small vessels of intermediate villi. (Right) Many of the villous capillaries ⮕ are also filled with neuroblastoma. This could reduce the ability of the placenta to oxygenate the fetus.

Neuroblastoma, NSE

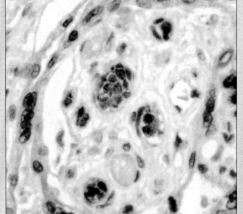

Metastatic Neuroblastoma, Synaptophysin

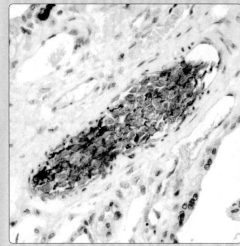

(Left) Intravascular neuroblastoma cells are weakly positive for NSE. (Right) Intravascular neuroblastoma cells are positive for synaptophysin.

TERMINOLOGY

Definitions

- Placental "metastasis"
  - Maternal malignancy within intervillous space
  - Fetal malignancy within villous vessels
  - Very rarely do cancer cells actually invade villous stroma as in true metastasis

ETIOLOGY/PATHOGENESIS

Maternal Tumors

- Malignant maternal tumor cells enter maternal bloodstream and are carried through decidual arteries into intervillous space
- < 0.1% of pregnant women have/develop malignancy, and only rarely does placental metastasis occur

Fetal Tumors

- Malignant fetal tumor cells enter fetal bloodstream and are carried through umbilical artery into villous circulation
- Extremely rare event

CLINICAL ISSUES

Presentation

- Many different tumors have been reported to metastasize to placenta, but occurrence very rare
  - Frequency of observed placental metastases depends on prevalence of tumor and propensity to metastasize
- Most common malignant maternal tumors with placental metastasis (in descending order of frequency)
  - Melanoma
  - Lymphoma/leukemia
  - Breast carcinoma
  - Lung carcinoma
  - Gastric adenocarcinoma
- Most common malignant fetal tumors with placental metastasis (in descending order of frequency)
  - Neuroblastoma
  - Lymphoma/leukemia
  - Hepatoblastoma
  - Melanoma
  - Sarcoma
  - Rhabdoid tumor
- Maternal history of malignancy usually known at birth
- Fetal mass be identified on ultrasound
  - Metastatic fetal tumors may present with nonimmune fetal hydrops
- Infants with large congenital melanocytic nevi may have intraplacental nevus cells; may be "rest" (not necessarily metastasis)
- Rare cases reported of mothers with placenta metastases from fetal neuroblastoma experiencing catecholamine-induced symptoms (sweating, flushing, palpitations)

Prognosis

- Maternal tumors
  - Increased risk of abruption &/or preterm delivery in setting of placental metastasis
  - Increased risk of fetal death in setting of maternal metastases to placenta
  - Neonates with maternally derived metastatic disease have extremely poor prognosis even when aggressively treated
- Fetal tumors
  - Fetal hydrops occurring in setting of malignant fetal tumor nearly always lethal
  - Fetal tumor metastasis to placenta may cause mirror syndrome in mother (preeclampsia in setting of fetal/placenta hydrops)
  - Massive amount of tumor in fetal vasculature may result in fetal demise due to hypoxia

MACROSCOPIC

General Features

- Metastatic maternal tumors
  - Melanoma may form pigmented nodules
  - Lymphoma (and less often, carcinoma) may form white nodules
- Metastatic fetal tumors
  - Large, pale, hydropic placenta (can exceed 1 kg)
  - Tumor emboli not usually visible grossly

MICROSCOPIC

Histologic Features

- Metastatic maternal tumors
  - Clusters of tumor cells within intervillous space, sometimes embedded within fibrinoid material
  - Tumor cells may invade villi (~ 1/2 of melanoma cases)
  - Rarely spread into fetal circulation (melanoma and leukemia/lymphoma)
  - Tumor cells either mimic primary neoplasm or simply appear as primitive small round blue cells
- Metastatic fetal tumors
  - Clusters of tumor cells within (often distended) fetal vessels and villous capillaries
  - Involvement may be diffuse or only very focal within sections
  - In rare cases, tumor cells infiltrate adjacent villous stroma
  - Spread into maternal circulation has not been reported

ANCILLARY TESTS

Immunohistochemistry

- Tumor-specific markers may help confirm/identify type of tumor

Genetic Testing

- Distinguishing fetal vs. maternal origin of metastatic tumor can be accomplished by PCR genotyping of short tandem repeats

DIFFERENTIAL DIAGNOSIS

Chronic Histiocytic Intervillositis

- Increased cellularity could be confused with maternal metastatic tumor
  - Monomorphic dense infiltrates of CD68(+) histiocytes, often with clinical history of recurrent reproductive failure or fetal growth restriction

Placental Diagnoses

Congenital Nevi

- Nevus cells from infants with large, congenital nevi may be mistaken for metastatic melanoma
  - Clinical history important
  - Molecular methods may be needed to distinguish fetal vs. maternal origin
- Stain like melanocytes (S100 and HMB45) within fetal villous stroma

Erythroblastosis Fetalis

- Clusters of circulating immature hematopoietic cells, usually erythroblasts
  - Immunohistochemistry can differentiate erythroblasts from potentially leukemic myeloblasts/lymphoblasts

Ectopic/Heterotopic Fetal Tissue

- Thought to result from aberrant migration of tissue during development with implantation into umbilical cord, chorionic plate, or chorionic villous parenchyma (usually proximal stem villi)
- Heterotopic fetal liver
  - Well-circumscribed, often pseudoencapsulated nodule in umbilical cord, chorionic plate, or villous parenchyma
  - Clusters of hepatocytes without portal tracts, central veins, or ductules (similar to postnatal hepatic adenoma)
  - May have associated hematopoiesis
  - Positive for cytokeratin AE1/AE3, HepPar1, AFP, and arginase-1; variable for glypican-3
- So-called "adrenal" heterotopia
  - Cleared cytoplasm and organization resembles zona glomerulosa of adult adrenal cortex
  - Usually hepatic in origin when studied with newer more specific antibodies

DIAGNOSTIC CHECKLIST

Pathologic Interpretation Pearls

- Clinical history or suspicion of maternal or fetal cancer is indication for gross and microscopic examination of placenta

- Relevant clinical history (e.g., maternal cancer or fetal mass on US) should raise suspicion and trigger thorough microscopic evaluation of placenta

SELECTED REFERENCES

1. Stonko DP et al: Ectopic fetal hepatic tissue in the placenta. Int J Gynecol Pathol. ePub, 2018
2. Saluja R et al: Ectopic liver within the placental parenchyma of a stillborn fetus. Pediatr Dev Pathol. 1093526617712640, 2017
3. Alomari AK et al: Congenital nevi versus metastatic melanoma in a newborn to a mother with malignant melanoma - diagnosis supported by sex chromosome analysis and Imaging Mass Spectrometry. J Cutan Pathol. 42(10):757-64, 2015
4. Mascelli S: A reliable assay for rapidly defining transplacental metastasis using quantitative PCR. Methods Mol Biol. 1160:125-31, 2014
5. Reif P et al: Metastasis of an undifferentiated fetal soft tissue sarcoma to the maternal compartment of the placenta: maternal aspects, pathology findings and review of the literature on fetal malignancies with placenta metastases. Histopathology. 65(6):933-42, 2014
6. Allen AT et al: Mirror syndrome resulting from metastatic congenital neuroblastoma. Int J Gynecol Pathol. 26(3):310-2, 2007
7. Alexander A et al: Metastatic melanoma in pregnancy: risk of transplacental metastases in the infant. J Clin Oncol. 21(11):2179-86, 2003
8. Baergen RN et al: Maternal melanoma metastatic to the placenta: a case report and review of the literature. Arch Pathol Lab Med. 121(5):508-11, 1997
9. Lynn AA et al: Disseminated congenital neuroblastoma involving the placenta. Arch Pathol Lab Med. 121(7):741-4, 1997

Metastatic Malignant Rhabdoid Tumor
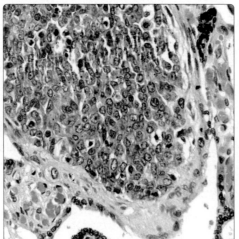

Metastatic Hepatoblastoma
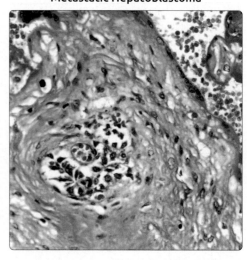

(Left) A sheet of metastatic large, epithelioid tumor cells is present within a distended fetal stem vessel in the placenta of a fetus with malignant rhabdoid tumor. (Right) A cluster of malignant small round blue cells is present in the placental vasculature of a fetus with congenital hepatoblastoma.

Metastatic Breast Cancer

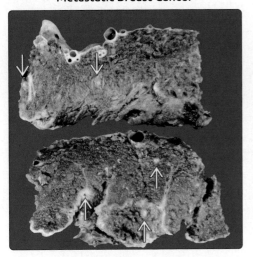

Metastatic Breast Cancer in Intervillous Space

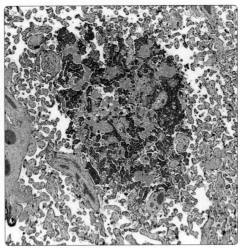

(Left) *Gross examination of placental cross sections from a mother with widely metastatic breast carcinoma shows multiple firm, yellow, 1- to 5-mm nodules* ➡ *scattered throughout the parenchyma.* (Right) *At low power, the nodules are seen microscopically to be composed of clusters of dark, amphophilic tumor cells within the maternal intervillous space, entrapping villi.*

Maternal Intervillous Space With Metastatic Breast Cancer

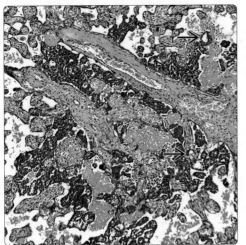

Necrosis in Metastatic Breast Cancer

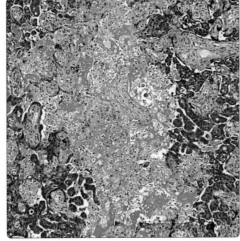

(Left) *At higher power, the tumor in the intervillous space is seen to be composed of sheets of darker, more cytologically atypical cells. Focally, primitive glandular structures can be appreciated* ➡. (Right) *In other areas, the tumor cells form nests and small trabecula with a central area of necrosis, forming a comedo-like pattern of intraductal breast carcinoma.*

Metastatic Lung Carcinoma

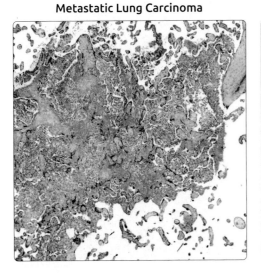

Metastatic Non-Small Cell Lung Carcinoma

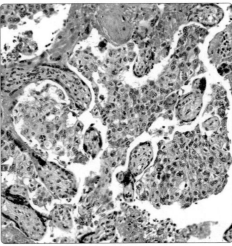

(Left) *A placenta from a mother with metastatic lung carcinoma contains multiple small foci of tumor involvement. The aggregates of intervillous tumor cells surround the villi, resulting in ischemia due to lack of maternal blood flow.* (Right) *Large sheets of metastatic lung carcinoma cells fill the intervillous space.*

Metastatic Melanoma

Maternal Metastatic Melanoma

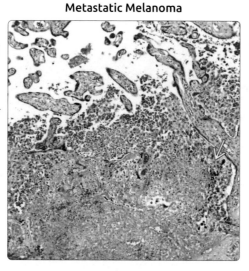

(Left) *A sheet of metastatic melanoma cells within the intervillous space shows broad areas of necrosis appreciable at low power. There is only focal melanin pigment ➡, which could be mistaken for hemosiderin in the presence of the necrosis.* **(Right)** *Metastatic maternal melanoma cells within the intervillous space are beginning to infiltrate villi. Melanin pigment is evident in some cells ➡.*

Metastatic Melanoma With Abundant Pigment

Metastatic Melanoma

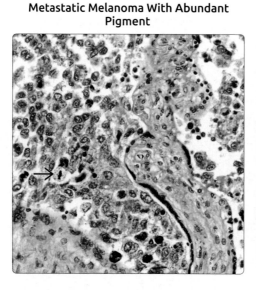
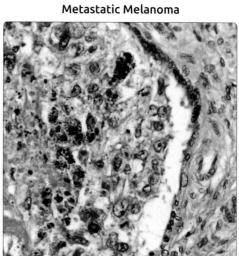

(Left) *A higher power view shows cytologically atypical melanoma cells, some of which are heavily pigmented. Rare mitotic figures are also present ➡.* **(Right)** *Coarse, brown melanin pigment is readily discernible within metastatic melanoma cells in the intervillous space of this placenta.*

Maternal T-Lymphoblastic Leukemia

Maternal T-Cell Leukemia, CD3

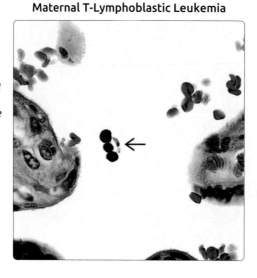
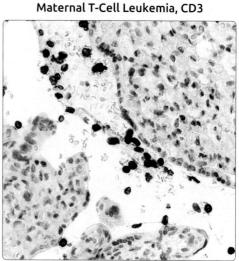

(Left) *A small cluster of circulating maternal T-lymphoblastic leukemia cells ➡ can be seen in the intervillous space.* **(Right)** *An immunostain for CD3, a T-cell marker, highlights the maternal leukemic cells in the maternal intervillous space. Additional, more-specific markers for the leukemia would be required to prove these are leukemic and not reactive T cells.*

Transient Myeloproliferative Disorder

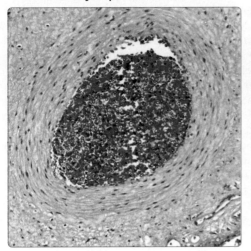

Trisomy 21

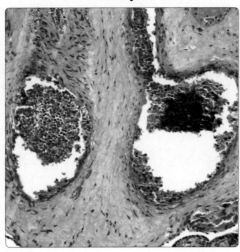

(Left) *A newborn baby with trisomy 21 had leukocytosis (186,000/uL) and was diagnosed with transient myeloproliferative disorder (transient abnormal myelopoiesis). A chorionic plate vessel contains numerous myeloblasts phenotypically indistinguishable from leukemic cells of acute myeloid leukemia.* (Right) *Fetal stem vessels in the same case are packed with immature myeloid cells. This can result in intrauterine hypoxia.*

Heterotopic Liver in Placenta

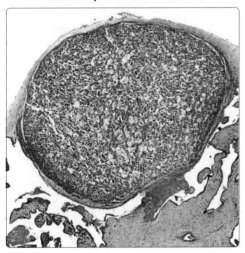

Ectopic Liver in Placenta

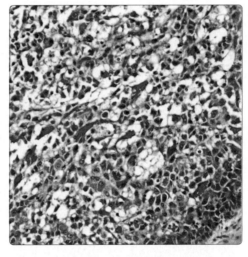

(Left) *A well-circumscribed and pseudoencapsulated nodule of benign hepatic tissue lies within a proximal stem villus just beneath the chorionic plate.* (Right) *At high power, the hepatocytes have a fetal appearance. The cells are polygonal with brightly eosinophilic cytoplasm and are arranged in vague cords. Portal tracts and bile ducts are not seen in this case. Foci of extramedullary hematopoiesis may be seen.*

Ectopic Liver AFP

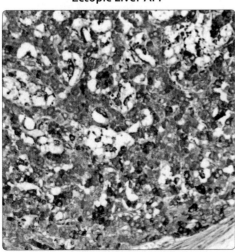

Nevus in Placental Villi

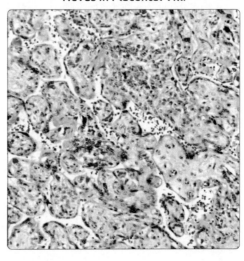

(Left) *The ectopic hepatocytes are strongly positive for AFP by immunohistochemistry.* (Right) *Benign nevus cells populate the villi of this placenta from an infant with a large, congenital, melanocytic nevus. Placental location can help distinguish this phenomenon from a maternal metastatic melanoma, which would be found in the maternal intervillous space.*

EPIDEMIOLOGY

Incidence

- Uterine tumors associated with delivered placenta are exceedingly rare
- Leiomyoma (fibroid) seen in 3-12% of pregnancies
  - Multiple and large leiomyomas associated with complications, such as prematurity
  - Commonly excised at cesarean section
  - Very rarely, leiomyoma remains attached to placenta with delivery

ETIOLOGY/PATHOGENESIS

Placental Tumor vs. Uterine Tumor

- Mesenchymal tumors of delivered placenta have historically been called "placental"; however, in all reported cases where molecular investigation was performed, they proved to be maternal in origin
- Decidua is of purely maternal origin
  - Endometrium under effect of pregnancy hormones

- Decidua present on membranes, basal surface, and within placental septa at base of parenchyma
- Endometrial lesion could be incorporated into any of these sites
- In some pregnancies, decidua is deficient and implantation may occur directly into uterine smooth muscle
  - More common in lower uterine segment, cornua, and after prior cesarean section
  - Uterine smooth muscle cells may be present adherent to basal plate or membranes
  - Associated with morbidly adherent placenta
- Tumors and tumor-like lesions of uterus may exist in pregnant uterus
  - Endometrial stromal lesions, endometrial polyp
  - Mesenchymal lesions, such as leiomyoma, inflammatory myofibroblastic tumor, rarely leiomyosarcoma
  - If these lesions are close enough to anchor to basal plate or membranous chorion, they may accompany placenta at delivery

(Left) *Vaginal delivery of this 6.8-cm fleshy mass followed delivery of a healthy neonate and placenta at term. On prenatal ultrasound, the mass resembled an accessory lobe of the placenta. (Courtesy S. Umetsu, MD and N. Ladwig, MD.)* (Right) *In contrast, this 1.5-cm tumor extends from the basal plate into the parenchyma, likely within a placental septum. (Courtesy S. Umetsu, MD and N. Ladwig, MD.)*

Gross Appearance of Inflammatory Myofibroblastic Tumor

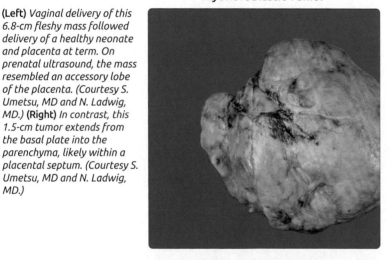

Intraplacental Inflammatory Myofibroblastic Tumor

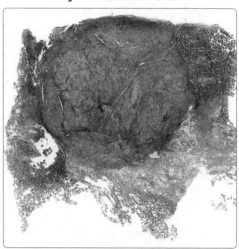

(Left) *Nitabuch fibrin ⊡ surrounds the margin of the tumor, continuous with the basal plate. Short tandem repeat genotyping confirmed that the tumor was maternal and did not arise from the (biparental) placenta. (Courtesy S. Umetsu, MD and N. Ladwig, MD.)* (Right) *Any maternal pathology of the endometrium could potentially be found in the decidua of the delivered placenta like this endometrial polyp. (Courtesy S. Umetsu, MD and N. Ladwig, MD.)*

Intraplacental Inflammatory Myofibroblastic Tumor

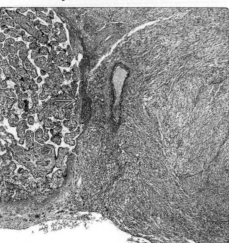

Endometrial Polyp in Membranous Decidua

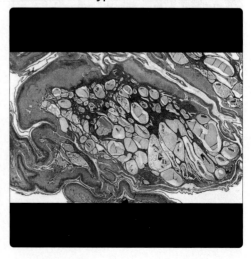

CLINICAL IMPLICATIONS

Imaging Findings

- Rounded mass of submucosal leiomyoma may appear to be intraplacental on ultrasound
- Lesions associated with membranes may resemble accessory (succenturiate) lobe, but no fetal vessels connect mass to placenta

Prognosis

- Leiomyoma, endometrial stromal nodule, endometrial polyp are benign lesions
- Endometrial stromal sarcoma, inflammatory myofibroblastic tumor have malignant potential
  - Patients managed with staging laparotomy, hysterectomy, and bilateral salpingo-oophorectomy as appropriate for diagnosis
  - Too few cases reported to ascertain any unique malignant potential in lesions delivered with placenta; none reported to date have behaved aggressively

MACROSCOPIC

Leiomyoma

- Well-circumscribed, firm nodule
- Usually presents attached to membranes; may be loosely associated with basal plate
- Whorled, fibrous cut surface as in leiomyoma of uterus

Inflammatory Myofibroblastic Tumor

- Fleshy, white nodule attached to basal plate; well circumscribed within parenchyma or attached to membranes

Endometrial Stromal Tumor

- Gray-white lesions of variable texture reportedly associated with disc margin or membranes
  - Case reported as endometrial stromal neoplasm well circumscribed in membranes
  - Case reported as endometrial stromal sarcoma involved fragmented bulky mass attached to margin of disc

MICROSCOPIC

Leiomyoma

- Intersecting fascicles of cytologically bland spindled cells with prominent eosinophilic cytoplasm
- Commonly undergo reactive/ischemic changes
  - Fibrosis/hyalinization, edema
- Ancillary studies usually not necessary for diagnosis

Inflammatory Myofibroblastic Tumor

- Composed mostly of spindled myofibroblasts with mixed inflammatory cell infiltrates
  - Areas with myxoid appearance on low power; variable cellularity with areas of tightly packed spindled cells
- Spindled cells show marked elongation of nucleus and cytoplasm
  - Nucleus has fine, evenly distributed chromatin with 1 or more nucleoli; nucleoli may be prominent
- Decidual-like cells described in placental inflammatory myofibroblastic tumor admixed with myofibroblasts
- May have degenerative changes and necrosis

- Immunohistochemistry: ALK-1 positive (in most cases), CD10 patchy positive, SMA positive, keratin negative, desmin negative, S100 positive, variable ER and PR staining
- FISH: *ALK* gene rearrangement may be demonstrated

Endometrial Stromal Tumors

- Extreme caution warranted in trying to make definitive diagnosis of endometrial stromal nodule or endometrial stromal sarcoma in this setting; molecular investigation for characteristic fusions should be considered
  - Cellular morphology is modified by effects of pregnancy (decidualization)
    - Impairs distinction of low-grade vs. high-grade cytology
    - May affect mitotic activity or induce necrosis
  - Relationship to uterus is disrupted in delivered placenta; difficult to assess tumor border
- Cases described as endometrial stromal tumor or sarcoma consisted mostly of polygonal to spindled cells in loose edematous matrix with admixed glands in one case report
- Immunohistochemistry: CD10, ER, and PR staining described in these lesions associated with placenta
- FISH, PCR: Molecular characterization of endometrial stromal tumors is rapidly evolving
  - Gene fusions include *JAZF1*, *SUZ12* (JJAZ1), *BCORL1*, and others

SELECTED REFERENCES

1. Heller DS et al: Endometrial stromal neoplasm in the placenta: report of a case and review of the literature. Int J Gynecol Pathol. 37(1):32-34, 2018
2. Ladwig NR et al: Inflammatory myofibroblastic tumor associated with the placenta: short tandem repeat genotyping confirms uterine site of origin. Am J Surg Pathol. 42(6):807-812, 2018
3. Mohammad N et al: ALK is a Specific Diagnostic Marker for Inflammatory Myofibroblastic Tumor of the Uterus. Am J Surg Pathol. ePub, 2018
4. Hand LC et al: Incidental leiomyosarcoma found at the time of cesarean hysterectomy for morbidly adherent placenta. Gynecol Oncol Rep. 20:127-130, 2017
5. Banet N et al: Inflammatory myofibroblastic tumor of the placenta: a report of a novel lesion in 2 patients. Int J Gynecol Pathol. 34(5):419-23, 2015
6. Ciavattini A et al: Number and size of uterine fibroids and obstetric outcomes. J Matern Fetal Neonatal Med. 28(4):484-8, 2015
7. Haltas H et al: Completely infarcted smooth muscle tumor of the placental membrane. J Obstet Gynaecol Res. 39(4):864-7, 2013
8. Murtoniemi K et al: Smooth muscle tumor of the placenta - an entrapped maternal leiomyoma: a case report. J Med Case Rep. 3:7302, 2009
9. Karpf EF et al: Endometrial stromal nodule embedded into term placenta. APMIS. 115(11):1302-5, 2007
10. Tarim E et al: Submucosal leiomyoma of the uterus incorporated into the fetal membranes and mimicking a placental neoplasm: a case report. Placenta. 24(6):706-9, 2003
11. Ernst LM et al: Intraplacental smooth muscle tumor: a case report. Int J Gynecol Pathol. 20(3):284-8, 2001
12. Katsanis WA et al: Endometrial stromal sarcoma involving the placenta. Ann Diagn Pathol. 2(5):301-5, 1998

ETIOLOGY/PATHOGENESIS

- ~ 20% of fetuses with placental mesenchymal dysplasia (PMD) have Beckwith-Wiedemann syndrome (BWS); at least subset have androgenetic/biparental mosaicism

CLINICAL ISSUES

- Suspected on US evaluation when placenta shows molar changes but fetus developing
- 1/2 of non-BWS fetuses with PMD have intrauterine growth restriction, 1/3 die in utero
- Fetus may be hydropic with anemia and thrombocytopenia

MACROSCOPIC

- Bulky, enlarged placenta with markedly dilated chorionic plate vessels
- Numerous gelatinous cysts in parenchyma

MICROSCOPIC

- Marked dilation of chorionic plate vasculature with mural hemorrhage, thrombi in some cases
- Stem villous cysts, abnormally enlarged villi with stromal and vascular proliferation
- Stem vessel obliteration, villous stromal/vascular karyorrhexis, and avascular villi of fetal vascular malperfusion
- Hypervascular villi similar to chorangiomatosis

TOP DIFFERENTIAL DIAGNOSES

- Partial hydatidiform mole
- Androgenetic/biparental mosaicism with component of complete hydatidiform mole

DIAGNOSTIC CHECKLIST

- Absence of trophoblastic proliferation distinguishes PMD from partial mole; partial moles are triploid
- Absence of trophoblastic proliferation and retention of p57 in villous cytotrophoblast excludes component of complete mole in androgenetic/biparental conceptions

Cysts in PMD

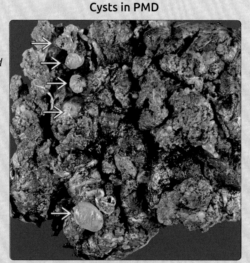

Villous Cysts in PMD

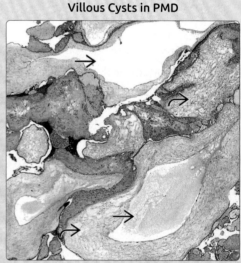

(Left) The diagnosis of placental mesenchymal dysplasia (PMD) is suspected on gross exam when presented with an enlarged, bulky placenta containing scattered, grape-like cysts ➡ within the parenchyma. (Right) Microscopic exam shows abnormal, large villi with cavernous cysts ➡ and loose, myxoid stroma ➡. Unlike molar villi, there is no cytotrophoblast proliferation.

Variable Amount of Cystic Change

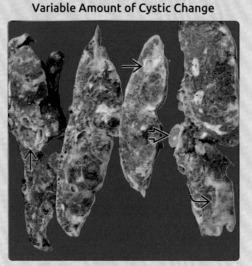

p57 Staining in PMD

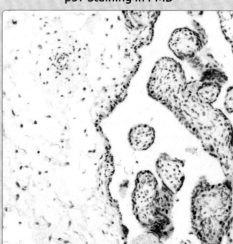

(Left) The amount of cyst formation ➡ and surface chorionic plate vessel dilation ➡ can be variable in PMD. Other placental pathologies such as fetal vascular malperfusion, infarcts ➡, and increased perivillous fibrin may also be present. (Right) p57 staining in PMD shows discordance, with expression in the cytotrophoblast but not the stroma. This often reflects the mosaicism of an androgenetic mesenchymal lineage (stroma) and biparental trophoblast lineage.

TERMINOLOGY

Abbreviations

- Placental mesenchymal dysplasia (PMD)

Synonyms

- Mesenchymal villous dysplasia, pseudopartial mole, placental mesenchymal hyperplasia

Definitions

- Abnormal placental development characterized by placentomegaly, stem-villous hydropic cyst formation, abnormal villous stroma, and fetal vessels
- Androgenetic: Chromosomes of entirely paternal origin, usually from endoreduplication of paternal genes with loss of maternal genome
- Androgenetic/biparental mosaic: Different cell lines with either androgenetic or biparental genomes admixed in tissues

ETIOLOGY/PATHOGENESIS

Imbalance of Paternal and Maternal Alleles

- Mesenchymal overgrowth of PMD due to excess of paternally expressed growth promoting genes, &/or absence of maternally expressed growth-restricting genes, reported abnormalities include
  - Chromosomal region 11p15.5 loss of heterozygosity, paternal uniparental disomy
    - Aberrant expression of *CDKN1C* (encodes p57/Kip2), *IGF2* genes in this region implicated in stromal overgrowth
  - Microdeletion in *GRB10* maternal allele (growth inhibitor gene)
  - Paternal uniparental disomy for chromosomes 6 and 14

Androgenetic/Biparental Mosaicism

- Complete androgenetic development results in complete hydatidiform mole
  - Complete mole resembles PMD but has trophoblastic hyperplasia, less villous stromal development, and usually no fetus
- At least a subset of PMD cases have androgenetic/biparental mosaicism
  - Line of cells carrying 2 copies of paternal genome with no maternal component give rise to some placental tissues
    - Amount of androgenetic cells is variable, explaining spectrum of changes in PMD, from minimal to severe
    - Trophoblast cell lineage is biparental, stromal cell lineage is androgenetic in PMD
  - Probably only minority of fetal somatic tissues have this abnormal androgenetic cell lineage, if any
    - Could explain association with some features of Beckwith-Wiedemann syndrome (BWS), or intrauterine growth restriction
    - Could explain preponderance of females as 46,YY fertilized eggs would not be viable
- Most cases diploid, though rare cases with chromosomal abnormalities confined to placenta, or fetus and placenta observed

BWS

- 20% of fetuses with PMD have BWS, characterized by macrosomia, organomegaly, hemihypertrophy, macroglossia, omphalocele, and increased risk of pediatric tumors including hepatoblastoma, Wilms tumor, adrenocortical carcinoma, gonadoblastoma, and brainstem glioma
  - Associated with abnormalities of chromosome 11p15 imprinting with loss of maternal allele expression
- Fetuses with BWS tend to be large for gestational age and have larger PMD placentas

CLINICAL ISSUES

Presentation

- Suspected on US evaluation when placenta shows molar changes but fetus developing
- > 80% of fetuses female, may have congenital hemangioma, hepatic mesenchymal hamartoma
- Fetus may be normally developed, small for gestational age, hydropic, or show changes of BWS
- Preeclampsia observed in some cases
- Serum HCG usually not elevated
  - Elevated HCG raises concern for mosaic conceptions with possible component of complete mole

Prognosis

- Child should be evaluated for possible BWS, given associated risk of malignancy
- Transient anemia and thrombocytopenia described in PMD with extensive hypervascularity (resembling chorangioma)
- ~ 1/3 of reported cases had fetal demise

IMAGING

Ultrasonographic Findings

- Large, thick placenta with multicystic, hyperechoic foci, with fetus
  - Differential diagnosis includes partial mole, complete mole with fetus, large chorangioma or subchorionic thrombus (Breus mole)
  - Color Doppler US shows stained glass appearance due to abundant blood flow
    - Complete mole has little blood flow

MACROSCOPIC

General Features

- Bulky, enlarged placenta with variably dilated, varicose-like, chorionic plate vessels
- Parenchyma shows grape-like cysts, and regions of tan gelatinous-appearing foci may be found in otherwise spongy red-brown villous parenchyma
- Excessively long, hypercoiled umbilical cord in subset of cases

MICROSCOPIC

Histologic Features

- Chorionic plate vasculature
  - Marked dilation with mural hemorrhage, thrombi in some cases
- Stem villi

- o Cysts, stromal overgrowth, abnormal vasculature
- o Thrombi and changes of fetal vascular malperfusion
- o Hypervascular villi similar to chorangiomatosis
- Distal villi
  - o Abnormal hypocellular stroma in subpopulation
  - o Fetal vascular malperfusion with stromal vascular karyorrhexis and avascular villi

ANCILLARY TESTS

Immunohistochemistry

- p57/KIP2 staining preserved in trophoblast, but lost in villous stroma of dysplastic villi
  - o Maternally expressed protein; staining absent in androgenetic cells or other conditions with loss of maternal allele

Genetic Testing

- Short tandem repeat (STR) marker genotyping may yield complex results, with excess of paternal alleles in androgenetic/biparental mosaicism

DIFFERENTIAL DIAGNOSIS

Partial Hydatidiform Mole

- Share cystic villi and presence of normally developed villi
- PMD lacks characteristic trophoblast proliferation around abnormal villi seen in partial mole
- Partial hydatidiform mole associated with diandric triploidy

Androgenetic/Biparental Mosaicism With Component of Complete Hydatidiform Mole

- Common differential earlier in pregnancy (< 20 weeks)
- Trophoblastic proliferation in subset of villi, with characteristic loss of p57 expression in cytotrophoblast and stroma
- Cases with recognizable foci of complete mole should be followed as gestational trophoblastic disease, not PMD
  - o Risk of gestational trophoblastic disease associated with mosaic conceptions with 20% complete molar component
- May have elevated maternal serum HCG

DIAGNOSTIC CHECKLIST

Clinically Relevant Pathologic Features

- PMD easily recognized cause of fetal and neonatal morbidity and mortality
- ~ 20% of PMD cases associated with BWS in neonate

Pathologic Interpretation Pearls

- Absence of trophoblastic proliferation distinguishes PMD from partial mole
- Be wary of any trophoblastic proliferation suspicious for mole, androgenetic/biparental mosaic conceptions with component of complete mole need to be recognized and get appropriate follow-up

SELECTED REFERENCES

1. Stampone E et al: Genetic and epigenetic control of CDKN1C expression: importance in cell commitment and differentiation, tissue homeostasis and human diseases. Int J Mol Sci. 19(4), 2018
2. Linn RL et al: Placental mesenchymal dysplasia without fetal development in a twin gestation: a case report and review of the spectrum of androgenetic biparental mosaicism. Pediatr Dev Pathol. 18(2):146-54, 2015
3. Pawoo N et al: Placental mesenchymal dysplasia. Arch Pathol Lab Med. 138(9):1247-9, 2014
4. Lewis GH et al: Characterization of androgenetic/biparental mosaic/chimeric conceptions, including those with a molar component: morphology, p57 immmnohistochemistry, molecular genotyping, and risk of persistent gestational trophoblastic disease. Int J Gynecol Pathol. 32(2):199-214, 2013
5. Ulker V et al: Placental mesenchymal dysplasia: a rare clinicopathologic entity confused with molar pregnancy. J Obstet Gynaecol. 33(3):246-9, 2013
6. Hoffner L et al: P57KIP2 immunostaining and molecular cytogenetics: combined approach aids in diagnosis of morphologically challenging cases with molar phenotype and in detecting androgenetic cell lines in mosaic/chimeric conceptions. Hum Pathol. 39(1):63-72, 2008
7. Kaiser-Rogers KA et al: Androgenetic/biparental mosaicism causes placental mesenchymal dysplasia. J Med Genet. 43(2):187-92, 2006
8. Pham T et al: Placental mesenchymal dysplasia is associated with high rates of intrauterine growth restriction and fetal demise: a report of 11 new cases and a review of the literature. Am J Clin Pathol. 126(1):67-78, 2006
9. Jauniaux E et al: Perinatal features associated with placental mesenchymal dysplasia. Placenta. 18(8):701-6, 1997
10. Lage JM: Placentomegaly with massive hydrops of placental stem villi, diploid DNA content, and fetal omphaloceles: possible association with Beckwith-Wiedemann syndrome. Hum Pathol. 22(6):591-7, 1991

Abnormal Villous Stroma in PMD

Hypervascular Villi of PMD

(Left) *More normal-sized villi may show stromal overgrowth with abnormal, small vessels ➡. Note that there is no trophoblastic proliferation around the abnormal villi.* (Right) *Other cases may show striking hypervascular villi. The hypervascular villi in PMD differ from usual chorangioma and chorangiomatosis. Capillaries are more loosely arranged and sinusoidal. The stroma may be abnormally cellular with degenerative changes.*

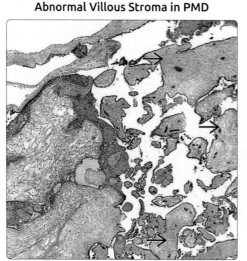

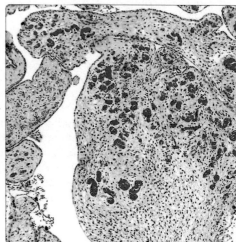

Chorionic Plate Vessels in PMD

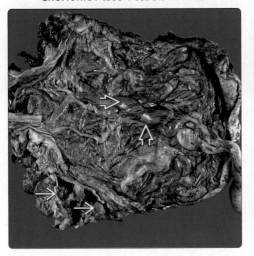

Dilated Chorionic Plate Veins

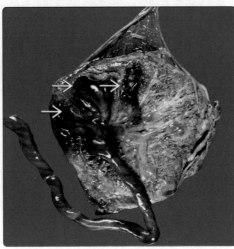

(Left) Grossly, PMD is characterized by molar-like cysts of stem villi ➡ and a variable degree of chorionic plate vessel dilatation. In this image, a chorionic plate vein is abnormally dilated ➡. (Right) This PMD placenta shows marked dilation of chorionic plate vasculature ➡ (in this case, veins). (Courtesy S. Kostadinov, MD.)

Chorionic Plate Vessels in PMD

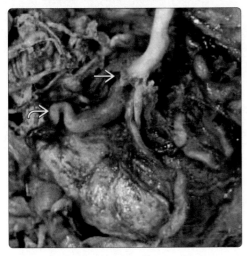

Thrombi In Chorionic Plate Vessel

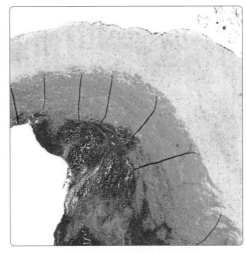

(Left) The chorionic plate vasculature ➡ may become cirsoid, or worm-like in PMD. In this case, the cord had a furcate insertion ➡ with the abnormal vessels branching before being tethered in the chorionic plate. (Right) The abnormal vasculature of PMD frequently contains thrombi. Other changes of fetal vascular malperfusion, such as villous stromal karyorrhexis and avascular villi, may also be seen.

Stem Vessel Obliteration in PMD

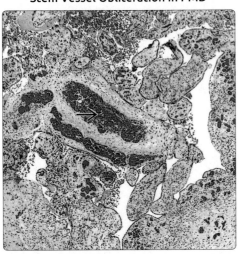

Distal Villi in PMD

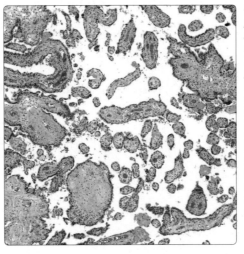

(Left) The abnormal vascular proliferation in PMD often shows changes of fetal vascular malperfusion. Thrombus formation ➡ is present in a larger vessel. Neonates with PMD may have a transient but severe coagulopathy, which could be related to the hypervascularity or frequent thrombi. (Right) Distal villi may show only very subtle changes in the stroma. In general, these distal villi show increased stromal cellularity with fewer sinusoidal capillaries.

SECTION 3
Placental Evaluation in Special Circumstances

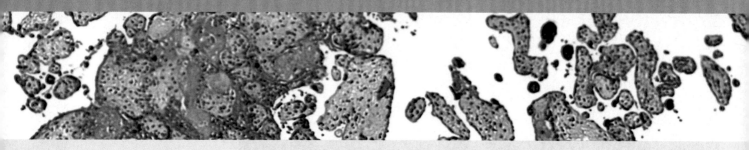

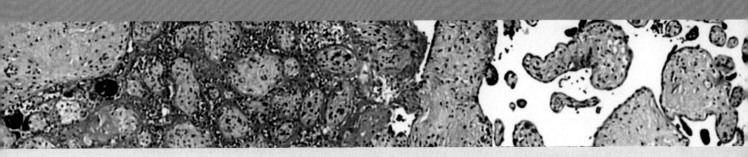

Multiple Gestations

Maternal Complications Of Pregnancy

TERMINOLOGY

Definitions

- Pregestational diabetes
  - Type 1DM, incidence, 0.2-0.5% of pregnancies
  - Type 2DM, incidence, 3-5% of pregnancies
- Gestational diabetes (GDM)
  - Hyperglycemia first detected during pregnancy, incidence 5-14%
    - Risk increases 2.6x for obese women and 4x with morbid obesity
    - Increased incidence in nonwhite race/ethnicity, 18%
- Prediabetes
  - Glucose levels higher than normal but below levels diagnostic for diabetes
  - No consensus criteria for diagnosis in pregnancy
- Diabetic embryopathy
  - Congenital malformations in fetus of diabetic mother
- Diabetic fetopathy
  - Disorders of fetal development in fetus of diabetic mother arising in 2nd and 3rd trimester

Diagnostic Criteria for Gestational Diabetes

- Criteria for diagnosing GDM have been highly variable over time and across countries
- WHO criteria revised in 2013 using International Association of Diabetes and Pregnancy Study Groups criteria
  - GDM is diagnosed when 1 or more of the following results are recorded at any time during pregnancy
    - Fasting plasma glucose levels 5.1-6.9 mmol/L (92-125 mg/dL)
    - 1-hour oral glucose tolerance test values ≥ 10.0 mmol/L (180 mg/dL) after 75-g oral glucose load
      - Usually performed at 24-28 weeks, may be earlier in women with obesity or previous diagnosis of GDM
    - 2-hour oral glucose tolerance test values between 8.5 and 11.0 mmol/L (153-199 mg/dL) after 75-g oral glucose load

Subtypes of Gestational Diabetes

- A1DM, controlled by diet and exercise

- A2DM, requires oral hypoglycemics and/or insulin for control
- White classification of diabetes
  - Class A
    - Abnormal glucose tolerance test at any age or of any duration, treated by diet therapy only
  - Class B
    - Maternal onset at age 20 years or older, duration of < 10 years
  - Class C
    - Maternal onset at age 10-19 years or duration of 10-19 years
  - Class D: Maternal onset before 10 years of age, duration > 10 years, benign retinopathy or hypertension (not preeclampsia)
    - D1: Onset before age 10 years
    - D2: Duration over 20 years
    - D3: Macrovascular disease (calcification of vessels of leg)
    - D4: Microvascular disease (retinopathy); hypertension (not preeclampsia)

ETIOLOGY/PATHOGENESIS

Diabetic Embryopathy

- Generally attributed to poor glucose control in early pregnancy
- Can also occur in tight glucose control
- Metabolic and hormonal milieu likely affects epigenetics during development
  - Diabetes is associated with increased oxidative stress, especially in 1st trimester

Diabetic Fetopathy

- Macrosomia occurs when placental capacity to store excess fetal glucose is exceeded
  - Accelerated fetal growth begins at 24 weeks but is markedly increased after 34 weeks
- Adiposity and organomegaly with fetal macrosomia
  - Increased levels of insulin-like growth factor 1 (IGF-1) in fetus

Choriangiosis in Diabetes

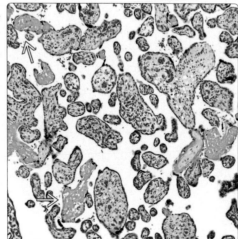

Delayed Villous Maturation

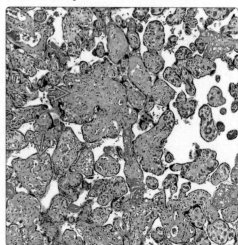

(Left) This placenta weighed 790 g at 35 weeks and showed significant hypervascularity, consistent with chorangiosis. There is also an increase in villi that have fibrinoid necrosis ➡. Both of these are commonly associated with diabetes. (Right) Villi from pregnancies complicated by diabetes or obesity may show delayed villous maturation. These villi are enlarged with few vasculosyncytial membranes compared to more normal villi. Some villi are hypervascular ➡; others appear hypovascular ➡.

- – Direct relationship between level of IGF-1 and fetal weight with or without diabetes
- Fetal glucose from maternal blood exceeds demand, so it is stored in liver and other fetal tissues
  - o Via GLUT1 transporter in placental vessels
  - o Excess glucose is stored in liver and other fetal tissues and transported back to placenta for storage
  - o Macrosomia occurs when placental capacity to store glucose is exceeded
- Active transport of amino acids across placenta is normally increased during last 6 weeks, variably increased in GDM and obesity
- Rapid transport of lipids across placenta and increased lipogenesis allow for increased accumulation of adiposity near term; increased in diabetes
- Leptin, a peptide hormone specifically expressed in adipose tissue, is increased in pregnancy and obesity

Placental Transport of Glucose

- Fetus is completely dependent upon glucose transport from maternal blood across trophoblast membranes
- Gluconeogenesis does not occur in fetal liver until 34-37 weeks
- Placenta utilizes 60% of uterine uptake of glucose
- Hypoxia increases glucose utilization by placenta
- In utero hyperglycemia results in fetal hyperinsulinemia

CLINICAL IMPLICATIONS

Maternal Complications of Diabetes

- Frequent spontaneous abortion, especially for type 1 diabetics
  - o Up to 4% of stillbirths are due to diabetes
- Polyhydramnios due to fetal hyperglycemia, osmotic diuresis, and increased fetal urination
- 5x increased risk for prematurity
- Preeclampsia
- Increased cesarean section rate
- Diabetic ketoacidosis during pregnancy
  - o 1-10% incidence during pregnancy
  - o 30% of cases occur as presenting symptom of diabetes
  - o Ketoacids cross placenta
  - o 9-25% fetal loss
- GDM usually resolves within 6 weeks after delivery
  - o 50% will develop type 2 diabetes over 20-30 years

Fetal Complications of Diabetes

- Diabetic embryopathy with congenital malformations, usually with preexisting diabetes
  - o Cardiac anomalies
    - – Transposition of great vessels, ventricular septal defect, atrial septal defect, tetralogy of Fallot
  - o Caudal regression syndrome is rare (extreme form is sirenomelia), but minor sacral abnormalities seen in 16%
    - – Rare but almost unique to diabetes
    - – Agenesis of sacrum and lumbar spine
    - – Hypoplasia of lower extremities
    - – May also have anal atresia, hypospadias, diaphragmatic hernia, and omphalocele
  - o Neural tube defect
  - o Genitourinary, gastrointestinal, and skeletal anomalies
- Diabetic fetopathy with macrosomia

- o Increased risk of birth trauma, such as shoulder dystocia, cephalohematoma
- o Increased risk for childhood obesity
- o Increased risk for late fetal demise, after 36 weeks
- Neonatal complications
  - o Fetal diabetic cardiomyopathy
    - – Hypertrophic cardiomyopathy, 20% mortality
      - □ 40-50% show significant thickening of interventricular septum up to 6 mm
      - □ Usually resolves within a week, but may persist for months
      - □ Fiber disarray, hydropic change, and myocyte hypertrophy
    - – Dilated cardiomyopathy
      - □ Occurs in less than 10%
      - □ Usually associated with severe hypoglycemia and acidosis
      - □ Focal myofiber necrosis
  - o Increased respiratory distress
    - – Lung immaturity, as insulin inhibits production of surfactant, which lags 2 weeks behind
    - – Pulmonary hypertension
  - o Renal vein thrombosis
  - o Hypoglycemia due to hyperinsulinemia
    - – 8-14% develop hypoglycemia during first 2-4 hours due to marked drop in glucose, which was previously available from maternal blood
    - – Increased number and size of fetal islets that continue to produce excess insulin
    - – Increase in size of islets is generally proportionate to fetal overgrowth and severity of maternal diabetes
  - o Hyperbilirubinemia due to polycythemia
  - o Pyloric stenosis
  - o Hypocalcemia with decreased bone mineralization; cardiac dysfunction
  - o Hypomagnesemia
  - o Hepatomegaly, 2x normal size due to increased glycogen, steatosis, and extramedullary hematopoiesis
  - o Adrenal glands, 2x normal
  - o Increased risk of type 2 diabetes later in life
  - o Increased incidence of behavior or intellectual deficits

Maternal Obesity Without Diabetes

- Incidence increasing: 50% of pregnant women are overweight prior to conception and 24% obese
- Results in similar complications, except caudal regression not seen
- Placental abnormalities may be more prevalent with female fetuses
- Placental features may be worse with increasing grade of obesity
- Increased risk of intrauterine fetal demise with each week of expectant management after 34 weeks
  - o Delivery by 38 weeks may minimize perinatal mortality
  - o Have to balance benefit of delivery in early term period with risk of neonatal respiratory distress

MACROSCOPIC

General Features

- Placental pathology in diabetes is variable

○ Placenta is normal in ~ 50% of cases
○ Features tend to segregate into cases with fetal overgrowth and cases characterized by maternal vascular malperfusion
○ Variability may be due to type of diabetes, duration of diabetes, different treatments, and comorbidities, such as maternal obesity or preeclampsia
○ Cases with fetal macrosomia include
  – All forms of diabetes
  – Nondiabetic mother with prepregnancy obesity (BMI > 30)
  – Mother with excessive weight gain during pregnancy
○ Features of maternal vascular malperfusion seen with
  – Preexisting maternal cardiovascular or renal disease
  – Hypertension
  – Longstanding type 1 diabetes
• Gross placental findings with fetal macrosomia
○ Placentomegaly
  – Weight > 90th percentile for age
  – Placenta appears bulky, greater in diameter, thickness, and weight
  – Increase in placental weight is greater than that of fetal weight, resulting in decreased fetal:placental weight ratio
  – Seen in all types of diabetes, especially type 2 diabetes mellitus; also seen in obesity (prepregnancy BMI > 30) and women with excessive weight gain during pregnancy
○ Thick umbilical cord with increased Wharton substance
• Gross placental findings with maternal hypertension
○ Placenta may be small for gestational age
○ Infarcts
• Single umbilical artery
○ 3-5% of diabetic placentas; 1% in nondiabetics

MICROSCOPIC

General Features

• Delayed villous maturation
○ Especially with GDM, maternal obesity, excessive weight gain during pregnancy
• Villous edema
○ Can be difficult to discern from delayed villous maturation or prematurity
○ Predominantly affects basal villi with increased stromal fluid
○ May see karyorrhexis of individual vessels in hypovascular-appearing villi, suggestive of fetal vascular malperfusion
• Chorangiosis
○ Especially with pregestational diabetes, types 1 and 2
○ Capillary bed has greater total length, branching, volume and surface area
• Increased fetal nucleated red blood cells, ~ 2x normal
○ Erythropoietin levels are higher, red blood cell mass is increased
• Fetal vascular malperfusion
○ May reflect hyperviscosity associated with increased red blood cell production
○ Seen in 10% of diabetic placentas
• Increased fibrinoid necrosis of terminal villi

○ Affecting more than 3% of terminal villi (some authors suggest > 10% of villi at term)
• Changes of maternal vascular malperfusion
○ Decidual arteriopathy, especially hypertrophic vasculopathy
○ Distal villous hypoplasia
○ Infarcts
○ Microscopic chorionic pseudocysts (extravillous trophoblast cysts)
• Basal and paraseptal intervillous thrombi
○ Appear more related to stasis of maternal blood than fetal-maternal hemorrhage
○ May be more common in GDM than pregestational diabetes

SELECTED REFERENCES

1. Tieu J et al: Screening for gestational diabetes mellitus based on different risk profiles and settings for improving maternal and infant health. Cochrane Database Syst Rev. 8:CD007222, 2017
2. Yao R et al: The risk of perinatal mortality with each week of expectant management in obese pregnancies. J Matern Fetal Neonatal Med. 1-8, 2017
3. Basnet KM et al: Prevalence of intervillous thrombi is increased in placentas from pregnancies complicated by diabetes. Pediatr Dev Pathol. 19(6):502-505, 2016
4. Huynh J et al: Type 1, type 2 and gestational diabetes mellitus differentially impact placental pathologic characteristics of uteroplacental malperfusion. Placenta. 36(10):1161-6, 2015
5. Persson M et al: Maternal overweight and obesity and risks of severe birth-asphyxia-related complications in term infants: a population-based cohort study in Sweden. PLoS Med. 11(5):e1001648, 2014
6. Starikov R et al: Comparison of placental findings in type 1 and type 2 diabetic pregnancies. Placenta. 35(12):1001-6, 2014
7. Crane JM et al: Maternal and perinatal outcomes of extreme obesity in pregnancy. J Obstet Gynaecol Can. 35(7):606-11, 2013
8. Salbaum JM et al: Responses of the embryonic epigenome to maternal diabetes. Birth Defects Res A Clin Mol Teratol. 94(10):770-81, 2012
9. Zhang Q et al: Synergistic regulation of p53 by Mdm2 and Mdm4 is critical in cardiac endocardial cushion morphogenesis during heart development. J Pathol. 228(3):416-28, 2012
10. Higgins M et al: Clinical associations with a placental diagnosis of delayed villous maturation: a retrospective study. Pediatr Dev Pathol. 14(4):273-9, 2011
11. Daskalakis G et al: Placental pathology in women with gestational diabetes. Acta Obstet Gynecol Scand. 87(4):403-7, 2008
12. Fetita LS et al: Consequences of fetal exposure to maternal diabetes in offspring. J Clin Endocrinol Metab. 91(10):3718-24, 2006
13. Jauniaux E et al: Villous histomorphometry and placental bed biopsy investigation in type I diabetic pregnancies. Placenta. 27(4-5):468-74, 2006
14. Evers IM et al: Placental pathology in women with type 1 diabetes and in a control group with normal and large-for-gestational-age infants. Placenta. 24(8-9):819-25, 2003
15. Mayhew TM et al: Maternal diabetes mellitus is associated with altered deposition of fibrin-type fibrinoid at the villous surface in term placentae. Placenta. 24(5):524-31, 2003

Fetal Vascular Malperfusion and Gestational Diabetes

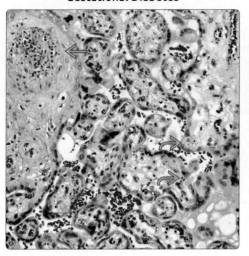

Increased NRBC in Fetal Vessels

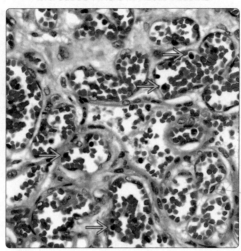

(Left) These villi show stem vessel obliteration ⇥ and a subtle villous stromal/vascular karyorrhexis ⇥ in this placenta from a pregnancy complicated by gestational diabetes. (Right) Diabetes in pregnancy, as well as hypoxia, stimulate fetal erythropoiesis, with increased NRBC ⇥ appearing in the blood. NRBC may be quantified in 10 40x fields of mature distal villi. Most mature placentas have < 1 NRBC. > 10 NRBC in 10 HPF is associated with significant fetal morbidity and increased NRBC count from the neonatal CBC (> 2.5 x 103/mm3).

Chorionic Trophoblast Microcysts

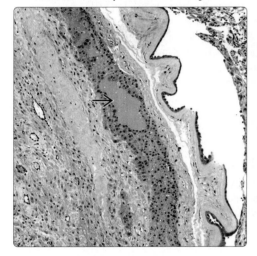

Intervillous Thrombus

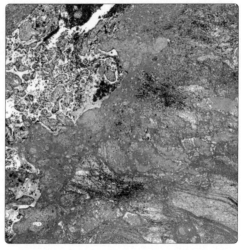

(Left) Chorionic trophoblast microcysts ⇥ are frequently seen in the membranes in placentas from mothers with gestational diabetes. (Right) Intervillous thrombi are more frequent in placentas from pregnancies complicated by diabetes, especially cases of gestational diabetes.

Macrosomia, Diabetic Fetopathy

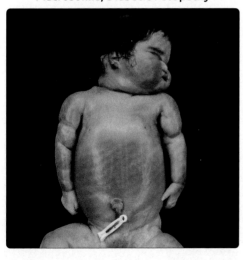

Caudal Regression Syndrome, Diabetic Embryopathy

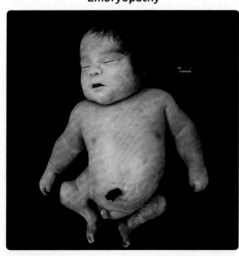

(Left) There is significant increase in body weight, with most of the increase noted in the chest and shoulder area. This contributes to the risk for shoulder dystocia. (Right) This shows classic increased chest adiposity of an infant of a diabetic mother. The vertebra were absent below T7. The sacrum was absent. The lower extremities in a frog-like position is characteristic of caudal regression.

TERMINOLOGY

Synonyms

- Excessive placental weight
- Large placenta for gestational age
- Placental overgrowth
- Placental hypertrophy

Definitions

- Macroscopic diagnosis based on comparison of placental weight to normative values for given gestational age
  - May be applied to any placental weight > 90th percentile
- May be more strictly defined as absolute singleton placental weight > 800 g at any gestational age

ETIOLOGY/PATHOGENESIS

Associated With Fetal Macrosomia

- Placental weight generally correlates with birth weight
- Fetal macrosomia variably defined as birth weight > 4,000 g or 4,500 g

Secondary to Pathological Processes

- Maternal conditions
  - Maternal diabetes, metabolic syndrome or obesity
  - Syphilis
  - Severe anemia
- Fetal conditions
  - Hydrops of any etiology
  - Severe anemia
    - Chronic fetal-maternal transfusion
    - Rh alloimmunization
  - Aneuploidy
  - Metabolic storage disorders with placental involvement
- Placental conditions
  - Chorangiosis
    - Terminal villous hypervascularity most often associated with diabetes
  - Placental mesenchymal dysplasia (PMD)
    - May be associated with overgrowth syndromes or fetal aneuploidy
  - Hydatidiform moles: Complete hydatidiform mole (CHM) and, rarely, partial hydatidiform mole (PHM)
    - Excess paternal gene expression drives placental overgrowth
  - Chorangioma
    - Placental hemangioma

CLINICAL IMPLICATIONS

Clinical Presentation

- Abnormal results of maternal serum screening tests
  - Marked elevations of hCG in CHM
  - Villous edema and fetal hydrops are associated with elevated maternal serum α-fetoprotein
- In association with fetal macrosomia, can present with related perinatal risk factors
  - Preterm labor and delivery
  - Arrest of labor secondary to cephalopelvic disproportion
  - Shoulder dystocia
- Placenta uses 40% of oxygen from uterus and is maintained during periods of reduced uterine oxygen supply
  - Placentomegaly has been associated with signs/symptoms of acute antenatal hypoxia
    - Low Apgar scores
    - Respiratory distress syndrome
    - Neurologic abnormalities
    - Intrauterine or perinatal death
- Association with polyhydramnios increases risk for preterm delivery
- Diagnosis of placentomegaly may raise clinical concern for previously undiagnosed maternal diabetes

Clinical Risk Factors

- Maternal diabetes, usually with poor glucose control
- Associated fetal conditions, including hydrops, aneuploidy, overgrowth syndromes, and infection
- Risk of maternal gestational trophoblastic neoplasm after CHM

Imaging Findings

- Ultrasound findings

(Left) Assessment of placental size is relative to gestational age. Both of these placentas are from 38-weeks gestation. The placenta on the left weighed 710 g and is slightly pale. The placenta on the right weighed 414 g, which is normal for gestational age. (Right) The maternal surface of this 918-g placenta at 32 weeks is pale and boggy with accentuation of the cotyledons. It was friable upon handling. The fetus had a cardiac mass resulting in fetal hydrops.

Placentomegaly

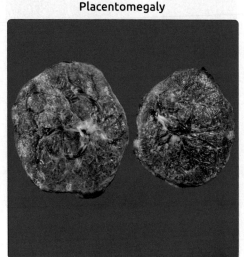

Placentomegaly Secondary to Edema

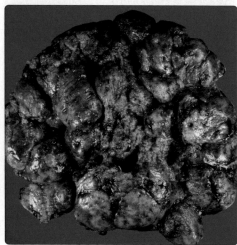

- o General enlargement or thickening of disc, > 3.3-4.0 cm
- o Hypoechoic or cystic spaces, including vesicles in CHM
- o Mass lesion with blood flow, chorangioma
- o Dilated, tortuous chorionic plate vessels in PMD
- o Associated fetal anomalies in aneuploidy or lack of fetus in CHM

MACROSCOPIC

General Features

- Size
  - o Disc weight > 90th percentile for gestational age
  - o Disc weight > 800 g in singleton placenta
  - o Placenta of unusually large diameter (> 22 cm) without abnormally increased weight should be carefully examined for other features suggestive of placenta membranacea
    - Abnormally thin and large placenta with all or most fetal membranes covered by chorionic villi

Specimen Handling

- Documentation of placental weight is standard component of placental examination
  - o Obtain prior to fixation, as immersion in formaldehyde fixative can increase weight by 5-10%
  - o Normograms are based on trimmed weight of disc following removal of free membranes, umbilical cord (to within 2 cm of insertion), and loosely adherent blood clot
  - o Prolonged fresh storage results in minimal weight loss due to evaporation and leakage of blood/serum
    - Accentuated in hydropic or edematous placentas
- Routine sections of villous parenchyma should be examined microscopically to evaluate for potential underlying pathology contributing to increased weight
- Photographic documentation of unusual features

Anatomic Features

- Specific macroscopic features of primary pathological processes/diagnoses
  - o Villous edema due to any cause, including hydrops fetalis, infection, metabolic storage disorders, mass lesions, and fetal anemia
    - Generalized parenchymal pallor
    - Boggy with increased friability
    - Placental hydrops may cause edema of umbilical cord, resulting in increased diameter and translucency
  - o Maternal diabetes
    - May be pale due to villous edema or plethoric due to fetal polycythemia
    - Increased friability
  - o PMD and overgrowth syndromes, including Beckwith-Wiedemann syndrome
    - Chorionic plate vessels with aneurysmal dilation and thrombosis
    - Focally enlarged stem villi with cyst and vesicle formation
  - o Hydatidiform moles
    - Diffuse vesicles, up to 2 cm in CHM, increased volume of tissue
    - Vesicles < 1 cm and affecting < 20% of villous parenchyma in PHM, rarely enlarged placenta
  - o Chorangioma

  - Mass lesion, firm homogeneous, sometimes with infarction
- Placentas affected by maternal anemia and diabetes may have no structural or gross abnormalities, besides increased weight

MICROSCOPIC

General Features

- Histopathological features relate to parenchymal alterations of primary process, including
  - o Maternal diabetes
    - Delayed villous maturation with increased villous width and prominent cytotrophoblast layer
    - Villous hypervascularity, including chorangiosis
    - Increased fetal nucleated red blood cells
  - o Villous edema
    - Increased villous width
    - Clearing of villous stroma with "floating" Hofbauer cells
    - Abnormal, scalloped villous contours in cases of extensive edema
    - Separation of trophoblastic layer from underlying stroma
  - o PMD
    - Enlarged stem villi with stromal overgrowth, vascular proliferation (chorangiomatosis), and areas of cystic degeneration or sinusoid formation
    - Distal villi may appear immature and may exhibit chorangiosis
  - o CHM
    - Homogeneous villous enlargement with cisterns containing karyorrhectic debris
    - Cytotrophoblast, intermediate trophoblast, and syncytiotrophoblast proliferation
    - Atypia of invasive trophoblasts at implantation site
  - o Metabolic storage disorders
    - Variable vacuolization of trophoblasts, stromal cells, endothelium, or amnion depending on specific disorder
    - Cases involving trophoblasts demonstrate diffuse thickening of trophoblast layer
    - Stromal cells usually have fine vacuolization and foamy appearance as opposed to clear spaces surrounding cells found in villous edema

SELECTED REFERENCES

1. Fadl S et al: Placental imaging: normal appearance with review of pathologic findings. Radiographics. 37(3):979-998, 2017
2. Pawoo N et al: Placental mesenchymal dysplasia. Arch Pathol Lab Med. 138(9):1247-9, 2014
3. Nayeri UA et al: Systematic review of sonographic findings of placental mesenchymal dysplasia and subsequent pregnancy outcome. Ultrasound Obstet Gynecol. 41(4):366-74, 2013
4. Treacy A et al: Delayed villous maturation of the placenta: quantitative assessment in different cohorts. Pediatr Dev Pathol. 16(2):63-6, 2013
5. Hecht JL et al: Reference weights for placentas delivered before the 28th week of gestation. Placenta. 28(10):987-90, 2007
6. Carter AM: Placental oxygen consumption. Part I: in vivo studies–a review. Placenta. 21 Suppl A:S31-7, 2000

Placentomegaly Associated With Fetal Cardiac Anomaly

(Left) *This large (795-g), diffusely homogeneous placenta was associated a fetal cardiac anomaly. There is often an increase in the number of intervillous hematomas ➡ in these large placentas.* **(Right)** *Marked hypervascularity is frequently associated with large placentas and diabetes. Chorangiosis is diagnosed when there are 10 villi with 10 or more vessels at 10x power in 3 different areas of the placenta.*

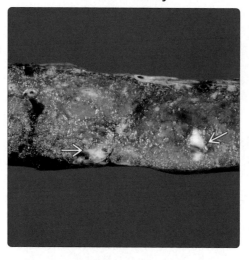

Chorangiosis With Diabetes

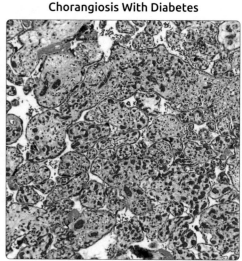

Placental Septal Cysts With Beckwith-Wiedemann Syndrome

(Left) *Placenta shows generalized pallor of the parenchyma and 2 macroscopic cysts ➡. The placenta weighed 882 g, and the neonate was diagnosed postnatally with Beckwith-Wiedemann syndrome.* **(Right)** *Beckwith-Wiedemann syndrome, infant of diabetic mother, and chronic fetal anemia due to hemolysis are all associated with increased size of pancreatic islets and nucleomegaly.*

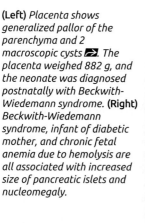
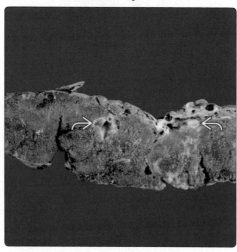

Pancreas With Enlarged Islet and Nucleomegaly

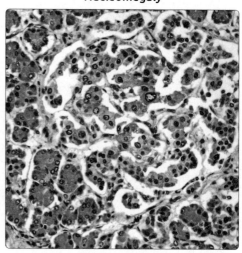

Erythroblastosis

(Left) *Increased numbers of erythroblasts ➡ may be present in cases of severe fetal anemia from any cause. Note that many of the fetal vessels are also empty, suggesting a low hematocrit.* **(Right)** *H&E shows villous edema with increased villus width and clear spaces containing "floating" Hofbauer cells ➡ in a 503-g placenta at 32 weeks from a pregnancy complicated by hydrops and polyhydramnios.*

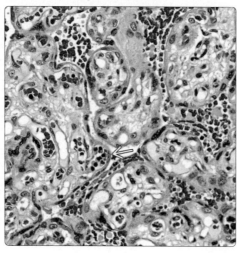

Villous Edema

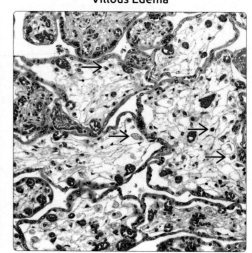

Ultrasound of Large Chorangioma

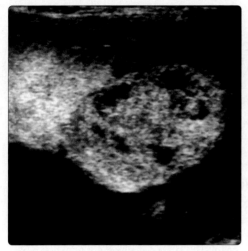

Chorangioma

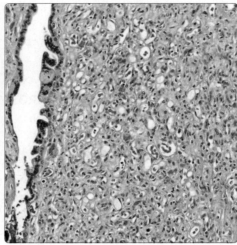

(Left) *Large chorangiomas are frequently associated with high cardiac output failure and fetal hydrops.* **(Right)** *The placental chorangioma is a capillary hemangioma covered by a trophoblastic layer. Spontaneous infarction may occur in utero with resolution of fetal hydrops. Laser ablation of the feeding vessel may be necessary.*

PMD With Thrombosed Chorionic Plate Vessel

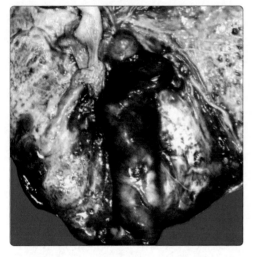

Chorionic Vessel Thrombosis

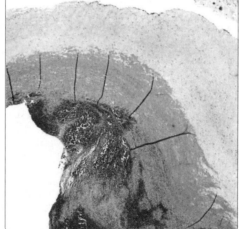

(Left) *Chorionic plate angiomatous abnormality is seen in most placentas with mesenchymal dysplasia. The aneurysmally dilated and tortuous vessels are prone to thrombosis. The placenta is generally huge, weighing over 1,000 g.* **(Right)** *Thrombosed chorionic plate vessel is shown in this case of placental mesenchymal dysplasia (PMD).*

Stem Vessels and Chorangiomatosis in PMD

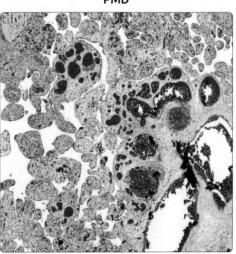

Chorangiomatosis

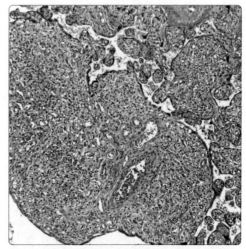

(Left) *PMD is often accompanied by chorangiomatosis, characterized by marked hypercapillarization of all stem vessels.* **(Right)** *Chorangiomatosis may be seen focally around large chorangiomas, a "field effect" of hypervascularity.*

Delayed Villous Maturation

TERMINOLOGY

- "Delayed villous maturation" now replaces terms "distal villous immaturity" and "villous maturation defect"
- Defined as areas of immature-appearing villi (at least 10 villi) demonstrating poor vasculosyncytial membrane formation, centrally placed capillaries, and continuous villous cytotrophoblast

ETIOLOGY/PATHOGENESIS

- Placental functional defect due to paucity of vasculosyncytial membranes with inefficient gas and nutrient exchange, decreased fetal tolerance for hypoxia, and other acute stress

CLINICAL ISSUES

- Commonly associated with maternal diabetes, prediabetes, obesity, excessive weight gain in pregnancy
- Less commonly associated with chronic variable umbilical cord obstruction, fetal chromosomal abnormalities
- Usually clinically silent with increased risk of perinatal mortality
- Risk of recurrent stillbirth

MACROSCOPIC

- Decreased fetoplacental weight ratio
- Placenta may be large for gestational age or pale appearing

MICROSCOPIC

- Monotonous villi with decreased vasculosyncytial membranes, centrally placed capillaries, continuous cytotrophoblast layer, and increased stromal cellularity and connective tissue

DIAGNOSTIC CHECKLIST

- Correlate villous maturation with gestational age
- Assess degree of vasculosyncytial membrane formation
- Diagnosis not recommended at < 34-weeks gestation
- Significance of focal vs. diffuse involvement not known

(Left) *This low-power image demonstrates delayed villous maturation in an 800-g placenta at 36-weeks gestation with monotonous villi with increased diameter for the gestational age and incomplete terminal villous maturation.* **(Right)** *These enlarged distal villi display a continuous trophoblast layer ⬌, increased stromal cellularity ⬌, and centrally located capillaries with poor vasculosyncytial membrane formation for the gestational age of 36 weeks.*

Delayed Villous Maturation at 36 Weeks

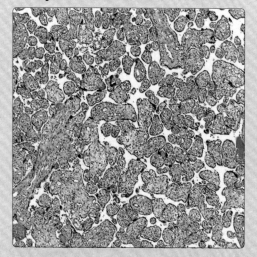

Delayed Villous Maturation at 36 Weeks

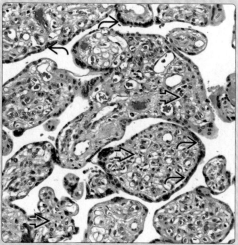

(Left) *Scanning EM studies by Kaufmann and colleagues illustrate the 3D appearance of normal villous branching. Secondary stem villi branch into a tertiary stem ⬌ and mature intermediate villi ⬌ with outpouchings of distal villi ⬌ rich in sinusoidal capillary coils.* **(Right)** *In delayed maturation, the normal tapering seen with villous arborization is less prominent, and outpouchings of terminal villi are larger and less well defined.*

3D Reconstruction of Normal Villous Branching

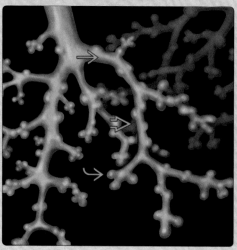

3D Structure of Delayed Maturation

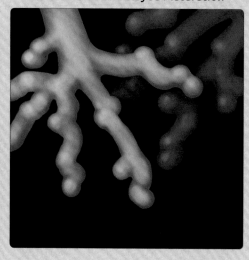

TERMINOLOGY

Abbreviations

- Delayed villous maturation (DVM)

Synonyms

- DVM, distal villous immaturity, villous maturation defect

Definitions

- Areas of immature-appearing villi comprised of at least 10 abnormal villi demonstrating poor vasculosyncytial membrane formation, centrally placed capillaries, continuous cytotrophoblast
  - At least 30% of parenchyma of at least 1 full-thickness slide should be involved

ETIOLOGY/PATHOGENESIS

Potential Etiologic Mechanisms

- Exact mechanism unclear; hypotheses include
  - Excessive growth factors or nutrients (e.g., diabetic pregnancies, maternal obesity) favoring continued growth of tertiary stem villi over maturation of distal villi
  - Alterations in fetal blood flow (stasis, decreased pressure) inducing stromal-vascular remodeling
  - Genetic abnormalities leading to abnormal villous development

Effect on Placental Function

- Paucity of vasculosyncytial membranes leads to inefficient gas and nutrient exchange, decreased fetal tolerance for hypoxia, and other acute stress

CLINICAL ISSUES

Epidemiology

- Incidence
  - Occurs in 1-6% of pregnancies

Presentation

- Commonly associated with maternal diabetes, prediabetes, obesity, excessive weight gain in pregnancy
- Less commonly associated with chronic variable umbilical cord obstruction, fetal chromosomal abnormalities
- May be clinically silent with lack of prenatal and US markers

Prognosis

- Associated with increased perinatal mortality
  - Increased risk of fetal death at > 37 weeks
    - Up to 5% risk of recurrent stillbirth
  - Mildly increased risk of early neonatal death

Fetal/Neonatal Characteristics

- Altered fetal growth; may see high or low birth weight for age
- Associated with admission to neonatal care units

MACROSCOPIC

General Features

- Decreased fetoplacental weight ratio
- Disc may be large for gestational age
- Decreased vascularization with relatively increased stroma may result in pallor
- Umbilical cord may be thick, hypercoiled

MICROSCOPIC

Histologic Features

- Distal villi show increased diameter for age, continuous cytotrophoblast and decreased syncytial knotting, variable capillary density with poor vasculosyncytial membrane formation and centrally placed vessels, and increased stromal cellularity and connective tissue

Associated Features

- Increased nucleated fetal red blood cells due to acute hypoxia
- Other villous vascular lesions, such as chorangiosis, chorangiomatosis, edema, or foci of avascular villi
- Subtle foci of vascular karyorrhexis involving some but not all capillaries in villi of DVM (fetal vascular malperfusion)

DIFFERENTIAL DIAGNOSIS

Age-Appropriate Villous Immaturity

- Requires familiarity with normal villous maturation

Chorangiosis

- Increased villous size with markedly increased capillary density
- Vasculosyncytial membranes present

DIAGNOSTIC CHECKLIST

Pathologic Interpretation Pearls

- Diagnosis not recommended at < 36-weeks gestation
- Villous abnormality present in at least 30% of 1 full-thickness section
- Assess degree of vasculosyncytial membrane formation
- Grading schema proposed in Amsterdam Placental Workshop Consensus Statement
  - Focal: Lesion present in 1 full-thickness slide only
  - Diffuse: Lesion present in 2 or more full-thickness slides

SELECTED REFERENCES

1. Lahti-Pulkkinen M et al: Placental morphology is associated with maternal depressive symptoms during pregnancy and toddler psychiatric problems. Sci Rep. 8(1):791, 2018
2. Khong TY et al: Sampling and definitions of placental lesions: Amsterdam Placental Workshop Group Consensus Statement. Arch Pathol Lab Med. 140(7):698-713, 2016
3. El-Tarhouny SA et al: Placental growth factor and soluble Fms-like tyrosine kinase 1 in diabetic pregnancy: a possible relation to distal villous immaturity. Histol Histopathol. 29(2):259-72, 2014
4. Treacy A et al: Delayed villous maturation of the placenta: quantitative assessment in different cohorts. Pediatr Dev Pathol. 16(2):63-6, 2013
5. Higgins MF et al: Clinical and ultrasound features of placental maturation in pre-gestational diabetic pregnancy. Early Hum Dev. 88(10):817-21, 2012
6. Redline RW: Distal villous immaturity. In Clarke B et al: Diagnostic histopathology. Oxford: Elsevier/Medicine Publishing. 18(5): 189-94, 2012
7. Higgins M et al: Clinical associations with a placental diagnosis of delayed villous maturation: a retrospective study. Pediatr Dev Pathol. 14(4):273-9, 2011
8. de Laat MW et al: Hypercoiling of the umbilical cord and placental maturation defect: associated pathology? Pediatr Dev Pathol. 10(4):293-9, 2007
9. Stallmach T et al: Rescue by birth: defective placental maturation and late fetal mortality. Obstet Gynecol. 97(4):505-9, 2001

TERMINOLOGY

Abbreviations

- Preeclampsia (PE)

Definitions

- Chronic hypertension (CHTN): Systolic pressure ≥ 140 mm Hg &/or diastolic ≥ 90 mm Hg
  - Present prior to pregnancy or at < 20-weeks gestation
  - Persisting beyond 6-12 weeks postpartum
- Gestational or pregnancy-induced hypertension (PIH): Systolic pressure ≥ 140 mm Hg &/or diastolic ≥ 90 mm Hg
  - New onset at ≥ 20-weeks gestation and resolves by 12-weeks postpartum
  - Absence of proteinuria or other features of PE
- PE: Systolic pressure ≥ 140 mm Hg &/or diastolic ≥ 90 mm Hg usually with proteinuria
  - New-onset hypertension at ≥ 20-weeks gestation
    - Early-onset or preterm PE (EOPE): Onset of PE < 34-weeks gestation
  - Proteinuria may or may not be present
  - PE with severe features
    - PE with signs of maternal organ dysfunction
    - Hemolysis, elevated liver enzymes, low platelets (HELLP)
  - Eclampsia defined as new-onset general seizures in setting of PE

EPIDEMIOLOGY

Incidence

- Hypertensive disorders affect up to 10% of pregnancies worldwide
  - Increased rates in industrialized countries
  - Increasing incidence of PE and EOPE
  - Increased risk among African Americans and Hispanics in USA
- PE affects 2-8% of pregnancies
  - Rare progression to HELLP syndrome and eclampsia
  - Up to 40% of women with CHTN will have superimposed PE

Mortality

- PE is leading cause of maternal mortality, worldwide

ETIOLOGY/PATHOGENESIS

Genetic Predisposition

- Combined effect of multiple gene variants/polymorphisms
  - Increased risk of PE in 1st-degree relatives
  - Increased risk of PE with some combinations of paternal HLA and maternal decidual NK-cell immunoglobulin receptor genes
  - Increased risk of PE in nonnative populations at high altitudes (e.g., individuals of European descent in Peru)

Immune Mechanisms

- Altered interaction of maternal immune cells and HLA expressed on trophoblast
  - Decreased tolerance to fetal/placental expressed paternal antigens

Pathogenesis of Maternal Morbidity

- Angiogenic factors elaborated by trophoblast
  - Healthy placenta promotes anticoagulation and vasodilation
  - Altered factors in PE procoagulant and vasoconstriction
  - Release of apoptotic debris and extracellular vesicles into maternal circulation
- Factor imbalance in PE leads to antiangiogenic state
  - Excess placental production of soluble fms-like tyrosine kinase-1 (sFLT1) and soluble endoglin (sEng)
    - SFLT1 also increased in trisomy 13, multiple gestations, molar pregnancy
    - Increased sEng leads to decreased nitric oxide production
  - sFLT1 decreases bioactive placental growth factor and vascular endothelial growth factor (VEGF)
    - VEGF inhibition leads to endothelial dysfunction
  - Elevated sFLT1 and sEng precedes clinical signs/symptoms of PE
  - Increasing sFLT1 level correlates with disease severity

Multiple Infarcts in Preeclampsia

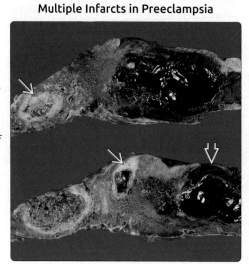

Infarction Hematoma

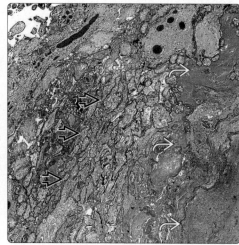

(Left) This small placenta has multiple infarcts of variable age, including infarction hematomas, as most commonly seen in preterm preeclampsia (PE). Pale, white infarcts ➡ are generally ≥ 7 days old, whereas red infarcts ➡ are more recent (2-3 days). (Right) This image from one of the older infarcts in the same case demonstrates hemorrhage ➡ in the center of the villous infarct ➡, a feature associated with an increased incidence of poor perinatal outcome.

- Resulting endothelial dysfunction and increased oxidative stress
  - Vasoconstriction with end-organ ischemia
  - Endothelial injury with increased thrombosis
  - Glomerular endotheliosis with decreased GFR, decreased renal blood flow and proteinuria

Pathogenesis of Placental Findings

- First there is abnormal placental implantation, which leads to decreased placental perfusion by 50-70%
  - Incomplete adaptation of spiral arteries, maternal decidual arteriopathy
  - While these findings are common to preterm PE, they may also be seen in preterm birth or intrauterine growth restriction without PE
- Decreased perfusion leads to placental hypoxia, which promotes release of factors that inhibit trophoblast differentiation
- Oxidative stress and damage from ischemia/reperfusion contribute to inflammation and apoptosis
  - Secondary ischemic changes such as infarcts and altered villous growth and maturation
  - Maternal inflammatory response

CLINICAL IMPLICATIONS

Clinical Presentation

- PE/eclampsia
  - May be asymptomatic at onset
  - Most cases also have proteinuria
    - Proteinuria documented on 2 random specimens 6 hours apart
    - Mild: ≥ 100 mg/dL (trace or 1 positive dipstick) urine protein levels or ≥ 300 mg protein in 24-hour collection
    - Severe: ≥ 5,000 mg protein in 24-hour collection
  - Additional symptoms
    - Edema and increased weight gain
  - Severe features
    - Severe hypertension with SBP ≥ 160 mm Hg &/or DBP ≥ 110 mm Hg
    - CNS symptoms of persistent headache or visual changes
    - Pulmonary edema
    - Platelet count < 100,000/mL
    - Renal insufficiency with creatinine > 1.1 mg/dL or doubling from baseline
    - Liver enzymes increased to ≥ 2x normal upper limit
    - Epigastric, right upper quadrant, pain
  - Increased risk of preterm labor, delivery, and abruption
  - Fetal growth restriction with severe features and EOPE
  - Symptoms typically resolve within 48 hours post partum
  - Some women develop symptoms in the postpartum period only
- HELLP syndrome
  - Variant of PE with severe features
  - Confirmed hemolysis
    - Abnormal peripheral smear (burr cells, schistocytes), bilirubin ≥ 1.2 mg/dL, LDH > 600 IU/L, decreased haptoglobin
  - Elevated liver enzymes and decreased platelet count

- Complications include
  - Eclampsia with generalized tonic-clonic seizures
    - Can occur post partum
  - Other CNS complications
    - Visual impairment from retinopathy or cortical blindness
    - Hemorrhagic stroke
    - Encephalopathy
  - Liver dysfunction and failure
  - Significant bleeding
    - Disseminated intravascular coagulation with placental abruption
    - Rupture of hepatic capsule
    - Postpartum hemorrhage
  - Adult respiratory distress syndrome, severe pulmonary edema
  - Renal dysfunction and severe acute kidney injury
  - Maternal death
    - Findings at autopsy include
      - Glomerular endotheliosis
      - Hepatic necrosis, zone 1

Diagnosis

- Based on clinical criteria as above
- Potential preclinical markers of PE
  - Decreased β-hCG and increased PAPP-A in 1st-trimester maternal serum screening
  - Impaired renal function with
    - Increased serum uric acid, creatinine, or proteinuria
  - Abnormal uterine artery Doppler velocimetry
    - Persistent early diastolic notch at > 24 weeks
  - Ongoing research for predictive biomarkers

Clinical Risk Factors

- Maternal age ≥ 40 years
- Prior PE or family history
- Obesity BMI ≥ 35
- Primiparity or long interpregnancy interval (> 10 years)
- Preexisting maternal disease
  - CHTN
  - Pregestational diabetes, especially type 1
  - Renal disease
  - Collagen vascular disease, lupus, anticardiolipin antibody
  - Thrombophilia, protein C, protein S
- In vitro fertilization
- Multiple gestations or hydatidiform mole

Prognosis

- 10% worldwide perinatal and neonatal mortality
- Adverse outcomes increased in CHTN with superimposed PE
- Fetal complications associated with
  - Growth restriction/low birth weight in severe and EOPE
    - Asymmetric with preservation of head/brain growth
  - Sequelae of prematurity
    - Necrotizing enterocolitis
    - Hypoxic brain injury
    - Chronic neonatal lung disease
    - Retinopathy of prematurity
  - Other effects of placental insufficiency
    - Oligohydramnios

- – Potential neurocognitive delay
- – Abruption
- – Fetal death
- Maternal sequelae
  - ○ Risk of recurrence in future pregnancies
    - – Increased risk with severe and EOPE (25%)
  - ○ Increased lifetime risk of disease
    - – Persistent, CHTN
    - – Ischemic heart disease
    - – Cerebrovascular disease
    - – Renal disease
    - – Metabolic disease and type 2 diabetes
    - – Thromboembolism
    - – Nonresolved neurologic disease including impaired vision

Treatment and Prevention

- Published guidelines to control blood pressure
- Expectant management to balance risks of prematurity and maternal welfare
  - ○ Weekly maternal assessments of symptoms and BP
  - ○ Antenatal steroids for preterm delivery (< 37-weeks gestation)
    - – Maximizes fetal lung maturity and may protect fetal CNS
- Prompt delivery with increasing severity
  - ○ Maternal magnesium sulfate for severe features
    - – Seizure prophylaxis
    - – Fetal neuroprotection
- Potential benefit of preventive low-dose aspirin after 12-weeks gestation and low-molecular-weight heparin

MACROSCOPIC

General Features

- Size
  - ○ Small-for-gestational-age placenta in severe and EOPE
    - – Defined as < 10th percentile
  - ○ Term PE may be within normal range or even larger than expected
  - ○ Rarely hydropic

Common Gross Findings

- Infarcts
  - ○ Extensive (> 5% of placenta) in severe and EOPE
  - ○ Large, central, and multiple of variable ages, more common in EOPE
    - – Examination after fixation may enhance chronologic dating
      - ☐ Older/remote infarcts appear pale/tan
      - ☐ Recent infarcts appear more congested/red
- Retroplacental &/or marginal hematomas (placental abruption)

Specimen Handling

- Obtain trimmed weight after removal of free membranes and cord
- Routine sectioning with attention to sampling maternal vessels
  - ○ Basal plate biopsies (superficial shallow wedge sections)
  - ○ 2 membrane rolls, include placental margin
- Describe gross lesions

- ○ Location, quantity, and appearance
- ○ Size, include 2 maximal dimensions per lesion
- ○ Estimate percentage of total parenchyma affected
- Submit additional sections to characterize lesions at interface with nonlesional parenchyma

MICROSCOPIC

Changes Associated With Early-Onset or Preterm Preeclampsia

- Decidual arteriopathy
  - ○ Persistence (in basalis) or mural hypertrophy of smooth muscle, fibrinoid necrosis, foamy macrophages, thrombosis, perivascular lymphoid infiltrates
- Distal villous hypoplasia and accelerated villous maturation
- Increased syncytial knots for age (Tenney-Parker change)
- Villous agglutination and infarcts
- Increased perivillous fibrin

Other Changes Associated With Preeclampsia

- Uneven villous maturation
- Increased number and proliferation of basal extravillous cytotrophoblasts
- Increased multinucleate trophoblast cells in decidua basalis
- Proliferation and prominence of villous cytotrophoblasts
- Thickened trophoblast basement membrane (highlighted by PAS stain)
- > 3% of villi with fibrinoid necrosis
- Increased frequency of findings attributable to fetal vascular malperfusion

Term Placenta With Preeclampsia

- May be completely normal
- Mild findings of accelerated villous maturation
- May see hypertrophic decidual arteriopathy in membrane rolls

SELECTED REFERENCES

1. Aouache R et al: Oxidative stress in preeclampsia and placental diseases. Int J Mol Sci. 19(5), 2018
2. Chisholm KM et al: Classification of preterm birth with placental correlates. Pediatr Dev Pathol. 1093526618775958, 2018
3. Sutton ALM et al: Hypertensive disorders in pregnancy. Obstet Gynecol Clin North Am. 45(2):333-347, 2018
4. Giannakou K et al: Genetic and non-genetic risk factors for pre-eclampsia: umbrella review of systematic reviews and meta-analyses of observational studies. Ultrasound Obstet Gynecol. ePub, 2017
5. Khong TY et al: Sampling and definitions of placental lesions: amsterdam placental workshop group consensus statement. Arch Pathol Lab Med. 140(7):698-713, 2016
6. Hod T et al: Molecular mechanisms of preeclampsia. Cold Spring Harb Perspect Med. 5(10), 2015
7. Stark MW et al: Histologic differences in placentas of preeclamptic/eclamptic gestations by birthweight, placental weight, and time of onset. Pediatr Dev Pathol. 17(3):181-9, 2014
8. Rana S et al: Angiogenic factors in diagnosis, management, and research in preeclampsia. Hypertension. 63(2):198-202, 2014
9. Lo JO et al: Hypertensive disease of pregnancy and maternal mortality. Curr Opin Obstet Gynecol. 25(2):124-32, 2013
10. Redline RW et al: Maternal vascular underperfusion: nosology and reproducibility of placental reaction patterns. Pediatr Dev Pathol. 7(3):237-49, 2004

Acute Infarct

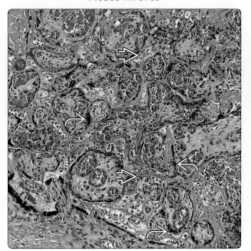

Remote Infarct

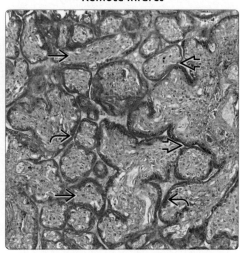

(Left) *This very acute infarct shows apoptotic inflammatory debris ⊟ in the partially collapsed maternal intervillous space and smudged, pyknotic syncytiotrophoblast nuclei ⊟.* **(Right)** *The intervillous space is collapsed in remote infarcts resulting in villi abutting adjacent villi ⊟. The villous trophoblast lining is nonviable with loss of cellular features ⊟. The villous stroma ⊟ becomes progressively avascular and fibrotic.*

Vascular Fibrinoid Necrosis and Atheroma

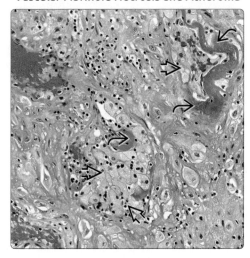

Atheroma in Decidua Parietalis

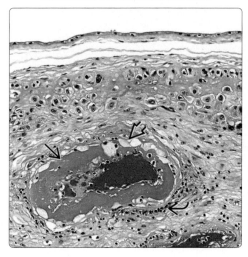

(Left) *Maternal spiral arteries demonstrate fibrinoid necrosis of the vessel walls ⊟ and marked accumulation of foamy macrophages ⊟ or atheroma formation. There is also a mild increase in lymphocytes in the decidua.* **(Right)** *A section from the free membranes shows acute atheroma within a maternal vessel of the decidua parietalis. There is fibrinoid necrosis ⊟, a cuff of surrounding lymphocytes ⊟, and there are foamy macrophages ⊟.*

Incomplete Maternal Vascular Adaptation

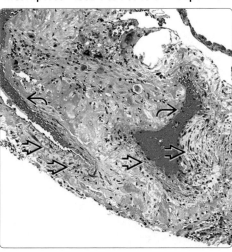

Fibrinoid Necrosis and Thrombosis

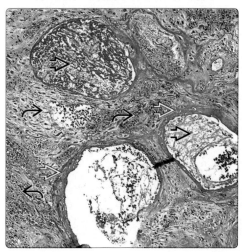

(Left) *These maternal spiral arteries ⊟ are incompletely adapted for pregnancy w/ persistent mural smooth muscle ⊟ in a 250-g placenta at 36 weeks w/ multiple infarcts. PE complicated pregnancy in a woman w/ history of deep venous thrombosis.* **(Right)** *Recent thrombosis ⊟ complicates fibrinoid necrosis ⊟ of maternal spiral artery in a 290-g placenta at 35 weeks from pregnancy w/ PE. The adjacent decidua is necrotic ⊟. Thrombi may be associated with antiphospholipid solids.*

Decidual Arteriopathy

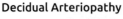

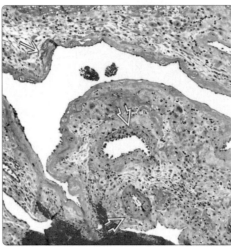

Vascular Mural Hypertrophy Decidua Parietalis

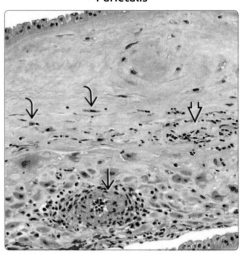

(Left) *Multiple spiral arteries are present in this section. One shows appropriate adaptation ➡ while the others have residual smooth muscle ➡ with increased chronic inflammation.* **(Right)** *A section of the free membranes shows a maternal vessel ➡ with mural hypertrophy; the vessel is also surrounded by a cuff of lymphocytes. Lymphocytes ➡ are also present in the adjacent chorion, as well as pigmented macrophages ➡.*

Chronic Deciduitis in Preeclampsia

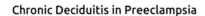

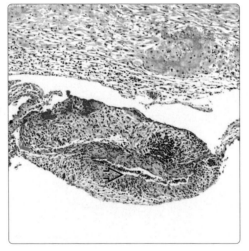

Accelerated Villous Maturation

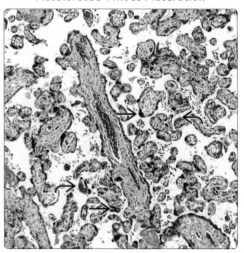

(Left) *Chronic inflammation is frequently increased in the placenta with PE. This placenta shows marked lymphocytic perivasculitis of a maternal spiral artery ➡ at the basal plate.* **(Right)** *This preeclamptic placenta shows accelerated villous maturation for 28-weeks gestation with predominance of small distal villi with vasculosyncytial membranes ➡ and prominent syncytial knots ➡.*

Distal Villous Hypoplasia

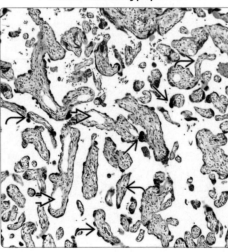

Villous Agglutination

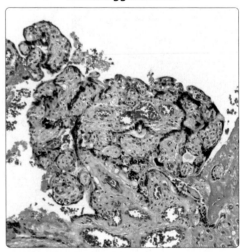

(Left) *Distal villous hypoplasia, an extreme form of accelerated maturation, is characterized by linear villous profiles ➡, paucity of distal villi, and prominent syncytial knots ➡. Markedly dilated stem vessels ➡ are associated with abnormal umbilical artery Doppler flow.* **(Right)** *Villous agglutination refers to isolated groups of villi that appear stuck together; it is frequently seen in placentas with other features of maternal malperfusion.*

Preeclampsia and Related Hypertensive Disorders

Exaggerated Syncytial Knots

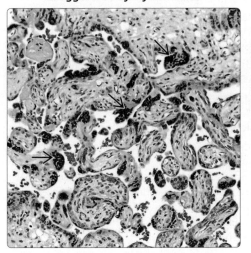

Villous Fibrinoid Necrosis

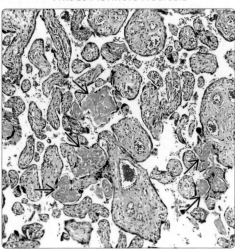

(Left) *Exaggerated syncytial knots, or Tenney-Parker change, is characterized by enlarged knots* ⊟ *containing many syncytiotrophoblast nuclei with condensed nuclear chromatin. This change may be seen in preterm PE and adjacent to infarcts.* (Right) *PE is associated with an increased number of villi with fibrinoid necrosis* ⊟. *The villi are completely or partially replaced by fibrinoid material and maintain an outer covering of syncytiotrophoblast.*

Trophoblast in Superficial Implantation

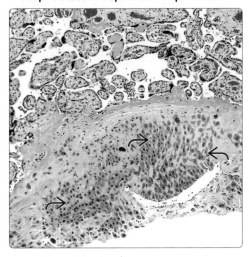

Multinucleated Invasive Trophoblast

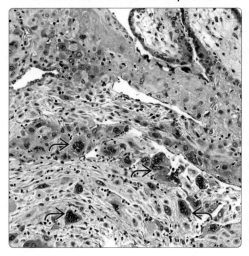

(Left) *PE has been attributed to a failure of trophoblast cells to effectively invade uterine tissues and facilitate vascular remodeling, termed "superficial implantation." This is supported by increased number of invasive trophoblasts* ⊟ *remaining at the basal plate later in gestation.* (Right) *Fusion of invasive trophoblast to form multinucleate cells* ⊟ *generally occurs at the end of trophoblast migration. Frequent multinucleate trophoblasts in the basal decidua also suggests abnormal implantation.*

Large Retroplacental Hematoma Abruption

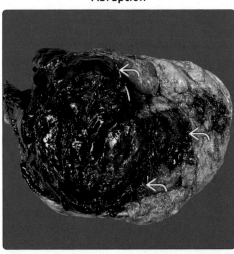

Villous Stromal Hemorrhage

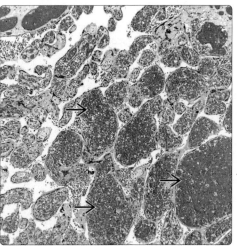

(Left) *PE increases the risk of placental abruption. An acute retroplacental hematoma* ⊿ *occupies at least 50% of the maternal surface, a feature associated with increased risk of fetal mortality.* (Right) *Acute abruption with retroplacental hematoma causes loss of blood flow to the intervillous space. A living fetus can become hyperdynamic and intravillous stromal hemorrhage* ⊟ *occurs due to rupture of the villous capillaries.*

TERMINOLOGY

Definitions

- Macroscopic diagnosis based on comparison of placental weight to normative values for given gestational age
  - Variably defined by weight below 10th, 5th, or 3rd percentile
  - Significant pathology more likely in weights below 5th or 3rd percentile

Synonyms

- Placental undergrowth
- Underweight placenta
- Placental growth restriction
- Placental hypoplasia
- Placental insufficiency

ETIOLOGY/PATHOGENESIS

Generalized Growth Impairment With Normal Villous Morphology

- Constitutional small size due to ethnic/genetic variation
- Secondary to maternal disease
- Confined placental mosaicism
  - Discrepant karyotypic or molecular genetic abnormality (e.g., loss of heterozygosity) present in placenta, absent in fetus
  - Occurs in 1-2% of pregnancies
  - Subcategorized as types 1, 2, or 3
    - Type 1 mosaicism confined to trophoblast
    - Type 2 mosaicism confined to villous stroma
    - Type 3 mosaicism involves trophoblast and stromal cells
  - Type 3 most associated with placental growth impairment

Placental Growth Impairment With Villous Maldevelopment

- Fetal and placental aneuploidy with dysmorphic villi
- Early-onset maternal malperfusion with distal villous hypoplasia

Secondary Pathology Associated With Loss of Functional Parenchyma

- Chronic maternal malperfusion with villous infarcts &/or villous sclerosis
- Chronic obstructed fetoplacental perfusion
- Parenchymal inflammation, infectious &/or idiopathic
- Extensive intervillous fibrinoid deposition

CLINICAL IMPLICATIONS

Clinical Risk Factors

- Maternal disease associated with fetal growth restriction and small placenta
  - Hypertensive disorders, including preeclampsia
    - Most common cause of small placenta and fetal growth restriction
  - Autoimmune disorders
  - Thrombophilic disorders
  - Severe malnutrition, poor weight gain during pregnancy
  - Tobacco use during pregnancy
    - Placental weight:birth weight ratio relatively increased
- Prior pregnancy affected by condition with known risk of recurrence
  - Early onset &/or preeclampsia with severe features
  - Massive perivillous fibrin deposition/maternal floor infarct
  - High-grade chronic villitis/villitis of unknown etiology
  - Chronic histiocytic intervillositis

Clinical Presentation

- Correlates with low fetal weight/fetal growth restriction
  - Risk of preterm birth with associated increased morbidity
    - Necrotizing enterocolitis
    - Hypoxic brain injury
    - Chronic neonatal lung disease
    - Retinopathy of prematurity
  - Increased long-term morbidity for neonate
    - Obesity, diabetes, ischemic heart disease
  - Associated features of congenital infections

Placental Size Differences at 37-Weeks Gestation

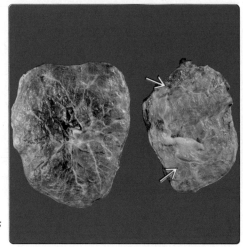

(Left) Assessment of placental size is relative to gestational age. These placentas from 37 weeks are visibly discordant in size with the placenta on the right being small for gestational age. Notably, the smaller placenta also shows a magistral pattern of fetal chorionic vessels ➡. (Right) A markedly small placenta weighed only 174 g at 36 weeks with a maximal diameter of 13 cm and was composed of dysmorphic villi; the pregnancy was complicated by fetal holoprosencephaly. The cord is also thin and hypercoiled.

Small-for-Gestational-Age Placenta

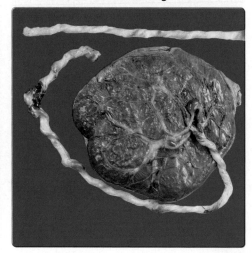

- – Cytomegalovirus (CMV) most common
  - o Oligohydramnios
- Fetal indications for preterm delivery
  - o ↑ fetal morbidity and mortality with abnormal Doppler velocimetry
- Fetal intolerance to labor
- Intrauterine fetal demise or stillbirth
  - o Increased risk independent of fetal birth weight

MACROSCOPIC

General Features

- Size
  - o Trimmed disc weight < 10th, 5th, or 3rd percentile
    - – Fetoplacental ratio may be maintained with low placental weight and low birth weight
  - o Decreased maximum disc diameter
    - – Variable depending on gestational age
  - o Decreased disc thickness
    - – 1.5-2.5 cm expected at viable gestational age
  - o Decreased placental volume

Specimen Handling

- Standard exam, including trimmed weight of disc following removal of umbilical cord and extraplacental membranes
  - o Weight should be obtained in fresh state, as fixation may increase weight as much as 10%
- Routine sections to include lesions plus samples of maternal vessels
  - o Basal plate biopsies (wedge sections or en face of maternal surface)
  - o 2 membrane rolls for identification of maternal decidual vasculopathy
- Tissue for cytogenomic analysis
  - o Consider in cases of severe growth restriction otherwise unexplained or discrepant prenatal testing
    - – Fresh tissue for conventional karyotype
    - – Frozen or formalin-fixed, paraffin-embedded tissue acceptable for FISH or CGH
    - – ≥ 3 distinct samples to assess for site- or tissue-specific mosaicism
- Consider photographic documentation of unusual anatomic features and macroscopic lesions

Anatomic Features

- Pale, firm parenchyma due to extensive inflammation or fibrin deposition
- Macroscopic lesions associated with maternal malperfusion
  - o Villous infarcts
  - o Abruption/retroplacental hematoma
- Variably associated umbilical cord features
  - o Velamentous insertion
  - o Short cord length, < 32 cm at term
  - o Hypercoiled, coiling index > 0.3 coils/cm
  - o Single umbilical artery

MICROSCOPIC

Villous Maldevelopment

- Distal villous hypoplasia
  - o Sparse, small distal villi
  - o Decreased capillaries per villous section

- o Frequent thin, elongated villous profiles
- o ↓ distal villi:tertiary stem villi ratio
- Dysmorphic features
  - o Irregular villous contours with poor branching
  - o Stromal trophoblast inclusions and stromal karyomegaly
  - o Abnormal villous capillary patterns
  - o Focal trophoblast hyperplasia

Lesions With Decreased Functional Reserve

- Features associated with maternal malperfusion
  - o Increased syncytial knots
  - o Villous agglutination
  - o Increased perivillous fibrin deposition
  - o Villous infarction
  - o Decidual arteriopathy
    - – Acute atherosis and fibrinoid necrosis
    - – Mural hypertrophy in decidua parietalis
    - – Incomplete remodeling with persistent smooth muscle
- Patterns of inflammation
  - o Chronic villitis of unknown etiology, lymphohistiocytic infiltrate
    - – High-grade lesions with foci of > 10 affected villi
    - – May have associated loss of fetal capillaries
    - – Associated basal villitis chronic villitis/intervillositis, chronic deciduitis, and chronic chorioamnionitis
  - o Chronic lymphoplasmacytic villitis
    - – Associated with stromal fibrosis, calcifications, and hemosiderin
    - – Consider CMV with ancillary viral testing, as CMV inclusions are rare
  - o Active chronic villitis with polymorphous infiltrate and villous necrosis
    - – Herpes simplex virus and varicella-zoster virus inclusions may be rare
  - o Chronic histiocyte intervillositis
    - – May be associated with perivillous fibrin deposition
- Extensive avascular villi with fetal vascular malperfusion
- Massive perivillous fibrin deposition in intervillous space

SELECTED REFERENCES

1. Levy M et al: Can placental histopathology lesions predict recurrence of small for gestational age neonates? Reprod Sci. 1933719117749757, 2018
2. Hirashima C et al: Independent risk factors for a small placenta and a small-for-gestational-age infant at 35-41 weeks of gestation: an association with circulating angiogenesis-related factor levels at 19-31 weeks of gestation. J Obstet Gynaecol Res. 43(8):1285-1292, 2017
3. McNamara H et al: Risk factors for high and low placental weight. Paediatr Perinat Epidemiol. 28(2):97-105, 2014
4. Hutcheon JA et al: Placental weight for gestational age and adverse perinatal outcomes. Obstet Gynecol. 119(6):1251-8, 2012
5. Toutain J et al: Confined placental mosaicism and pregnancy outcome: a distinction needs to be made between types 2 and 3. Prenat Diagn. 30(12-13):1155-64, 2010
6. Cox P et al: Pathological assessment of intrauterine growth restriction. Best Pract Res Clin Obstet Gynaecol. 23(6):751-64, 2009
7. Yong PJ et al: Placental weight in pregnancies with trisomy confined to the placenta. J Obstet Gynaecol Can. 31(7):605-10, 2009
8. Hecht JL et al: Reference weights for placentas delivered before the 28th week of gestation. Placenta. 28(10):987-90, 2007
9. Kalousek DK et al: Confined placental mosaicism. J Med Genet. 33(7):529-33, 1996
10. Pinar H et al: Reference values for singleton and twin placental weights. Pediatr Pathol Lab Med. 16(6):901-7, 1996

(Left) *This placenta weighed 123 g at 31-weeks gestation and demonstrates multiple lesions, including perivillous fibrin deposition ⮑ and extensive avascular villi ⮑. The pregnancy was complicated by maternal Sjögren syndrome and complete fetal heart block.* **(Right)** *Perivillous fibrin deposition consists of amorphous eosinophilic material ⮑ filling the intervillous space, which results in entrapped, nonfunctional villi ⮑. Gross exam may have a nodular or diffuse pattern.*

Maternal Autoimmune Disease

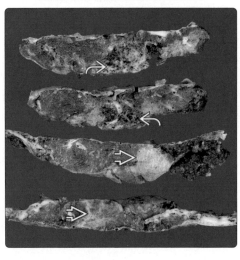

Perivillous Fibrin Deposition

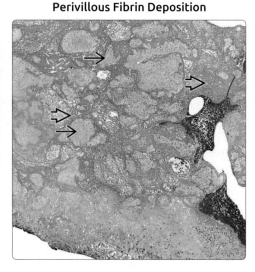

(Left) *H&E demonstrates extensive avascular villi with complete loss of fetal capillaries ⮑ and obliteration of stem villous vessels ⮑. This was related to poor fetal blood flow in the setting of congenital heart block.* **(Right)** *High-grade lymphocytic villitis, with confluent focus of inflamed villi, was identified in this placenta that weighed just 252 g at 38-weeks gestation. This H&E also shows loss of villous capillaries, collapse of the intervillous space with villous agglutination, and trophoblast injury ⮑.*

Avascular Villi Due to Fetal Vascular Malperfusion

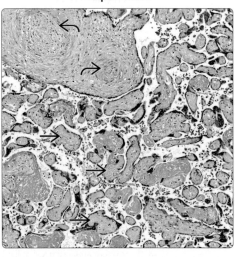

High-Grade Chronic Villitis

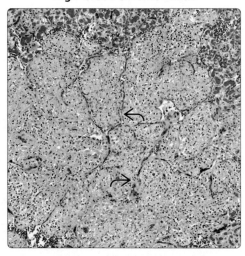

(Left) *The presence of plasma cells ⮑ in cases of villitis should increase clinical suspicion for an infectious etiology, as seen in this case of confirmed congenital cytomegalovirus infection. Inclusions are usually very rare.* **(Right)** *In cases of chronic histiocytic intervillositis, the inflammatory infiltrate involves the intervillous space ⮑ with sparing of the villi ⮑. The infiltrate is predominantly composed of maternal monocytes. This lesion can recur in subsequent pregnancies.*

Lymphoplasmacytic Villitis

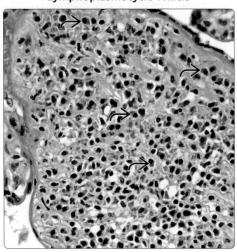

Chronic Histiocytic Intervillositis

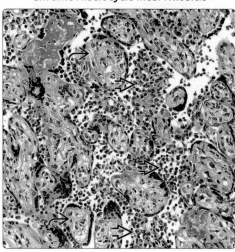

Infarcts With Maternal Vascular Malperfusion

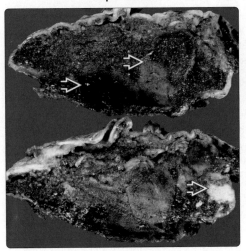

Villous Infarct

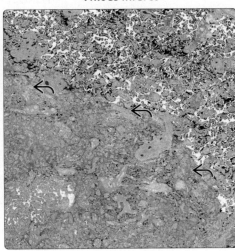

(Left) Multiple infarcts of variable age ⊳ are demonstrated in this 104-g placenta from a pregnancy complicated by maternal hypertension, resulting in stillbirth at 23-weeks gestation. (Right) H&E demonstrates the microscopic appearance of a villous infarction ↪ with collapse of the intervillous space and loss of functional parenchyma. The center of the infarct shows minimal residual nuclear basophilia.

Villous Agglutination

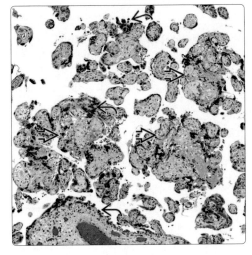

Distal Villous Hypoplasia

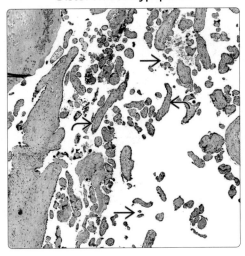

(Left) H&E demonstrates microscopic features of chronic maternal malperfusion, including villous agglutination ⇉ and prominent syncytial knots ↗. The affected villi are nearly avascular. (Right) Distal villous hypoplasia is characterized by sparse, small, thin distal villi ↪ with elongated villous profiles ↗. This altered villous growth pattern occurs in the setting of early-onset maternal vascular malperfusion.

Dysmorphic Villi

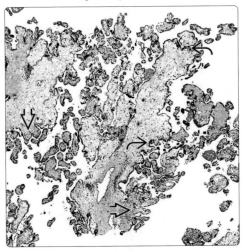

Dysmorphic Villi

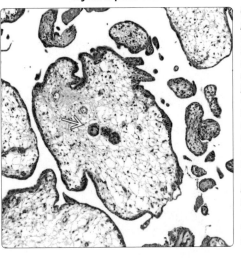

(Left) Small placenta from a pregnancy with multiple fetal anomalies, including holoprosencephaly, demonstrates dysmorphic villi, characterized by dual villous populations, irregular villous contours ↗, loose mesenchymal stroma, poor vascularity, and minimal branching ↗. (Right) Dual villous populations show large hydropic and small fibrous villi. Trophoblast pseudoinclusions ⇉ are consistent with irregularity of villous shape. These features are often seen with chromosomal or malformation syndromes.

TERMINOLOGY

- Distal villous hypoplasia (DVH): Decrease in number and diameter of distal villi in relation to surrounding stem villi
  - Villi appear more mature than expected for gestational age
- Focal DVH: Involves at least 30% of parenchyma on 1 slide
- Diffuse DVH: Involves at least 30% of parenchyma on > 1 slide

CLINICAL ISSUES

- Seen in fetal growth restriction, ± preeclampsia
- When combined with fibrinoid necrosis of individual villi, strongly associated with absent end-diastolic flow in umbilical arteries on Doppler studies

MACROSCOPIC

- No specific gross features of DVH, placenta usually small for age

MICROSCOPIC

- Small, widely spaced, elongate, thin villi with increased syncytial knots
- Increased empty maternal intervillous space
- Few capillaries per villous cross section

TOP DIFFERENTIAL DIAGNOSES

- Small distal villi normally present beneath chorionic plate, in placental periphery, and adjacent to infarcts
  - DVH diagnosis requires 30% of appropriately sampled parenchyma to be affected (not exclusively subchorionic or peripheral)

DIAGNOSTIC CHECKLIST

- Villi appear "too mature" for gestational age
- Even in term placenta, villi are too small for normal development
- Placenta and fetal growth are small for age

Small Villi of DVH in Cross Section

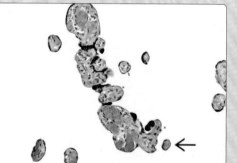

Elongated Thin Villi of DVH

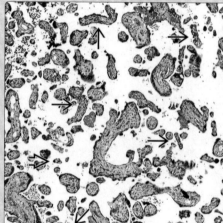

(Left) In distal villous hypoplasia (DVH), villi are sparsely distributed and very small, often accommodating only a single capillary ➡. There may also be a paucity of intermediate villi between the stem and terminal villi. (Right) At low-power magnification, the elongate, thin villous profiles ➡ are striking, as well as the increased white space dotted by minute terminal villi ➡ and syncytial knots. Diffuse DVH involves > 30% of parenchyma on more than 1 slide.

DVH in 2nd Trimester

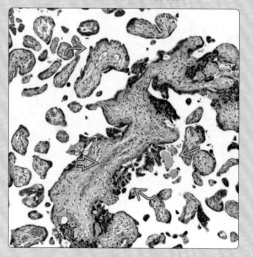

Absent End-Diastolic Flow on Umbilical Artery Doppler Studies

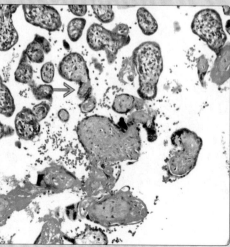

(Left) This 19-weeks-gestation placenta shows occlusion of a stem vessel ➡ imposed upon evolving DVH. Intense villous sprouting ➡ is present with wave-like syncytial knots. Fibrinoid necrosis of individual villi ➡ is also seen. (Right) Normally there is continued forward flow through the umbilical arteries during diastole. DVH and fibrinoid necrosis ➡ results in less vascular distribution to accept fetal blood resulting in absent or reversed end-diastolic umbilical artery flow.

TERMINOLOGY

Abbreviations

- Distal villous hypoplasia (DVH)

Synonyms

- Deficiency of intermediate villi, peripheral villous hypoplasia, villous hypermaturity, accelerated maturation

Definitions

- Paucity of distal villi in relation to surrounding stem villi
  - Distal villi of DVH are thin, elongated, with increased syncytial knots
  - Features must be seen in lower 2/3 of thickness of parenchyma and involve at least 30% of 1 full-thickness parenchymal slide
- May be focal (limited to 1 slide) or diffuse (> 1 slide)

ETIOLOGY/PATHOGENESIS

Abnormal Villous Development

- Predominance of nonbranching angiogenesis over branching angiogenesis
  - Yields long, slender profiles with few capillaries per cross section
- Associated with maternal vascular malperfusion
  - Most commonly seen in severe fetal growth restriction, ± preterm preeclampsia
  - Intervillous oxygen pressures are high
    - Proposed that DVH yields sparse villous mass less able to extract maternal blood oxygen compared to normally developed villi; DVH causing intervillous hyperoxia
    - Termed postplacental hypoxia instead of uteroplacental hypoxia because of decreased villous uptake of oxygen
  - Placental hyperoxia hypothesis suggests high maternal oxygen pressures disrupt VEGF-mediated regulation of villous angiogenesis
    - Proposes that hyperoxia is cause rather than result of DVH
  - May be early adaptation to maternal malperfusion (underperfusion, higher pressure and inconstant perfusion)
    - Villi maximize potential for oxygen exchange prematurely with formation of vasculosyncytial membranes
    - Adaptation is at cost of further branching angiogenesis and number of villi

CLINICAL ISSUES

Epidemiology

- Strongly associated with severe intrauterine growth restriction (IUGR)
  - This clinical setting constitutes 10% of high-risk pregnancies
  - Severe cases of diffuse DVH with fibrinoid necrosis of villi associated with absent end diastolic umbilical artery flow on Doppler studies
- DVH found in 36% of early preterm placentas, usually indicates preterm birth for IUGR or preeclampsia with severe features

- Increased incidence with maternal smoking

Prognosis

- High fetal and neonatal morbidity and mortality
- Associated with pulmonary hypertension and bronchopulmonary dysplasia in neonate

MACROSCOPIC

General Features

- Diffuse DVH almost always in small-for-gestational-age placenta
- Thin umbilical cord
- Often 1 or more infarcts

MICROSCOPIC

Histologic Features

- Small, widely spaced distal villi with few capillaries per villus cross section
- Frequent elongated, thin villous profiles
- Stem villi appear relatively close together compared to normal parenchyma
- Often accompanied by small, regular projections of syncytium from surface (wave-like syncytial knots, or serrated appearance)

DIFFERENTIAL DIAGNOSIS

Physiologic Small Distal Villi

- Terminal villous distribution varies nonuniformly
- DVH is normally present beneath chorionic plate and at placental periphery
- For DVH diagnosis, 30% of appropriately sampled parenchyma must be affected, not just subchorionic or peripheral villi

Small Distal Villi Adjacent to Infarcts

- May reflect same pathophysiology of maternal vascular malperfusion

DIAGNOSTIC CHECKLIST

Pathologic Interpretation Pearls

- Familiarity with this finding normally found beneath chorionic plate facilitates recognition elsewhere
- Villi appear too mature for gestational age
- Even in term placenta, villi are too small

SELECTED REFERENCES

1. Khong TY et al: Sampling and definitions of placental lesions: Amsterdam Placental Workshop Group consensus statement. Arch Pathol Lab Med. 140(7):698-713, 2016
2. Mukherjee A et al: The placental distal villous hypoplasia pattern: interobserver agreement and automated fractal dimension as an objective metric. Pediatr Dev Pathol. 19(1):31-6, 2016
3. Mestan KK et al: Placental pathologic changes of maternal vascular underperfusion in bronchopulmonary dysplasia and pulmonary hypertension. Placenta. 35(8):570-4, 2014
4. Spinillo A et al: Placental histopathological correlates of umbilical artery Doppler velocimetry in pregnancies complicated by fetal growth restriction. Prenat Diagn. 32(13):1263-72, 2012

DVH

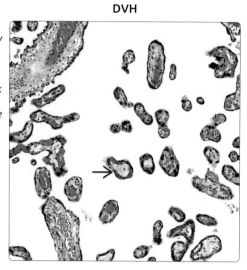

Normal Intermediate Villi

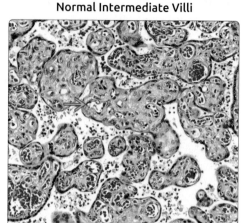

(Left) *Branching angiogenesis is reduced in DVH, yielding few capillaries per villous cross section. Note the fully developed vasculosyncytial membranes* ⊟ *in this 24-week gestation placenta, a markedly hypermature feature for this age.* (Right) *In comparison, normal villi at 24 weeks are larger, with numerous central capillary profiles not approaching the syncytiotrophoblast layer* ⊟. *Branching and nonbranching angiogenesis continue together in normal development.*

DVH Stem Villi

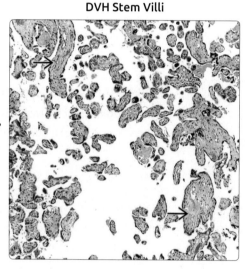

Normal Immature Intermediate Villi

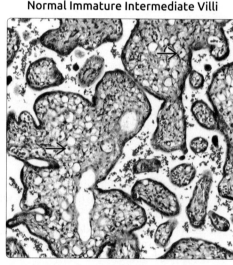

(Left) *Larger villi of DVH have more collagenous tissue in their cores* ⊟ *compared to those normally seen at this gestational age (30 weeks). Absent are the numerous immature intermediate villi normally present at this age.* (Right) *Immature intermediate villi are abundant in normal late 2nd-/early 3rd-trimester placentas. They have abundant reticular stroma, containing Hofbauer cells* ⊟ *in rounded spaces. They are normally present in the center of mature lobules but absent in areas of DVH.*

Wave-Like Syncytial Knots

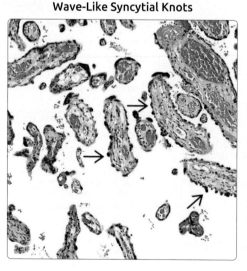

Normal Syncytiotrophoblast in Immature Placenta

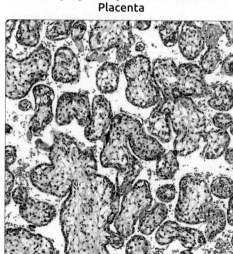

(Left) *Other features often seen with DVH are regular polypoid projections of syncytial knots from the villous surface* ⊟. *Their appearance on electron microscopy led to the term wave-like because of their continuity across the surface.* (Right) *In this 29-weeks-gestation placenta, there is almost no syncytial knotting. The amount of knotting increases with gestational age. Wave-like syncytial knots suggest abortive attempts at villogenesis with extensive sprouting.*

Distal Villous Hypoplasia

3D Structure of Villous Tree in DVH

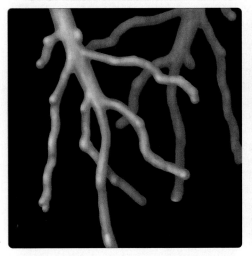

Normal 3D Villous Branching

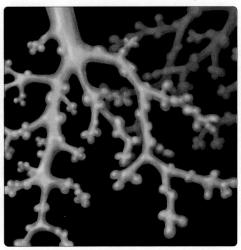

(Left) *Scanning EM of villi in DVH suggests branching stops at the level of intermediate villi. The histology resembles terminal villi (small profiles, high capillary:villus area ratio, and vasculosyncytial membranes), but capillaries are less coiled, yielding many forms with only a pair of capillaries.* (Right) *Normal placental development includes a balance of branching and nonbranching angiogenesis. Intermediate villi connect stem villi to multiple series of terminal villi.*

Physiologic DVH-Like Histology

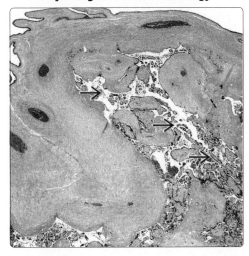

Physiologic DVH-Like Histology

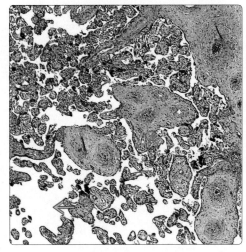

(Left) *Villi beneath the chorionic plate commonly show features of DVH ➡. This subchorionic region has the most sluggish and inconsistent maternal perfusion. Blood must travel from the basal plate to the subchorionic space, where it will have progressively less oxygen.* (Right) *A focal region of the mature placenta, often at the periphery of a lobule, can also resemble DVH ➡. DVH should involve 30% of the parenchyma for diagnosis. This avoids overcalling the feature in the normal variation of villous morphology.*

DVH Histology Adjacent to Infarct

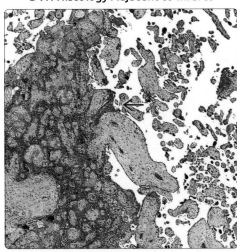

Decidual Arteriopathy

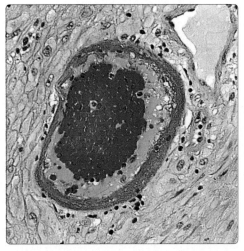

(Left) *Villi adjacent to infarcts ➡ often show DVH. This likely represents the common pathophysiology of poor maternal perfusion and also the location of the villi at the periphery of a lobule.* (Right) *DVH often accompanie decidual arteriopathy in the preterm placenta from preeclamptic mothers. The failure of the maternal vasculature to appropriately remodel early in pregnancy underlies the chronic malperfusion of the placenta, giving rise to DVH.*

Decidual Arteriopathy

TERMINOLOGY

- Decidual arteriopathy (replaces previous terminology of "maternal decidual vasculopathy")

ETIOLOGY/PATHOGENESIS

- Results from failure of normal vascular remodeling for pregnancy

CLINICAL ISSUES

- Incidence
  - Occurs in < 1% of uncomplicated pregnancies
  - More frequent in pregnancies associated with fetal growth restriction ± preeclampsia

MICROSCOPIC

- Subtypes of decidual arteriopathy diagnosed in membranous decidua or basal plate/decidua basalis
  - Mural hypertrophy: Arterial/arteriolar wall thickness > 1/3 of vessel diameter (membranous decidua or decidua basalis)
  - Fibrinoid necrosis: Muscular wall is replaced by fibrin, ± foam cells (membranous decidua or decidua basalis)
  - Acute atherosis: Fibrinoid necrosis of vessel wall with numerous subendothelial and intramural foamy macrophages (membranous decidua or decidua basalis)
- Subtypes of decidual arteriopathy diagnosed in basal plate/decidua basalis only
  - Absence of spiral artery remodeling: Failure of normal physiologic conversion of basal spiral arteries during pregnancy (basal plate/decidua basalis)
    - Only assess in central 2/3 of disc where remodeling occurs most consistently
    - Small basilar branches of the spiral arteries, do not adapt for pregnancy
  - Persistence of endovascular trophoblast in 3rd trimester
- Decidual arteriopathy associated with small placentas, infarcts, distal villous hypoplasia

Normal Maternal Vessels in Membranous Decidua

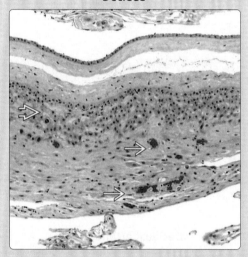

(Left) These small maternal arteries ⇨ do not become invaded by intermediate trophoblasts ⇉ but do become thinner during pregnancy as a result of hormonal changes. (Right) In contrast, vessels with mural hypertrophy ⇨ have thick walls (> 30% of diameter). This feature may be seen in the membranous decidua or in the decidua basalis.

Mural Hypertrophy

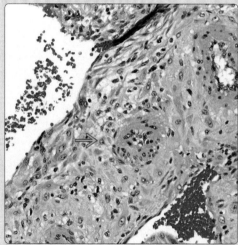

Mural Hypertrophy Progressing to Fibrinoid Necrosis

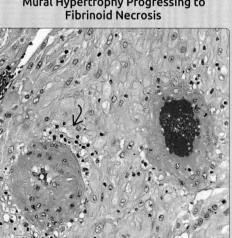

(Left) The endothelium and vascular smooth muscle cells of these vessels are degenerating as mural hypertrophy progresses to fibrinoid necrosis. Note the cuff of perivascular lymphoid cells ⇗, a common feature with decidual arteriopathy. (Right) In acute atherosis, the media is replaced by thick, glassy fibrin with numerous mural foamy histiocytes (foam cells).

Acute Atherosis

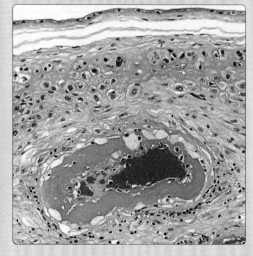

TERMINOLOGY

Abbreviations

- Decidual arteriopathy (DA)

Synonyms

- Maternal decidual vasculopathy (previous terminology)

Definitions

- Subtypes of DA diagnosed in membranous decidua or basal plate/decidua basalis
  - Mural hypertrophy: Arterial/arteriolar wall thickness > 1/3 of vessel diameter (membranous decidua or decidua basalis)
  - Fibrinoid necrosis: Muscular wall is replaced by fibrin, ± foam cells (membranous decidua or decidua basalis)
  - Acute atherosis: Fibrinoid necrosis of vessel wall with numerous subendothelial and intramural foamy macrophages (membranous decidua or decidua basalis)
  - Arterial thrombosis: Usually seen in decidua basalis with fibrinoid necrosis
- Subtypes of DA diagnosed in basal plate/decidua basalis only
  - Absence of spiral artery (SA) remodeling: Failure of normal physiologic conversion of basal SA during pregnancy (central 2/3 of placental disc)
  - Persistence of endovascular trophoblast in 3rd trimester

ETIOLOGY/PATHOGENESIS

Decidual Arteriopathy

- Cause unclear
  - Failure to remodel may be due to dysfunctional early uterine NK-cell/trophoblast interactions at implantation site
  - Evolution of fibrinoid necrosis may be due to ischemia, endothelial damage from circulating factors such as s-Flt1 and sEng, aberrant Th1 responses, or susceptibility of unremodeled muscular vessels to effects of late pregnancy
- Perivascular lymphocytes (chronic perivasculitis) may accompany any of these changes

Absence of SA Remodeling

- Trophoblast cells normally remodel preplacental SA in decidua basalis and underlying myometrium
- Spiral arteries that do not remodel are susceptible to fibrinoid necrosis and acute atherosis
  - Includes all membranous decidual vessels, and basal vessels that did not remodel
- Small basilar branches of spiral arteries at decidua basalis do not undergo adaptation (including arcuate arteries)

Mural Hypertrophy

- SA and veins throughout decidua have attenuation of vascular smooth muscle early in pregnancy
- When SA thinning fails, vessels remain thick
  - Associated with preexisting vascular disease such as hypertension and diabetes
- May be evident in cases that otherwise have appropriate trophoblast-mediated remodeling in decidua basalis
- Progresses to fibrinoid necrosis in some cases, usually with small-for-age fetal growth ± preeclampsia

- Vascular smooth muscle fragments on desmin staining
- Endothelial cells swell, begin to see CD34, CD31 granular staining in media

Fibrinoid necrosis

- Smooth muscle is degenerated with minimal desmin staining, regular nuclei of vascular smooth muscle replaced by fibrin
- Granular staining of CD34 and CD31 in media is pronounced
- Foam cells (foamy macrophages) may or may not be present adjacent to or within vessel wall

Acute Atherosis

- Advanced stage of fibrinoid necrosis with subendothelial and mural foam cells
  - May be late effort to remodel vessels, immune-mediated effect, or effect of other soluble factor
- Despite name and appearance, pathogenesis is not related to atherosclerosis

Persistence of Endovascular Trophoblast in 3rd Trimester

- Endovascular trophoblast is normal in 1st and 2nd trimester, over time trophoblastic cells invade vessels and no longer persist in the lumen
- Reason for their presence in 3rd trimester is unclear, possibilities include
  - Delay of remodeling process
  - Increased production of extravillous trophoblast from anchoring villi
  - Inhibited migration down vessel and through wall

CLINICAL ISSUES

Epidemiology

- Incidence
  - Occurs in < 1% of uncomplicated pregnancies
  - More frequent in pregnancies with fetal growth restriction with or without preeclampsia
    - Fibrinoid necrosis, acute atherosis most common in SGA with preeclampsia and abnormal Dopplers of umbilical vessels

Prognosis

- Associated with recurrent indicated preterm birth

MACROSCOPIC

General Features

- DA is not visible grossly
  - Large thrombi of decidual vessels may be seen on gross exam

Sections to Be Submitted

- Membranous decidua
  - 2 rolls of membranous decidua with chorioamnionic membranes improves detection of decidual arteriopathy
  - If membranous chorion has separated from decidua, SA may be absent
- Basal plate decidua
  - When maternal vascular malperfusion is suspected, submit cassette of multiple wedge sections from central 2/3 of disc basal surface

Associated Gross Features

- Small-for-gestational-age trimmed placenta weight, infarcts, thin umbilical cord

MICROSCOPIC

Absence of SA Remodeling

- Presence of smooth muscle in SA of central 2/3 of basal decidua
  - Thinned muscular arteries are normal in membranous decidua and peripheral basal plate
  - Very small muscular arteries at basal plate are basilar branches of SA and do not undergo adaptation

Mural Hypertrophy

- Abnormally thickened SA in membranous decidua or decidua basalis

Fibrinoid Necrosis

- Loss of vascular smooth muscle integrity progressing to replacement of smooth muscle with fibrin
- ± foam cells near vessel or in wall

Acute Atherosis

- Fibrinoid necrosis of muscular wall of SA with foamy macrophages beneath endothelium or in wall
  - Can be seen in any muscular SA of membranous decidua and basal decidua, including margin

Persistence of Endovascular Trophoblast in 3rd Trimester

- Accumulation of EVT within vessel at basal plate or decidua

Other Abnormalities of SA Not Recognized as DA

- Small caliber: Basal plate/decidual SA may remain small with delicate media, appropriate transformation should yield large lumens with fibrinoid and EVT in vessel wall
- Necrosis of basal plate/decidua basalis SA with decidual necrosis
- Mural lymphocytes in transformed decidual vessel
  - May see paucity of mural trophoblast and scattered lymphocytes

Associated Microscopic Findings With DA

- Dense perivascular lymphoid infiltrates in decidua, distal villous hypoplasia, increased syncytial knots, infarcts

ANCILLARY TESTS

Immunohistochemistry

- Desmin and CD34 staining can help identify evolution of fibrinoid necrosis if unfamiliar with histology

DIFFERENTIAL DIAGNOSIS

Mimics

- Entrapped villi in basal fibrin with muscular fetal vessels mimic muscular maternal vessels in basal plate
- Normal early vascular remodeling in 1st-trimester placenta can resemble mural hypertrophy
  - Use caution when calling these early processes pathologic
  - Acute atherosis recognized in early spontaneous abortion associated with systemic lupus erythematosus

DIAGNOSTIC CHECKLIST

Pathologic Interpretation Pearls

- Understanding normal vascular remodeling is key to appreciating DA

SELECTED REFERENCES

1. Hecht JL et al: Revisiting decidual vasculopathy. Placenta. 42:37-43, 2016
2. Khong TY et al: Sampling and definitions of placental lesions: Amsterdam Placental Workshop Group consensus statement. Arch Pathol Lab Med. 140(7):698-713, 2016
3. Stevens DU et al: Decidual vasculopathy in preeclampsia: lesion characteristics relate to disease severity and perinatal outcome. Placenta. 34(9):805-9, 2013

Remodeled Vessels in Decidua Basalis

Retained Vascular Smooth Muscle

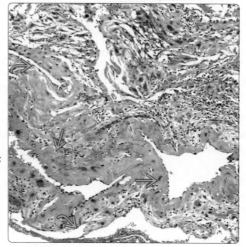
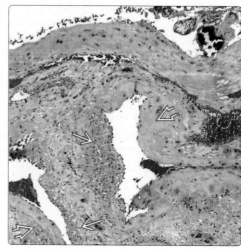

(Left) Remodeled spiral arteries ⇨ show replacement of media with fibrin and frequent mural trophoblast. Their coiled arrangement aids recognition. Veins ⇨ also show loss of smooth muscle, but less fibrin, and only occasional trophoblast near the endothelium. (Right) Incomplete remodeling of the maternal spiral arteries in the decidua basalis is shown in this field by residual thick smooth muscle ⇨ involving a portion of the wall, while a portion of the vessel has normally adapted ⇨.

Endovascular Trophoblast

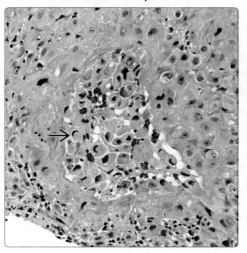

Endovascular Trophoblast

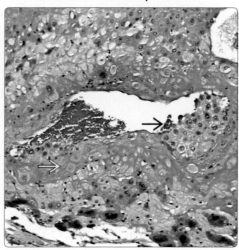

(Left) *This 1st-trimester spiral artery is filled with invasive trophoblast ➡, forming a plug. The occlusion may have a role in protecting the conceptus from the pressure and oxygen tension of arterial blood. Endovascular trophoblast is normal in the 1st and 2nd trimesters.* (Right) *This remodeled vessel shows persistence of endovascular trophoblast cells ➡. The presence of endovascular trophoblast in the 3rd trimester is a feature of decidual arteriopathy. There is a normal amount of fibrinoid ➡.*

Decidual Arteriopathy

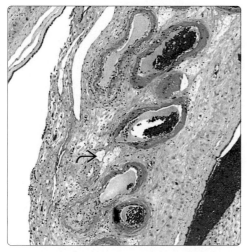

Thrombosis in Decidual Arteriopathy

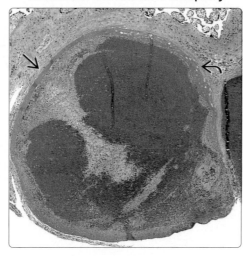

(Left) *Mural hypertrophy, fibrinoid necrosis and acute atherosis are most easily identified in membrane rolls. Routine sampling of 2 membrane rolls increases the likelihood of detection. The lesions are on a spectrum; fibrinoid necrosis with and without foam cells ➡ is seen here.* (Right) *This large, thrombosed basal plate vessel shows fibrinoid necrosis ➡ with foamy histiocytes ➡.*

Necrotic Vessels With Decidual Necrosis

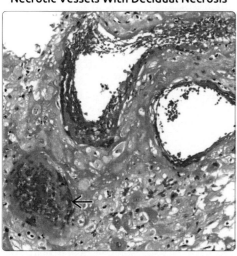

Fibrin at Basal Plate Vessel Openings

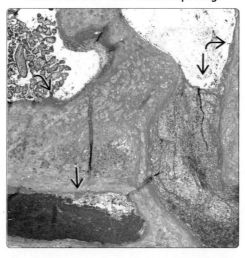

(Left) *Vessels in a region of necrotic decidua may be difficult to interpret. The vessels suggest fibrinoid necrosis ➡, but it is unclear if these changes preceded, or are the result of, decidual necrosis.* (Right) *Fibrin may accumulate at the openings of maternal vessels ➡ in the basal plate at term, continuous with Rohr's fibrinoid ➡. These are likely sites of venous drainage. They can be difficult to distinguish from fibrinoid necrosis; no other changes of malperfusion are seen.*

Infarcts

TERMINOLOGY

- Infarct: Ischemic tissue necrosis of villous parenchyma due to maternal vascular malperfusion
- Marginal infarct: Infarct located within acute angle of disc margin, ~ 1 cm of disc margin
- Infarction hematoma: Infarct with rounded hemorrhage in center of lesion

CLINICAL ISSUES

- Marginal infarcts seen in healthy term deliveries, associated with older maternal age
- Multiple central infarcts associated with small-for-gestational-age fetal growth, severe preeclampsia
- Extensive infarction associated with neonatal asphyxia and fetal demise

MACROSCOPIC

- Placenta is often small for age
- Recent infarct: Dark red, firm lesion

- Subacute to remote infarct: Pale, tan, firm area with granular consistency
- Infarction hematoma: Rounded hematoma surrounded by rim of firm parenchyma
- Infarcts at disc margin often have associated intervillous fibrin comprising gross lesion

MICROSCOPIC

- Early: Collapse of intervillous space with cessation of maternal perfusion, smudging of syncytiotrophoblast nuclei ± neutrophils in intervillous space
- Remote: Intervillous fibrin/fibrinoid deposits between pale ghosts of necrotic villi
- Infarction hematoma: Round focus of hemorrhage surrounded by infarcted villi
- Infarcts associated with other changes of maternal vascular malperfusion: Decidual arteriopathy, distal villous hypoplasia, accelerated villous maturation, placental abruption

---

Early Ischemic Change

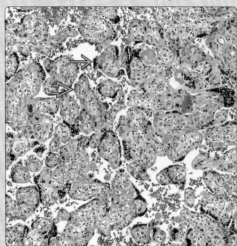

Early Infarct

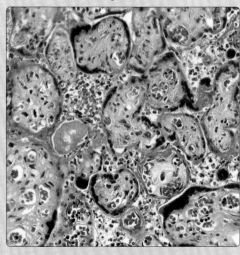

(Left) *In an early infarct, the syncytiotrophoblast nuclei appear smudged ⇨ and the cytoplasm eosinophilic ⇨. There is collapse of the intervillous space, as villi are in close proximity to one another. Grossly, these foci may be darker red and firm.* (Right) *In this early infarct, the syncytiotrophoblast layer is variably smudged-appearing and necrotic. The villi are too close together (collapse of the intervillous maternal blood space). Scattered degenerating neutrophils are seen in the intervillous space.*

Evolving Infarct

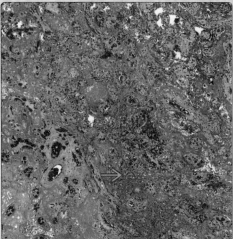

Remote Infarct

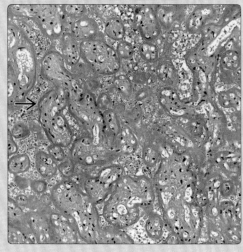

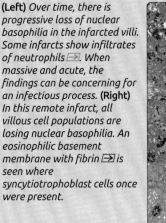

(Left) *Over time, there is progressive loss of nuclear basophilia in the infarcted villi. Some infarcts show infiltrates of neutrophils ⇨. When massive and acute, the findings can be concerning for an infectious process.* (Right) *In this remote infarct, all villous cell populations are losing nuclear basophilia. An eosinophilic basement membrane with fibrin ⇨ is seen where syncytiotrophoblast cells once were present.*

TERMINOLOGY

Synonyms

- Infarction hematoma, rounded intraplacental hematoma, microabruption

Definitions

- Infarct: Ischemic tissue necrosis of villous parenchyma due to maternal vascular malperfusion
  - Marginal infarct: Infarct located within acute angle of disc margin, ~ 1 cm of disc margin
  - Infarction hematoma: Infarct with rounded hemorrhage in center of lesion

ETIOLOGY/PATHOGENESIS

Ischemic Injury

- Maternal spiral arteries bring oxygenated blood to intervillous space bathing villi
- Thrombosis or occlusion of spiral artery causes infarct, associations include
  - Absence of spiral artery remodeling with persistence of smooth muscle
  - Decidual arteriopathy with thrombosis
    - Antiphospholipid antibody syndrome
  - Maternal thrombophilia, preexisting vascular disease (hypertension, diabetes), cocaine use

CLINICAL ISSUES

Presentation

- Single infarcts seen in 2-12% of placentas, not all studies included histologic documentation
  - May be seen in healthy term deliveries, associated with older maternal age at 1st pregnancy
  - Uncommon in 2nd-trimester placenta
- Placentas with central infarcts and multiple infarcts are associated with small-for-gestational-age fetal growth and increased severity of preeclampsia symptoms
- Associated with onset of preeclampsia < 30 weeks

Prognosis

- Due to extensive placental reserve, small infarcts and those at placental margins may be of no clinical significance
  - Single, marginal infarcts may be seen in normal, healthy term deliveries
- Central infarcts, larger infarcts, multiple infarcts, and preterm infarcts are pathologic
  - Associated with fetal growth restriction &/or abnormal umbilical Doppler indices, preterm preeclampsia
  - Infarction of > 30% of placental parenchyma is associated with neonatal asphyxia, intrauterine growth restriction, and fetal demise
- Grossly identified infarcts were associated with increased risk of hypoxic-ischemic encephalopathy with development of cerebral palsy in study from Western Australia Cerebral Palsy Register

Associated Placental Findings

- Changes of maternal vascular malperfusion, including small-for-gestational-age placental growth, decidual arteriopathy, distal villous hypoplasia, accelerated villous maturation, placental abruption

MACROSCOPIC

General Features

- Recent infarcts are dark red and firm
- As they age, infarcts lose fetal hemoglobin and become increasingly yellow, then tan-gray to white, remain firm
- Infarcts at disc margin often have associated intervillous fibrin comprising the gross lesion
- Infarction hematomas are rounded intraplacental hemorrhages ± rim of firm, infarcted parenchyma on gross exam

MICROSCOPIC

Histologic Features

- Early: Collapse of intervillous space with cessation of maternal perfusion, smudging of syncytiotrophoblast nuclei ± neutrophils in intervillous space
- Subacute: Progressive loss of nuclear basophilia
- Remote: Intervillous fibrin/fibrinoid deposits between pale ghosts of necrotic villi
- Infarction hematoma shows round focus of hemorrhage surrounded by infarcted villi
  - Hematoma and infarcted villi may show recent, subacute, or remote features

DIFFERENTIAL DIAGNOSIS

Excessive Perivillous Fibrin Deposition

- Localized excess of perivillous fibrin has gross and histologic overlap with infarcts
- If > 50% of lesion is intervillous fibrin, may diagnose excessive perivillous fibrin deposition and not infarct
  - Marginal infarcts and excessive perivillous fibrin are often both present in same gross lesion

Massive Perivillous Fibrin Deposition/Maternal Floor Infarction

- Infarcted basal villi with increased perivillous fibrin may be maternal floor infarction, correlate with gross exam
- Villous stroma may remain viable in massive perivillous fibrin deposition with intact fetal vessels; over time, villi become ghost-like, often with proliferation of extravillous trophoblast in fibrin

Intervillous Thrombus

- May have similar gross appearance, microscopically distinct
  - Clotted blood in intervillous space, often lamellated, displacing chorionic villi

SELECTED REFERENCES

1. Bendon RW: Nosology: infarction hematoma, a placental infarction encasing a hematoma. Hum Pathol. 43(5):761-3, 2012
2. Blair E et al: Placental infarction identified by macroscopic examination and risk of cerebral palsy in infants at 35 weeks of gestational age and over. Am J Obstet Gynecol. 205(2):124, 2011
3. Fitzgerald B et al: Rounded intraplacental haematomas due to decidual vasculopathy have a distinctive morphology. J Clin Pathol. 64(8):729-32, 2011
4. Vinnars MT et al: The severity of clinical manifestations in preeclampsia correlates with the amount of placental infarction. Acta Obstet Gynecol Scand. 90(1):19-25, 2011
5. Becroft DM et al: Placental infarcts, intervillous fibrin plaques, and intervillous thrombi: incidences, cooccurrences, and epidemiological associations. Pediatr Dev Pathol. 7(1):26-34, 2004

Chronologic Dating on Gross Exam

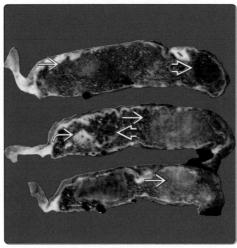

Multiple Central Infarcts

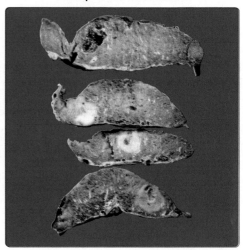

(Left) *Macroscopic aspect of multiple infarcts in the placenta of a mother with preeclampsia who had a stillborn fetus is shown. Varying ages of infarcts are present as red ⇥ (recent), tan ⇥ (intermediate), and white ⇥ (old).* (Right) *This placenta was from a case of severe, preterm preeclampsia with fetal growth restriction. While single small infarcts at the disc margin are common, multiple larger infarcts are pathologic.*

Extensive Infarction

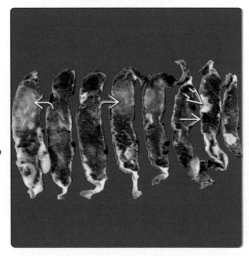

Infarction Hematoma

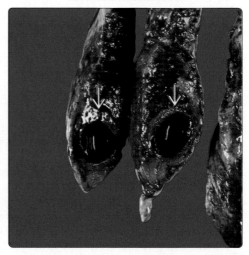

(Left) *These multiple infarcts are from a case with fetal demise. Most of the parenchyma is infarcted. The lesions progress from recent (dark red) ⇥ through subacute (progressively tan) ⇥ to remote (white) ⇥. (DP: Placenta.)* (Right) *Infarction hematoma ⇥ is often seen with poor Apgar scores. Some authors attribute the lesion to reperfusion of infarcted parenchyma; others note an association with decidual arteriopathy and similarity to abruption (so-called microabruption). (DP: Placenta.)*

Infarction Hematoma

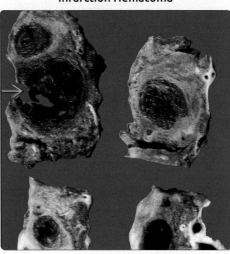

Infarction Hematoma

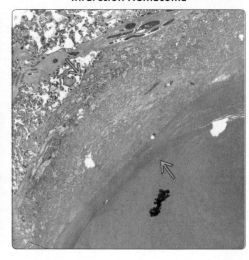

(Left) *This placenta had multiple infarction hematomas. Focally, the largest lesion communicates with the basal plate ⇥. These lesions are important to recognize on gross exam.* (Right) *A rim of infarcted parenchyma ⇥ surrounds a rounded, central hematoma. The blood degenerates over time and lacks characteristic layering of blood and fibrin as seen in intervillous thrombi.*

Villous Agglutination

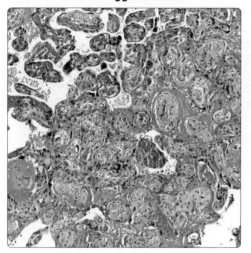

Microscopic Infarct

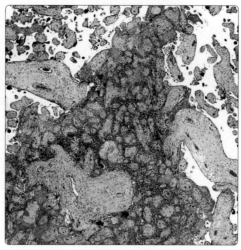

(Left) There is a continuum between villous agglutination and microscopic infarcts. Either term could be used to describe this focus. **(Right)** This larger lesion contains > 100 villi and is more appropriately termed a microscopic infarct (if not identified grossly).

Microabruption

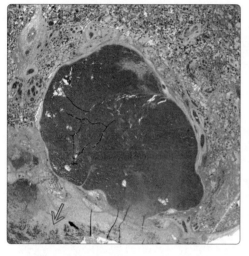

Infarction Over Retroplacental Hemorrhage

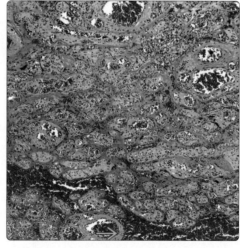

(Left) Infarction hematoma resembles a placental abruption that is confined to a region within the placental parenchyma, instead of a broader separation of the placenta from the decidua basalis. Both processes share infarction of parenchyma overlying the lesion. Decidual leukocytoclastic necrosis is seen deep to the lesion ➡. **(Right)** Parenchyma shows recent infarction overlying a retroplacental hematoma ➡ that covered 30% of the maternal surface.

Maternal Vessels Beneath Infarct

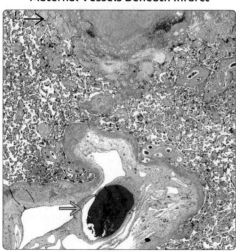

Other Changes Adjacent to Infarcts

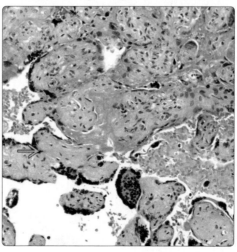

(Left) The occluded vessel is rarely seen beneath an infarct ➡, as the lesion is often deeper in the placental bed than the basal plate decidua. In this focus, a spiral artery ➡ appears distended with layering of fibrin, suggestive of thrombosis. **(Right)** Areas of chronic villitis or avascular villi ➡ may be seen immediately adjacent to infarcts. These avascular villi should not be diagnosed as fetal vascular malperfusion; the changes are secondary to the adjacent infarct.

TERMINOLOGY

- Trophoblast cysts
  - Pools of extracellular matrix material surrounded by extravillous trophoblast (EVT)
  - Found in sites where EVT accumulate and proliferate
    - Cellular chorion of membranes
    - Base of chorionic plate
    - Placental cell islands, septa
    - Basal plate
- May be macroscopic or microscopic (e.g., microcysts)

ETIOLOGY/PATHOGENESIS

- Accompany proliferations of EVT
- Contents are related to placental matrix-type fibrinoid

CLINICAL ISSUES

- **Membranous trophoblast microcysts**
  - Associated with conditions of uteroplacental hypoxia, including preeclampsia, gestational diabetes

- Require ≥ 3 foci to report, significance is unclear without other changes of uteroplacental malperfusion
- **Chorionic plate and septal trophoblast cysts**
  - Associated with delivery at high altitude (preplacental hypoxia)
  - Large cysts on chorionic plate surface (> 4.5 cm) associated with intrauterine growth restriction
  - Associated with massive increased perivillous fibrin (maternal floor infarction)

MICROSCOPIC

- Cysts of homogeneous, colloidal appearing pink fluid lined by EVT cells
- Clotting seen where cyst contents are in contact with maternal blood

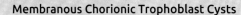

Membranous Chorionic Trophoblast Cysts

Septal Cyst

(Left) Membranous chorionic trophoblast cysts accompany a proliferation of extravillous trophoblast (EVT). Small trophoblast cells ➡ with variably vacuolated cytoplasm surround microscopic pools of eosinophilic fluid ➡. (Right) Cysts ➡ in the septa and decidua basalis may appear more irregular. The secreted product is believed to play a role in solidifying the placental architecture.

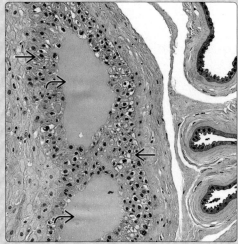

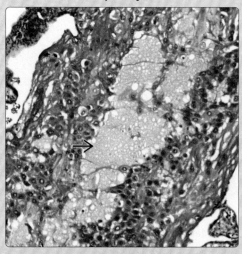

Grossly Visible EVT Cyst in Chorionic Plate

EVT Proliferations Near Infarct

(Left) This cyst was seen on gross examination of the chorionic plate. It expands the chorionic plate extending from just under the amnion to the bottom. (Right) EVT proliferations often accompany older infarcts ➡ and may be associated with localized fluid/extracellular matrix production ➡. In this case, the substance appears more like cyst contents than fibrin deposition.

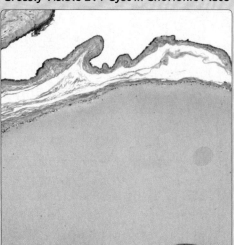

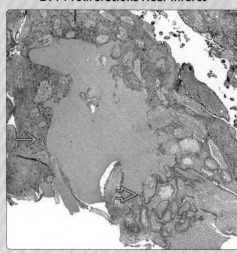

TERMINOLOGY

Abbreviations

- Extravillous trophoblast (EVT)

Synonyms

- Trophoblast microcysts and microscopic chorionic pseudocysts
- Chorionic cysts and subchorionic cysts
- Cell island trophoblast cysts and X-cell cysts

Definitions

- Pools of matrix-type fibrinoid material produced by surrounding EVT
- May be macroscopic or microscopic (e.g., microcysts)
- Found in sites where EVT proliferate
  o Cellular chorion of membranes, chorionic plate, basal plate, cell islands, and septa

ETIOLOGY/PATHOGENESIS

Occurrence With Extravillous Cytotrophoblast Proliferations

- Function of fluid production is unknown
- Proliferations in basal plate postulated as sign of superficial implantation
- Linked to uteroplacental hypoxia

Degenerative Change vs. Secretory Product

- Assumed to be degenerative until recently
- Contents resemble placental matrix-type fibrinoid
  o Usually secreted without polarity, surrounding individual EVT cells
  o Considered "glue" anchoring placenta to maternal floor

CLINICAL ISSUES

Epidemiology

- Incidence
  o Membranous trophoblast microcysts
    – Reported incidence varies greatly
    – 4-5% of placentas selected for pathologic evaluation
    – 18% of unselected placentas from predominantly uncomplicated term births
  o Chorionic trophoblast cysts of basal plate: 5-7% of term placentas
  o Septal and cell island trophoblast cysts: 17% of mature placentas

Clinical Implications

- **Membranous trophoblast microcysts**
  o Associated with conditions of maternal malperfusion, including preeclampsia
    – At least 3 foci of membranous microcysts, chorionic plate, or cell island cysts
  o Associated placental findings: Changes of uteroplacental malperfusion
- **Chorionic plate and septal trophoblast cysts**
  o Associated with delivery at high altitude (preplacental hypoxia)
  o Large cysts (> 4.5 cm) near umbilical cord insertion are associated with intrauterine growth restriction
    – May compromise blood flow in fetal chorionic plate vasculature
  o Associated with massive increased perivillous fibrin deposition (maternal floor infarction)
    – Large (> 4.5 cm) and numerous cysts

MACROSCOPIC

General Features

- Membranous trophoblast microcysts are grossly inapparent
- Chorionic trophoblast cysts are frequently large and visible on chorionic plate
  o May have blood-tinged contents when large
- Septal and cell island trophoblast cysts in parenchyma may be visible on gross cut section

MICROSCOPIC

Membranous Trophoblast Microcysts

- Cysts of homogeneous, colloidal-appearing pink fluid in cellular chorion of free membranes
- Lined by epithelioid-appearing chorionic trophoblast

Chorionic Plate Trophoblast Cysts

- Arise from EVT on intervillous space side of chorionic plate
- Can elevate overlying fetal vasculature; can extend beneath amnion
- Often have admixed blood, can communicate with intervillous space

Septal and Cell Island Trophoblast Cysts

- Cysts appear similar to membranous chorionic microcysts but larger
- Septal cysts may have associated decidual stromal cells of septa

DIFFERENTIAL DIAGNOSIS

Regressed Villi

- Remnants of villi that initially covered entire gestational sac in 1st trimester (chorion laeve)
  o Similar size as chorionic microcysts, also often rimmed by chorionic trophoblast
  o Usually have residual polygonal stromal cells
    – Chorionic microcysts may contain macrophages but no polygonal cells
  o Regressed villi lack homogeneous appearance of chorionic microcysts

Endometrial Glands

- May have similar proteinaceous fluid as chorionic microcysts
- Located deeper in membranous decidua and are not continuous with chorionic trophoblast

SELECTED REFERENCES

1. Stanek J: Membrane microscopic chorionic pseudocysts are associated with increased amount of placental extravillous trophoblasts. Pathology. 42(2):125-30, 2010
2. Soma H et al: Characteristics of histopathological and ultrastructural features of placental villi in pregnant Nepalese women. Med Mol Morphol. 38(2):92-103, 2005
3. Vernof KK et al: Maternal floor infarction: relationship to X cells, major basic protein, and adverse perinatal outcome. Am J Obstet Gynecol. 167(5):1355-63, 1992

Membranous Chorionic Microcysts

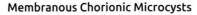
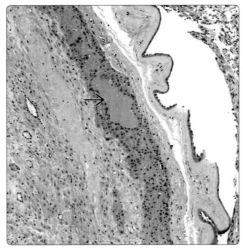

(Left) *Trophoblast microcysts in the membranes are shown. Pools of eosinophilic substance ➡ in the membranous chorion are visible at low power. The cyst content can appear dense, like colloid in the thyroid.* **(Right)** *The cyst fluid often appears more dense in the membranes than in other trophoblast cyst locations. The associated membranous chorionic trophoblast often show cleared cytoplasm, suggestive of glycogen on PAS staining.*

Membranous Chorionic Microcysts

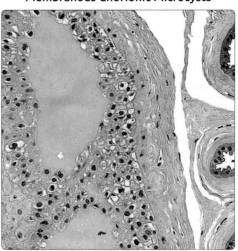

Membranous Chorionic Microcysts

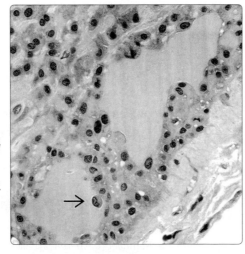

(Left) *Higher power examination shows the homogeneity of the cysts in the membranous chorion. Occasional trophoblast cells ➡ may appear within the lumen, which reflects the irregular contour of the cysts.* **(Right)** *The closest mimic of trophoblast cysts in the membranes are regressed villi. These may also be surrounded by trophoblast ➡. Unlike the cysts, they have an internal stroma and are not fluid filled. They are most numerous near the insertion of the membranes on the disc.*

Regressed Chorionic Villi

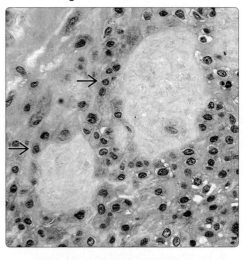

Endometrial Glands in Basal Decidua

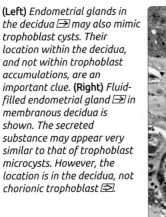
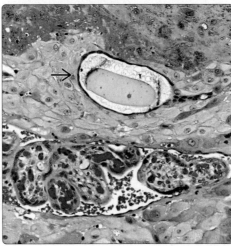

(Left) *Endometrial glands in the decidua ➡ may also mimic trophoblast cysts. Their location within the decidua, and not within trophoblast accumulations, are an important clue.* **(Right)** *Fluid-filled endometrial gland ➡ in membranous decidua is shown. The secreted substance may appear very similar to that of trophoblast microcysts. However, the location is in the decidua, not chorionic trophoblast ➡.*

Endometrial Glands in Membranous Decidua

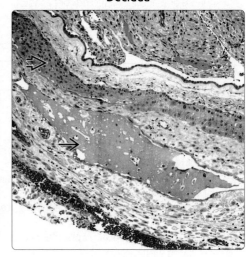

Chorionic Plate Cyst

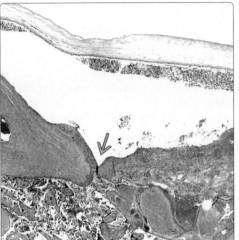

Grossly Evident Chorionic Plate Cyst

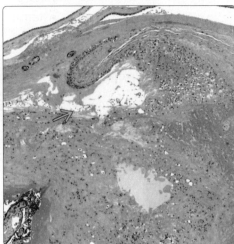

(Left) *This chorionic plate cyst had bloody contents. Microscopic examination shows communication ⇒ with the intervillous maternal blood space.* (Right) *This large cyst ⇒ showed dark brown contents suggestive of blood on gross exam. The EVT associated with the cyst are in continuity with an underlying septum. The blood is likely maternal.*

EVT Pleomorphism in Cyst Beneath Chorionic Plate

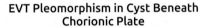
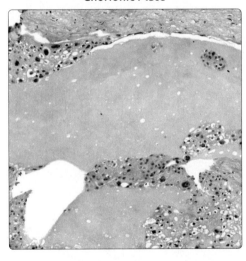

Septal Cysts

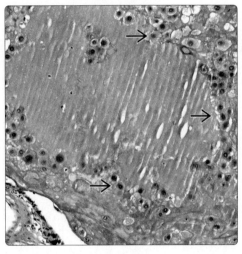

(Left) *Microcysts in the membranes are uncommonly associated with EVT pleomorphism. In this case, cyst fluid is associated with a proliferation of EVT beneath the chorionic plate, with reactive pleomorphism. Changes of uteroplacental malperfusion were extensive in this placenta.* (Right) *This EVT cyst is seen at the tip of a septum, just below the chorionic plate. The cyst appears less well circumscribed by trophoblast ⇒.*

Basal Plate Microcysts

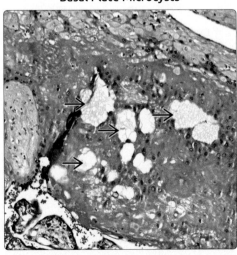

Basal Plate Microcysts

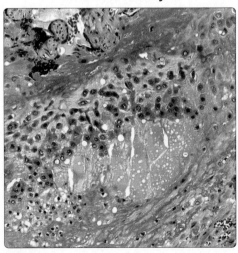

(Left) *Trophoblast cysts ⇒ in the basal plate are shown. Abundant matrix-type fibrinoid from these trophoblast cells, together with blood-type fibrin from the maternal circulation, bond together elements of the basal plate and adhere the placenta to the underlying decidua.* (Right) *EVT associated with cysts typically remain epithelioid appearing, lacking the marked cytomegaly that can be seen with reactive EVT proliferations.*

CLINICAL ISSUES

- Laminar decidual necrosis
  - More common in pregnancies complicated by hypertensive disorders in one study; suggested association with acute hypoxia
  - Frequent in normal term deliveries in another study
- Diffuse decidual leukocytoclastic necrosis
  - Associated with indicated preterm (23- to 32-weeks gestation) and recurrent indicated preterm birth
  - Associated with preeclampsia and poor fetal growth
  - Not associated with spontaneous preterm birth and chorioamnionitis

MACROSCOPIC

- Not usually identified grossly unless extensive or associated with old hemorrhage
- Identified in decidua capsularis of membrane rolls
- Seen in basal plate decidua of full-thickness parenchyma sections or basal plate wedge sections

MICROSCOPIC

- Laminar decidual necrosis
  - Loss of nuclear basophilia of decidual stromal cells and vessels in band-like pattern involving at least 10% of membrane roll
- Diffuse decidual leukocytoclastic necrosis
  - Similar to laminar necrosis but with residual karyorrhectic nuclear debris
  - Should involve 30% of represented decidua

TOP DIFFERENTIAL DIAGNOSES

- Mimics include excessive matrix-type fibrin in membranes
- Decidual leukocytoclastic necrosis with marginal abruption preterm can be difficult to distinguish from acute chorioamnionitis and abruption
  - Look for inflammation at other sites characteristic of amniotic fluid infection to differentiate these processes

(Left) In laminar decidual necrosis (LDN), the membranous decidua ➡ shows loss of nuclear basophilia. The amnion ➡ and cellular chorion ➡ are viable with normal nuclear basophilia. (Right) In decidual leukocytoclastic necrosis (DLN), the neutrophilic infiltrates ➡ can be prominent, raising concern for amniotic fluid infection. Chorioamnionitis and DLN can occur together; careful inspection of the membranes is required to exclude chorioamnionitis.

Laminar Decidual Necrosis

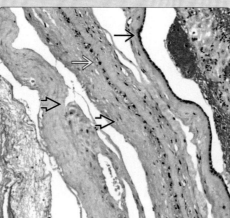

Decidual Leukocytoclastic Necrosis

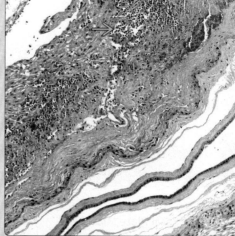

(Left) Thick white material ➡ seen behind the membranes of this placenta represents decidual necrosis. (Right) This cesarean hysterectomy specimen shows linear restriction of LDN ➡ to a band of decidua just below the chorion ➡ of the membranes. No significant inflammation is seen.

Gross Appearance of Decidual Necrosis

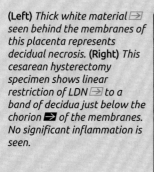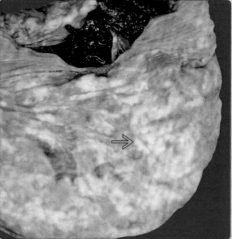

Geographic Restriction of Laminar Decidual Necrosis

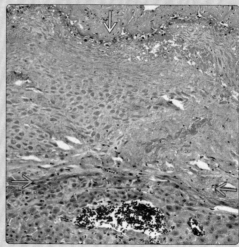

TERMINOLOGY

Abbreviations

- Laminar decidual necrosis (LDN)
- Decidual leukocytoclastic necrosis (DLN)

Synonyms

- Decidual degeneration, bland decidual necrosis

Definitions

- LDN: Coagulative necrosis of decidua
- DLN: Coagulative necrosis of decidua with residual karyorrhectic nuclear debris and degenerating neutrophils

ETIOLOGY/PATHOGENESIS

Laminar Decidual Necrosis

- Cause is unclear; hypotheses include
  - Ischemia from maternal vascular malperfusion, or premature promotion of parturition
  - Physiologic degeneration of membranous decidua in preparation for parturition

Decidual Leukocytoclastic Necrosis

- Etiology unknown, as in LDN
  - Intact or karyorrhectic neutrophils may be present
    - Located on decidual side only
    - Likely reacting to necrotic tissue
    - Not associated with amniotic fluid infection
    - Not associated with spontaneous preterm rupture of membranes
- Small foci of DLN are commonly seen in LDN

CLINICAL ISSUES

Epidemiology

- Incidence
  - LDN
    - Reported incidence varies greatly
    - 6% of placentas selected for pathologic evaluation in one study, 18% of unselected placentas (predominantly uncomplicated deliveries at term)
  - DLN
    - ~ 25% of early preterm births (23- to 32-weeks gestation); 2% of term placentas

Implications

- LDN
  - More common in pregnancies complicated by hypertensive disorders in one study
  - Frequent in normal term deliveries in another study
  - Seen in all cases of abruption preterm in another study
- DLN
  - Diffuse DLN of basal decidua associated with medically indicated preterm birth (23- to 32-weeks gestation) and recurrent indicated preterm birth
    - With preeclampsia and poor fetal growth
  - No association with spontaneous preterm birth and chorioamnionitis
  - Often seen with marginal abruption in preterm placenta, can be difficult to tell if inflammation is part of DLN or chorioamnionitis
- **Significance is controversial**

  - Newly described entities in literature
  - Data for significance of LDN as isolated finding is less convincing
    - Unclear if LDN is normal physiologic process at term
    - May be more significant in preterm placentas
  - Data for diffuse DLN from Alabama Preterm Birth Study suggests stronger association with maternal malperfusion in early preterm births

MACROSCOPIC

General Features

- Not usually identified grossly unless extensive or associated with old hemorrhage

Sections to Be Submitted

- Membranous decidua included with 2 membrane rolls
- Basal plate decidua of full-thickness parenchyma sections or basal plate wedge sections

MICROSCOPIC

Laminar Decidual Necrosis

- Loss of nuclear basophilia in decidual stromal cells and vessels in band-like pattern beneath chorion of membranes
  - Quantitative criteria not universally established; suggested: Involvement of at least 10% of membrane roll
- May accompany recent or remote hemorrhage; may be seen in basal decidua

Decidual Leukocytoclastic Necrosis

- Similar to laminar decidual necrosis but with residual karyorrhectic nuclear debris
  - Suggested: For diagnosis of diffuse DLN, need involvement of at least 30% of sampled basal decidua
- Often with associated microfocal hemorrhages and hemosiderin deposition
- Often present adjacent to infarct or microabruption

DIFFERENTIAL DIAGNOSIS

Matrix-Type Fibrin in Membranes

- Low power resembles "band of pink" seen in LDN, interspersed residual chorionic villi prove this not decidual lesion

SELECTED REFERENCES

1. Chisholm KM et al: Classification of preterm birth with placental correlates. Pediatr Dev Pathol. 1093526618775958, 2018
2. Bendon RW et al: Reassessing the clinical significance of chorionic membrane microcysts and linear necrosis. Pediatr Dev Pathol. 15(3):213-6, 2012
3. Stanek J: Placental membrane laminar necrosis and chorionic microcysts. Pediatr Dev Pathol. 15(6):514-6, 2012
4. Goldenberg RL et al: The Alabama Preterm Birth Study: diffuse decidual leukocytoclastic necrosis of the decidua basalis, a placental lesion associated with preeclampsia, indicated preterm birth and decreased fetal growth. J Matern Fetal Neonatal Med. 20(5):391-5, 2007
5. Stanek J et al: Laminar necrosis of placental membranes: a histologic sign of uteroplacental hypoxia. Pediatr Dev Pathol. 8(1):34-42, 2005
6. Salafia CM et al: Placental pathologic features of preterm preeclampsia. Am J Obstet Gynecol. 173(4):1097-105, 1995

Laminar Decidual Necrosis

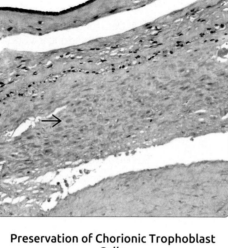

Decidual Vessels in Laminar Decidual Necrosis

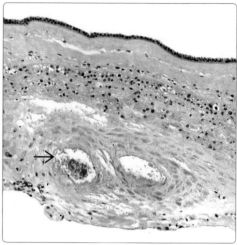

(Left) *Ghosts of decidual stromal cell nuclei ➡ are barely visible in the membranous decidua of LDN. The overlying chorion and amnion are unaffected.* (Right) *Maternal spiral arterioles ➡ in the membranous decidua undergo a similar bland necrosis.*

Preservation of Chorionic Trophoblast Cells

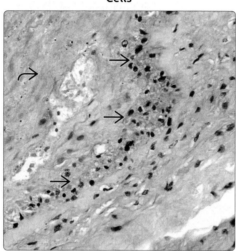

Fibrin in Chorion

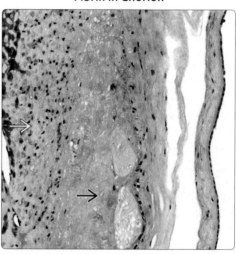

(Left) *Viable chorionic trophoblast cells ➡ are distinct from the subjacent necrotic decidua ➡. The histology suggests ischemic necrosis of the decidua, but why it only affects the maternal decidual cells (and not trophoblast or amnion) is unclear.* (Right) *Excessive fibrin ➡ can mimic laminar decidual necrosis. The matrix-type fibrin is a product of chorionic trophoblast. Note that viable decidua ➡ is present, and there are no ghost cells.*

Fibrin and Residual Villi

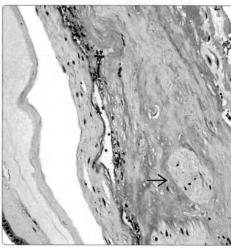

Fibrin Mimic of Laminar Decidual Necrosis

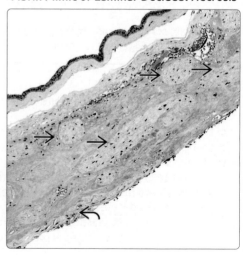

(Left) *Excessive matrix-type fibrin and fibrin from previous membranous hemorrhage mimic LDN. Note residual villi ➡ in the center of the fibrin. True LDN would be located deep to this layer. Residual villi are not present in the membranous decidua layer.* (Right) *Excessive matrix-type fibrin and hemorrhage mimic LDN. Only a small portion of true decidua ➡ is present in this field. Note that residual villi ➡ of the chorion are present.*

Fibrin Deposition in Membranes

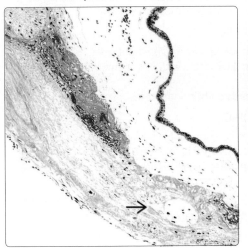

Fibrin vs. Laminar Decidual Necrosis

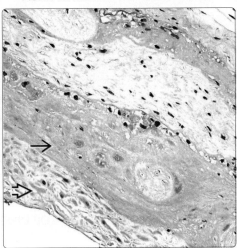

(Left) *Low-power examination suggests laminar decidual necrosis. However, the presence of residual villi ➡ in the "band of pink" confirms the presence of excessive matrix-type fibrin.* (Right) *Excessive fibrin ➡ is present adjacent to laminar necrosis of the decidua. The fibrin appears more homogeneous, as it is an extracellular product, compared with the individual decidual stromal cells of LDN that have lost nuclear basophilia ➡.*

Decidual Leukocytoclastic Necrosis

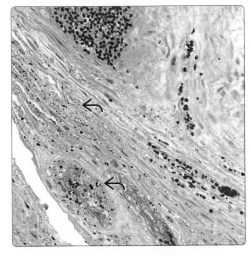

Decidual Leukocytoclastic Necrosis

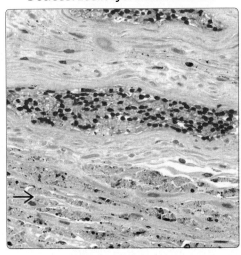

(Left) *DLN in the decidua basalis is characterized by karyorrhectic nuclear dust ➡ along with ghost cells. Karyorrhectic cells often include occasional intact neutrophils, likely reacting to necrotic tissue.* (Right) *The density of nuclear debris ➡ suggests that a leukocytic infiltrate is present. DLN may coexist with chorioamnionitis. Amniotropic inflammation should be sought elsewhere to diagnose amniotic fluid infection.*

Decidual Leukocytoclastic Necrosis

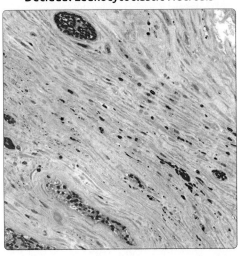

Old Decidual Necrosis

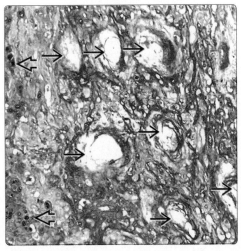

(Left) *Some findings suggest that DLN may be a marker of poor placental perfusion. It often accompanies placental abruption. Microbial studies are usually negative.* (Right) *Outlines of a maternal spiral artery ➡ are seen in this region of necrotic decidua basalis. Viable trophoblast cells ➡ are present. This finding appears more remote than LDN or laminar necrosis and may be a part of basal plate formation.*

ETIOLOGY/PATHOGENESIS

- Local injury to chorionic villi is common; fetal-maternal hemorrhage (FMH) is usually stopped by perivillous fibrin deposition
- Acute villous injury with loss of villous integrity may be due to trauma from falls, motor vehicle accidents

CLINICAL ISSUES

- Minute-volume FMH common, not clinically significant
- Massive FMH presents as decreased fetal movement, sinusoidal fetal heart rate pattern, hydrops, and fetal demise
  - Volume and rate of blood loss affect fetal outcome
- Kleihauer-Betke (KB) acid elution test
  - Maternal red blood cells (RBC) lose ability to take up stain, fetal RBC preserved on stain
- Flow cytometry detection of fetal RBC
  - More accurate than KB but less widely available
  - Detects HbF in fetal RBC with monoclonal antibody

- Percentage of fetal RBC from 2,000 cell count is translated to volume of fetal blood lost from FMH

MACROSCOPIC

- Pale parenchyma in acute significant FMH
- Hydropic pale placenta with Kline hemorrhages in chronic FMH
- Intervillous thrombi in some cases

MICROSCOPIC

- Villous edema/dysmaturity (delayed villous maturation) with increased NRBC in fetal circulation
- Diffusely edematous villi in chronic FMH, foci of villous injury with adjacent intervillous NRBC (fetal blood)
- NRBC in intervillous thrombi indicate fetal blood

TOP DIFFERENTIAL DIAGNOSES

- Fetal anemia due to hemolytic disease of newborn, parvovirus B19, or CMV

Fetal-Maternal Hemorrhage

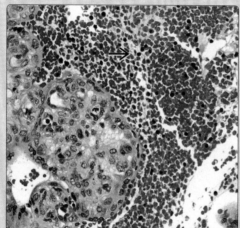

Pallor

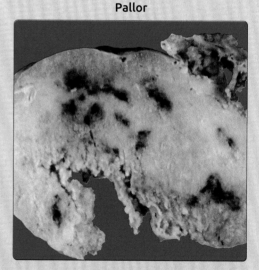

(Left) *Fetal-maternal hemorrhage (FMH) is due to leakage of fetal blood into the maternal intervillous blood space. Fetal blood is rich in nucleated red blood cells (NRBC). Most nucleated cells in the intervillous space here are fetal NRBC ➡.* (Right) *Pallor on gross exam is the most consistent finding with significant FMH. The dark red color normally seen in the mature placenta is due to fetal blood in the villous parenchyma. Fetal anemia leads to pallor.*

Erythroblastosis

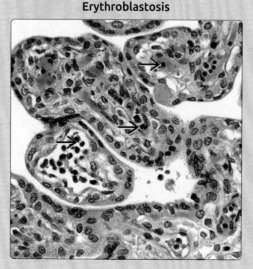

Villous Edema and Fetal Anemia

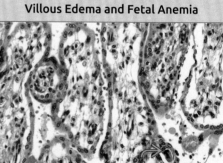

(Left) *Erythroblastosis in a case of severe fetal anemia due to FMH is shown. Rare NRBC have irregular nuclei with buds ➡, a sign of stressed hematopoiesis.* (Right) *Edematous villi are enlarged and pale. Delayed villous maturation has similar features, making distinction between the 2 processes difficult. The fetal capillaries contain mainly NRBC ➡ in this case of severe fetal anemia. A circulating megakaryocyte ➡ is also seen.*

TERMINOLOGY

Abbreviations

- Fetal-maternal hemorrhage (FMH)

Synonyms

- Rounded intraplacental hematoma, infarction hematoma, and microabruption
- Massive subchorial thrombus, subchorionic thrombohematoma, and Breus mole

Definitions

- FHM: Passage of fetal blood from fetal circulation into maternal circulation
- Massive FMH: Clinically significant FMH resulting in fetal morbidity and mortality
- Hematoma, thrombohematoma, and thrombus
  - Imaging literature uses term hematoma; terms thrombohematoma and hematoma are more common in European placental literature; term thrombus more common in USA
  - All of these terms refer to abnormal collection of blood within, behind, or adjacent to placenta
    - Lesions that consist mostly of fibrin with little residual RBC are often called subchorionic or intervillous thrombi
- Kline hemorrhages
  - Foci of FMH, microscopically evident by presence of fetal blood in intervillous space, grossly seen in placentas of chronic FMH as small foci of hemorrhage in otherwise pale hydropic placenta

ETIOLOGY/PATHOGENESIS

Loss of Villous Integrity

- Fetal blood is confined in chorionic villi
  - Vasculosyncytial membrane of mature distal villi is most vulnerable site for rupture
  - Microscopic injury to chorionic villi is common; ongoing fetal hemorrhage is stopped by perivillous fibrin deposition
- Acute villous injury
  - Due to trauma from falls, motor vehicle accidents
  - Due to acute placental abruption

Abnormal Placental Architecture

- Massive FMH reported with chorangioma, in situ choriocarcinoma
  - Large chorangiomas present higher risk for massive FMH

Poor Maternal Clotting at Foci of Villous Injury

- Perivillous fibrin deposition at site of villous injury stops ongoing FMH
- Maternal-fetal ABO compatibility associated with higher risk of significant FMH in one study

Venous Obstruction

- FMH with fetal demise rarely reported with umbilical vein thrombosis

No Known Precipitating Event

- In majority of cases of severe FMH

CLINICAL ISSUES

Epidemiology

- Incidence
  - Some degree of FMH occurs in as many as 75% of pregnancies
    - In > 90% of cases, amount of fetal hemorrhage is small with < 0.1 mL of blood transferred
    - 1 in 1,146 liveborns have transferred volume of ≥ 80 mL of blood to maternal circulation
    - 1 in 2,813 liveborns have transferred volume of ≥ 150 mL
  - Massive FMH is more frequent in pregnancies complicated by stillbirth, fetal distress, or neonatal anemia
    - ~ 60% of cases with these complications have evidence of FMH ≥ 150 mL
    - Stillbirth due to FMH most common near term, ~ 37 weeks
      - Coincides with full-villous arborization and formation of vasculosyncytial membranes in placenta
    - Rate of stillbirth attributed to FMH constant over past 25 years
  - Massive subchorial thrombus found in 1/1,500 placentas submitted for pathologic examination

Presentation

- Massive FMH
  - Decreased fetal movement (27% of cases)
  - Sinusoidal fetal heart rate pattern lacking accelerations in late disease
  - Fetal hydrops in prolonged severe anemia
  - Fetal tachycardia with increased middle cerebral artery peak velocity blood flow on Doppler studies if fetus can compensate for acute loss
  - Maternal transfusion reaction in some cases after acute massive FMH
- Massive subchorial thrombus
  - Originally described with intrauterine fetal demise (IUFD) only
  - Can occur in liveborn, recognized on ultrasound
  - IUFD and liveborn commonly preterm

Laboratory Tests

- Kleihauer-Betke (KB) acid elution test
  - Most widely available method
  - Maternal blood smear is washed in acid, adult hemoglobin of maternal RBC is removed, fetal hemoglobin of fetal RBC is preserved
  - Subsequent staining with Shepard method shows rose pink fetal cells in background of pale "ghost" maternal RBC
  - Percentage of fetal RBC from 2,000 cell count is translated to volume of fetal blood lost from FMH
  - Number of factors can affect KB test leading to inaccurate estimate of FMH volume, including increased hemoglobin F (HbF)-containing cells of maternal origin
    - Confounding in mothers with hemoglobinopathy
  - Maternal-fetal ABO incompatibility leads to lower volume of fetal RBC detected, due to rapid lysis in maternal bloodstream

– Elevated maternal AFP consistent with fetomaternal hemorrhage in this setting

- Flow cytometry detection of fetal RBC
  - More accurate than KB but less widely available
  - Can detect fetal RBC based on larger size
  - Detects HbF in fetal RBC with monoclonal antibody
  - Can differentiate maternal F cells from fetal RBC with carbonic anhydrase (CA)
    – Adult F cells are HbF(+)/CA[bright (+)]; fetal RBC are HbF[bright (+)]/CA(-)

Treatment

- In utero transfusions may help anemic fetus
  - Exchange transfusion and multiple transfusions may be necessary for ongoing FMH

Prognosis

- Volume and rate of blood loss affect fetal outcome
  - Sudden loss of smaller volumes may be catastrophic with sudden demise or ischemic organ injury
  - Slow loss of larger volumes allows time for fetus to compensate
    – May develop fetal hydrops with ongoing anemia
- Massive subchorial thrombus
  - Normal umbilical artery Doppler waveform associated with in utero survival

MACROSCOPIC

General Features

- Placenta may be grossly normal in acute FMH
- Pallor due to fetal anemia most common gross feature
- Hydropic placenta with prolonged FMH
  - Enlarged, bulky, pale, and friable villous parenchyma
  - Amnion often shredded
  - Minimal fibrin deposition on cut section
  - Numerous small Kline hemorrhages
- Intervillous thrombus
  - Usually rhomboid or triangular
  - Commonly reflects FMH but not all intervillous thrombi associated with FMH
    – Maternal blood usually does not clot in intervillous space unless stagnant
  - Differentiate from infarcts with central hemorrhagic necrosis (infarction hematoma)
  - Differentiate from extension/dissection of retroplacental maternal hemorrhage near basal plate, septa, or chorionic plate
- Massive subchorial thrombus
  - One study requires subchorial thrombus to measure 1 cm in thickness and occupy at least 50% of fetal surface
  - Attributed to large vessel FMH
  - Differentiate from nodular accumulations of subchorionic fibrin, hemorrhage into extravillous trophoblast cysts of chorionic plate or septa

MICROSCOPIC

Hydropic Placenta With Kline Hemorrhages

- Numerous small breaks in vasculosyncytial membranes associated with adjacent intervillous extension of fetal blood

- Numerous nucleated red blood cells (NRBC) in intervillous space without significant clot formation
- Usually with diffusely edematous villi, containing little fetal blood

Intervillous Thrombus

- Angular collections of clotted blood in intervillous space laterally displacing chorionic villi
  - Lamellations common
- Presence of NRBC indicates fetal blood component
  - NRBC: Precursor erythroid lineage cell
    – Common constituent of fetal blood, especially in times of stress or anemia, rare in maternal circulation
- Confirm fetal blood component with immunoperoxidase stain for HbF
  - May remain positive in older hemorrhage wherein NRBC have degenerated

Massive Subchorial Thrombus

- Very large intervillous thrombus underlying chorionic plate, displacing chorionic villi downward

Delayed Villous Maturation

- Most common finding in cases of FMH detected by flow cytometry
  - Difficult to distinguish delayed villous maturation from edema; some term change edema/dysmaturity
- Associated with increased NRBC in fetal circulation
- Persistence of villus immaturity described after successful treatment of fetal anemia with in utero transfusion

DIFFERENTIAL DIAGNOSIS

Other Causes of Fetal Anemia

- Immune-mediated hemolytic disease of newborn, Parvovirus B19 or CMV

DIAGNOSTIC CHECKLIST

Clinically Relevant Pathologic Features

- Pallor, villus edema/dysmaturity, and increased fetal NRBC have strongest association with significant FMH
- Identification of fetal NRBC in intervillous thrombi confirms FMH
  - May not be clinically significant
- Chronic FMH may lack true thrombi
  - Placentas are pale and hydropic due to fetal anemia
  - Numerous NRBC seen near villi in intervillous space
- Intervillous thrombi associated with positive KB but not with magnitude of hemorrhage

Pathologic Interpretation Pearls

- FMH is considered common cause of fetal morbidity and mortality that is often overlooked
  - Placental examination may be 1st opportunity to recognize causative role of FMH

SELECTED REFERENCES

1. Dana M et al: Fetal hemoglobin in the maternal circulation - contribution of fetal red blood cells. Hemoglobin. 1-3, 2018
2. Lewis NE et al: Placental pathologic features in fetomaternal hemorrhage detected by flow cytometry. Pediatr Dev Pathol. 20(2):142-151, 2017
3. Ravishankar S et al: Placental findings in feto-maternal hemorrhage in livebirth and stillbirth. Pathol Res Pract. 213(4):301-304, 2017

Intravillous Hemorrhage

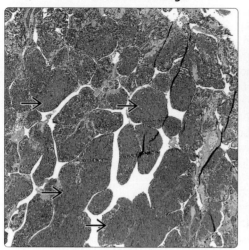

Intervillous Thrombus

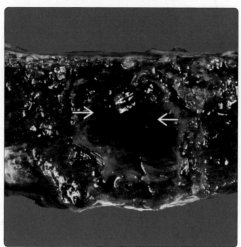

(Left) Retroplacental hemorrhage (acute abruption) and trauma may cause acute FMH due to massive bruising of the chorionic villi. Extensive intravillous hemorrhage ➡ yields fragile sacs of fetal blood ready to burst. Acute venous obstruction may cause the same change. (Right) Intervillous thrombi commonly have angular contours. Lines of Zahn ➡ identify this lesion as a true thrombus vs. an unclotted collection of maternal blood (i.e., flow void).

Older Intervillous Thrombus

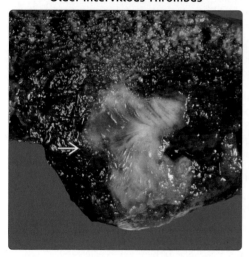

Massive Subchorionic Thrombus

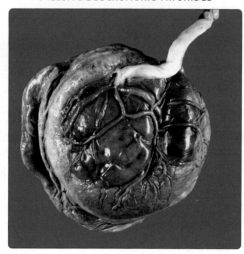

(Left) Older intervillous thrombus ➡ has more fibrin deposition. Intact fetal NRBCs are not likely to be found in older lesions. Immunohistochemistry for fetal hemoglobin F may be useful to confirm FMH when clinically indicated. (Right) Massive subchorionic thrombus is historically termed a Breus mole. The gross differential for these lesions includes hemorrhage into a massive chorionic cyst. Both conditions may represent significant fetal hemorrhage if the lesions are found to contain fetal blood.

Intraplacental Choriocarcinoma

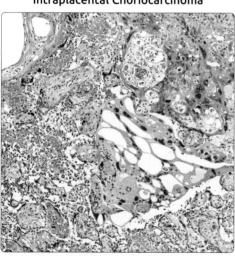

Chorangioma

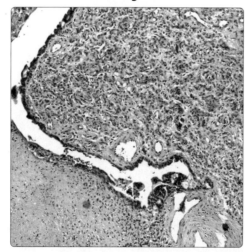

(Left) Intraplacental choriocarcinoma may also present with significant FMH. The presence of FMH does not necessarily mean the tumor has spread to the fetus. (Right) Large chorangiomas are associated with significant FMH. These highly vascular placental tumors may contain a large amount of fetal blood.

TERMINOLOGY

Abbreviations

- Fetal growth restriction (FGR)
- Intrauterine growth restriction (IUGR)
- Small for gestational age (SGA)

Definitions

- FGR = IUGR = SGA
  - Moderate: Weight < 10th percentile for GA
  - Severe: Weight < 3rd percentile for GA
- Low birth weight can be due to prematurity, IUGR, or both
  - Low birth weight: < 2,500 g
  - Very low birth weight: < 1,500 g
  - Extremely low birth weight: < 1,000 g
- Premature: < 36 completed weeks of gestation
- Placental insufficiency: Critical reduction of placental exchange capacity

EPIDEMIOLOGY

Incidence

- Term infants with IUGR: 10% by definition
  - Using normative data for developed countries shows 23% of births in developing countries are IUGR
- Preterm infants with IUGR: 9-22% of preterm births

Gender

- Female infants tend to weigh slightly less than male infants

ETIOLOGY/PATHOGENESIS

General Overview

- Adequate fetal growth depends on adequate supply of oxygen and nutrients to fetus
- IUGR is associated with
  - Maternal factors
    - Maternal medical disease (hypertension 20-30%), renal disease, uterine abnormalities
    - Pregestational diabetes, autoimmune disorders (lupus, antiphospholipid antibody)
    - Hypoxemia (high altitude, cardiac abnormality, anemia), toxic exposure (smoking alcohol, drugs)
  - Fetal factors
    - Genetic diseases; aneuploidy, triploidy, single-gene disorders, 5-20%
    - Confined placental mosaicism with few or no pathologic changes in placenta, 16%
    - Malformations without identifiable genetic marker, 1-2%
    - Infection, 5-10%
    - Multiple gestations, 3%
      - Twin-twin transfusion syndrome associated with IUGR in donor twin
      - Selective FGR of one twin due to unequal placental share or cord abnormality
      - Higher multiples, in utero crowding
  - Placental factors
    - Fetal growth is dependent upon adequate maternal-placental blood flow, placental-fetal blood flow, and villous permeability
    - IUGR is more likely associated with lesions that are chronic, multiple, or single but affecting significant amount of parenchyma

CLINICAL IMPLICATIONS

Imaging Findings

- Low estimated fetal weight
- Small abdominal circumference for age, abnormal head:abdominal circumference ratio (HC:AC), abnormal femur length:abdominal circumference ratio (FL:AC)
- Low amniotic fluid index/oligohydramnios

Umbilical Artery Doppler

- Considered test of placental well-being
- Normal Doppler
  - Development of terminal villi with increased vascularity and thinning of stem vessels, results in normal reduction of placental resistance with increasing GA
  - Fetoplacental system is low resistance with continuous forward flow throughout cardiac cycle

Avascular Villi Due to Fetal Vascular Malperfusion

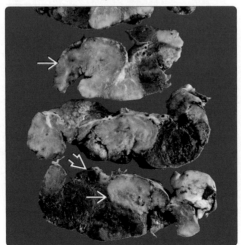

Multiple Infarcts of Different Ages

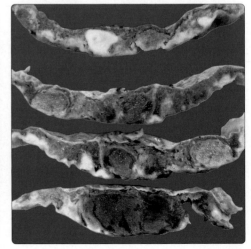

(Left) Placental causes of intrauterine growth restriction (IUGR) generally affect large areas of the parenchyma. The areas of villous pallor ➡ occupy > 50% of the parenchyma. Histologically, they were avascular villi secondary to thrombi within the chorionic plate ➡ and stem vessels. (Right) This is the characteristic appearance of preterm preeclampsia. The infarcts vary from white to red and occupy > 30% of the villous tissue. These babies are severely growth restricted and have high morbidity and mortality.

- Abnormal Doppler indicates rise in peripheral placental resistance, due to 30-70% reduction in villous gas exchange area
  - ↑ S/D ratio: Large diameter but thin placenta, poor vascularity, thick muscular or loss of stem vessels, and acute umbilical vasculitis
  - Absent (AEDF) or reversed end diastolic flow (REDF): Oligohydramnios, small diameter but thick placenta, marginal or velamentous cord insertion, thin cord, decreased size of umbilical vein, abnormalities of stem vessels, circumvallate membranes, infarcts > 10%, accelerated maturation, decreased numbers of villi and decreased capillaries, increased perivillous fibrin deposition, villous stromal hemorrhage, chronic villitis
    - AEDF: Vessel medial hyperplasia with luminal obliteration or thrombus, meconium associated smooth muscle injury
    - REDF: Poorly vascularized terminal villi, villous stromal hemorrhage, and thin, vein-like ectatic stem vessels

Complications

- Term infants
  - Perinatal asphyxia, meconium aspiration, persistent pulmonary hypertension, developmental delay
- Preterm infants
  - Neonatal death, necrotizing enterocolitis, respiratory distress syndrome, bronchopulmonary dysplasia, pulmonary hemorrhage, pulmonary hypertension, postnatal growth failure, developmental delay
- IUGR may be antecedent to adult disease
  - Linked to hypertension, coronary artery disease, hyperlipidemia, and diabetes mellitus

EVALUATION OF FGR

Fetal Evaluation

- Fetal body weight percentile
- Fetal:placental weight ratio
  - Increases with ↑ GA = ~ 7:1 at term; ratio > 9-10:1 suggests placental insufficiency
- Ponderal index (PI): Measure of leanness of infant calculated as relationship between weight and height: Birth weight (g)/length (cm)^3 x 100
  - PI < 10th percentile reflects fetal malnutrition, PI < 3rd percentile reflects severe fetal wasting
- Symmetric vs. asymmetric fetal body growth
  - Symmetric: Reduction in both body weight and head circumference, attributed to reduced growth potential
    - 20-30% of IUGR, generally early onset
      - Intrinsic fetal abnormalities, malformations, genetic syndromes, chromosomal abnormalities or infection
    - Growth curves parallel to percentiles throughout pregnancy
  - Asymmetric: Reduction in body weight with normal head size and preservation of brain growth, attributed to reduced nutrient and oxygen supply
    - 70-80% of IUGR, generally late onset, majority are due to chronic placental abnormalities
    - Growth curves falls below percentiles in second 1/2 of pregnancy

Placental Evaluation

- Placental weight
  - Most chronic placental lesions resulting in IUGR are associated with low placental weight
- Umbilical cord
  - Chronically obstructive umbilical cord lesions: Knots, single umbilical artery, hypercoiling, excessive length, velamentous and marginal insertion
  - Thin umbilical cord (< 0.8 cm in diameter as measured off of slide)
- Chorionic plate vessels
  - Magistral vascular distribution with velamentous and marginal cord insertion with less branching and fewer vascular trees
  - Fetal vascular malperfusion; thrombosis or obliteration
- Stem villous vessels
  - Proximal chronic villitis
  - Fetal vascular malperfusion; thrombosis or obliteration
- Membranes and chorionic plate
  - Remote retromembranous hemorrhage
  - Diffuse chorioamniotic hemosiderosis
    - Associated with circumvallate insertion of membranes, chronic marginal hemorrhage (chronic abruption)
  - Amnion nodosum (feature of severe and prolonged oligohydramnios)
  - Chronic chorioamnionitis associated with high-grade chronic villitis
  - Maternal decidual vasculopathy in utero placental malperfusion
- Chorionic villi
  - Accelerated maturation, distal villous hypoplasia
  - Multiple infarcts
  - High-grade chronic villitis ± fetal vascular obstruction
  - Avascular villi as part of fetal vascular malperfusion
- Intervillous space
  - Massive subchorionic thrombus (Breus mole)
  - Chronic histiocytic intervillositis
  - Massive perivillous fibrin deposition

SELECTED REFERENCES

1. Levytska K et al: Placental pathology in relation to uterine artery doppler findings in pregnancies with severe intrauterine growth restriction and abnormal umbilical artery doppler changes. Am J Perinatol. 34(5):451-457, 2017
2. Junaid TO et al: Fetoplacental vascular alterations associated with fetal growth restriction. Placenta. 35(10):808-15, 2014
3. Mifsud W et al: Placental pathology in early-onset and late-onset fetal growth restriction. Fetal Diagn Ther. 36(2):117-28, 2014
4. Baergen RN: Placental Pathology, An Issue of Surgical Pathology Clinics. Philadelphia: Elsevier, 2013
5. Cox P et al: Pathological assessment of intrauterine growth restriction. Best Pract Res Clin Obstet Gynaecol. 23(6):751-64, 2009
6. Redline RW: Placental pathology: a systematic approach with clinical correlations. Placenta. 29 Suppl A:S86-91, 2008

Placental Evaluation in Special Circumstances

Partial Hydatidiform Mole

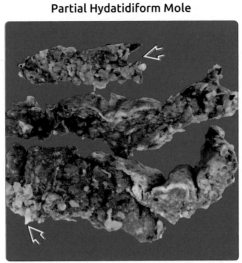

Partial Hydatidiform Mole

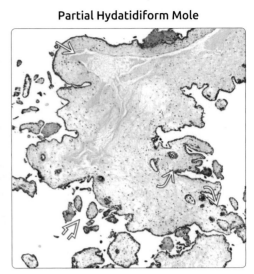

(Left) This midgestation placenta shows focal vesicles ⮞ involving ~ 20% of the villi. Diandric triploidy results in severe IUGR and partial molar features in the placenta. (Right) The partial mole has a dual villous population with large hydropic villi with central cisterns ⮞ and smaller fibrotic villi ⮞. The irregular shape of the villi results in the trophoblastic pseudoinclusions ⮞.

Triploidy With Asymmetric IUGR

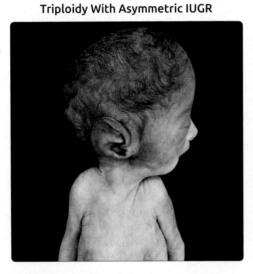

Symmetric IUGR and Trisomy 18

(Left) Digynic triploidy is associated with a very small nonmolar placenta and severe asymmetric IUGR. (Right) Trisomy 18 is generally associated with severe but symmetric IUGR, which is in part due to a very small placenta. Note the clinched fists due to overlappping fingers.

Massive Perivillous Fibrin Deposition

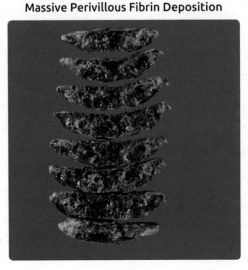

Severe IUGR With Osteopenia

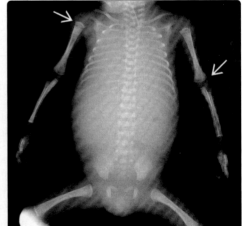

(Left) This placenta shows the characteristic features of massive perivillous fibrin deposition (MPVFD). The intervillous space is occupied with firm, net-like fibrin deposition that prevents maternal-fetal exchange and leads to placental insufficiency. (Right) IUGR can be so severe in MPVFD that ultrasound will show significant shortening of the long bone growth, raising the possibility of dwarfism. The epiphyses are flared ⮞, and the bones are significantly osteopenic, which can result in bowing of the femurs.

Dilated Stem Vessels With Preeclampsia

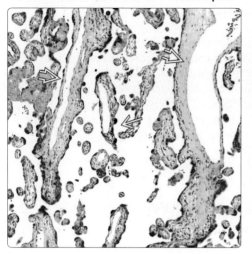

Decidual Arteriopathy

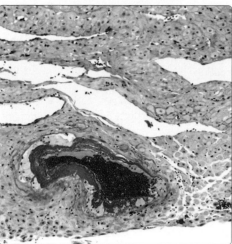

(Left) *Preterm preeclampsia is usually associated with severe IUGR. Umbilical artery Doppler studies are commonly used to monitor the fetus for optimum delivery outcome. Reversed end diastolic flow is commonly associated with small villi, exaggerated "serrated" syncytial knots ➡, and dilated vein-like stem vessels ⇥.* (Right) *Maternal arteries in the membranous decidua are commonly abnormal in preterm preeclampsia and may show atheroma formation.*

High-Grade Villitis With Stem Vessel Obliteration

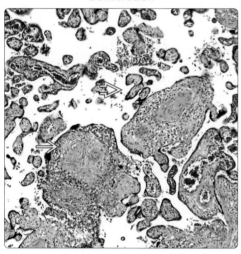

High-Grade Fetal Vascular Malperfusion

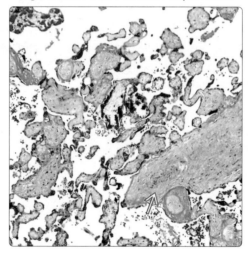

(Left) *Villitis of unknown etiology is usually found in the 3rd trimester. High-grade VUE can be associated with IUGR, especially when there is associated fetal vascular malperfusion, as seen here with stem vessel obliteration ⇥ and avascular villi ⇥.* (Right) *Large areas of avascular villi are secondary to obliteration of larger vessels ⇥ upstream in the fetal vascular tree.*

Lymphoplasmacytic Villitis Due to CMV

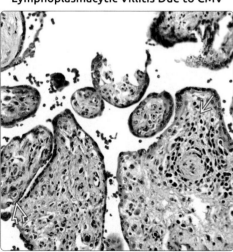

Chronic Histiocytic Intervillositis

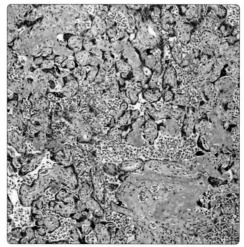

(Left) *CMV is the most common virus transmitted to the fetus. It commonly results in IUGR in the 2nd trimester. Plasmacytic villitis ⇥ should always raise the concern for CMV. Viral inclusions ⇥ may be hard to find.* (Right) *Chronic histiocytic intervillositis is associated with IUGR and has a strong recurrent potential. Macrophages/histiocytes fill the intervillous space and compromise maternal-fetal exchange. Perivillous fibrin deposition often increased.*

TERMINOLOGY

Definitions

- Preterm birth: Delivery prior to 37-weeks gestation
- Late preterm birth: Delivery from 34- to 37-weeks gestation
- Preterm labor (PTL): Regular contractions with cervical change prior to 37-weeks gestation
- Preterm premature rupture of membranes (PPROM): Spontaneous rupture of membranes prior to 37-weeks gestation and > 1 hour before onset of contractions

Clinical Categories of Premature Birth

- Spontaneous preterm births
  - PTL with intact membranes (40-45%)
  - PPROM (25-30%)
- Indicated preterm births (30-35%)
  - Maternal indications
    - Preeclampsia/eclampsia
    - Clinical placental abruption
    - Other medically indicated causes (thyroid disease, asthma, diabetes mellitus, primary hypertension, maternal neoplasm necessitating chemotherapy, sepsis, sickle cell crisis)
  - Fetal indications
    - Intrauterine growth restriction
    - Fetal distress (nonreassuring fetal heart tracing)
    - Other indicated causes (oligohydramnios, twin-twin transfusion syndrome, fetal amniotic band syndrome, absent or reversed umbilical artery end-diastolic flow)

EPIDEMIOLOGY

Incidence

- 10-15% of births are prior to 37-weeks gestation
- 3.5% of births are prior to 34-weeks gestation
- Multiple gestations are at increased risk
  - Account for 15-20% of preterm births

ETIOLOGY/PATHOGENESIS

Potential Causes

- Intrauterine infection: Reflected in changes of intrauterine inflammation/infection
- Uteroplacental malperfusion/ischemia: Reflected in changes of maternal vascular malperfusion
- Uterine overdistension/stretching: As in twin gestations
- Uterine anomalies
- Immune-mediated processes: Reflected in chronic villitis, chronic chorioamnionitis, and chronic histiocytic intervillositis
- Stress (nutritional, social)
- Endocrine disorders

CLINICAL IMPLICATIONS

Perinatal Mortality

- Accounts for 75% of perinatal mortality

Increased Morbidity

- Neonatal morbidities
  - Respiratory distress syndrome
  - Necrotizing enterocolitis
  - Intraventricular hemorrhage
  - Retinopathy of prematurity
- Accounts for > 50% of long-term morbidity
  - Neurological deficits
  - Blindness
  - Deafness
  - Chronic lung disease

PLACENTAL FINDINGS IN PRETERM BIRTH

Amniotic Fluid Infection Sequence

- Maternal inflammatory response
  - Acute subchorionitis and acute chorioamnionitis
- Fetal inflammatory response
  - Umbilical arteritis, umbilical phlebitis, and chorionic plate vasculitis

Acute Chorioamnionitis

Fetal Inflammatory Response

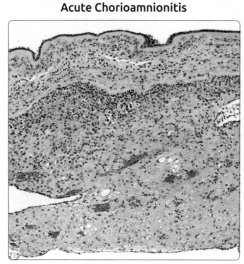
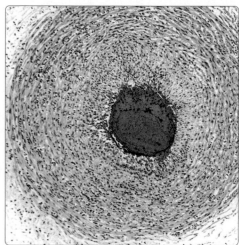

(Left) Acute chorioamnionitis is a frequent cause of spontaneous preterm birth, including preterm premature rupture of membranes and preterm labor. It is a maternal inflammatory response to amniotic fluid infection. (Right) Fetal inflammatory response syndrome is associated with amniotic fluid infection and has significant neonatal morbidity. It is histologically reflected in severe umbilical arteritis and chorionic plate vasculitis.

- Severe histologic umbilical vasculitis and chorionic plate vasculitis are associated with fetal inflammatory response syndrome with multisystem organ involvement in neonate
- More frequent and severe in early preterm birth
- Often seen in spontaneous preterm birth, including PPROM and PTL
- Associated with placental abruption

Maternal Vascular Malperfusion

- Gross placental features
  - Small placental size
  - Infarctions
- Microscopic features
  - Decidual arteriopathy
  - Distal villous hypoplasia
  - Infarcts
- Identified in many placentas in preterm birth (both spontaneous and indicated causes)
  - More frequent in maternal &/or fetal indicated causes for preterm birth, including preeclampsia and intrauterine growth restriction

Chronic Inflammation

- Gross features
  - Pale granular foci seen with extensive parenchymal involvement
- Microscopic features
  - Chronic chorionitis and chorioamnionitis
  - Basal chronic villitis
  - Parenchymal chronic villitis
- Chronic chorioamnionitis seen in cases of late spontaneous preterm birth
- Infectious chronic villitis and chronic deciduitis can be seen in cases of PTL
- Infectious chronic villitis and chronic villitis of unknown etiology can cause fetal intrauterine growth restriction with indicated preterm birth
- Chronic villitis of unknown etiology, chronic chorioamnionitis, and chronic villitis with obliterative vasculopathy associated with late preterm birth

- Chronic villitis with obliterative vasculopathy associated with severe intrauterine growth restriction and perinatal morbidity
- Chronic histiocytic intervillositis more often seen in early preterm births for fetal indications of intrauterine growth restriction

Fetal Vascular Malperfusion

- Gross placental features
  - Large vessel thrombosis
- Microscopic features
  - Large vessel thrombosis
  - Villous damage (avascular villi or stromal vascular karyorrhexis)
- Not common in prematurity, associated with late preterm birth for fetal indications
- Associated with intrauterine growth restriction due to loss of functional placental parenchyma
- Increased risk in infant for neurologic sequelae

Maternal Hemorrhage

- Gross placental features
  - Retroplacental or marginal hemorrhage/hematoma
- Microscopic features
  - Diffuse chorioamniotic hemosiderosis in chronic abruption
  - Infarcts, acute ischemic changes of villous placenta in acute abruption
  - Frequently show laminar decidual necrosis or decidual leukocytoclastic necrosis

SELECTED REFERENCES

1. Chisholm KM et al: Classification of preterm birth with placental correlates. Pediatr Dev Pathol. 2018 [ePub ahead of print]
2. Catov JM et al: Neonatal outcomes following preterm birth classified according to placental features. Am J Obstet Gynecol. 216(4):411.e1-411.e14, 2017
3. Faye-Petersen OM: The placenta in preterm birth. J Clin Pathol. 61(12):1261-75, 2008
4. Goldenberg RL et al: Epidemiology and causes of preterm birth. Lancet. 371(9606):75-84, 2008

Chronic Abruption

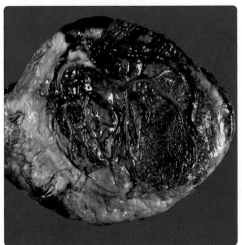

Distal Villous Hypoplasia

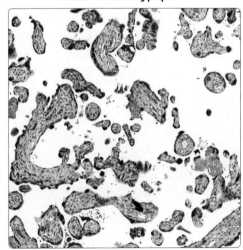

(Left) *Chronic abruption with diffuse chorioamniotic hemosiderosis is associated with preterm birth. There is old hemorrhage at the margin with circumvallate membranes.* (Right) *Distal villous hypoplasia indicates chronic uteroplacental malperfusion. It is seen in indicated preterm birth for preeclampsia or fetal growth restriction, often with abnormal umbilical Doppler waveforms.*

Placenta Accreta

ETIOLOGY/PATHOGENESIS

- Nearly all associations with placenta accreta relate to absence or deficiency of endometrium available for decidualization

CLINICAL ISSUES

- Risk increased significantly with ≥ 2 cesarean deliveries (CDs) and with anterior placenta previa
- Placenta will not spontaneously separate, and attempts to do so can result in massive hemorrhage or uterine inversion
- Incidence of maternal mortality is ~ 4% with high risk of hemorrhage and disseminated intravascular coagulopathy

MICROSCOPIC

- Normal implantation: Decidua is present between basal plate and myometrium
  - Invasive trophoblasts normally invade through endometrium and into inner 1/3 of myometrium
  - Villi may extend into maternal veins at basal plate

- Placenta accreta
  - Villi and uterine smooth muscle interface with only fibrin and invasive trophoblast, no intervening decidua
  - Absent decidualized endometrium, myometrium not thinned
- Placenta increta
  - Villi and uterine smooth muscle interface with only fibrin and invasive trophoblast, no intervening decidua
  - Absent decidualized endometrium, thinned myometrium
- Placenta percreta
  - Placental tissues only contained by uterine serosa, rarely invades into surrounding organs
- Occult placenta accreta
  - Uterine smooth muscle cells adherent to basal plate without intervening decidua
  - Distinguish myometrial from vascular smooth muscle

Cesarean Hysterectomy Accreta

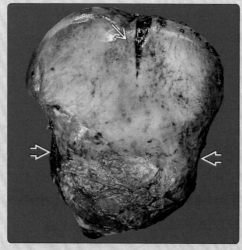

Cesarean Hysterectomy Placenta Accreta

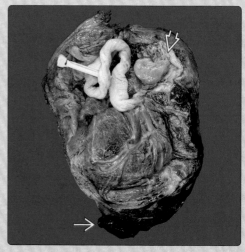

(Left) Postpartum hysterectomy uterus, with an anterior fundal hysterotomy incision ➡, shows a markedly thinned, bulging lower uterine segment ➡ with an in situ placenta. Prominent serosal vasculature is present along with anterior fibrous adhesions. (Right) Bivalved uterus shows placenta previa, covering the cervical os with a blood clot ➡. There is abundant remote retromembranous hemorrhage ➡, which is a common finding associated with accreta.

Placenta Accreta/Increta Gross

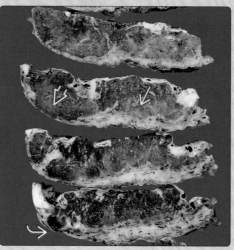

Placenta Accreta

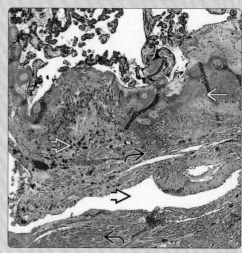

(Left) Serial sections show a myometrium of variable thickness. Thinned areas of myometrium imply placenta increta. Microscopic examination showed areas of both accreta ➡ and increta ➡. A fibrous plaque ➡ is present in the area of increta. (Right) Section from an area of accreta shows Nitabuch fibrinoid ➡ and invasive trophoblasts ➡, immediately adjacent to myometrium ➡ without intervening decidua. Spaces noted are dilated uterine veins ➡ that are normally present.

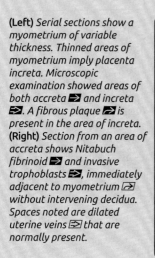

TERMINOLOGY

Synonyms

- Morbidly adherent placenta and "placenta creta"
  - Encompasses accreta (75%), increta (18%), and percreta (7%)

Definitions

- Placenta accreta: Villi and basal fibrin adhere to myometrium without decidual layer
  - Accreta has been described by some as focal (involving 1 cotyledon), partial (involving > 1 cotyledon), or complete (involving all cotyledons)
- Placenta increta: Thinned myometrium with villi extending into myometrium
- Placenta percreta: Absent myometrium with villi extending through myometrium
  - Usually confined by uterine serosa
  - Obstetricians use term percreta to imply extension beyond uterus
  - Percreta extending beyond uterus is mostly into bladder, which may present with blood in urine
- Occult placenta accreta: Presence of uterine smooth muscle cells on basal surface of delivered placenta with no intervening decidua between villi and myometrium
- Morbidly adherent placenta: Intervention beyond spontaneous delivery or simple manual extraction necessary
- Retained placenta: Placenta that has not detached within 30 minutes of delivery
- Placenta previa: Placental disc either partially or completely covers internal cervical os; incidence 0.3-1.3% with 25% having accreta
- Uterine window: Thinned area of myometrium, usually anterior in area of previous hysterotomy, not associated with implantation site
- Decidua: Hormonally transformed endometrial stromal cells
  - Acts as physical and immunologic barrier and has ability to shed with parturition
- Basal plate fibrin
  - Nitabuch fibrin: Lies between invasive trophoblasts and decidua
  - Rohr fibrin: Lies between maternal intervillous space and invasive trophoblasts
  - At term, Nitabuch and Rohr fibrin are essentially single layer

ETIOLOGY/PATHOGENESIS

Deficiency of Decidua

- Nearly all associations with placenta accreta relate to absence or deficiency of endometrium available for decidualization
  - Previous cesarean delivery (CD)
    - Most cases of accreta have history of previous CD
    - Risk increases after ≥ 2 prior CDs
    - History of prior CD with current low-lying placenta increases from 3% after 1 CD to 67% after 5 or more CDs
  - Other previous uterine instrumentation
    - Increased risk after any uterine surgery, including myomectomy, curettage, or endometrial ablation
    - Scarring after procedure may affect abundance of endometrium able to be decidualized
  - Implantation in lower uterine segment (placenta previa)
    - Many cases of placenta accreta are associated with placenta previa
    - Decidua is less prominent in lower uterine segment
  - Implantation in other uterine regions deficient in decidua
    - Uterine cornu of fallopian tubes, over submucosal leiomyoma
- Other proposed etiologies include increased invasiveness of trophoblast, abnormal smooth muscle, or differences in immunologic milieu, but all of these factors could also relate to absence of decidua

CLINICAL ISSUES

Epidemiology

- Incidence
  - Placenta creta has increased from 1/10,000 in 1960s to 1/500 deliveries now, paralleling increase in CDs
    - Increased risk in advanced maternal age, hypertensive disorders, smoking
    - Incidence of placenta previa 0.3-1.3% (previous uterine surgery, smoking, cocaine, advanced maternal age, multiparity, multifetal pregnancy)
    - Increased incidence with in vitro fertilization, especially with cryopreserved embryos

Presentation

- Morbidly adherent placenta
  - Placenta accreta is now being diagnosed prior to delivery by ultrasound (US) and magnetic resonance (MR) imaging
  - Commonly associated with low-lying placenta or placenta previa and antepartum hemorrhage
  - Postpartum hemorrhage with delayed placental separation and inability to manually remove placenta
  - Placenta accreta can occur in 1st trimester
- Occult placenta accreta
  - May present with delayed placental separation or need to manually remove placenta
  - More common in preterm placentas (10%) vs. term (1%)
    - Seen in preeclampsia, premature rupture of membranes, preterm labor, abruption; most of these are also associated with prematurity

Laboratory Tests

- Biologic markers, such as cell-free fetal DNA and placental mRNA have been tested; MS-AFP, PAPP-A are elevated in women with accreta, none are sensitive or specific enough to be useful as screening tool

Natural History

- Placenta will not spontaneously separate, and attempts to do so can result in massive hemorrhage or uterine inversion

Treatment

- Surgical approaches
  - Cesarean hysterectomy, often with fundal hysterotomy, for delivery of baby

- o Focal accreta may be treated with local resection or curettage after vaginal or CD
- Conservative management
  - o Some have advocated leaving placenta in place and postpartum methotrexate
    - – Increased risk for sepsis, thrombosis, renal failure, or late postpartum hemorrhage
  - o Embolization of beads or Gelfoam
  - o Ligation of uterine or hypogastric arteries
  - o Allows some women to have successful subsequent pregnancies

Prognosis

- Maternal morbidity: ~ 4% of cases of placenta creta are fatal
  - o High risk of antenatal and intrapartum hemorrhage and disseminated intravascular coagulopathy
  - o 40% chance of requiring transfusion of > 10 units of red blood cells
  - o Attempts at placental removal may significantly increase bleeding
  - o Risk for uterine inversion following attempted removal of adherent placenta
- Neonatal morbidity is primarily due to prematurity or maternal bleeding, planned delivery 34-35 weeks
- Recurrence risk after occult placenta accreta
  - o Little significance with subsequent pregnancies if there was no problem delivering placenta with index pregnancy
  - o Increased risk for morbidly adherent placenta in subsequent pregnancy if there was delayed placental separation or manual removal of placenta in index pregnancy (25-30%)
  - o Increased risk for morbidly adherent placenta in subsequent pregnancy when large areas or multiple foci of myometrium are present in index pregnancy
    - – Increased risk with increased thickness of myometrium adherent to placenta
  - o Risk for occult placenta accreta in subsequent pregnancy nearly 50%

IMAGING

Ultrasonographic Findings

- US diagnostic in most cases, improved by addition of Doppler
- Loss of clear zone hypoechoic area between placenta and myometrium thought to represent decidua basalis, low predictive value
- Presence of bridging vessels, crossing interface from bladder to uterus, subplacental hypervascularity
- Myometrium < 2 mm thick
- Normal border between bladder and myometrium is echogenic and smooth, accreta is associated with interruptions, bulging with increased vascularity
- Round, smooth, placental lacunae sensitive for diagnosis of accreta midgestation
  - o Associated with turbulent flow
  - o Pathologic correlate to this US finding is unknown

MR Findings

- MR is more sensitive for diagnosis of placenta creta and more accurate
  - o Thickened, dark nodular contour of placenta-uterine interface with extension of dark bands within placenta
  - o Mass effect of placenta on uterus causing outward bulge
  - o Heterogeneous placental signal on T2-weighted sequences with large placental lakes or vessels
  - o Most useful 24-30 weeks, before uterus gets too distended

MACROSCOPIC

General Features

- Placenta is frequently abnormally shaped (bilobation, accessory lobes) with velamentous cord insertion in placenta accreta
- Cesarean hysterectomy specimen
  - o External appearance
    - – Uterus is boggy with prominent vessels on serosal surface, usually in lower uterine segment
    - – Rarely, portion of bladder is resected with uterus
      - □ May have portions of bladder wall smooth muscle within fibrous adhesions; rarely, portion of bladder is resected to prevent tearing
    - – Inferior resection margin may be irregular in supracervical hysterectomy
    - – Recent hysterotomy incision
  - o Uterus is bivalved along coronal plane revealing placenta in situ
    - – Note where placenta implants
      - □ May see partial or complete placenta previa, often associated with remote or recent hematoma
    - – Section through placenta in situ to identify greatest depth of implantation
      - □ Myometrium is thinned in area of abnormal implantation
- Delivered placenta
  - o Morbidly adherent placenta may be removed in pieces
    - – Disc may be fragmented
    - – Disrupted basal plate
    - – Missing cotyledons
  - o Occult placenta accreta is generally not recognized grossly

Sections to Be Submitted

- Cesarean hysterectomy specimen
  - o Submit sections from area of thinnest myometrium
  - o Submit sections of prior hysterotomy scar if identified
  - o Submit normal-appearing placenta-uterus interface for comparison
  - o Submit membrane/decidua attachment sites
  - o Submit standard section from umbilical cord and placenta
  - o Additional sections from uterine cervix, leiomyomas, etc.
- Basal plate examination for occult placenta accreta
  - o Thin sections from basal plate, submitted on edge to detect amount of any myometrium attached
  - o Sections from areas adjacent to disrupted maternal surface and near maternal arteries have the highest yield

MICROSCOPIC

Histologic Features

- In normal implantation, villi are separated from myometrium by basal plate (Rohr and Nitabuch fibrin with invasive trophoblasts) and decidualized endometrium
  - Invasive trophoblasts normally invade through endometrium and into inner 1/3 of myometrium; this is not accreta
  - Villi may normally extend into maternal veins at basal plate; this is not accreta
- Placenta accreta
  - Villi and uterine smooth muscle interface with only basal plate fibrin and invasive trophoblast, no intervening decidua
    - Nitabuch fibrin may be normal, thin, or absent
    - Normal invasive trophoblasts
    - Normal myometrial muscle
    - Increased chronic inflammation at basal plate, lymphocytes, and plasma cells
  - Increased retromembranous, subchorionic, and intervillous hemorrhage
- Placenta increta
  - Villi and uterine smooth muscle interface with only basal plate fibrin and invasive trophoblast, no intervening decidua
    - Nitabuch fibrin may be normal, thin, or absent
    - Invasive trophoblasts may be decreased
    - Myometrium still present, although thin; some have described myocyte injury
    - Increased chronic inflammation at basal plate and superficial myometrium
- Placenta percreta
  - No residual myometrium, villi generally confined to serosa but can extend into surrounding structures, particularly bladder
    - Nitabuch fibrin may be thin
    - Invasive trophoblasts often significantly diminished
    - Increased chronic inflammation at basal plate and serosa
    - Maternal vessels in serosa may show adaptation for pregnancy
- Occult placenta accreta
  - Variable amount of uterine smooth muscle cells adherent to basal plate fibrin without intervening decidua
    - Increased incidence of acute retroplacental hemorrhage described in one study
- Placenta accreta in D&C specimens
  - Very difficult diagnosis to make due to lack of orientation of placenta/myometrium fragments
- Implantation onto cesarean scar
  - Pale-staining area of elastosis with myofiber disarray, may be evidence of poor wound healing

DIFFERENTIAL DIAGNOSIS

Placenta Increta vs. Normal Thinning of Myometrium

- Normally thinned myometrium in lower uterine segment
- Compare thickness of muscle at same level on side opposite implantation

  - Tissues may be too disrupted in supracervical postpartum hysterectomy to distinguish

Occult Placenta Accreta vs. Vascular Smooth Muscle

- Distinguish myometrial from vascular smooth muscle at implantation site
  - Vascular smooth muscle from maternal decidual veins is normally present

DIAGNOSTIC CHECKLIST

Pathologic Interpretation Pearls

- Placenta accreta is primarily due to absence of decidualized endometrium

SELECTED REFERENCES

1. Ernst LM et al: Placental pathologic associations with morbidly adherent placenta: potential insights into pathogenesis. Pediatr Dev Pathol. 20(5):387-393, 2017
2. Roeca C et al: Pathologically diagnosed placenta accreta and hemorrhagic morbidity in a subsequent pregnancy. Obstet Gynecol. 129(2):321-326, 2017
3. Wyand R et al: Association of retroplacental blood with basal plate myofibers. Pediatr Dev Pathol. 1093526617741071, 2017
4. Cramer SF et al: Placenta accreta and placenta increta: an approach to pathogenesis based on the trophoblastic differentiation pathway. Pediatr Dev Pathol. 19(4):320-33, 2016
5. Endler M et al: Macroscopic and histological characteristics of retained placenta: a prospectively collected case-control study. Placenta. 41:39-44, 2016
6. Goh WA et al: Placenta accreta: diagnosis, management and the molecular biology of the morbidly adherent placenta. J Matern Fetal Neonatal Med. 29(11):1795-800, 2016
7. Jauniaux E et al: Accreta placentation: a systematic review of prenatal ultrasound imaging and grading of villous invasiveness. Am J Obstet Gynecol. 215(6):712-721, 2016
8. Linn RL et al: Adherent basal plate myometrial fibers in the delivered placenta as a risk factor for development of subsequent placenta accreta. Placenta. 36(12):1419-24, 2015
9. Lyell DJ et al: Maternal serum markers, characteristics and morbidly adherent placenta in women with previa. J Perinatol. 35(8):570-4, 2015
10. McDonagh M et al: The invasive phenotype of placenta accreta extravillous trophoblasts associated with loss of E-cadherin. Placenta. 36:645-51, 2015
11. Comstock CH et al: The antenatal diagnosis of placenta accreta. BJOG. 121(2):171-81; discussion 181-2, 2014
12. Hull AD et al: Placenta accreta and postpartum hemorrhage. Clin Obstet Gynecol. 53(1):228-36, 2010
13. Stanek J et al: Occult placenta accreta: the missing link in the diagnosis of abnormal placentation. Pediatr Dev Pathol. 10(4):266-73, 2007

(Left) *In normal implantation, a layer of fibrin* ⮕ *and gray decidua is discerned grossly between villous tissue and myometrium.* **(Right)** *Microscopically, normal implantation shows Nitabuch fibrinoid* ⮕ *overlying normal decidualized endometrium* ⮕. *The presence of invasive trophoblasts* ⮕ *in the underlying endomyometrium is physiologic and not evidence of placenta accreta.*

Normal Implantation, Gross

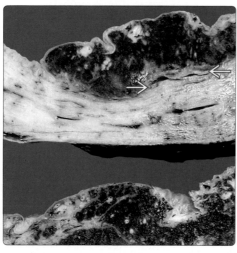

Basal Plate of Normal Implantation

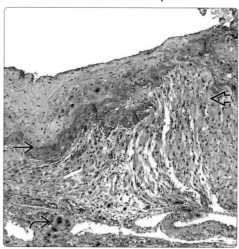

(Left) *In contrast to the extravillous trophoblasts of the basal plate, the trophoblasts of the chorion laeve* ⮕ *do not invade into the myometrium. Decidua capsularis* ⮕ *is present between the fetal membranes and myometrium* ⮕. **(Right)** *The presence of villi in basal plate veins* ⮕ *is a normal finding. It should not be interpreted as placenta accreta.*

Normal Membrane Attachment

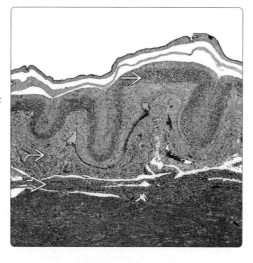

Villous Extension Into Basal Plate Veins

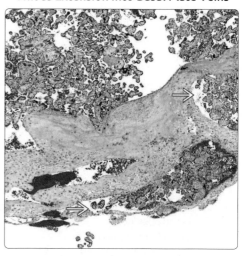

(Left) *The presence of the normal decidua* ⮕ *is highlighted by a vimentin immunohistochemical stain. Decidual stromal cells are strongly vimentin positive.* **(Right)** *Pancytokeratin stain highlights the villous syncytiotrophoblasts and the invasive trophoblasts* ⮕ *in the decidualized endometrium. Invasive trophoblasts in the endometrium and inner myometrium are a normal feature of implantation.*

Normal Implantation Site Vimentin

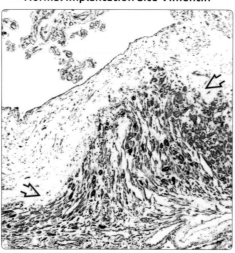

Normal Implantation Site Cytokeratin

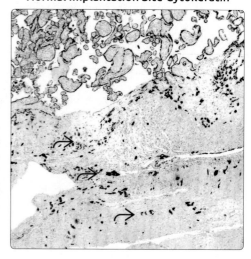

Placenta Percreta Bladder Mucosa

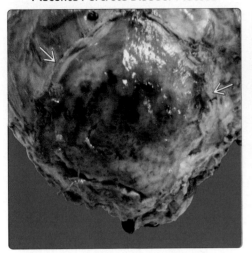

Placenta Percreta Bladder Muscle

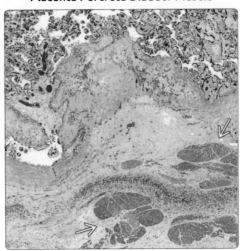

(Left) *A portion of the bladder* ➡ *was intentionally resected at the time of the cesarean hysterectomy to reduce the risk of tearing the bladder due to marked fibrous adhesions. This type of cystostomy is easier to repair than a ragged tear.* (Right) *Placenta percreta is most often anterior in the lower uterine segment in the area of a prior hysterotomy. Adhesions between the uterus and bladder are common. Occasionally, a portion of the bladder wall* ➡ *will be resected during lysis of anterior adhesions.*

Placenta Percreta Bladder Wall

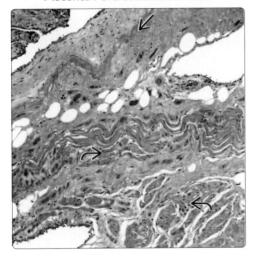

Placenta Increta With Chronic Inflammation

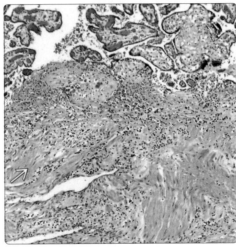

(Left) *In this section taken from an area of placenta percreta, fibrinoid at the base of the placenta* ➡ *is adjacent to omental adipose tissue and bundles of smooth muscle* ➡ *from the bladder.* (Right) *Abnormal implantation is frequently associated with an increased number of lymphocytes and plasma cells extending into the adjacent myometrium* ➡.

Placenta Increta With Abnormal Maternal Vessels

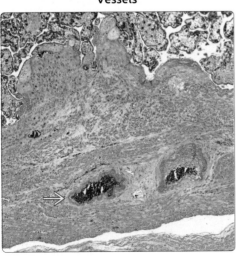

Abnormal Maternal Serosal Vessels in Placenta Percreta

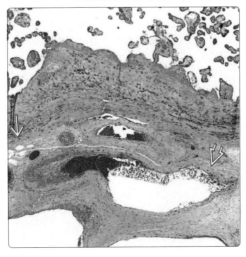

(Left) *Maternal vessels at the implantation site of placenta creta frequently show fibrin* ➡ *in the walls, fibroblast proliferation, and chronic inflammation. These are changes similar to those of decidual arteriopathy.* (Right) *These abnormal vessels are serosal, as evidenced by the presence of adipose tissue* ➡ *between the implantation and the vessel. Under normal circumstances, these serosal vessels do not undergo any adaptative changes during pregnancy. Invasive trophoblasts* ➡ *can be seen in the vessel wall.*

315

(Left) *Cesarean hysterectomy for placenta accreta commonly shows a fundal-sutured hysterotomy incision* ➡ *with a thin, bulging lower uterine segment* ⇥. *The prominent vessels seen through the serosa indicate the location of the placental tissue.* **(Right)** *Bivalving the uterus shows that the placenta completely covers the internal cervical os* ➡, *demonstrating complete placenta previa.*

Cesarean Hysterectomy Fundal Hysterotomy

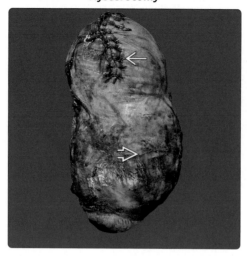

Cesarean Hysterectomy Placenta Previa Accreta

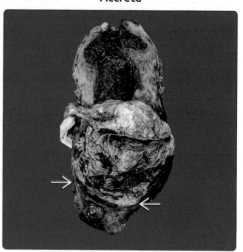

(Left) *Section of placenta previa shows the basal plate of placenta* ➡ *adjacent to the endocervical mucosa* ➡. *Placenta accreta frequently complicates implantation in the lower uterine segment, as there is insufficient decidua at this anatomic site.* **(Right)** *Hysterectomy from a 14-weeks-gestation cervical pregnancy is shown. There is marked destruction of the cervix and lower uterine segment. Umbilical cord is seen extending from the cervix.*

Placenta Previa

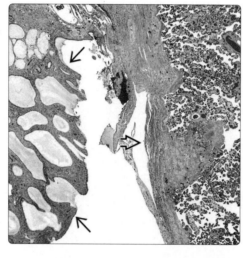

Cervical Implantation With Accreta

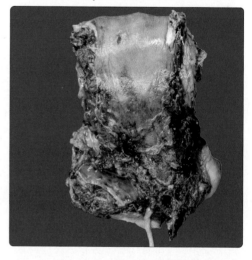

(Left) *Placenta was morbidly adherent in the fundus. The previous endometrial ablation removed the cells capable of forming decidua. Pregnancy rarely occurs after ablation, but when it does, there is a high incidence of accreta.* **(Right)** *Bivalved postpartum hysterectomy specimen shows the placental bed of a cornual placenta increta with thinned myometrium* ➡ *and marked hemorrhage. The placenta has been removed.*

Fundal Placenta Accreta

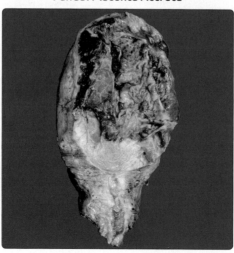

Cornual Placenta Increta, Gross

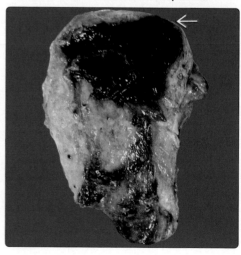

Placenta Increta/Perceta Fibrinoid Plaques

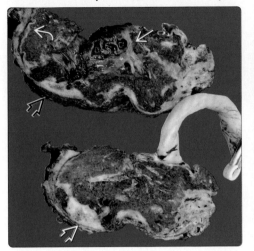

Placenta Percreta With Plaque

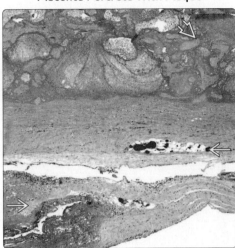

(Left) *The uterus with in situ placenta has been serially sectioned, showing multiple fibrin plaques* ➡. *The presence of plaques on imaging has been associated with percreta* ➡. *A subchorionic hematoma* ➡ *has cystic degeneration. Normal Nitabach fibrin and normal separation is noted at the margin* ➡. **(Right)** *There is complete absence of the myometrium; however, no placental tissue extends beyond the confines of the uterus. Fibrous adhesions* ➡ *are present. The fibrin plaque* ➡ *has a few entrapped villi.*

Uterine Window, Gross

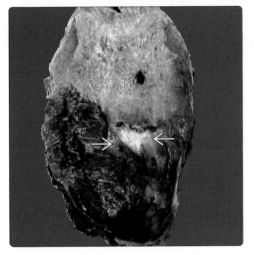

Uterine Window

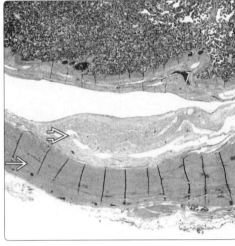

(Left) *Anterior 1/2 of a cesarean hysterectomy uterus shows a low-lying placenta with diffuse increta. A "uterine window"* ➡ *is in the area of a previous hysterotomy incision. This may happen without placenta accreta and may be the site of uterine scar dehiscence or uterine rupture.* **(Right)** *The myometrium* ➡ *is extremely thinned, but there is appropriate decidualized endometrium* ➡ *at this implantation site associated with a uterine window.*

Absent Decidua Parietalis

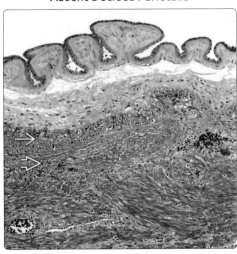

Multiple Accessory Lobes, Gross

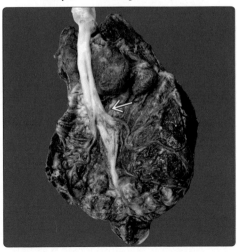

(Left) *With placenta accreta, there is often a diffuse paucity or absence of decidualized endometrium, not just at the implantation site. In the membranes* ➡, *chorion laeve is directly apposed to the myometrium* ➡ *without any decidua.* **(Right)** *Placenta creta is often associated with bilobation or accessory lobes. The cord is furcate and inserted* ➡ *between placental lobes.*

Placenta Accreta-Delivered Placenta, Gross

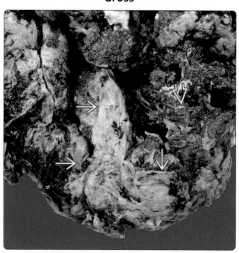

Occult Placenta Accreta-Basal Plate Myofibers

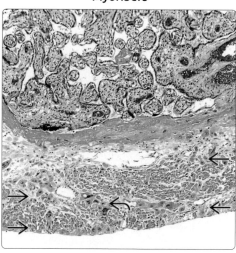

(Left) *Maternal surface of placenta has an unusually large area of attached myometrium ➡. Placenta was able to be delivered without significant hemorrhage. This finding may be termed occult placenta accreta. Notice the adjacent surface ➡ is ragged, a feature suggesting tissue left in the uterus.* **(Right)** *Section of a term placenta has a large amount of attached myometrium ➡ and occult placenta accreta. Normal Nitabuch fibrinoid is present with normal invasive trophoblasts ➡ and no decidua.*

Incomplete Maternal Surface

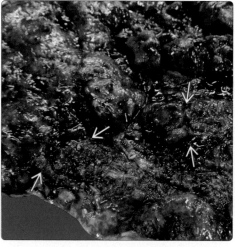

Occult Placenta Accreta-Basal Plate Myofibers

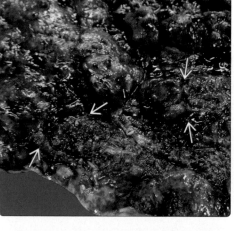

(Left) *When the placenta has been manually delivered, there may be tearing of the maternal surface. Sections taken from the interface of the shiny intact surface with the ragged, torn surface ➡ will increase recovery of occult placenta accreta.* **(Right)** *The usual appearance of occult placenta accreta is only a few myometrial smooth muscle fibers ➡. Invasive trophoblasts ➡ are also noted, but there is a significant deficiency of decidualized endometrial cells ➡.*

Normal Implantation With Basal Plate Vascular Smooth Muscle

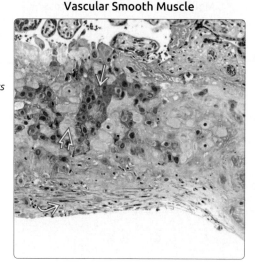

Normal Implantation Site With Vascular Smooth Muscle

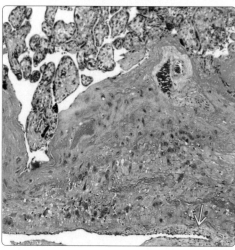

(Left) *Thin, wispy smooth muscle fibers ➡ may be seen at the basal plate. They are generally vascular in origin. This is a normal implantation site with invasive trophoblasts ➡ and decidual cells ➡.* **(Right)** *Normal implantation site also has a dilated vein at the base, which is easier to distinguish as vascular in origin due to the plump endothelial cells ➡.*

Partially Delivered Placenta Accreta

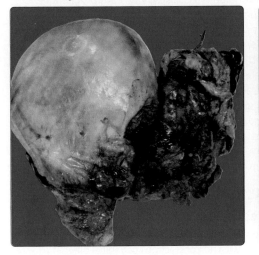

Partial Uterine Resection With Focal Placenta Accreta

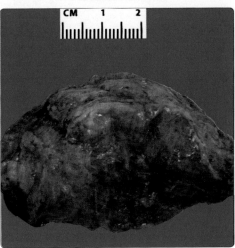

(Left) *Unsuspected placenta accreta was found when the placenta could not be completely removed after cesarean delivery for placenta previa.* (Right) *Conservative surgical management of focal placenta accreta yielded in a full-thickness resection of the uterus and area of accreta.*

D&C Specimen for Retained Placenta

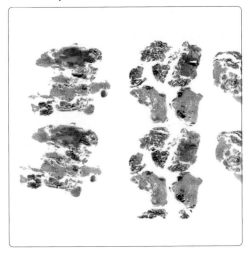

D&C Specimen With Placenta Accreta

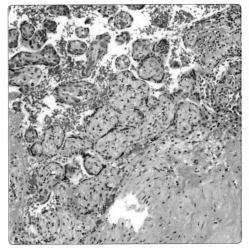

(Left) *The multiple fragments of unoriented tissue and blood clot makes the diagnosis of placenta accreta difficult in a D&C sample. It may be necessary to submit the entire tissue component (not the clot) to identify focal accreta.* (Right) *D&C was performed due to persistent bleeding 2 days post vaginal delivery. Villous tissue is present without decidua. The villi have chronic inflammation but are viable because they retain their attachment to the implantation site.*

D&C Specimen for Retained Placenta

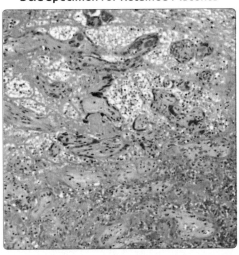

Curettage 4 Weeks Postpartum

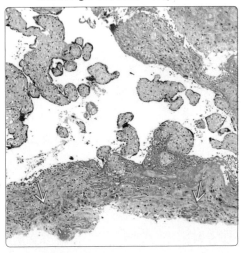

(Left) *This is another area of the same curettage specimen, which contains devitalized villi and fibrin, consistent with a portion of retained, but detached, placenta.* (Right) *Patient had a cesarean delivery 4 weeks prior to presentation with vaginal bleeding. A curettage specimen contained portions of well-oriented placenta with chronic inflammation and avascular villi. There is basal smooth muscle ➡ without decidua- placenta accreta.*

1st-Trimester Pregnancy Loss

TERMINOLOGY

Definitions

- 1st trimester: Up to 13 weeks, 6 days of gestation
- Embryo: Development from conception to end of 10th week post last menstrual period (LMP)
- Spontaneous abortion: Previable pregnancy loss due to genetic, developmental, placental, or infectious etiologies

EPIDEMIOLOGY

Incidence

- 10-20% of recognized pregnancies result in pregnancy loss, most commonly in 1st trimester
  - 100 per 1,000 pregnancies at 4-7 weeks post LMP
  - 70 per 1,000 pregnancies at 8-11 weeks post LMP

ETIOLOGY/PATHOGENESIS

Chromosomal Abnormalities

- Account for 40-70% of 1st-trimester spontaneous abortions
- Mostly numerical abnormalities, few structural
  - 40-70% of cases are aneuploid (usually differs from normal number of chromosomes by 1)
    - Most common are trisomies 16, 22, 21, and 15; trisomies are associated with maternal age > 35 years
    - Monosomy X is also common
  - 24-40% of cases are polyploid (> 2 sets of chromosomes)
  - 4-8% of cases are structural abnormalities
    - Unbalanced translocations and inversions; often reflect abnormal parental chromosomes
- Chromosomal microarray analysis reveals submicroscopic abnormalities, such as copy number variants and single nucleotide polymorphisms
  - These changes do not appear to be associated with advanced maternal age
  - Will not detect some balanced chromosome rearrangements or low-level mosaicism

Other Factors

- Maternal conditions associated with early pregnancy loss
  - Autoimmune disorders, antiphospholipid antibodies
  - Endocrinopathy (i.e., diabetes, obesity, luteal-phase defects, polycystic ovary syndrome)
  - Uncontrolled chronic illness
  - Thrombophilia
  - Severe acute illness (e.g., pneumonia, appendicitis)
  - Infection (rare): *Listeria*, *Toxoplasma*, herpes simplex virus, coxsackievirus, cytomegalovirus
  - Uterine anomalies (intrauterine adhesions, uterine septum, and leiomyomata)
- Teratogen exposure and smoking/drug use

CLINICAL IMPLICATIONS

Clinical Presentation

- Missed abortion: Nonviable pregnancy, usually detected incidentally, with no contractions or vaginal bleeding
- Incomplete abortion: Nonviable pregnancy with cervical dilation and passage of blood or tissue
- Blighted ovum: Obstetric term describing preembryonic loss (5-6 weeks post LMP) composed of gestational sac containing no embryonic structures
- Embryonic loss: Embryo detected with no cardiac activity (6-10 weeks, 6 days post LMP)

Treatment

- Surgical
  - Dilation and curettage (D&C); vacuum aspiration: Electric or manual
- Pharmacologic
  - Misoprostol (prostaglandin E1 analog)
- Expectant monitoring
  - Complete expulsion may take up to 1 month

(Left) *Intact sac contains a macerated embryo. Growth appears organized. Subchorionic hemorrhage ➡ is present, a common finding with 1st-trimester pregnancy loss. (From DP: Placenta.)* (Right) *The subchorionic hematoma is a combination of recent and remote hemorrhage. It is present in the retromembranous region, more often than at the basal plate.*

Subchorionic Hemorrhage

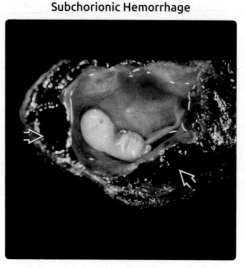

Subchorionic Hematoma

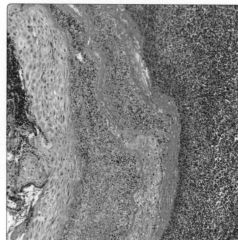

MACROSCOPIC

General Features

- Pathologic examination of 1st-trimester spontaneous abortion specimens should confirm intrauterine pregnancy and provide possible clues as to cause of pregnancy loss
  - Ability to accomplish these objectives may be limited by specimen contents
    - ~ 40% of specimens consist of decidua and blood clot ± fragmented chorionic sac and no embryo
    - Even if embryo/fetus is noted on ultrasound, there is rarely grossly identifiable tissue after suction evacuation

Components of Gross Exam

- After measuring specimen, partition sample into decidua, implantation site decidua, and gestational sac
  - Implantation site decidua is tan-pink to yellow and has more resistance than nonimplantation site decidua
    - Decidual tissues are frequently hemorrhagic; nearly impossible to define retroplacental hemorrhage in 1st trimester
    - Subchorionic hematoma, as seen on ultrasound, may be hemorrhage on free membranes
  - Note if gestational sac is intact or ruptured
    - If intact, note presence or absence of embryo or yolk sac
    - Identify presence or absence of umbilical cord root
  - Note villous morphology: Sparse or lush, blunted or stringy ± vesicular changes
  - If no placental elements are seen, floating specimen in saline or water facilitates better visualization
- If embryo is present, note following characteristics
  - Crown-rump length (may not have any discernible cephalocaudal differentiation)
    - Embryo size < expected for menstrual age may reflect growth disorganization (GD) due to chromosomal abnormalities or embryonic demise at earlier developmental age
    - Embryonic "nubbin" (< 10-mm tissue mass without discernible developmental characteristics) has high incidence of chromosomal abnormalities (60-80%)
    - Differentiate abnormal embryo from yolk sac by positioning of yolk sac between amnion and chorion
  - Evidence of cephalocaudal differentiation (e.g., presence or absence of retinal pigment)
  - Presence of GD (failure to acquire expected anatomic features for age or asynchronous development of features)
    - Expected developmental characteristics defined for age and embryonic length
    - Easiest to assess in fetus (> 30 mm); difficult but not impossible in embryo
    - Abnormal embryos with GD are 3x as likely to have chromosomal abnormality
  - Localized anatomic defects associated with specific chromosomal abnormalities
    - Monosomy X: Delayed limb development, encephalocele

- Triploidy: Neural tube defects, facial clefting, delayed upper and lower limb development, fused 3rd and 4th fingers and toes, midline or symmetric subectodermal hemorrhage
    - Trisomy 13: Facial clefting, holoprosencephaly, polydactyly
    - Trisomy 14, trisomy 15: Facial clefting, delayed limb development
  - Isolated anatomic anomalies, such as neural tube defects or cleft palate, may be found with significance similar to that of older fetus
- Sections to be submitted
  - Villous parenchyma
  - Implantation site decidua

Ancillary Studies

- Consider submission of chorionic plate or villous tissue for molecular karyotype or routine cytogenetics
  - Chromosomal microarray analysis recommended by ACOG and Society for Maternal Fetal Medicine
    - Detects submicroscopic changes in addition to large changes of chromosomes
    - Should obtain informed consent from parent to order
    - Fresh; formalin-fixed; or formalin-fixed, paraffin-embedded tissue can be submitted for chromosomal microarray array
  - Especially useful in recurrent pregnancy loss or in cases of morphologically normal embryo
  - Submit embryonic tissue if it appears viable

Categories of Growth Disorganization

- GD system describes embryonic development in spontaneous abortion
- GD1: Intact, empty sac (no embryo)
- GD2: Nodular embryo, cannot distinguish cranial from caudal end
- GD3: Cylindrical embryo, can distinguish cranial end with retinal pigment
- GD4: Recognizable embryonic development with delayed or abnormal development based upon expected features for crown-rump length

MICROSCOPIC

Confirming Intrauterine Pregnancy

- Identification of implantation site decidua
  - Need "invasive" extravillous cytotrophoblast, maternal vascular remodeling, and deposition of fibrinoid in decidua
  - Confirms intrauterine pregnancy even when villi are not identified
- Identification of villi
  - Be cautious if only rare villi or isolated syncytiotrophoblasts are found without implantation site decidua (cannot exclude villous migration from tubal pregnancy)

Distinguishing Hydropic Degeneration From Hydatidiform Mole

- No excessive villous trophoblastic proliferation in hydropic degeneration
  - Trophoblast proliferation is appropriately confined to poles of anchoring villi

Placental Evaluation in Special Circumstances

- o Trophoblast layer typically appears thin and atrophic in early embryonic death with extensively hydropic villi
- p57 (KIP2) immunostaining helpful in hydropic degeneration vs. complete mole

Estimating Time of Embryonic Demise
- Hydropic swelling of villi
  - o Fluid transferred from trophoblast into stroma of early noncollagenized villi accumulates with no vasculature to absorb it
  - o Hydropic villi are extensive in very early embryonic loss ("blighted ova"); often before 6.5 weeks post LMP with no fetal erythroblasts [nucleated red blood cells (NRBC)]
  - o Later embryonic death associated with mixture of hydropic and fibrotic villi
- Fibrosis of villi
  - o Usually seen in embryonic loss after 7-8 weeks post LMP, when villous fibroblasts are more abundant
- Percentage of NRBC in fetal vasculature
  - o Erythroid elements persist in linear arrangements even though endothelial cells degenerate quickly after embryonic demise
  - o Hemangioblastic foci rich in erythroblasts develop in chorionic plate and villi from 6 weeks post LMP
  - o Nearly all fetal villous RBC are NRBC from 6.5-9.0 weeks post LMP
  - o NRBC are rapidly replaced with nonnucleated RBC from hepatic hematopoiesis from 9-12 weeks post LMP as embryonic circulation is established, connecting placental vascular network with embryo
  - o < 5% of fetal erythrocytes are nucleated after 12 weeks post LMP

Villous Changes in Pregnancy Loss With Normal Karyotype
- Chronic villitis, plasma cell deciduitis, and chronic histiocytic intervillositis are all associated with recurrence
- Massively increased perivillous fibrin deposition with extravillous trophoblast proliferation associated with recurrence
  - o Increased perivillous fibrin without extravillous trophoblast proliferation, seen with embryonic demise after 8-12 weeks
    - Due to blood clotting and prolonged retention; lacks clinical significance of massive perivillous fibrin deposition
- Heavy acute inflammation: Acute chorioamnionitis is uncommon in 1st trimester

Villous Morphology Associated With Abnormal Karyotype
- Dysmorphic changes described in association with karyotypic abnormalities but have limited sensitivity and specificity
  - o Irregularity of villous shape with trophoblastic pseudoinclusions
  - o Stromal cell cytomegaly or hypercellular stroma
  - o Only changes of complete and partial hydatidiform moles have significant reproducibility

Other Microscopic Changes
- Spontaneous abortion specimens show less physiologic conversion of spiral arteries for pregnancy compared to therapeutic abortion specimens
  - o Spiral arteries may appear patent when they should normally be occluded by trophoblast
    - Unclear if this is primary cause of pregnancy loss; may be due to chromosomally abnormal trophoblast cells and poor remodeling
- Decidua frequently shows hemorrhage, necrosis, and focal acute inflammation, reflecting physiology of abortion
  - o Chronic inflammation may be associated with implantation problems
- Acute villitis, abscess formation, granulomas, or viral cytopathic changes are consistent with infection

FINAL DIAGNOSIS REPORTING
Clinical Data
- Gestational age by LMP
- Procedure that produced specimen (D&C, vacuum, spontaneous passage)

Data From Pathologic Exam
- Components present
  - o Gestational sac (ruptured or intact) or fragments of amnion/chorion
  - o Embryo (with crown-rump length, status of anatomic development), if present (or note if absent)
  - o Presence and status of villi (e.g., edema, fibrosis), associated pathology
  - o Implantation site decidua and maternal vessels

Diagnostic Comment
- Note likely retention period based upon evaluation of villous features, especially percentage of NRBC
- Correlate with results of chromosomal microarray or cytogenetics when available

SELECTED REFERENCES
1. Sahoo T et al: Comprehensive genetic analysis of pregnancy loss by chromosomal microarrays: outcomes, benefits, and challenges. Genet Med. 19(1):83-89, 2017
2. Aplin JD et al: Hemangioblastic foci in human first trimester placenta: distribution and gestational profile. Placenta. 36(10):1069-77, 2015
3. Dhillon RK et al: Additional information from chromosomal microarray analysis (CMA) over conventional karyotyping when diagnosing chromosomal abnormalities in miscarriage: a systematic review and meta-analysis. BJOG. 121(1):11-21, 2014
4. Waters BL et al: Significance of perivillous fibrin/oid deposition in uterine evacuation specimens. Am J Surg Pathol. 30(6):760-5, 2006
5. Redline RW et al: Prevalence of developmental and inflammatory lesions in nonmolar first-trimester spontaneous abortions. Hum Pathol. 30(1):93-100, 1999
6. Kalousek DK: Clinical significance of morphologic and genetic examination of spontaneously aborted embryos. Am J Reprod Immunol. 39(2):108-19, 1998
7. Kohut KG et al: Decidual and placental histologic findings in patients experiencing spontaneous abortions in relation to pregnancy order. Am J Reprod Immunol. 37(3):257-61, 1997
8. van Lijnschoten G et al: The value of histomorphological features of chorionic villi in early spontaneous abortion for the prediction of karyotype. Histopathology. 22(6):557-63, 1993
9. Szulman AE: Examination of the early conceptus. Arch Pathol Lab Med. 115(7):696-700, 1991
10. Novak R et al: Histologic analysis of placental tissue in first trimester abortions. Pediatr Pathol. 8(5):477-82, 1988

Embryonic Development

Crown-Rump Length (mm)	Days After Ovulation	Stage	Main External Feature	Placenta
	0-2	1	Fertilized egg	
	2-4	2	Morula	
	4-6	3	Blastocyst	
0.1		4	Bilaminar embryo	
0.2-0.4	6-15	5	Bilaminar embryo with yolk sac	
		6	Trilaminar embryo with primitive streak	Mesenchyme from primitive streak migrates to inner surface of trophoblast, early primary villous formation begins
0.4-1.0	15-17	7	Trilaminar embryo with notochordal process	
1.0-1.5	18-20	8	Primitive pit and notochordal canal formed	
1.5-2.0	20-22	9	Deep neural groove; 1st somites present; heart tubes begin to fuse	
2-3	22-24	10	Neural folds begin to fuse; heart begins to beat; embryo is straight; 4-12 pairs of somites	
3.4	24-26	11	Rostral neuropore closing; embryo slightly curved; 13-20 pairs of somites	
4.5	26-30	12	Upper limb buds appear; caudal neuropore closed; tail appearing	
5-6	28-32 (~ 6 weeks post LMP)	13	4 pairs of branchial arches; lower limb buds appear; tail present; 30 somites	Hemangioblastic foci seen in primary chorionic plate and villi with nucleated RBC
6-7	31-35	14	Lens pits and nasal pits visible; optic cups present	
7-10	35-38	15	Hand plates formed; lens vesicles and nasal pits prominent	Erythropoiesis begins in liver
10-12	37-42	16	Foot plates formed; nasal pits face ventrally; pigment visible in retina	
12-14	42-44 (~ 8 weeks post LMP)	17	Finger rays appear; auricular hillocks developed; upper lip formed	Nonnucleated RBC appear in placental fetal vessels
14-17	44-48	18	Toe rays and elbow region appear; eyelids are forming; ambiguous genital tubercle seen	Nonnucleated RBC comprise 10% of placental fetal vessel RBC at 9 weeks post LMP
16-20	48-51	19	Trunk elongating and straightening; midgut herniation into umbilical cord	Progressive replacement of nucleated erythroblasts with nonnucleated RBC
20-22	51-53	20	Fingers distinct but webbed; scalp vascular plexus appears	
22-24	53-54	21	Fingers free and longer; toes still webbed	
24-28	54-56	22	Toes free and longer; eyelids and external ear more developed	
28-30	56-60 (~ 10-11 weeks post LMP)	23	Head more rounded; fusing eyelids	By 12 weeks post LMP, only 5% nucleated erythroblasts persist

LMP = last menstrual period; RBC = red blood cells.

Kalousek DK: Clinical significance of morphologic and genetic examination of spontaneously aborted embryos. Am J Reprod Immunol. 39(2):108-19, 1998; Szulman AE: Examination of the early conceptus. Arch Pathol Lab Med. 115(7):696-700, 1991; Aplin JD et al: Hemangioblastic foci in human first trimester placenta: Distribution and gestational profile. Placenta. 36(10):1069-77, 2015.

Embryo in Amniotic Sac

(Left) *This large amniotic sac has a very small, malformed embryo* ⇨ *that was found to have trisomy 13. The white structure overlying the fetus is the involuted yolk sac* ⇨. (Right) *The embryo from the large gestational sac shows midline clefting* ➡ *and delayed limb development* ➡. *Cytogenetics revealed trisomy 13.*

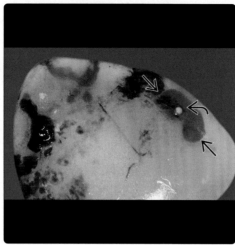

GD4 Embryo With Abnormal Development

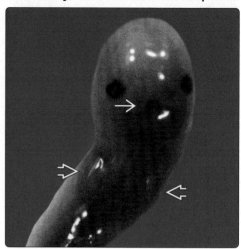

Embryo With Ectopia Cordis

(Left) *Gestational sac from a 1st-trimester spontaneous abortion shows a fetus with ectopia cordis* ➡. *There is also a midline facial cleft* ➡. (Right) *Embryo has a severe abdominal wall defect* ⇨, *allowing the entire abdominal contents to extrude into the amniotic sac, and also extrophy of the bladder* ⇨. *Asymmetry of the lower extremities indicates that this is likely a limb/body wall malformation.*

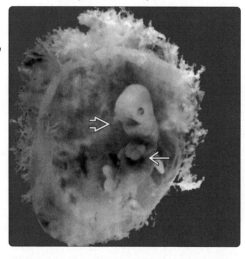

Embryo With Abdominal Wall Defect

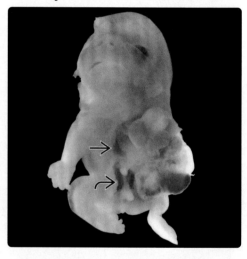

Neural Tube Defect

(Left) *Embryo (days 44-46) with an open neural tube defect* ⇨ *and encephalocele* ⇨ *is shown. The neural tube is completely closed at day 28. (From DP: Placenta.)* (Right) *This 11-weeks-gestation fetus has Turner syndrome (monosomy X). There is a large cystic hygroma of the neck* ➡ *and massive hydrops. (From DP: Placenta.)*

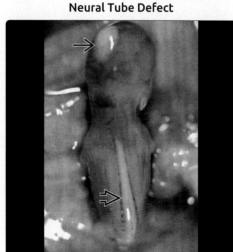

Nuchal Cystic Hygroma, 45,X

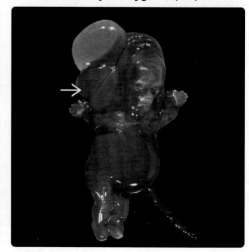

Villi With Hydropic Degeneration

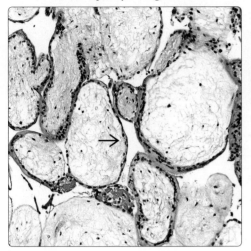

Abnormal Villous Morphology

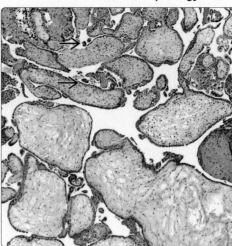

(Left) *Hydropic degeneration is a common finding with blighted ovum. The villi are nearly avascular with lightly staining stroma. The syncytiotrophoblast layer is thin and atrophic* ⇨. **(Right)** *The mixture of hydropic and fibrous-appearing villi is usually found later in 1st-trimester embryonic demise and may be associated with chromosomal abnormalities. Syncytiotrophoblast sprouts* ⇨ *may be seen as a normal feature of early placental growth.*

100% Nucleated Red Blood Cells

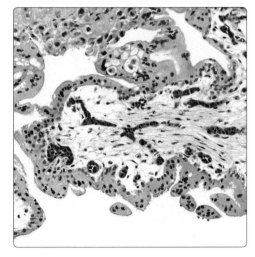

11-Weeks-Gestation Villi

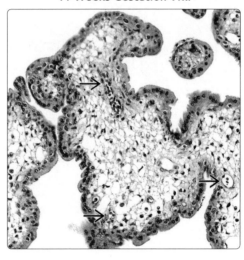

(Left) *The percentage of nucleated red blood cells in the villous capillaries helps date the embryonic age at demise. At 7 weeks (seen here), all of the erythrocytes are enlarged, nucleated forms arising from the yolk sac. The villous red blood cells persist even after capillaries degenerate.* **(Right)** *Villi from 11-weeks gestation (post last menstrual period) show more admixed nonnucleated red blood cells* ⇨. *By this age, more nonnucleated red blood cells are seen, presumably from hepatic hematopoiesis.*

Chronic Histiocytic Intervillositis

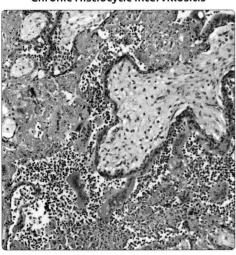

Massive Perivillous Fibrin Deposition

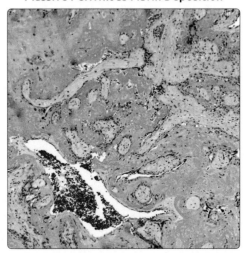

(Left) *H&E shows chronic histiocytic intervillositis of unknown etiology in a 1st-trimester spontaneous abortion specimen. This disorder has a high recurrence risk for future pregnancies.* **(Right)** *Massive perivillous fibrin deposition is most often diagnosed in the 2nd or 3rd trimester. In recurrent cases, it may be seen as early as 8 weeks. Prolonged retention of the tissues is associated with a nonspecific increase in perivillous fibrin.*

Triploid Macerated Fetus

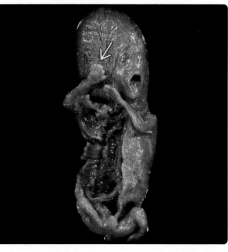

Partial Hydatidiform Mole

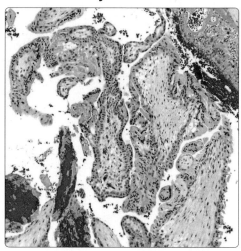

(Left) *It would be easy to overlook the abnormal fusion of the 2nd and 3rd fingers* ➡ *on the hands of this severely macerated triploid fetus.* **(Right)** *Subtle syncytiotrophoblast proliferation is present in a partial hydatidiform mole (PHM). It may be necessary to review multiple slides of villous tissue in order to find all of the features to diagnose a PHM.*

Very Early Complete Hydatidiform Mole

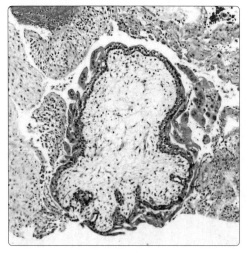

Implantation Trophoblasts of Complete Hydatidiform Mole

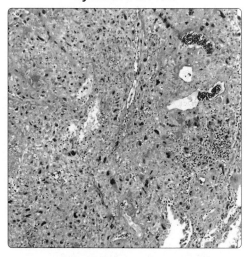

(Left) *Subtle villous irregularity, circumferential trophoblast proliferation, and stromal karyorrhexis are consistent with a complete hydatidiform mole (CHM).* **(Right)** *The invasive trophoblasts at the implantation site of a CHM usually shows significant nuclear hyperchromasia and enlargement. In the 1st trimester, this may be a useful clue to the diagnosis of CHM when villous vesicles and trophoblast proliferation are subtle.*

Stromal Intermediate Trophoblasts

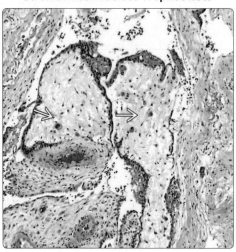

Normal Invasive Trophoblasts

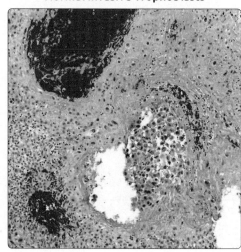

(Left) *The presence of intermediate trophoblasts in the villous stroma* ➡ *is one of the features often associated with chromosomally abnormal conception.* **(Right)** *Implantation site trophoblasts normally invade into the decidua and maternal spiral arteries. They are significantly smaller and less hyperchromatic than the trophoblasts from a CHM.*

Normal-Appearing Embryo

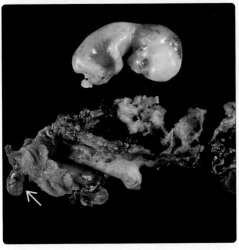

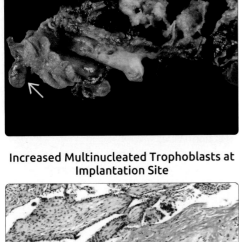

Yolk Sac and Disorganized Embryonic Tissue

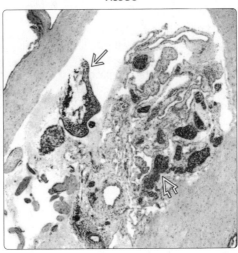

(Left) The embryo is nonmacerated and structurally normal. Occasional villi are present next to pink decidual tissues with admixed blood clot. Rare vesicular villi ➡ may be present, often with villi in the chorion laeve; care is taken to exclude a possible PHM. (Right) There may only be an irregular portion of disorganized embryonic tissue ➡ in 1st-trimester loss. There is abundant hematopoiesis ➤ within the adjacent yolk sac.

Increased Multinucleated Trophoblasts at Implantation Site

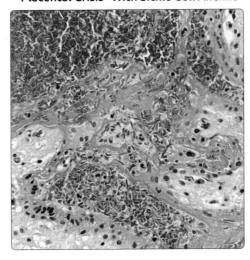

"Placental Crisis" With Sickle Cell Anemia

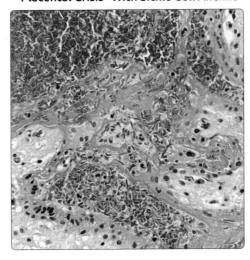

(Left) The large number of multinucleated invasive trophoblasts at the implantation of this pregnancy suggests abnormal implantation as a possible cause of pregnancy loss. (Right) The intervillous space may be a site of sickle cell crisis with thrombosis and ischemia, as in other organs. It is a low oxygen tension site, and sickled cells will frequently be seen in both sickle cell disease and sickle cell trait. Note the presence of villous ischemia and fibrin deposition associated with the sickled red blood cells.

Septic Abortion

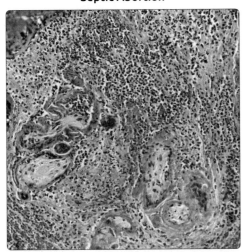

Chronic Chorioamnionitis

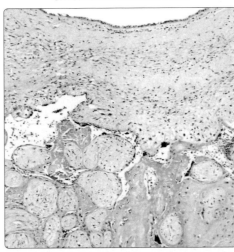

(Left) Acute chorioamnionitis is uncommon in the 1st trimester. Although some acute inflammation is present in most spontaneous abortions, this case has an extensive infiltrate, which is suggestive of the cause of pregnancy loss. (Right) Chronic inflammation is uncommon in the 1st trimester. This case had inflammation in the chorionic plate, villi, and at the basal plate. Immunohistochemistry for CD3 can be helpful to tell T-lymphocytes from immature stroma cells.

CONTENT

Scope of Discussion

- Placental and fetal findings in 2nd-trimester fetal demise (gestational age: 13 weeks and 6 days through 27 weeks and 6 days)
- Findings after termination of pregnancy for fetal anomalies

TERMINOLOGY

Definitions

- Stillbirth: Refers to in utero demise of potentially viable fetus (generally after 20-weeks gestation)
- Miscarriage: Lay term, usually refers to in utero demise of previable fetus (generally before 20-weeks gestation)

EPIDEMIOLOGY

Incidence

- Intrauterine fetal demise (IUFD) is relatively uncommon in 2nd trimester
  ○ 1-5% of pregnancies are lost at 13- to 19-weeks gestation
  ○ 0.3% of pregnancies are lost at 20- to 27-weeks gestation

ETIOLOGY/PATHOGENESIS

Infection

- Ascending infection, chorioamnionitis (amniotic fluid infection sequence): 40-60% of 2nd-trimester fetal deaths
  ○ Organisms, group B *Streptococcus*, *Neisseria gonorrhoeae*, *Gardnerella* spp., *Mycoplasma/Ureaplasma*, *Fusobacterium* spp.
- Hematogenous infection
  ○ TORCH infections: *Toxoplasma gondii*, other (syphilis, varicella-zoster virus, parvovirus B19), rubella, cytomegalovirus (CMV), herpes simplex virus (HSV)

Fetal Chromosomal Abnormalities

- 24% of 2nd-trimester fetal deaths

Placental Insufficiency

- Placenta is unable to support further life of fetus due to loss of functional parenchyma
  ○ Maternal vascular malperfusion evidenced by small placenta, infarcts, distal villous hypoplasia, and decidual arteriopathy
    – Usually occurs after 23-weeks gestation and is often associated with severe preeclampsia, intrauterine growth restriction (IUGR)
  ○ Massively increased perivillous fibrin deposition, associated with IUGR
  ○ Extensive chronic inflammation
    – Chronic villitis in 2nd trimester is uncommon and more likely to be infectious
    – Chronic histiocytic intervillositis
  ○ Acute or chronic placental abruption

Impaired Fetal-Placental Perfusion

- Umbilical cord abnormalities
  ○ Nuchal or body entanglement, knots, amniotic bands, or excessively long and hypercoiled cord, strictures
- Fetal vascular malperfusion (often in association with cord lesions above)
  ○ Differentiate from changes of fetal vascular involution after fetal demise

Fetal-Maternal Hemorrhage

- Acute fetal-maternal hemorrhage (FMH) may have few findings other than relative pallor of parenchyma
- Fetal hydrops, edematous villi lacking fetal erythrocytes, nucleated red blood cells (NRBC) in intervillous space ± intervillous thrombi seen with chronicity

Maternal Conditions

- Cervical incompetence
- Uncontrolled chronic illness (e.g., diabetes, hypertension, autoimmune disease)
- Trauma (e.g., motor vehicle accident, physical abuse)
- Teratogen exposure and smoking/drug use
- Thrombophilia

In Utero Demise Due to Chorioamnionitis

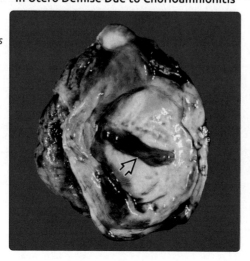

Necrotizing Acute and Subacute Chorioamnionitis

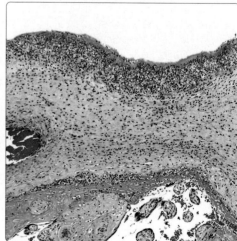

(Left) This late 2nd-trimester placenta shows a purulent amniotic surface & membranes characteristic of subacute necrotizing chorioamnionitis. The umbilical cord is edematous & congested ➡. (DP: Placenta.) (Right) Subacute necrotizing chorioamnionitis is typically seen in the 2nd trimester and usually associated with infection of up to 2 weeks. It may be associated with premature birth or fetal demise.

- Müllerian duct and uterine anomalies, uterine septa or bicornuate uterus

Amniotic Band Syndrome

- Rupture of amniotic sac, usually before fusion with chorion in 1st trimester
  o Amniotic sheets may attach to skin of skull or face, resulting in disruptions
  o Limb/body wall complex refers to contiguity of amnion with some portion of body wall, typically abdomen (early defect in morphogenesis)
  o Bands may constrict extremities &/or cord in otherwise normally developed fetus

CLINICAL IMPLICATIONS

Clinical Presentation

- Loss of fetal movement
- Vaginal bleeding
- Abdominal cramping
- Absence of fetal heartbeat

Imaging Findings

- US may identify ≥ 1 fetal anomaly
- Placental and umbilical cord lesions are less commonly identified

Procedures

- Dilation and evacuation (D&E): Fetus and placenta are fragmented
- Induction of labor: Less commonly performed; intact fetus is delivered

MACROSCOPIC

General Features

- Most institutions require consent for examination of intact fetus > 20-weeks gestation; some require consent for dissection of intact fetus at any gestational age
- According to American Board of Pathology, autopsy of fragmented fetuses from pregnancy terminations for malformations or genetic disease fulfills autopsy requirements, provided standard protocol is used for examination
- Majority of 2nd-trimester IUFD or termination of pregnancy specimens are fragmented after D&E
  o D&E specimen: Surgical pathology specimen requiring pathologic examination
    – Autopsy may be requested
  o Use of standardized template improves ability to find causes of IUFD
  o Surgical pathology exam should confirm that all major fetal skeletal parts are present
    – Retention of fetal part in uterus is uncommon but may have associated maternal morbidity
  o Placenta and cord examination should be performed as thoroughly as possible
    – Especially useful in cases of unexplained IUFD
  o Anomalies identified on US are variably confirmed on pathologic examination
    – CNS malformations almost never confirmed due to disruption of brain tissues

- Genitourinary anomalies frequently confirmed as intact kidneys and bladder are readily identified
- Cardiac malformations are variably confirmed, expertise in dissection along lines of flow is useful: Intracardiac potassium chloride injection with fetal termination yields macerated heart tissue; difficult to assess
- Abnormalities of extremities (e.g., polydactyly, ectrodactyly) usually confirmed
- Neural tube defects variably confirmed; sac is usually disrupted, but bony defects remain identifiable

- Intact organs are weighed, appropriate growth for age is assessed with normative tables
  o Tables available that take into account degree of tissue maceration
  o Tables available for weight of formalin-fixed fetal organs
- Sections to be submitted
  o Sections of umbilical cord, membranes, chorionic plate, and placental parenchyma should be submitted as for intact placenta
  o Fetal lung and cross sections of fetal stomach and gastrointestinal tract aid in confirming amniotic fluid infection sequence as cause of fetal demise
  o Fetal heart, liver, and kidney are useful for dating in utero demise-to-delivery interval and confirming pathology (e.g., renal cystic disease)
- Intact fetus is evaluated with same approach as used in standard autopsy
  o Document anomalies of anatomic development
  o Posterior approach with exposure of cervical spinal cord and posterior fossa useful for documenting CNS malformations (e.g., Dandy-Walker and Arnold-Chiari)
- Ancillary studies
  o Skin or placental samples for cytogenetics or chromosomal microarray
    – Most useful with fetal anomalies
    – Chromosomal microarray recommended by American College of Obstetricians and Gynecologists (ACOG) on all IUFD
  o In cases of fetal growth restriction with no identifiable cause, consider genomic evaluation of placenta for confined placental mosaicism
    – 4 samples from different regions of placenta sampled for karyotype (fresh tissue) or chromosomal microarray (fresh, formalin-fixed, or formalin-fixed, paraffin-embedded tissue)
  o Microbiology cultures may be performed on placental and fetal tissues if clinically desired
  o Specimen radiographs useful in suspected skeletal dysplasia, fetal anomalies and some cases of IUGR

Artifacts

- Intact, late, 1st- or early 2nd-trimester fetuses (gestational ages 9-16 weeks) may show artifactual dislocation of CNS tissue into soft tissue of retroperitoneum, neck, shoulders, buttocks, pelvis
  o May mimic tumor on gross exam

Findings Compatible With Specific Chromosomal Abnormalities on Dilation & Evacuation Examination

Chromosomal Abnormality	Gross Finding
Monosomy X (Turner syndrome)	Fetal hydrops, prominent dorsal edema of hands and feet, coarctation of aorta
Trisomy 18	Overlapping fingers, rocker-bottom feet, polydactyly
Trisomy 13	Severe craniofacial abnormalities, including holoprosencephaly, midline cleft lip, abnormal skull base, polydactyly, splenopancreatic fusion, and heart defects
Trisomy 21	Wide space between 1st and 2nd toes, clinodactyly, single palmar crease, heart defects, and duodenal atresia
Triploidy	Syndactyly of 3rd and 4th digits

From Ernst LM et al: Pathologic examination of fetal and placental tissue obtained by dilation and evacuation. Arch Pathol Lab Med 137:326-337; 2012.

MICROSCOPIC

Placenta, Cord, and Membranes

- Look for evidence of amniotic fluid infection; special stains for organisms may be considered
- Look for fetal thrombi and organizing changes of fetal vascular malperfusion; correlate with gross umbilical cord findings
- Look for villous parenchymal processes, e.g., chronic villitis, chronic histiocytic intervillositis, massive perivillous fibrin deposition
- Look for changes of uteroplacental malperfusion, e.g., distal villous hypoplasia, villous agglutination, infarcts
- Look for evidence of hematogenous infection
  - Plasmacytic chronic villitis, viral inclusions in CMV infection; correlate with fetal organ histology, confirm with immunohistochemistry or PCR
  - Fetal erythroblastosis with intranuclear inclusions and hydrops in parvovirus B19 infection
- Look for evidence of FMH
  - Pallor of placenta and fetal organs in acute FMH
  - Extensive villous edema, erythroblastosis, intervillous NRBC, with chronicity
  - Correlate with maternal Kleihauer-Betke or flow cytometry for fetal hemoglobin studies for fetal-maternal transfusion

Fetal Organs

- Evaluate lungs and stomach/gastrointestinal tract lumen for aspirated or swallowed neutrophils in amniotic fluid infection sequence
- Liver and adrenal glands useful for identification of viral inclusions of CMV and HSV
- Heart, lung, kidney, and liver autolysis useful for estimating in utero demise-to-delivery interval
- Kidney especially useful in estimating gestational age
- Specific anomalies such as cystic kidneys may be further classified

CHECKLIST FOR EVALUATION OF DILATION & EVACUATION SPECIMEN

Fetus

- Separate fetal tissues from placental and decidual tissues
- Measure foot length for assessment of growth
- Confirm skeletal parts are complete

- Note degree of maceration (dull, tan skin and dehydrated tissue in prolonged retention after fetal demise)
- Examine tissues for anatomic anomalies other than procedure-related disruption
  - Head (usually collapsed with fragments of cranium)
  - Face
    - Note presence and any abnormalities of eyes, ears, nose, mouth, and palate
    - Ear position is difficult to assess in young &/or fragmented fetus, but cleft palate is easily identified
  - 4 extremities
    - Fingers, palmar creases (develop in early 2nd trimester), toes, foot length
  - Fragments of rib and vertebral column
  - External genitalia
    - Urethral groove closes in male by 12 weeks, develops into labia in female
  - Internal genitalia (identified in 40% of D&E specimens)
  - Loose organs
    - Heart, lungs, GI tract, liver, and kidneys are nearly always identified
    - Adrenal glands are found in majority of specimens
    - Pancreas, spleen, and thymus are found in < 50% of specimens

Placenta

- Placental tissues should be examined as completely as possible and standard tissue submitted for microscopic examination

Disposition of Specimen

- Determined by state law and hospital policy; hospital disposal often acceptable for < 20-week fetus
- Family may request burial or cremation of intact or disrupted fetal remains at any gestational age

SELECTED REFERENCES

1. Ernst LM et al: Pathologic examination of fetal and placental tissue obtained by dilation and evacuation. Arch Pathol Lab Med. 137(3):326-37, 2013
2. Hauerberg L et al: Correlation between prenatal diagnosis by ultrasound and fetal autopsy findings in second-trimester abortions. Acta Obstet Gynecol Scand. 91(3):386-90, 2012
3. Gambhir PS et al: Chronic umbilical cord entanglements causing intrauterine fetal demise in the second trimester. Pediatr Dev Pathol. 14(3):252-4, 2011
4. Maroun LL et al: Autopsy standards of body parameters and fresh organ weights in nonmacerated and macerated human fetuses. Pediatr Dev Pathol. 8(2):204-17, 2005

Anomalous Fetus With Exencephaly

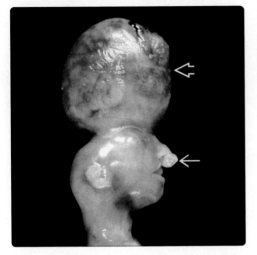

Bowel Calcifications in Fetal Demise

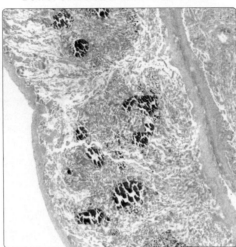

(Left) *This intact fetus with trisomy 13 has a cleft lip and palate ➡ and exencephaly ➡. In the fragmented fetus, facial clefting may still be identified, as well as fragments of skin overlying the exencephalic brain tissue. (DP: Placenta.)* (Right) *Aneuploidy is associated with echogenic bowel on prenatal US, which is most likely the result of these block-like calcifications within the bowel contents. These are preserved even with severe maceration.*

Alobar Holoprosencephaly

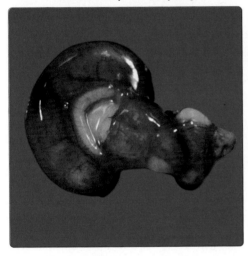

Anomalies in Trisomy 13

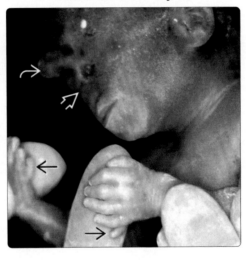

(Left) *Alobar holoprosencephaly is characteristic of trisomy 13 and triploidy. Malformations such as this, hydrocephalus, Dandy-Walker, lissencephaly, and polymicrogyria are only rarely identifiable in dilation & evacuation (D&E) specimens.* (Right) *This fetus with trisomy 13 has postaxial polydactyly ➡. There is also cyclopia with incomplete fusion of the eyes ➡ and proboscis ➡ that is usually associated with alobar holoprosencephaly.*

Anomalies in Trisomy 18

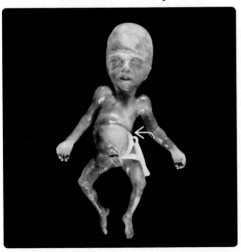

Fetal Hydrops

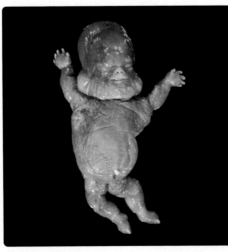

(Left) *This fetus with trisomy 18 has a large omphalocele ➡. Omphalocele and gastroschisis are only variably identifiable in the fragmented fetus of a D&E procedure.* (Right) *Marked fetal edema may be associated with Turner syndrome (monosomy X), trisomy 21 (as in this case), or erythroblastosis fetalis and parvovirus B19 infection.*

Placental Evaluation in Special Circumstances

Anencephaly

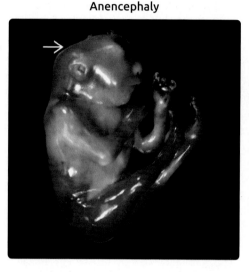

Thanatophoric Dysplasia

(Left) In contrast to other CNS malformations, anencephaly ➡ usually can be confirmed in D&E specimens. Upper extremities show flexion contractures and lower extremities fixed extension, consistent with arthrogryposis. (DP: Placenta.) (Right) Thanatophoric dysplasia is the most common lethal chondrodysplasia. This type of fetus should always be x-rayed, and multiple bones should be decalcified for microscopic examination including calvarium, vertebra, and femurs.

Congenital Diaphragmatic Hernia

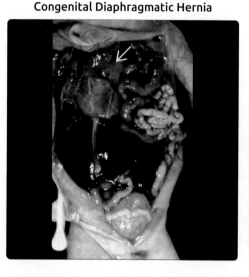

Gastroschisis

(Left) Diaphragmatic hernia is seen with the majority of the intestines occupying the left chest, shifting the heart to the right. The hypoplastic left lung ➡ is pushed to the right. Presence of the liver in the left chest is associated with more severe pulmonary hypoplasia. (DP: Placenta.) (Right) This fetus shows extrusion of bowel loops through a defect ➡ in the abdominal wall (gastroschisis). The defect is usually to the left of the umbilical cord.

Adrenal Situs in Renal Aplasia

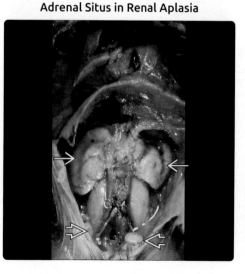

Amnion Nodosum

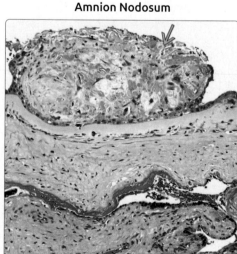

(Left) Bilateral renal agenesis is associated with severe pulmonary hypoplasia and oligohydramnios. In the absence of kidneys, the adrenal glands ➡ assume a flattened configuration in the retroperitoneum, which on US may be mistaken for kidneys. The testes ➡ are seen within the abdominal cavity. (Right) Amnion nodosum ➡ is seen in renal agenesis, due to prolonged oligohydramnios with accumulation of amniotic fluid debris.

Examination of the Dilation & Evacuation Specimen

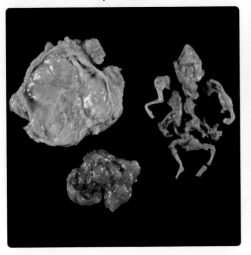

Confirming Anomalies in the Dilation & Evacuation Specimen

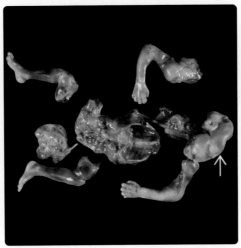

(Left) Surgical pathology examination of D&E tissues starts with separation into fetal, placental, and decidual parts. (Right) Anencephaly ➡ is one of the few CNS abnormalities identifiable in fragmented fetuses. Cranium is usually collapsed in D&E fetus to allow removal with extensive disruption of brain tissues. In anencephaly, head may be delivered intact.

Amputation Due to Amniotic Bands

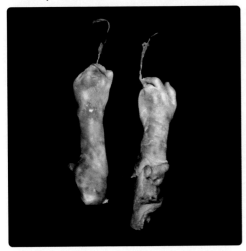

Ectrodactyly

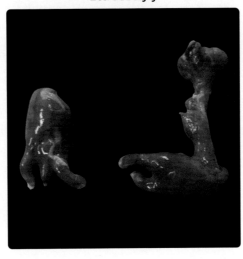

(Left) These upper extremities show multiple amputations of the fingers with attached bands, due to early amnion rupture. (Right) These upper extremities show severe abnormalities of the fingers and radii. The DDx includes numerous syndromes, such as VATER, Holt-Oram, and Roberts-SC phocomelia. Careful documentation of anomalies allows the surgical pathologist to work together with medical geneticists in establishing a diagnosis for the family.

Osteogenesis Imperfecta

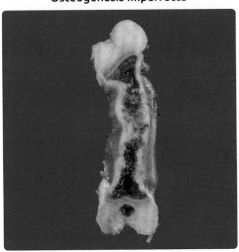

Histology of Osteogenesis Imperfecta

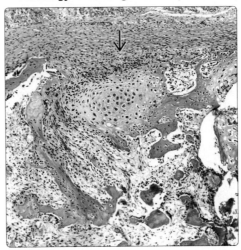

(Left) This femur from a fetus with osteogenesis imperfecta shows the crinkled bone appearance caused by multiple cortical fractures. (Right) The histology of osteogenesis imperfecta type II shows disrupted cortical bone with a nodule of cartilage ➡ and irregularly oriented trabecular bone, consistent with a healing fracture.

Placental Evaluation in Special Circumstances

333

Cord Constriction Due to Amniotic Bands

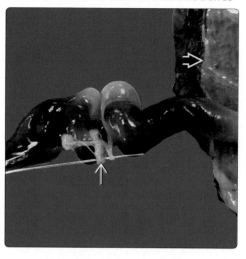

Chorion Nodosum

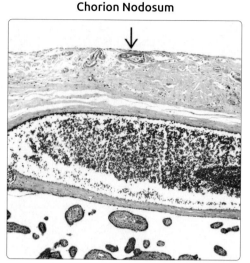

(Left) *Amniotic bands ➡ may also constrict the umbilical cord, causing fetal demise. Note the opacity of the chorionic plate ➡ due to thickening of the denuded chorion.* (Right) *Chorion nodosum occurs after prolonged rupture of the amnion. There is thickening of the chorion, which has embedded amniotic fluid debris ➡.*

IUFD Due to Excessively Long, Hypercoiled Cord With Strictures

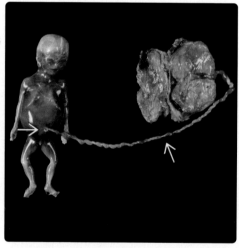

Fetal Vascular Malperfusion

(Left) *The cord is long and hypercoiled with strictures ➡. Fetuses with this condition may become hydropic, as suggested by the swollen abdomen in this case.* (Right) *Umbilical cord compromise is a mechanism of fetal vascular malperfusion. This stem vessel has fibroblast proliferation and extravasation of red blood cells, an early change of stem vessel obliteration. In this field, there are also avascular villi ➡. Focality and temporal heterogeneity of the changes helps distinguish them from involution after fetal demise.*

Fetal Vascular Malperfusion

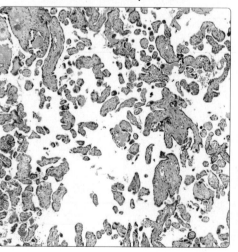

Subchorionic Hematoma

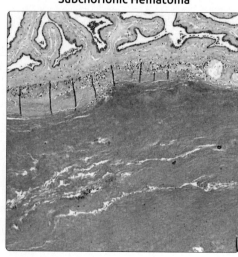

(Left) *Fetal vascular malperfusion may cause growth restriction, premature birth, or in utero death. Image shows distal villous hypoplasia with small, poorly vascularized villi and exaggerated syncytial knots. These changes are often associated with preterm preeclampsia.* (Right) *Vaginal bleeding and finding of hematoma on US increases risk of pregnancy complications. Image shows residua of a subchorionic hematoma noted on early US. Longstanding hemorrhage may show hemosiderin-laden macrophages in the chorion.*

Chronic Histiocytic Intervillositis

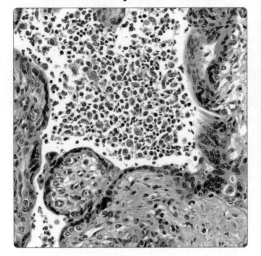

Massive Perivillous Fibrin Deposition

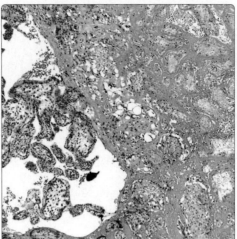

(Left) *Chronic histiocytic intervillositis is a cause of recurrent pregnancy complications with intrauterine growth restriction and fetal loss. It is associated with maternal autoantibodies.* (Right) *Massive perivillous fibrin deposition is associated with severe intrauterine growth restriction and fetal demise. It also has a significant risk for recurrence. Preserved villi are surrounded by placental matrix-type fibrin with abundant extravillous trophoblast embedded in the fibrin. With time the villi become necrotic.*

Chronic Villitis

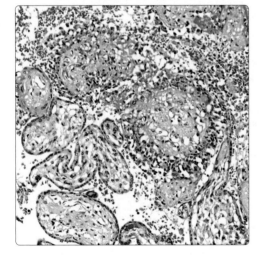

Cytomegalovirus

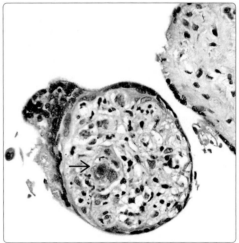

(Left) *Chronic villitis of unknown etiology is less common in the 2nd trimester; infection should be strongly considered, especially with fetal demise.* (Right) *CMV infection, characterized by owl-eyed viral inclusions* ⊡.

Storage Changes in Galactosialidosis

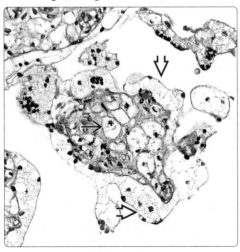

Dysmorphic Villi

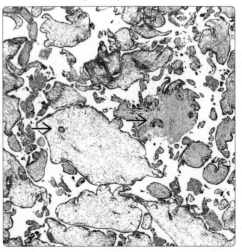

(Left) *The placenta may also contain clues to genetic disorders of the fetus. Villi from this fetus with galactosialidosis show massive vacuolization of the syncytiotrophoblast* ⊡ *and Hofbauer cells* ⊡. (Right) *Dysmorphic villi are frequently associated with chromosomal abnormalities. The villi show marked variation in size and shape. There are large edematous villi and small fibrotic villi. Irregular contours result in formation of trophoblast pseudoinclusions* ⊡.

TERMINOLOGY

Definitions

- Demise or stillbirth of fetus after 24 weeks of pregnancy

EPIDEMIOLOGY

Incidence

- 0.3% of pregnancies are lost at 24- to 40-weeks gestation

ETIOLOGY/PATHOGENESIS

General

- Fetal demise may result from multiple additive maternal, fetal, and placental processes
- Conditions associated with fetal demise are similar to those causing intrauterine growth restriction (IUGR), premature birth, and significant neonatal morbidity
  - These unfortunate outcomes are on same biologic continuum
  - Delayed villous maturation is an exception: Not associated with IUGR or prematurity but significant contributor to late fetal demise

Placental Causes of Fetal Demise

- Subacute and chronic processes
  - Increased fetal growth in 3rd trimester imposes further demands on placental function
    - Compromised placenta may be unable to meet those demands
    - Placenta with delayed villous maturation unable to meet needs of near-term fetal physiology
  - Subacute/chronic conditions
    - Maternal vascular malperfusion characterized by small placenta, infarcts, distal villous hypoplasia, decidual arteriopathy
    - Extensive chronic villitis (usually villitis of unknown etiology)
    - Massively increased perivillous fibrin deposition

- Fetal vascular malperfusion with single umbilical artery, marginal, velamentous, or furcate cord insertion, hypercoiled cord
- Complications of twin or higher order birth gestations (twin-twin transfusion, small placental share)
- Prolonged amniotic fluid infection
- Chronic fetal-maternal transfusion
- Acute processes
  - Placental abruption
  - Acute umbilical cord obstruction
    - May be caused by umbilical cord prolapse, cord rupture, kinking/compression, thrombosis
    - Also acute-on-chronic exacerbation of a nuchal/limb/body cord entanglement due to increased fetal growth and physical changes in intrauterine environment with labor
  - Ruptured vasa previa
  - Massive fetal-maternal hemorrhage
  - Acute amniotic fluid infection (fetal outcome may depend upon virulence of microorganism)

Maternal Factors

- Uncontrolled chronic illness
  - Obesity, especially BMI > 40
  - Hypertension; preeclampsia; hemolysis, elevated liver enzymes, low platelets (HELLP) syndrome
    - May show changes of abruption &/or maternal vascular malperfusion in placenta
  - Diabetes, especially pregestational diabetes
  - Systemic lupus erythematosus and other immunologic conditions
  - Postterm pregnancy
- Severe acute illness
  - Maternal sepsis, acute pneumonia, pyelonephritis, appendicitis, diabetic ketoacidosis
- Incompetent cervix
  - May show changes of amniotic fluid infection
- Uterine leiomyomata
- Alcohol, smoking, drug use, and teratogen exposure

Severe Acute Chorioamnionitis

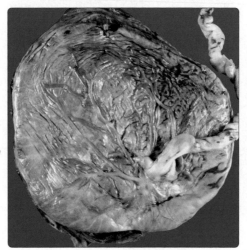

Delayed Villous Maturation

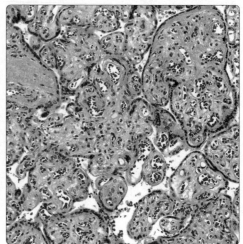

(Left) *Severe acute chorioamnionitis, as seen in this case with purulent membranes, can be a cause of premature birth of a sick baby or 3rd-trimester fetal demise. The processes are on a continuum.* (Right) *Delayed villous maturation is associated with late fetal demise. The lack of sufficient vasculosyncytial membranes in distal villi impairs gas and nutrient exchange.*

- Trauma (e.g., motor vehicle accident, physical abuse, etc.), uterine rupture
- Thrombophilia
  o Factor V Leiden, protein S deficiency, and prothrombin G20210A mutation

Fetal Factors

- Syndromes and single malformations account for ~ 10% of stillbirths; these include chromosomal abnormalities
  o Chromosomal abnormalities
    – 4% of 3rd-trimester stillbirths are due to aneuploidy
    – Majority have characteristic dysmorphic features and malformations
  o Anatomic malformations
    – Congenital heart defects (CHD) most common; recurrence risk in subsequent pregnancies is 2-3%
    – 25-33% of CHDs have syndromic features, 5-10% have chromosomal defects, 3% are attributed to single gene defects
    – Neural tube defects, renal abnormalities, congenital diaphragmatic hernia are less common
- Developmental disruptions, dysplasias, and metabolic disorders comprise < 5% of stillbirth causes
  o Metabolic/storage diseases are very rare
  o Severe fetal anemia with hydrops
    – 30% die in utero
    – Hydrops occurs once critical level of anemia is reached (hematocrit of < 15%)
- Congenital tumors
  o Most commonly sacrococcygeal teratoma, usually associated with hydrops due to high-output failure
- Complications of twinning
  o Twin-to-twin transfusion, acardiac twinning, conjoined twins

MACROSCOPIC

General Features

- Placental examination is essential to determine cause of fetal demise
  o While fetal autopsy is ideal for thorough investigation, placental exam identifies cause of fetal demise more frequently than autopsy or cytogenetics
    – Placenta yields cause of death in up to 35% of stillbirths; may be only source for diagnosis in 16%
- Careful attention to umbilical cord pathology is warranted
  o Portions of umbilical cord may be submitted for cultures or other laboratory studies
    – If possible, these should be retrieved for pathologic examination after necessary samples are obtained

MICROSCOPIC

General Features

- Placental findings in stillbirth are similar to those associated with IUGR or premature birth with exception of delayed villous maturation

Infection

- Ascending infection
  o Amniotic fluid infection sequence

  – Maternal inflammatory response: Acute or subacute chorioamnionitis
  – Fetal inflammatory response: Umbilical vasculitis, chorionic plate vasculitis
  – Frequent cause of postterm in utero demise (after 41-weeks gestation)
- Hematogenous infection: Chronic villitis and intervillositis
  o Chronic villitis in 3rd trimester is usually due to idiopathic maternal immune response
  o ~ 5% of cases are due to infections (especially cytomegalovirus)
    – Fetus may have hydrops

Maternal Vascular Malperfusion

- Often associated with maternal hypertensive conditions, preeclampsia
- Acute retroplacental hemorrhage
- Chronic marginal abruption
- Small placenta with multiple infarcts, distal villous hypoplasia, accelerated villous maturation, increased syncytial knots
- Decidual arteriopathy

Fetal Vascular Malperfusion

- Umbilical cord pathology
  o Includes gross abnormalities, such as
    – Single umbilical artery
    – Abnormal insertion
    – Hypercoiling
    – Obstruction
    – Thrombi
  o Proposed criteria for diagnosis of umbilical cord compromise as cause of stillbirth
    – Dilated fetal vessels (vascular ectasia to ≥ 4x diameter of adjacent muscular vessel)
    – Thrombi of fetal muscular vessels [organized thrombi, organizing thrombi, and loss of endothelial integrity with bridging strands of fibrous connective tissue and extravasation of endothelial cells (fibromuscular sclerosis)]
    – Focal or regional presence of avascular villi or villous stromal karyorrhexis
    – Familiarity with vascular involutional changes after fetal demise is essential for proper utilization of proposed criteria, as similar changes may be due to demise alone

Delayed Villous Maturation

- Associated with late in utero demise
  o After 37 weeks
- Associated with gestational diabetes, maternal obesity, hypercoiled umbilical cords
- Villi are larger with poor vasculosyncytial membrane formation
  o Increased CD15 expression in villous vasculature similar to developing placenta

Other Placental Pathologies

- Uncommon causes of fetal demise but important to recognize as placental cause of death with potential for recurrence

Probable and Possible Causes of Stillbirth

Category	24-27 Weeks	28-31 Weeks	32-36 Weeks	≥ 37 Weeks	Entire 3rd Trimester
Placental disease (~ 50% due to maternal vascular malperfusion)	36%	25%	27%	25%	28%
Infection (fetus, placenta, or mother)	8%	6%	8%	12%	8%
Fetal/genetic structural abnormality	11%	14%	18%	13%	14%
Maternal medical complications (including gestational diabetes, antiphospholipid antibody syndrome)	10%	4%	8%	11%	8%
Hypertensive disorders (hypertension and preeclampsia)	16%	17%	10%	5%	12%
Umbilical cord abnormalities (cord prolapse, strictures, thrombi)	11%	6%	13%	14%	11%
Obstetric complications (abruption, multiple gestation, preterm labor/premature rupture of membranes, cervical insufficiency, chorioamnionitis)	19%	21%	17%	14%	18%
Other (hydrops, early amniotic rupture)	3%	6%	3%	2%	4%

All cases included complete placental examination, autopsy, and cytogenetics.

From Stillbirth Collaborative Research Network Writing Group: Causes of death among stillbirths. JAMA. 306(22):2459-68, 2011.

Placental Findings More Frequent in Stillbirth Compared to Livebirth

Placental Finding	24-31 Weeks	32-36 Weeks	≥ 37 Weeks
Single umbilical artery	Yes	Yes	Yes
Distal villous immaturity (placental maturation defect)	No	No	Yes
Chorionic plate vascular degenerative changes*	Yes	Yes	Yes
Retroplacental hematoma	Yes	Yes	No
Focal infarction	No	Yes	No
Multifocal infarction	No	Yes	No
Diffuse infarction	Yes	Yes	Yes
Massive perivillous fibrin deposition	No	Yes	No
Intraparenchymal thrombus	No	No	Yes
Chorionic plate thrombi	No	Yes	Yes
Focal avascular villi	Yes	No	Yes
Multifocal avascular villi	No	No	Yes
Diffuse avascular villi*	Yes	Yes	Data unavailable
Diffuse villous edema	No	No	Yes

*The frequency of these findings in stillbirth was significantly increased compared to livebirths of comparable gestational ages. Many pathologies are present in both preterm birth and in utero demise. *Chorionic plate vascular degenerative changes and diffuse avascular villi may occur as pathologic processes or as secondary findings after fetal demise.*

From Pinar H et al: Placental findings in singleton stillbirths. Obstet Gynecol. 123(2 Pt 1):325-36, 2014.

- o Massive perivillous fibrin deposition/maternal floor infarction
- o Chronic histiocytic intervillositis of unknown etiology
- o Extensive chronic villitis of unknown etiology

SELECTED REFERENCES

1. Page JM et al: Potentially preventable stillbirth in a diverse U.S. cohort. Obstet Gynecol. 131(2):336-343, 2018
2. Bukowski R et al: Altered fetal growth, placental abnormalities, and stillbirth. PLoS One. 12(8):e0182874, 2017
3. Page JM et al: Diagnostic tests for evaluation of stillbirth: results from the stillbirth collaborative research network. Obstet Gynecol. 129(4):699-706, 2017
4. Bodnar LM et al: Maternal prepregnancy obesity and cause-specific stillbirth. Am J Clin Nutr. 102(4):858-64, 2015
5. Pinar H et al: Placental findings in singleton stillbirths. Obstet Gynecol. 123(2 Pt 1):325-36, 2014
6. Gardosi J et al: Maternal and fetal risk factors for stillbirth: population based study. BMJ. 346:f108, 2013
7. Stillbirth Collaborative research network writing group: causes of death among stillbirths. JAMA. 306(22):2459-68, 2011
8. Pauli RM: Stillbirth: fetal disorders. Clin Obstet Gynecol. 53(3):646-55, 2010
9. Pinar H et al: Placenta and umbilical cord abnormalities seen with stillbirth. Clin Obstet Gynecol. 53(3):656-72, 2010
10. Parast MM et al: Placental histologic criteria for umbilical blood flow restriction in unexplained stillbirth. Hum Pathol. 39(6):948-53, 2008

Massive Placental Abruption

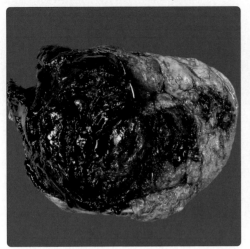

Histology of Acute Placental Abruption

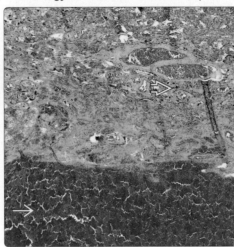

(Left) *Massive placental abruption is commonly associated with preeclampsia. Abruption of > 30-50% of the placental basal surface has a high fetal mortality rate.* (Right) *H&E shows acute retroplacental hemorrhage ➡ with overlying acute infarct. Infarction is evinced by collapse of the intervillous space and the smudged appearance of syncytiotrophoblast nuclei ⮞.*

Infarction Hematoma

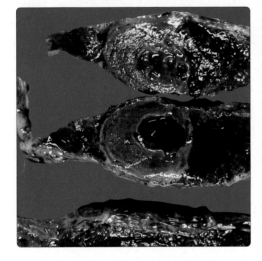

Multiple Infarcts

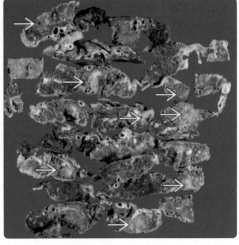

(Left) *This large subacute infarct with central hemorrhage (infarction hematoma) was associated with fetal demise. The clinical associations are similar to those of placental abruption.* (Right) *Multiple large or nonmarginal infarcts are seen in preeclampsia. They are associated with growth restriction, prematurity, and fetal demise. Gross photo shows numerous poorly circumscribed, tan foci ➡ in this placenta due to multiple remote infarcts. The placenta is often small for age.*

Distal Villous Hypoplasia

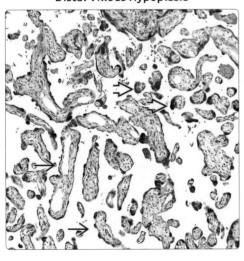

Acute Atherosis of Decidual Artery

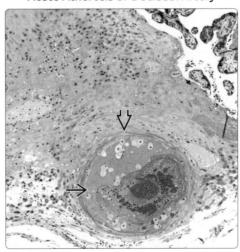

(Left) *Distal villous hypoplasia (accelerated villous maturation) is characterized by increased elongate slender villi ➡ and exaggerated syncytial knots ⮞ (Tenney-Parker change). The findings reflect longstanding maternal vascular malperfusion and are characteristic of preterm preeclampsia.* (Right) *Maternal vascular malperfusion in preterm preeclampsia is associated with decidual arteriopathy. Note the fibrin necrosis ➡ and foamy macrophages ⮞ in this spiral artery.*

(Left) *Close attention to cord lesions is essential in 3rd-trimester fetal loss. In this case associated with a nuchal cord, the looped portion of the cord is flattened and appears macerated ⇒. A thrombus is visible in a proximal chorionic plate vein ➡.* (Right) *Abrupt changes in cord color ⇒ may suggest vascular pathology, as in this severely hypercoiled cord. Hypercoiled cords are associated with both chronic fetal vascular malperfusion and delayed villous maturation.*

Umbilical Cord Pathology in Fetal Demise

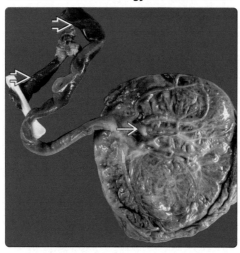

Hypercoiled Umbilical Cord

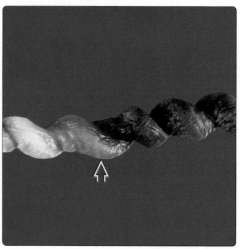

(Left) *A remote thrombus ➡ is visible in a chorionic plate vein.* (Right) *This chorionic plate vessel displays an organizing thrombus. Within the endothelial cushion, there is mural calcification ⇨ and subendothelial fibrin forming a fibrin cap ⇨. These changes are consistent with occlusion of flow in vivo and are usually associated with distal villous changes of fetal vascular malperfusion.*

Chorionic Plate Vessel Thrombus

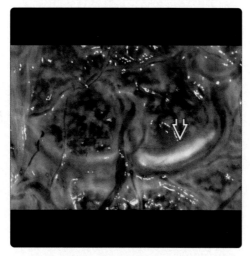

Fetal Vascular Malperfusion

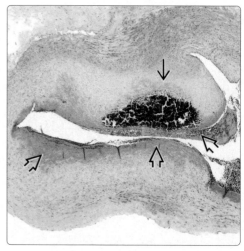

(Left) *Stem villous changes of fetal vascular malperfusion include organizing thrombi ⇨ as well as fibromuscular sclerosis ⇨ with fibroblast proliferation and red blood cell extravasation.* (Right) *Distal villi become avascular ⇨ with cessation of fetal perfusion. The syncytiotrophoblast layer remains intact and the intervillous space is preserved. This will occur throughout the placenta after prolonged in utero demise but regionally when due to malperfusion in vivo.*

Fetal Vascular Malperfusion

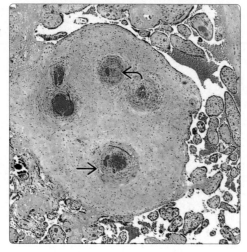

Avascular Villi of Fetal Vascular Malperfusion

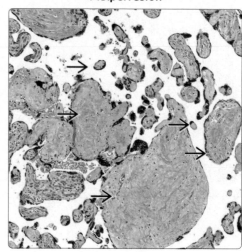

Pale and Bulky Placenta in Fetal-Maternal Hemorrhage

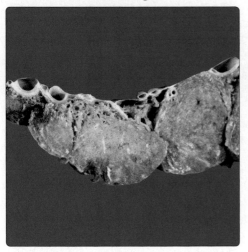

Fetal Anemia and Villous Edema

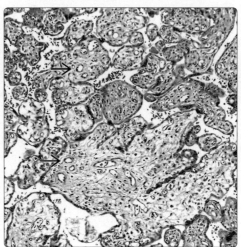

(Left) *A pale, bulky placenta with dilated chorionic plate vessels empty of blood is characteristic of chronic fetal-maternal transfusion. The fetus may be severely anemic. Intervillous hemorrhages with fibrin deposition, another feature of fetal-maternal hemorrhage, may be absent.* (Right) *These villi have dilated capillaries ⇒ that contain little blood. Villous edema ensues once the hematocrit becomes critically low.*

Choriangiosis

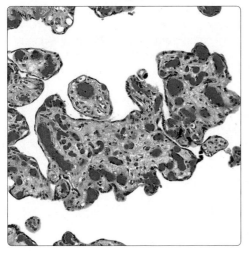

Chronic Villitis

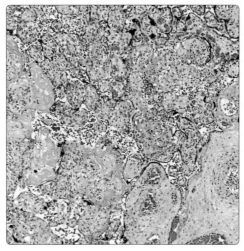

(Left) *Chorangiosis is characterized by hypervascular villi. The finding is associated with gestational diabetes and other conditions. Several maternal and fetal complications of diabetes can result in fetal demise.* (Right) *Chronic villitis may be sufficiently severe and diffuse to result in intrauterine fetal demise. Possible infectious causes should be excluded. The etiology is presumed to be an exaggerated maternal immune response to placental/fetal tissues in most cases.*

Massive Perivillous Fibrin Deposition

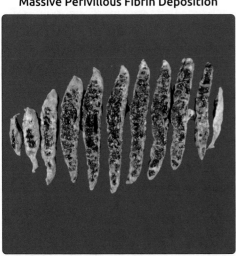

Massive Perivillous Fibrin Deposition

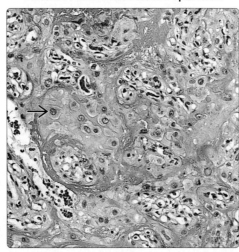

(Left) *Massive perivillous fibrin deposition is generally defined as > 30% placental involvement. It may be isolated to the maternal floor or diffuse throughout the placenta, as seen here.* (Right) *Massive perivillous fibrin deposition has bands of villi embedded in fibrin with extravillous cytotrophoblast cell proliferation ⇒. Normal-appearing villi are noted between the bands.*

TERMINOLOGY

Abbreviations

- Recurrent pregnancy loss (RPL)

Definitions

- Definitions vary
  - ≥ 3 consecutive pregnancy losses
  - ≥ 2 clinical miscarriages (not necessarily consecutive) characterized by ultrasound or histology

EPIDEMIOLOGY

Incidence

- Affects 1-5% of couples of reproductive age

Clinical Presentation

- Most RPLs occur in 1st trimester (58% before 12-weeks gestation vs. 3% after 12 weeks)
  - Both chromosomally normal and abnormal conceptions tend to be lost early in RPL

ETIOLOGY/PATHOGENESIS

Genetic Abnormalities

- Genetic testing of products of conception in RPL is most likely to reveal cause of loss in early pregnancy (< 12 weeks)
  - Methods include karyotype, array-CGH, quantitative fluorescent-PCR
    - Molecular methods have lower failure rates, as cells are not required to grow in culture
  - Identification of unbalanced rearrangements in products of conception identifies need for parental karyotype
    - Parental balanced translocation estimated to occur in 4-5% of recurrent miscarriages
  - In < 1% of cases does abnormality imply risk of affected child that would be live born in future pregnancy
  - ~ 2% will show pathogenic gene microdeletions or microduplications
- Conceptus is aneuploid in ≥ 50% of RPL with normal parental genetics, as in isolated pregnancy loss

- Women with RPL may be more tolerant of chromosomally abnormal conceptus after implantation
- Individual variant alleles of multiple genes are investigated as potential causes of RPL
  - Some appear linked with risk factors, such as obesity or thrombophilia

Uterine Anatomy

- Uterine anatomic pathology exists in 2-27% of women with RPL
  - Unicornuate or bicornuate uteri, septa
  - Asherman syndrome
  - Submucosal leiomyomata
- Poor uterine artery blood flow with higher resistance to flow in subendometrial region in luteal phase found in one ultrasound study

Maternal Thrombophilia

- Various thrombophilic factors are associated with RPL, but it is unclear if thrombosis is necessarily cause of pregnancy loss
- Lupus anticoagulant/antiphospholipid antibody (APL) in 4%
  - APLs may contribute to RPL in various ways, many of which are nonthrombotic
    - APLs bind trophoblast and impair their migration, cytokine, and hormone secretion; APLs induce inflammation
- Anticardiolipin antibodies in 15%
- Abnormal homocysteine/methylenetetrahydrofolate reductase in 14%
- Factor V Leiden mutations in 7-8% (homozygous or heterozygous with elevated active protein C resistance ratio)

Endocrine Abnormality

- Abnormal TSH in 7%
- Depressed midluteal progesterone in 17%
- Hyperprolactinemia in 6%
- Vitamin D deficiency in up to 47%
- Poorly controlled type 1 diabetes mellitus

Chronic Histiocytic Intervillositis

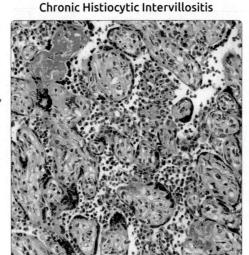

Chronic Villitis of Unknown Etiology

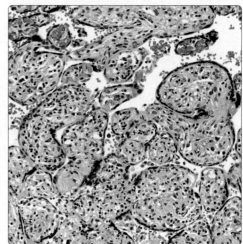

(Left) Chronic histiocytic intervillositis is an uncommon cause of recurrent pregnancy loss (RPL), but it is important for pathologists to recognize. Pregnancy loss may occur in any trimester and has a nearly 70% recurrence rate. (Right) Chronic villitis of unknown etiology is a relatively frequent finding in RPL. Focal lesions are likely insignificant, but extensive involvement impairs placental function.

Immune Dysregulation

- Idiopathic RPL comprises 50-60% of patients; likely due to immune abnormalities
  - Insufficient uterine decidual cell cytokine production for support of pregnancy
  - Past or subclinical infection may shift uterine environment to proinflammatory T-cell state (Th1) over pregnancy-supporting immune state
- Antiphosphatidylserine antibodies in 6%
- Lupus anticoagulant and anticardiolipin antibodies likely interfere with appropriate immune interactions that support pregnancy

Infection

- Positive cervical microbial cultures for *Chlamydia*, *Mycoplasma*, and *Ureaplasma* are seen in 15% of RPL patients, but similar results are found in women without RPL
  - Subclinical infection postulated as basis for proinflammatory uterine immune state in RPL
- Herpes simplex virus 2 and parvovirus B19 IgM seropositivity are more frequent in RPL patients than controls
- Group B *Streptococcus* can cause recurrent 2nd-trimester loss due to acute chorioamnionitis

Maternal Health

- Women with diabetes, obesity, chronic hypertension all may experience RPLs
- Environmental pollutants, phthalates may also increase risk of RPL

PLACENTAL EVALUATION

Embryo Loss

- Molecular genotyping recommended by ACOG (array-CGH, QF-PCR)
  - Karyotype also informative but higher rate of test failure
- Implantation site decidua may show lack of trophoblast-mediated remodeling of spiral arteries

- May see dysmorphic changes, such as irregular villous contours and stromal cell cytomegaly
- May see chronic histiocytic intervillositis even in 1st trimester

Fetal Loss

- More likely to have placental pathology; findings include
- Changes of maternal vascular malperfusion (SGA placental weight, infarcts, decidual arteriopathy)
  - Seen in maternal thrombophilia-related RPL and idiopathic RPL
    - May relate to incomplete transformation of uteroplacental vasculature for pregnancy, either due to immune dysregulation, genetic abnormalities, or thrombosis
- Changes of chronic inflammation
  - Likely reflect RPL due to abnormal immune environment, potential infectious causes should be excluded
  - Chronic villitis, plasma cell deciduitis
  - Chronic histiocytic intervillositis
- Increased perivillous fibrin deposition (more common in older gestations)
  - Damage to surface syncytiotrophoblast leads to excessive perivillous fibrin deposition
  - Seen in maternal thrombophilia-related RPL and APL RPL

SELECTED REFERENCES

1. Bahia W et al: Genetic variation in the progesterone receptor gene and susceptibility to recurrent pregnancy loss: a case-control study. BJOG. 125(6):729-735, 2018
2. Mansour GM et al: Uterine artery flow velocity waveform (FVW) type and subendometrial vascularity in recurrent pregnancy loss. J Matern Fetal Neonatal Med. 1-151, 2018
3. Jaslow CR et al: Diagnostic factors identified in 1020 women with two versus three or more recurrent pregnancy losses. Fertil Steril. 93(4):1234-43, 2010
4. Gun BD et al: The comparison of vessels in elective and spontaneous abortion decidua in first trimester pregnancies: importance of vascular changes in early pregnancy losses. Acta Obstet Gynecol Scand. 85(4):402-6, 2006
5. Boyd TK et al: Chronic histiocytic intervillositis: a placental lesion associated with recurrent reproductive loss. Hum Pathol. 31(11):1389-96, 2000

Decidual Arteriopathy

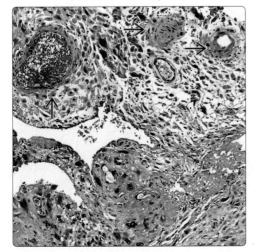

Group B *Streptococcus*

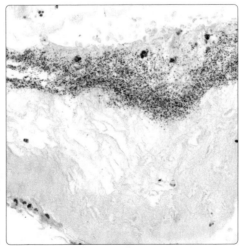

(Left) These decidua basalis spiral arteries ⊟ have not been remodeled for pregnancy. Maternal vascular malperfusion is a cause of RPL. (Right) Some women may have recurrent late pregnancy loss due to an incompetent cervix with complications of amniotic fluid infection. Group B Streptococcus can cause RPL. Enterouterine fistulae should also be considered in women with recurrent severe chorioamnionitis.

TERMINOLOGY

Definitions

- Intravascular karyorrhexis: Karyorrhexis of cells in lumen of placental fetal vasculature
  - Identifies short (6-48 hours) in utero demise-to-delivery interval
- Villous stromal-vascular karyorrhexis: Expansion of intravascular karyorrhexis to include karyorrhexis of endothelial and stromal cells in terminal villi
  - When localized, feature of fetal vascular malperfusion (FVM)
- Stem vessel luminal abnormalities: Loss of vessel integrity with loss of endothelium, fibrous septation of lumen, and RBC extravasation, resolving into several small irregular blood-filled spaces, often arrayed in circle at site of prior endothelium
  - Identifies short to intermediate (48 hours to 2 weeks) in utero demise-to-delivery interval
- Avascular villi: Fibrous-appearing villi with absent fetal vessels and viable syncytiotrophoblast layer
  - Identifies prolonged (> 2 weeks) in utero demise-to-delivery interval when extensive
  - When localized, feature of FVM

Synonyms

- Fetal vascular involutional or occlusive changes, luminal septation, fibromuscular sclerosis, and hemorrhagic endovasculitis/endovasculosis all describe similar histopathologic changes in large fetal vessels that are part of FVM in vivo
- Avascular villi and villous fibrosis
- Intravascular karyorrhexis and villous stromal-vascular karyorrhexis describe similar lesions on spectrum in terminal villi with karyorrhexis of intravascular cells preceding that of vessel wall and villous stroma

MACROSCOPIC

External Fetal Exam

- Characteristic changes accompany prolonged retention of fetus

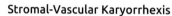

Stromal-Vascular Karyorrhexis

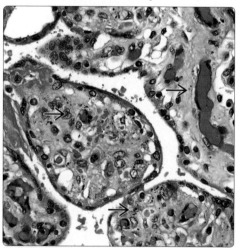

Stem Vessel Luminal Abnormalities With Demise

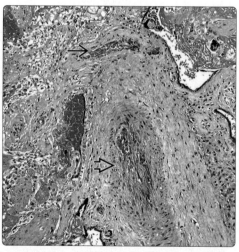

(Left) *Extensive karyorrhectic debris ⊡ is present in the villi. This is one of the earliest postdemise changes; it must be distinguished from in vivo pathology of fetal vascular malperfusion.* (Right) *The lumen of the larger vessel ⊡ shows loss of lumen integrity with fibroblast septation and small residual channels ⊡. This change is typical of an intermediate demise-to-delivery interval.*

Diffuse Avascular Villi

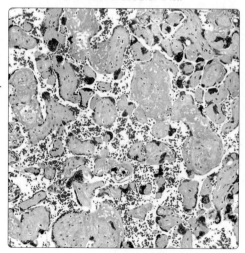

Mummification With Prolonged Demise

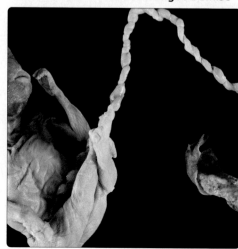

(Left) *Diffuse avascular villi are a late postdemise change, 2 weeks after fetal death. They may also be a feature of fetal vascular malperfusion. In fetal vascular malperfusion, the changes are regional; after remote demise, they are diffuse.* (Right) *"Mummification," as seen in this fetus, refers to the diffusely tan, wrinkled, dehydrated appearance. The fetus is often flattened. This demise was due to a hypercoiled cord with stricture.*

Estimation of In Utero Demise-to-Delivery Intervals

Features	Postdemise Interval	Sensitivity	Specificity	Positive Predictive Value
Placental Histology				
Intravascular karyorrhexis in small villous vessels of several different regions	≥ 6 hours	94%	100%	1.000
Multifocal (10-25%) stem vessel luminal abnormalities	≥ 48 hours	94%	100%	1.000
Extensive (> 25%) stem vessel luminal abnormalities	≥ 2 weeks	78%	98%	0.875
Extensive (> 25% of terminal villi) avascular villi	≥ 2 weeks	100%	93%	0.750
External Fetal Examination				
Desquamation < 1 cm	≥ 6 hours	86%	100%	1.000
Desquamation of face, back, or abdomen	≥ 12 hours	80%	100%	1.000
Desquamation of ≥ 5% of body surface	≥ 18 hours	80%	100%	1.000
Desquamation ≥ 2 of 11 zones*	≥ 18 hours	90%	92%	0.900
Mummification	≥ 2 weeks	100%	100%	1.000
Fetal Organ Histology				
Kidney: Loss of tubular nuclear basophilia in ≥ 1% of cells	≥ 4 hours	97%	89%	0.970
Liver: Loss of hepatocyte nuclear basophilia in ≥ 1% of cells	≥ 24 hours	100%	92%	0.890
Myocardium: Inner 1/2 loss of nuclear basophilia in ≥ 1% of cells	≥ 24 hours	94%	100%	1.000
Myocardium: Outer 1/2 loss of nuclear basophilia in ≥ 1% of cells	≥ 48 hours	100%	96%	0.910
Bronchus: Loss of epithelial nuclear basophilia in ≥ 1% of cells	≥ 96 hours	100%	97%	0.910
Liver: Loss of nuclear basophilia in 100% of cells	≥ 96 hours	91%	100%	1.000
GI tract: Loss of nuclear basophilia in 100% of cells	≥ 1 week	90%	100%	1.000
Adrenal: Loss of nuclear basophilia in 100% of cells	≥ 1 week	100%	100%	1.000
Trachea: Loss of chondrocyte nuclear basophilia in ≥ 1% of cells	≥ 1 week	89%	100%	1.000
Kidney: Loss of nuclear basophilia in 100% of cells of any type	> 4 weeks	100%	98%	0.880

The 11 zones are scalp, face, neck, chest, abdomen, back, arms, hand, leg, foot, and scrotum; data excerpted from Genest et al. In general, fetal hydrops or prolonged autopsy to delivery time may accelerate postmortem changes. The changes above are for evaluation of the 3rd-trimester fetus.

- o Early red-brown discoloration of cord stump and focal skin slippage suggests fetus has been dead at least 6 hours before delivery
- o Over time, progressively larger areas of body show skin slippage
- o Later change of mummification rarely seen in 3rd-trimester fetus
- Collapse of cranial contents, body flattening with prolonged retention

MICROSCOPIC

Distinguishing In Vivo Placental Pathology From Postdemise Changes

- Large vessel (chorionic plate, stem villous vessel) involutional changes after fetal demise are similar to changes of FVM
  - o Changes of fetal demise are diffusely distributed
    - − Only 10% of stem villi may be affected with short demise-to-delivery interval, but they are widely distributed
  - o In contrast, changes downstream of fetal thrombi are restricted to affected vascular tree
- Distal villous involutional changes after fetal demise are similar to changes of FVM

- o Changes of fetal demise are widespread; villi in any region may show these changes
  - − Widespread changes can also be seen with fetal heart failure or severe anemia
- o In contrast, changes due to focal process, such as chorionic plate vessel thrombosis or proximal chronic villitis, only affect villi downstream of lesion
- These changes were studied in 3rd-trimester placenta
  - o Similar large vessel changes occur in 2nd trimester
  - o Immature intermediate villi may have persistence of Hofbauer cells in stroma ± peripheral capillary net with subacute and prolonged demise

SELECTED REFERENCES

1. Jacques SM et al: Estimation of time of fetal death in the second trimester by placental histopathological examination. Pediatr Dev Pathol. 6(3):226-32, 2003
2. Genest DR et al: Estimating the time of death in stillborn fetuses: I. Histologic evaluation of fetal organs; an autopsy study of 150 stillborns. Obstet Gynecol. 80(4):575-84, 1992
3. Genest DR et al: Estimating the time of death in stillborn fetuses: III. External fetal examination; a study of 86 stillborns. Obstet Gynecol. 80(4):593-600, 1992
4. Genest DR: Estimating the time of death in stillborn fetuses: II. Histologic evaluation of the placenta; a study of 71 stillborns. Obstet Gynecol. 80(4):585-92, 1992

TERMINOLOGY

- Hypoxic-ischemic encephalopathy (HIE) ACOG/AAP criteria
  - Neonatal signs consistent with acute peripartum or intrapartum event in infant ≥ 35 weeks
  - Apgar score < 5 at 5 minutes
  - Umbilical artery pH < 7 &/or base deficit ≥ 12 mmol/L
  - Neuroimaging evidence of acute brain injury or MR consistent with hypoxia-ischemia
  - Multisystem organ failure/dysfunction

ETIOLOGY/PATHOGENESIS

- Maternal blood flow issues
  - Abruption, infarcts, maternal decidual vasculopathy
- Fetal blood flow issues
  - Umbilical cord abnormalities, ruptured vasa previa, FTV
- Villous permeability issues
  - Accelerated maturation, delayed maturation, chorangiosis, chronic villitis, perivillous fibrin deposition
- Meconium associated vascular necrosis

- Severe fetal anemia; fetal maternal transfusion, TTTS
- Chorioamnionitis with fetal vasculitis

IMAGING

- Patterns of HIE brain injury on MR
  - Watershed, parasagittal, white matter injury, due to partial prolonged asphyxia
    - Small placenta, infarcts, maternal decidual vasculopathy, chorioamnionitis and funisitis, delayed villous maturation, increased NRBC, severe fetal anemia, high-grade villitis, FTV
  - Basal ganglia, thalami, deep gray matter injury, due to acute profound asphyxia
    - Uterine rupture, placental abruption, cord prolapse, ruptured vasa previa, chronic villitis, chorioamnionitis
  - Total, both deep gray and white matter injury
    - Small and large placentas, chorioamnionitis, delayed villous maturation, moderate to severe increase in NRBC, chronic villitis, FTV

Central Retroplacental Hematoma

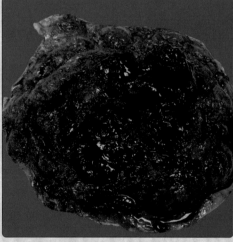

Retroplacental Hematoma Cross Section

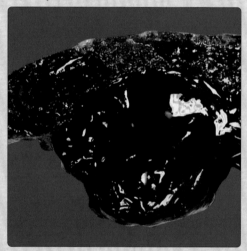

(Left) *Central retroplacental hematoma that occupies 50% of the maternal surface is considered massive and is associated with fetal morbidity and mortality.* (Right) *Cross section of the retroplacental hematoma with depression of maternal surface is shown. This is consistent with some passage of time between the hematoma formation and delivery.*

Retroplacental Hematoma

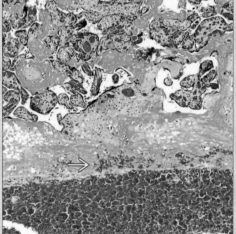

Villous Stromal Hemorrhage

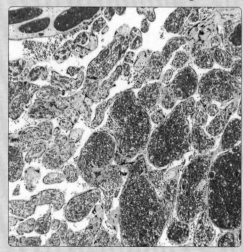

(Left) *H&E shows retroplacental hematoma with blood actively dissecting into the basal tissues ➡; this may be associated with clinical abruption. The overlying villi have acute ischemic changes with hypereosinophilia of the cytoplasm and hyperchromasia of the syncytiotrophoblasts.* (Right) *Villous stromal hemorrhage occurs as a result of abnormal placental separation. There is loss of blood pressure in the maternal intervillous space, and the fetus becomes hyperdynamic, resulting in rupture of the capillaries.*

TERMINOLOGY

Abbreviations

- Hypoxic-ischemic encephalopathy (HIE)

Synonyms

- Neonatal depression and asphyxia
- Fetal thrombotic vasculopathy and fetal vascular malperfusion

Definitions

- Hypoxia-decreased oxygen tension
- Ischemia-decreased blood flow
- HIE, ACOG/AAP criteria
  - Neonatal signs consistent with acute peripartum or intrapartum event in infant ≥ 35-weeks gestation
    - Apgar score of < 5 and 5 minutes
    - Umbilical artery pH < 7 &/or base deficit ≥ 12 mmol/L
    - Neuroimaging evidence of acute brain injury on MR consistent with hypoxia-ischemia
    - Multisystem organ failure/dysfunction
  - Type and timing of contributing factors consistent with acute peri- or intrapartum event
    - Sentinel event, immediately before or during labor and delivery (only present in 15-29%)
      □ Acute cord occlusion, fetal hemorrhage, early-onset bacterial sepsis, abruption, maternal cardiopulmonary arrest, uterine rupture
    - Fetal heart rate monitor pattern consistent with acute peri- or intrapartum event (bradycardia of < 60)
    - Neuroimaging studies consistent with etiology of acute peri- or intrapartum event
    - No evidence of other proximal or distal factors that could be contributing factors
      □ Identifiable etiologies, cerebral dysgenesis, trauma, coagulation disorders (hemorrhagic or thrombotic), infection, metabolic including hypoglycemia, or genetic disorders
    - Developmental outcome spastic quadriplegia or dyskinetic cerebral palsy (CP)
- CP
  - Nonprogressive congenital motor dysfunction with findings of spasticity, rigidity, or choreoathetosis
  - Incidence: 2.0-2.5/1,000 live births
  - Etiology heterogeneous
    - 28-36% due to prematurity
    - 10-20% due to CNS malformations
    - Genetic disorders affecting primary brain development
      □ 1-2% familial
      □ 14% have likely causative single-gene mutations and up to 31% have clinically relevant copy number variations
    - 8-10% due to birth asphyxia, which may be primary or secondary to preexisting pathology
    - Teratogenic insults, infection, toxins, dietary deficiency, inborn errors of metabolism
- Chronic hypoxia, >1 week prior to delivery
  - Increased perivillous fibrin, decreased placental weight, multiple foci of avascular villi, multiple foci of chronic villitis, circumvallate membrane insertion, hemosiderosis

- Subacute hypoxia, 6-12 hours prior to delivery
  - Acute chorioamnionitis with fetal vasculitis, organizing fetal vascular thrombi, abundant meconium-laden macrophages, meconium-associated vascular necrosis, retroplacental hemorrhage with overlying infarct

ETIOLOGY/PATHOGENESIS

Maternal Blood Flow Abnormalities

- Abruption, significant increase in bad outcome when > 50%
  - Arterial abruption, central, generally associated with maternal vasculopathy, preeclampsia
  - Venous abruption, marginal, may be associated with low-lying placenta
  - Abruption in extreme prematurity generally marginal and associated with chorioamnionitis and decidual necrosis
  - Abruption secondary to abdominal trauma, generally severe injury to maternal pelvis
  - Chronic abruption, chronic abruption-oligohydramnios syndrome, hemosiderosis, circumvallate membrane insertion
- Infarcts, indirect evidence of severe maternal vascular abnormalities
  - Placenta has good collateral circulation from maternal vessels
- Decidual arteriopathy may or may not be associated with clinical syndrome of preeclampsia
- Uterine rupture usually associated with placental abruption

Fetal Blood Flow Abnormalities

- Umbilical cord abnormalities; generally takes something other than just cord abnormality to result in HIE; increased risk for intrauterine growth restriction (IUGR), intrauterine fetal demise, and nonreassuring fetal heart tones
  - Abnormalities of insertion, knots, nuchal or body wraps, hypo- or hyperspiraling, length, decreased diameter
  - Acute cord compression associated with normal umbilical venous blood gas and large discrepancy between venous and arterial pH and base deficit
  - Tight nuchal cord may result in mild anemia due to obstruction of blood flow through vein from placenta to fetus
  - Limited information about cord length and outcome; short cords appear to be worse than long cords
  - Long cords associated with entanglements, nonreassuring fetal heart tones
  - Velamentous and marginal cord: Significantly higher complications
    - Velamentous insertion occurs in 1% of placentas
- Fetal thrombotic vasculopathy (FTV)
  - Most commonly associated with umbilical cord compression
  - Polycythemia and hyperviscosity; diabetes, recipient in twin-twin transfusion syndrome (TTTS)
  - Increased association with preeclampsia
  - Inherited hypercoagulability, rare
  - Fetal thromboemboli can occur, resulting in neonatal stroke, renal vein thrombosis
  - Increasing impairment with increasing placental involvement
- Endothelial injury resulting in thrombosis

- ○ Injury due to abnormal turbulent blood flow
- ○ Severe fetal inflammatory response, leads to necrosis and thrombus formation

Villous Permeability Issues

- Accelerated maturation
- Delayed maturation
- Chorangiosis
- Villitis
  - ○ Increased risk associated with high-grade villitis, especially when associated with FTV
  - ○ Maternal and fetal cytokine production is different from that associated with chorioamnionitis, maternal allograft rejection, and maternal anti-fetal graft-vs.-host disease
- Perivillous fibrin deposition
  - ○ Risk increased with > 10% villous involvement
  - ○ Massive perivillous fibrin deposition when > 30% of parenchyma involved; may primarily involve maternal surface

Meconium

- Meconium may be marker of stress
  - ○ Only 0.5% of babies with meconium-stained fluid develop CP
- Etiology, chorioamnionitis, decreased uteroplacental blood flow, or decreased fetal placental blood flow
- Presence of meconium may exacerbate other placental abnormalities
- Meconium-associated vascular necrosis has high incidence of HIE

Nucleated Red Blood Cells

- Nucleated red blood cells (NRBCs) increase secondary to many acute and chronic stimuli
  - ○ Hypoxia, ischemia, anemia, hypovolemia, acidosis, infection
  - ○ Increased in IUGR, preterm labor, preterm premature rupture of membranes, diabetes
- Degree of elevation of NRBC proportionate to degree of hypoxia
- NRBC release secondary to erythropoietin (EPO)
  - ○ EPO generation time: 4-5 hours
  - ○ NRBC emergence time: 24-36 hours afterward
  - ○ EPO production begins in kidney at 30 weeks
- NRBC increased prior to EPO, suggesting other mediators (IL-6, hypoxia-inducible factors-1 and -2, and TNF-α)
  - ○ Release from liver sinusoids

Severe Fetal Anemia

- Chronic fetal anemia (HCT < 35)
  - ○ Alloimmune hemolysis, chronic TTTS, viral infection
  - ○ Primary hemoglobinopathies (Barts), dyserythropoiesis
- Acute fetal anemia
  - ○ Severe acute blood loss results in hypovolemic shock
  - ○ Etiology
    - – 31% fetal maternal transfusion
    - – 26% ruptured vasa previa
      - □ 1/2,000-5,000 deliveries
      - □ Most associated with velamentous cord insertion but may also be marginal cord
      - □ Intramembranous blood vessels present with bilobation or accessory lobes

- – 8% acute twin-twin transfusion
- – 6% cord rupture
- – 6% hemolysis

Chorioamnionitis

- Evidence for causal or associative role of chorioamnionitis at term and CP controversial
  - ○ Inconsistent as to whether studying clinical chorioamnionitis or histologic chorioamnionitis
  - ○ Inconsistent in histologic definition of both maternal and fetal inflammatory response
  - ○ Chorioamnionitis at term usually not associated with acidosis
- Preterm infants have increased risk for white matter injury
  - ○ Especially with severe fetal inflammation and neonatal sepsis, presumably due to cytokine injury

CLINICAL ISSUES

Term Infants

- Prevalence of HIE 1-3/1,000 term births and incidence has not changed significantly even with advances in antenatal and intrapartum monitoring
- 15-29% secondary to sentinel event occurring during labor
- Prognosis
  - ○ Neonatal death
  - ○ 13% of term infants with HIE develop CP
  - ○ Worse prognosis with deep gray and total ischemic patterns
  - ○ Injury to posterior limb of internal capsule and basal ganglia associated with CP
  - ○ Thalamic injury associated with neurodevelopmental abnormalities
  - ○ 9% of term babies with intracranial hemorrhage develop CP

Preterm Infants

- Preterm infants can have HIE with brain injury similar to term babies
- Preterm infants more often have white matter injury, periventricular leukomalacia
  - ○ Neuronal and glial necrosis in periventricular regions; develops cysts or glial scar
  - ○ Prematurity leading cause of CP, accounting for 28-36% of cases
  - ○ Babies < 28 weeks have highest risk for CP
  - ○ 60-100% of infants with cystic periventricular leukomalacia will develop CP
  - ○ Association between chorioamnionitis with fetal inflammatory response and white matter injury

IMAGING

General Features

- Patterns of HIE brain injury on MR
  - ○ Watershed, parasagittal, white matter injury and may extend into cortical gray matter if insult severe enough
    - – 19-54% of HIE
    - – Associated with partial prolonged chronic hypoxic ischemia

- – Reduction of blood flow to brain, flow shunted from anterior to posterior circulation to maintain adequate perfusion of brainstem, cerebellum, and basal ganglia
- – Placental findings: Small placenta, infarcts, maternal decidual arteriopathy (IUGR), chorioamnionitis and funisitis (sepsis), delayed villous maturation, increased NRBC, severe fetal anemia, high-grade villitis, fetal vascular malperfusion
  - o Basal ganglia, thalami, deep gray matter injury, and perirolandic cortex
    - – 17-30% of HIE
    - – Profound acute, near total asphyxia
    - – Placental findings: Uterine rupture, placental abruption, cord prolapse, ruptured vasa previa, chronic villitis, chorioamnionitis
  - o Total, both deep gray and white matter injury
    - – 27-41% of HIE
    - – May be very severe injury or chronic injury with superimposed acute injury; hypoglycemia
    - – Placental findings: Small and large placentas, chorioamnionitis, delayed villous maturation, moderate to severe increased NRBC, chronic villitis, FTV
- • Cerebral infarcts due to ischemic stroke
  - o Fetal thrombi in placenta
- • Intracranial hemorrhage at term usually due to trauma, or vascular abnormality
  - o Neonatal alloimmune thrombocytopenia, rare
  - o CMV is common cause for hemorrhage and CP

MACROSCOPIC

General Features

- • Accurate placental weight should be obtained after removal of umbilical cord and free membranes
  - o Report should clearly state how placenta was weighed and whether fresh or fixed
  - o Low placental weight as isolated factor has small impact on neurologic outcome
  - o Abnormal placental weight may make fetus less able to tolerate stress or adverse events during labor
  - o Heavy placenta may also result in decreased tolerance to labor
- • Maternal vascular malperfusion
  - o May be associated with smaller than expected placenta and high fetal:placental weight ratio
  - o Small placentas usually have additional lesions
    - – Lesions may directly affect fetus
      - □ Note percentage of placenta involved
      - □ Note location, central or peripheral
    - – Lesions may be marker for underlying process
  - o Infarcts
    - – Marginal infarct usual finding in term placenta
    - – Central infarcts, infarcts > 2 cm, or multiple infarcts abnormal
    - – Red, pink, tan, and white over time but will retain fine, granular appearance
    - – Infarction hematoma, infarct with central hemorrhage
- • Fetal vascular malperfusion
  - o Umbilical cord issues

- – Velamentous or marginal insertion, significant risk for HIE
- – Intramembranous blood vessels, ± vasa previa; measure length of unprotected vessels and note whether intact, disrupted, or thrombosed
- – Thin cord, may appear wrinkled, due to loss of Wharton substance
- – Abnormal hyper- or hypocoiling, thrombosis, or strictures
- – Nuchal cord, may have flattening on one side, takes ~ 15 cm of cord to wrap around neck
- – True knots, document whether tight, and note differences in congestion from fetal side to placental side; place sections in different cassettes
- – Cord length, may not include sample sent for blood gases
  - o Chorionic plate vessels
    - – Arteries cross over veins, determination must be made on gross exam
    - – Recent thrombi may be dilated and firm; may have extravasation of hemoglobin into surrounding tissues
    - – Remote thrombi will appear white through vessel wall
  - o Stem vessels may appear dilated and thrombosed, usually surrounded by pale villi
- • Villous permeability issues
  - o Accelerated maturation, usually associated with small placenta, may or may not have infarcts
  - o Delayed maturation, usually associated with larger than expected placenta
  - o Chronic villitis, may have granular appearance due to clustering of inflamed villi
  - o Perivillous fibrin deposition; shiny bands of dense white tissue, extending vertically from base to chorionic plate, or may predominately involve maternal surface
    - – Document percentage of placental parenchymal &/or maternal surface involved
- • Meconium
  - o Light meconium, may only be slightly yellow to green
  - o Placentas with deeply stained membranes are most important
    - – Fresh meconium dark green, sitting on surface of membranes
    - – Chronic meconium becomes progressively brown to yellow over time
  - o Additional sections should be submitted from deeply stained umbilical cord
    - – Meconium-associated vascular necrosis may have ulcerated cord surface
- • Fetal anemia
  - o Severe fetal anemia will result in pale villi
  - o Chorionic plate vessels, may be dilated and appear empty, containing low hematocrit blood
  - o Placenta with acute fetal blood loss can appear normal

MICROSCOPIC

Histologic Features

- • Maternal vascular malperfusion
  - o Usually looking for surrogate markers of decreased uteroplacental blood flow
    - – Accelerated maturation

- – Infarcts
  - ▫ Zonation, central devitalized villi with collapsed intervillous space, peripheral perivillous fibrin, surrounding villi have exaggerated syncytial knots
  - ▫ Progressive loss of syncytiotrophoblast nuclear chromatin basophilia
  - ▫ Acute infarcts may have maternal neutrophil response
  - – Decidual arteriopathy, fibrinoid necrosis, subendothelial lymphocytes, retained vascular smooth muscle, foamy macrophages, thrombosis
  - ○ Abnormal chronic inflammation in decidua parietalis often surrounding maternal vessels, layer of lymphocytes at deep chorionic plate, chronic villitis, basal plate often with plasma cells
- Fetal vascular malperfusion
  - ○ Large vessel form
    - – Acute thrombosis associated with worse outcome
  - ○ Distal villous form
    - – Diffuse avascular villi or villi with stromal karyorrhexis (> 2 foci ≥ 15 villi in > 2 blocks) associated with poor outcome
  - ○ Umbilical cord accidents
    - – Histologic features suggestive of umbilical cord accident
      - ▫ Dilated fetal vessels, thrombosed fetal vessels, avascular or nearly avascular villi
- Villous permeability issues
  - ○ Accelerated maturation: Small villi, exaggerated syncytial knots, villous agglutination, terminal villous hypoplasia
  - ○ Delayed maturation: Large villi, loose reticular stroma with centrally placed capillaries and poorly formed vasculosyncytial membranes
  - ○ Chorangiosis, ≥ 10 terminal villi with ≥ 10 vessels, in at least 3 different areas
  - ○ Perivillous fibrin deposition
    - – Villi not devitalized but lose syncytiotrophoblast layer and eventually become avascular
    - – Villi embedded in fibrin that fills maternal intervillous space
    - – Chronic perivillous fibrin will have extravillous trophoblast proliferation
    - – May be associated with histiocytic intervillositis
  - ○ Villitis
    - – Lymphocytes or lymphohistiocytic infiltrate
    - – High grade; multiple foci on > 1 slide with > 10 contiguous inflamed villi
    - – Chronic villitis with stem vessel obliteration or avascular villi
- Meconium
  - ○ Fresh meconium may be seen lying free on amnion surface
  - ○ Chronic meconium implies meconium within macrophages; amnion, chorion, decidua
  - ○ No specific stain for meconium; some meconium stains well with H&E, while some only yields vacuolated macrophages
    - – Meconium is water soluble and may leach into storage fluid; meconium is light sensitive
  - ○ Meconium-associated muscle necrosis

- – Involves muscle on outer surface of umbilical arteries; surface amnion may be denuded or ulcerated
  - ▫ May also involve vein, but very rarely only vein
  - ▫ Must distinguish this from autolysis
  - ▫ May also involve chorionic plate vessels
- – Smooth muscle cytoplasm becomes hypereosinophilic with pyknotic nuclei
- – Meconium-laden macrophages will be present in cord substance
- – Frequently associated with acute fetal inflammatory reaction
- NRBCs
  - ○ Estimate > 10 NRBC/10 HPF in term placenta correlates with elevated peripheral blood NRBC
- Fetal anemia
  - ○ Acute fetal anemia
    - – Placenta may appear normal
  - ○ Subacute or chronic fetal anemia
    - – Fetus can equilibrate sudden blood loss within 4-6 hours
    - – Dilated, empty fetal vessels and increased nucleated red blood cells

DIAGNOSTIC CHECKLIST

Clinically Relevant Pathologic Features

- Always consider that acute blood loss at delivery could be fetal and examine placenta for disrupted fetal vessels

SELECTED REFERENCES

1. Shi Z et al: Chorioamnionitis in the development of cerebral palsy: a meta-analysis and systematic review. Pediatrics. 139(6), 2017
2. Cimic A et al: Meconium-associated umbilical vascular myonecrosis: correlations with adverse outcome and placental pathology. Pediatr Dev Pathol. 19(4):315-9, 2016
3. Frank CM et al: Placental pathology and outcome after perinatal asphyxia and therapeutic hypothermia. J Perinatol. 36(11):977-984, 2016
4. Nasiell J et al: Hypoxic ischemic encephalopathy in newborns linked to placental and umbilical cord abnormalities. J Matern Fetal Neonatal Med. 29(5):721-6, 2016
5. Chisholm KM et al: Fetal thrombotic vasculopathy: significance in liveborn children using proposed society for pediatric pathology diagnostic criteria. Am J Surg Pathol. 39(2):274-80, 2015
6. Executive summary: Neonatal encephalopathy and neurologic outcome, second edition. Report of the American College of Obstetricians and Gynecologists' Task Force on Neonatal Encephalopathy. Obstet Gynecol. 123(4):896-901, 2014
7. Harteman JC et al: Placental pathology in full-term infants with hypoxic-ischemic neonatal encephalopathy and association with magnetic resonance imaging pattern of brain injury. J Pediatr. 163(4):968-95.e2, 2013
8. Redline RW: Elevated circulating fetal nucleated red blood cells and placental pathology in term infants who develop cerebral palsy. Hum Pathol. 39(9):1378-84, 2008

Umbilical Cord Rupture

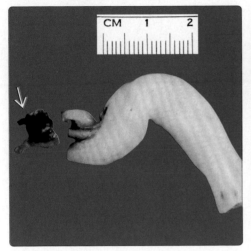

Avulsed Velamentous Cord Insertion

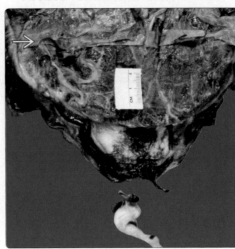

(Left) *Rupture of the umbilical cord, shown here, occurred with uncontrolled maternal expulsive effort resulting in severe fetal blood loss. The torn end* ➡ *has a clot and irregular vessels.* (Right) *Velamentous cord insertion with avulsion of the umbilical cord at the insertion into the membranes is shown. Clot formation is suggestive of some degree of chronicity. This was a dichorionic twin placenta* ➡*, which has an increased incidence of velamentous cord insertions of at least one twin.*

Furcate Cord Insertion

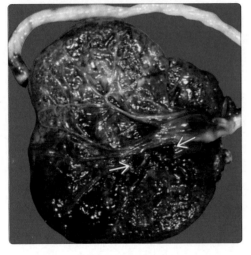

Disrupted Chorionic Plate Vessel

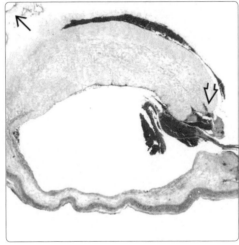

(Left) *This is a furcate cord insertion with division of multiple fetal vessels prior to entry onto the chorionic plate. There is disruption of one vessel at the chorionic plate surface* ➡*, associated with some fetal hemorrhage. The amnion has been stripped off.* (Right) *Disrupted chorionic plate vessel with focal fibrin clot formation* ➡ *is shown. The amnion is focally present* ➡*, and there is acute subamniotic hemorrhage.*

Cordocentesis Injury

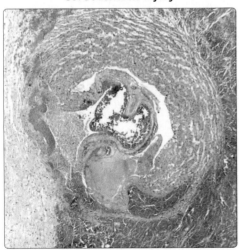

Umbilical Cord Prolapse

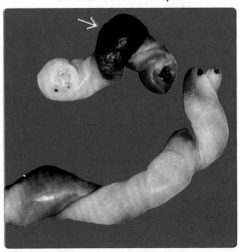

(Left) *Sudden decompensation of fetus occurred during cordocentesis. Section of the cord shows focal disruption of the vein wall with displacement of vascular smooth muscle into the lumen, associated with fibrin and perivascular hemorrhage.* (Right) *This is a section of umbilical cord from a previable fetus with recent fetal demise with cord prolapse. This hemorrhagic portion of cord* ➡ *was entrapped in the cervix. Generally, cord prolapse is brief and leaves no gross abnormalities.*

Thrombosis of Stem Vessel

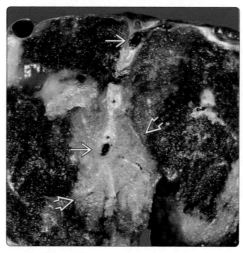

Stem Vessel With Early Obliteration

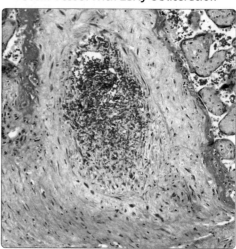

(Left) Thrombosis and dilation ➡ of a large fetal stem vessel is associated with pale, avascular villi ➡ that involves a vascular tree. This meets all the criteria for an umbilical cord accident. (Right) H&E of a large stem vessel shows fibroblast proliferation and extravasation of red blood cells with avascular villi.

Calcification in Thrombosed Stem Vessel

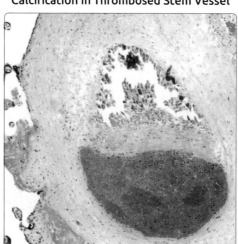

Avascular Villi

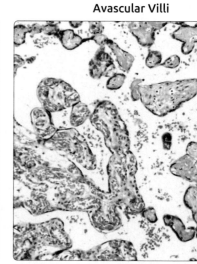

(Left) Thrombosed stem vessel with partial calcification is consistent with a more remote thrombus. (Right) Vascularized villi are seen adjacent to avascular villi, which have had blood flow disrupted in a upstream stem vessel.

Iron Staining in Avascular Villi

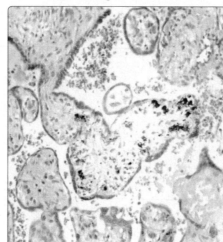

Early Villous Changes of Fetal Vascular Malperfusion

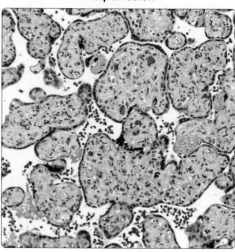

(Left) Variation of iron staining within Hofbauer cells is characteristic of progressive obliteration of the stem vessels, consistent with a premortem event. Adjacent villi have intact capillaries and no hemosiderin. (Right) Early villous changes of fetal thrombotic vasculopathy is demonstrated by stromal and vascular karyorrhexis with extravasated red blood cells.

Gross Appearance of Severe Fetal Anemia

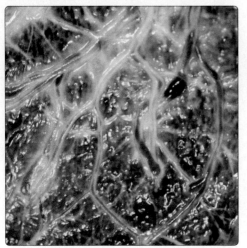

Equilibrated Fetal Anemia

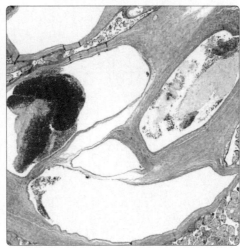

(Left) *This is the typical gross appearance of placenta with severe fetal anemia. The chorionic plate vessels contain low hematocrit blood but are not collapsed. The parenchyma is pale for a term gestation.* (Right) *H&E shows large stem vessels that are dilated and mostly empty or contain low hematocrit blood with scant fibrin deposition. This is characteristic of equilibrated fetal anemia.*

Fetal Maternal Transfusion

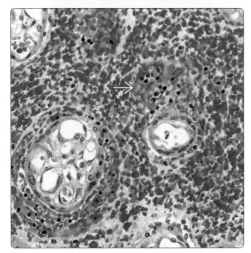

Fetal Maternal Transfusion With Hemoglobin F Staining Cells

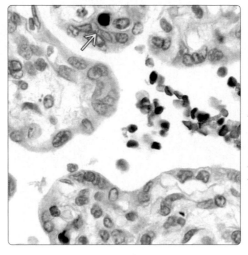

(Left) *Intervillous hemorrhage has a large number of nucleated red blood cells ➡ and can be a feature of fetal-maternal transfusion. Most intervillous hemorrhage is of maternal origin.* (Right) *Placenta associated with fetal-maternal transfusion stained with hemoglobin F shows the maternal intervillous space filled with fetal red blood cells. There are few residual fetal cells ➡ in the villous capillaries.*

Subacute Thrombosis of Umbilical Artery

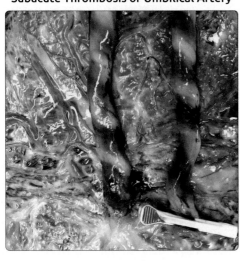

Acute Thrombosis of Umbilical Artery

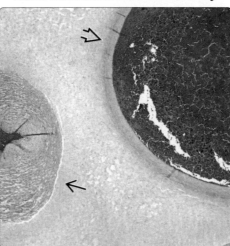

(Left) *This umbilical cord shows hemoglobin pigments that have extravasated out into the cord substance from a subacute thrombosis of one of the arteries. A more acute thrombus may not show any gross features.* (Right) *Compare the appearance of the normal ➡ and acutely thrombosed ➡ umbilical artery. This can be a very difficult diagnosis. Careful examination demonstrates the lack of viability of the vascular muscle in the thrombosed vessel.*

Placental Evaluation in Special Circumstances

Massive Perivillous Fibrin Deposition

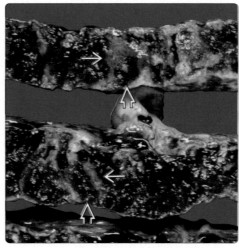

(Left) *Massive perivillous fibrin deposition within the placenta will usually be found in dense, shiny white bands ➡️ extending from the basal plate to the chorionic plate, as shown. Normal-appearing villi ➡️ may be seen between the bands, yielding a lacy appearance.* **(Right)** *Chronic perivillous fibrin deposition will have extratrophoblast proliferation ➡️ within the fibrin, as shown. The entrapped villi are viable with some retained syncytiotrophoblasts ➡️ and residual villous vessels ➡️.*

Chronic Perivillous Fibrin Deposition

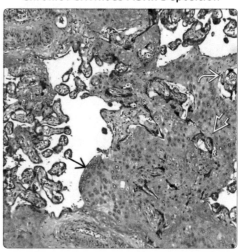

Remote Infarct

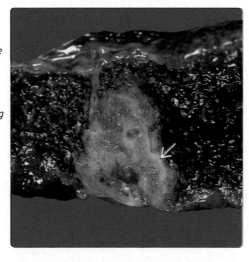

(Left) *This remote infarct is nonmarginal and wedge shaped. Cut surface shows residual fine granularity of the devitalized villi, which are surrounded by a thin rim of perivillous fibrin ➡️.* **(Right)** *Zonation of villous changes can be helpful in distinguishing an infarct from perivillous fibrin deposition. There are central devitalized villi ➡️, then a layer of villi with perivillous fibrin ➡️, with an outer layer of ischemic villi with exaggerated syncytiotrophoblastic knots ➡️.*

Infarct vs. Perivillous Fibrin Deposition

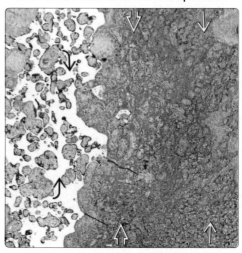

Remote Retroplacental Hematoma

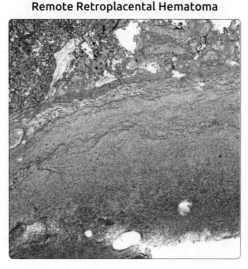

(Left) *Remote retroplacental hematoma is usually associated with a chronic abruption and may be associated with oligohydramnios and hemosiderosis of the membranes.* **(Right)** *A large number of hemosiderin-laden macrophages may be seen in the free and attached membranes and is usually associated with chronic abruption or a large, retromembranous hematoma. Iron stain may be necessary to distinguish hemosiderin from meconium.*

Hemosiderosis in Membranes

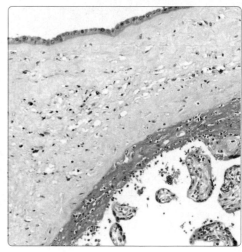

Distal Villous Hypoplasia

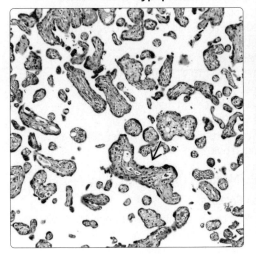

Delayed Villous Maturation

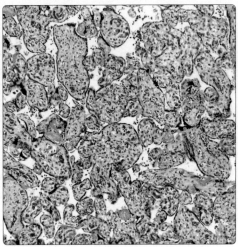

(Left) *Distal villous hyperplasia is characterized by small, elongated villi with exaggerated syncytial knots. A serrated appearance of the knots ⮕ is a frequent finding associated with preterm preeclampsia.* (Right) *Delayed villous maturation is characterized by large, hypercellular, and hypervascular villi with decreased vasculosyncytial membranes.*

Meconium-Associated Vascular Necrosis

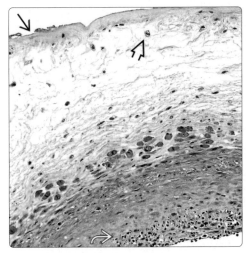

Meconium-Laden Macrophages in Membranes

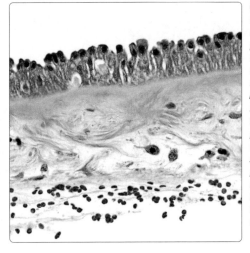

(Left) *H&E shows meconium-associated vascular necrosis, a rare occurrence due to prolonged exposure to heavy meconium. The surface amnion is degenerated ⮕. Meconium-laden macrophages ⮕ are present in the cord substance. The smooth muscle is hypereosinophilic with pyknotic nuclei. There is an acute vasculitis ⮕.* (Right) *Amnion from the chorionic plate contains a moderate number of darkly stained, meconium-laden macrophages. The amnion epithelium is reactive.*

Chronic Villitis With Obstructive Fetal Vasculopathy

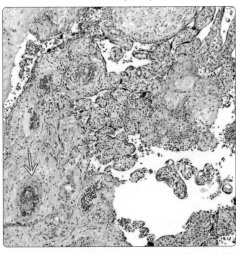

High-Grade Chronic Villitis

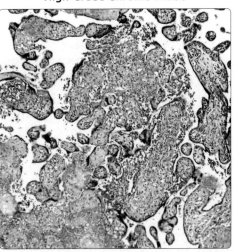

(Left) *Chronic villitis with obstructive vasculopathy of stem vessels ⮕ has been described as destructive villitis and may be associated with increased neonatal morbidity.* (Right) *High-grade chronic villitis is believed to be a maternal immune response to the placental tissues in most cases. Involvement of large areas (> 10 contiguous villi) on multiple slides qualifies this as high grade.*

TERMINOLOGY

Abbreviations

- Monochorionic monoamniotic (MCMA)
- Monochorionic diamniotic (MCDA)

EPIDEMIOLOGY

Incidence

- Least common form of twin placentation
- < 2% of all twin placentas are MCMA
- ~ 10-15% of monozygous twins are MCMA
- Assisted reproductive technologies have increased incidence of both monozygotic and dizygotic twins (although more so the latter)

ETIOLOGY/PATHOGENESIS

Development

- MCMA placentation occurs when blastocyst divides during 2nd week after fertilization
  - Blastocyst splitting during this time results in 2 fetuses but 1 placenta (1 chorion and 1 amnion)
- Acardiac twins
  - Theory 1
    - Primary developmental failure of heart in acardiac twin
  - Theory 2
    - Disruption of normal cardiac development because of hypoxia
  - Theory 3
    - Fertilization of polar body
  - Acardiac twin is supplied with deoxygenated blood through artery-artery anastomosis from pump twin
  - Vascular anastomoses occur during embryonic period and reversal of flow has been detected at 5- to 6-weeks gestation
  - Acardiac twin may be diagnosed as anencephalic or fetal demise until movement is detected
  - May be either MCMA or MCDA
- Conjoined twins

- Occurs with division of blastocyst after 13 days
- Vast majority are MCMA
  - MCDA placentation has been rarely documented, mostly with minimally conjoined abdomens
- Symmetric
  - Female predominance
  - Planes of failed division (fusion) are varied
- Asymmetric
  - Equal incidence in females and males
  - External: Parasitic twin
  - Internal: Fetus in fetu (fetiform teratoma), a.k.a. included twin

CLINICAL IMPLICATIONS

Clinical Risk Factors

- Monoamniotic twins have mortality rate of 10-40%
- Overall, twin pregnancies have higher rates of growth restriction, congenital anomalies, and all-cause morbidity/mortality
- Preterm delivery is nearly 100%
- Cord disorders
  - Umbilical cord entanglement
    - Disc insertion sites are usually close to each other
    - Cords are not separated by dividing membrane and intermingle
    - 1 cord wraps around neck or body of other twin in ~ 20% of cases
    - Cords wrap around each other in ~ 50-75% of cases
    - Entanglement usually occurs at < 24-weeks gestation when fetuses are smaller and have more room to move in amniotic sac
  - Anomalous cord insertion is more common in MCMA than in singleton placentas but less common than in MCDA placentas
  - Single umbilical artery (SUA; 2-vessel cord) more common than in MCDA twins or singletons, usually only affecting 1 twin
- Twin-twin transfusion syndrome

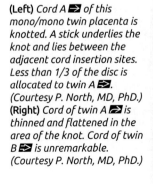

(Left) Cord A ➡ of this mono/mono twin placenta is knotted. A stick underlies the knot and lies between the adjacent cord insertion sites. Less than 1/3 of the disc is allocated to twin A ➡. (Courtesy P. North, MD, PhD.) (Right) Cord of twin A ➡ is thinned and flattened in the area of the knot. Cord of twin B ➡ is unremarkable. (Courtesy P. North, MD, PhD.)

Cord Entanglement

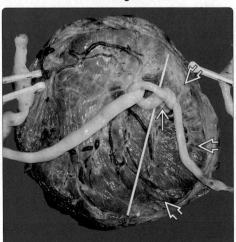

Cord Narrowing

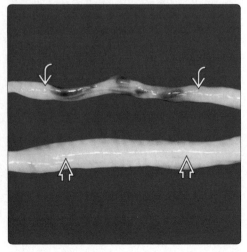

- Much less common and much less morbid in MCMA twins than in MCDA twins
  - Anastomoses are usually large caliber, bidirectional, and result in compensatory parenchymal changes
  - No intraamniotic pressure differences that could differentially alter blood flow
- Asymmetric growth
  - Usually **not** due to twin-twin transfusion
  - Contributing factors can include cord anomalies and discrepant placental mass
  - Discordant twins have increased risk of death
- Intrauterine death
  - Monochorionic twins have highest mortality rates of all twinning types
  - Many early demises show genetic and phenotypic abnormalities
  - Late demises can occur suddenly and without observable warning signs
    - May be due to sudden cord compromise
    - May be due to acute exsanguination of viable twin to demised twin through large caliber anastomoses
- Acardiac twinning (twin reversed arterial perfusion)
  - Incidence
    - 1 in 35,000 deliveries; 1% of monozygotic pregnancies
  - 40-50% are MCMA
  - Increased incidence of 3% in monozygotic triplet pregnancies
  - Acardiac twin loses its vascular connection to placenta and receives all blood supply from pump twin
  - Direct artery-artery and vein-vein anastomoses between cords
  - Acardiac twin receives blood through artery-artery anastomosis
  - 33-42% of acardiac twins have cord with single umbilical artery
    - Artery may enter directly into aorta of acardiac twin
    - Artery may be persistent vitelline artery rather than true umbilical artery
  - 33-50% of acardiac twins have chromosomal abnormalities
  - Acardiac twin has lethal malformation and pump twin has 50% mortality without treatment
  - Pump twin may have high-output failure, especially if acardiac twin is > 50% weight of pump twin
    - Fetoscopic laser coagulation or radiofrequency ablation of acardiac twin umbilical cord/anastomosis → 80% survival of pump twin
- Conjoined twins
  - Symmetric
    - Incidence: 1:30,000-100,000 births
    - F:M = 3:1
    - 28% die in utero, 50% die in neonatal period
    - Ability to surgically separate twins is based on anatomical arrangement and shared organs
  - Asymmetric (parasitic twins)
    - Incidence: ~ 1 in 1,000,000 births
    - May have high-output cardiac failure or significant disability depending on location and size
    - Generally can be resected
  - Fetus in fetu
    - May create vascular steal or mass effect

Imaging Findings

- Acardiac twin
  - Doppler US shows reversed blood flow in anastomosis to acardiac twin
  - Acardiac twin may be thought to be fetal demise until movement is detected

MACROSCOPIC

General Features

- MCMA placental membranes form single sac without dividing membrane
  - Carefully examine placental surface for amnion
    - Amnion may become stripped off surface during delivery, giving false appearance of absent dividing membrane
  - Umbilical cords may be inserted close to one another
  - Vascular anastomoses between placental territories of twins are always present
- Acardiac twin
  - Umbilical cords are close together or one may branch from the other
  - Acardiac twin umbilical cord is usually very short
  - Direct vascular connections between the 2 cords are present
  - Acardiac twin morphology varies
    - ~ 50% have some cardiac tissue, although nonfunctional
    - 68% acardius acephalus (no head development; often missing thoracic organs)
    - 15% acardius anceps (partial head development; often has most body parts and rudimentary organs)
    - Less common: Acardius amorphus (least differentiated, amorphous tissue) and acardius acormus (only head development)
    - Lower extremities are typically much more developed than upper extremities or head (except in acardius amorphus and acardius acormus)
    - Multiple malformations include intestinal atresia, imperforate anus, renal agenesis (usually no lung parenchyma)
- Conjoined twins
  - Symmetric
    - Most common forms are thoracoomphalopagus, ischiopagus, and dicephalus
    - 87% are joined front to front or side to side (ventral union)
    - 48% are joined rostral (dicephalus or cephalopagus, thoracopagus, omphalopagus)
    - 11% are joined caudal (ischiopagus)
    - 28% are joined lateral (parapagus, pelvis, and variable trunk)
    - 13% are joined back to back (dorsal union)
    - 5% are joined craniopagus (joined at cranial vault)
    - 2% are joined rachipagus (joined at vertebral column)
    - 6% are joined pygopagus (joined at sacrum)
  - Asymmetric, parasitic twins
    - Common sites are upper jaw, palate, basal skull, epigastrium, and back
    - Varying external and internal differentiation
  - Fetus in fetu

– Location: 75% upper retroperitoneum, 12.5% intracranial, 12.5% intrascrotal or testicular
– Degree of differentiation that exceeds teratoma; axial skeleton
– Some forms have umbilical cords and amniotic sac-like structures; rare chorionic villous tissue described

Specimen Handling

- Cords
  - Look for evidence of cord entanglement or communicating vessels between cord insertion sites
  - Note abnormal cord insertion patterns (marginal, velamentous, etc.)
  - Note number of umbilical arteries
  - Features suggestive of ongoing vascular compromise
    - Cord narrowing
    - Grooving (from knots or compression)
    - Thrombosis (from stasis and mural damage)
  - Cords from acardiac fetus will also vary
    - May be 2 cords with acardiac generally having SUA
    - May be 1 cord that branches
  - Cords from conjoined twins will vary depending on area of fusion
    - Fusion of abdomen will have 1 cord with 4, 5, or 6 vessels
- Chorionic plate vasculature
  - Measure and estimate relative disc surface area supplying each twin based on vascular network from each cord
  - Look for superficial vascular anastomoses (usually artery-artery), noting number and caliber
  - Injection studies (air, milk, or dye) may help identify superficial anastomoses, but their presence may or may not be clinically relevant
- Membranes
  - Examine membranes to confirm monoamniotic placentation; ensure that amnion is present over fetal surface
    - Disruption of membranes with stripped amnion commonly occurs during delivery of twins
  - Amniotic surface should be continuous and smooth between cord insertion site, without disruption or excess membranes (could be site of separated dividing membrane)
  - Amnion itself may peel up from fetal surface of disc and mimic dividing membrane
- Parenchyma
  - Note any differences in congestion between the 2 sides (suggesting blood flow issues)
- Sections
  - Each vascular geographic zone should be treated as separate entity with submission of standard sections from each

MICROSCOPIC

General Features

- Twin gestations in general are frequently premature
- Changes of uteroplacental malperfusion are not uncommon

- Increased incidence of fetal thrombotic vasculopathy associated with abnormal cord insertions &/or cord compromise

DIFFERENTIAL DIAGNOSIS

Monochorionic Diamniotic

- Pseudomonoamniotic placentation occurs with rupture of dividing membrane of MCDA placenta
  - Disruption may occur intentionally with septostomy treatment of twin-twin transfusion syndrome
  - Disruption may occur unintentionally during laser therapy for twin-twin transfusion syndrome
  - Spontaneous rupture may occur
  - Loss of dividing membrane creates single amniotic cavity with risk for cord entanglement
- Amnion may be stripped off fetal surface during delivery and dividing membrane may be missed

SELECTED REFERENCES

1. Moldenhauer JS et al: Diagnosis and management of complicated monochorionic twins. Clin Obstet Gynecol. 58(3):632-42, 2015
2. Paepe ME: Examination of the twin placenta. Semin Perinatol. 39(1):27-35, 2015
3. Lewi L et al: The vascular anastomoses in monochorionic twin pregnancies and their clinical consequences. Am J Obstet Gynecol. 208(1):19-30, 2013
4. Chalouhi GE et al: Specific complications of monochorionic twin pregnancies: twin-twin transfusion syndrome and twin reversed arterial perfusion sequence. Semin Fetal Neonatal Med. 15(6):349-56, 2010
5. Hack KE et al: Placental characteristics of monoamniotic twin pregnancies in relation to perinatal outcome. Placenta. 30(1):62-5, 2009
6. Aston KI et al: Monozygotic twinning associated with assisted reproductive technologies: a review. Reproduction. 136(4):377-86, 2008
7. Diehl W et al: Selective cord coagulation in acardiac twins. Semin Fetal Neonatal Med. 12(6):458-63, 2007
8. Dickinson JE: Monoamniotic twin pregnancy: a review of contemporary practice. Aust N Z J Obstet Gynaecol. 45(6):474-8, 2005
9. van den Wijngaard JP et al: Modelling the influence of amnionicity on the severity of twin-twin transfusion syndrome in monochorionic twin pregnancies. Phys Med Biol. 49(6):N57-64, 2004
10. Giménez-Scherer JA et al: Malformations in acardiac twins are consistent with reversed blood flow: liver as a clue to their pathogenesis. Pediatr Dev Pathol. 6(6):520-30, 2003
11. Roqué H et al: Perinatal outcomes in monoamniotic gestations. J Matern Fetal Neonatal Med. 13(6):414-21, 2003
12. Spitz L et al: Conjoined twins. JAMA. 289(10):1307-10, 2003
13. Umur A et al: Monoamniotic-versus diamniotic-monochorionic twin placentas: anastomoses and twin-twin transfusion syndrome. Am J Obstet Gynecol. 189(5):1325-9, 2003
14. De Paepe ME et al: Demonstration of placental vascular anatomy in monochorionic twin gestations. Pediatr Dev Pathol. 5(1):37-44, 2002
15. Van Allen MI et al: Twin reversed arterial perfusion (TRAP) sequence: a study of 14 twin pregnancies with acardius. Semin Perinatol. 7(4):285-93, 1983

Close Cord Insertions and Entanglement in MCMA

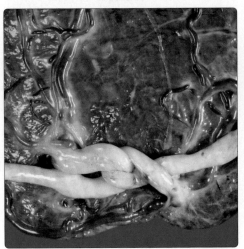

Complex Cord Entanglement

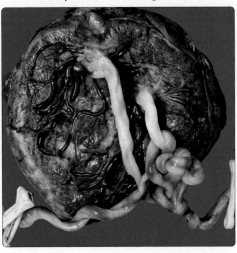

(Left) *Monochorionic monoamniotic (MCMA) twin placentas usually have cord insertions close to one another. The absence of a dividing membrane allows for cord entanglement.* (Right) *Severe cord entanglement in this MCMA placenta was fortunately associated with a good outcome for both twins.*

Cord Entanglement in MCMA Twins

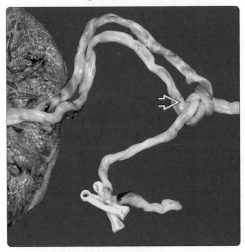

Fetal Demise Due to Cord Entanglements

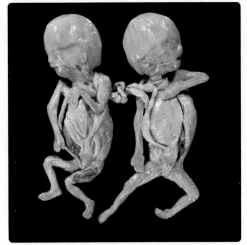

(Left) *A complex knot ⮊ has formed involving the midportions of both cords. Both twins did well.* (Right) *Multiple cord loops around the neck of each fetus with additional entanglements between the 2 cords are the obvious cause of 2nd-trimester fetal loss in this MCMA placenta.*

Vascular Anastomoses in Monochorionic Placenta

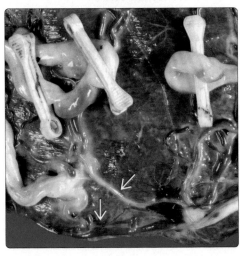

Dye Injection of Monochorionic Placenta

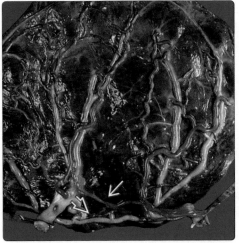

(Left) *Vascular anastomoses are always present in the MCMA placenta. Two superficial anastomoses ⮊ are seen in this placenta. The larger is an artery to artery, the smaller cannot be determined on this photograph.* (Right) *Injection with dye allows precise description of the various types of anastomoses in the same placenta. The 2 anastomoses are now more clearly identified as artery to artery (red) ⮊ and vein to vein (green) ⮊.*

Branched Umbilical Cords of Acardiac Twins

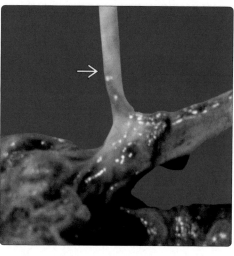

5-Vessel Umbilical Cord in Conjoined Twins

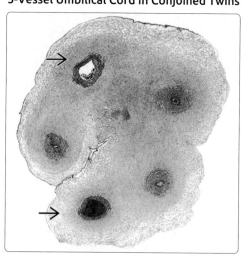

(Left) *Gross photograph shows a branched umbilical cord. The smaller 2-vessel cords ➡ of the acardiac twin anastomoses with the larger cord of the pump twin.* (Right) *The number of umbilical vessels may vary within the shared umbilical cord of conjoined twins. This cord has 3 arteries and 2 veins ➡, consistent with 1 of the twins having a single umbilical artery.*

Direct Cord Artery-to-Artery Anastomosis

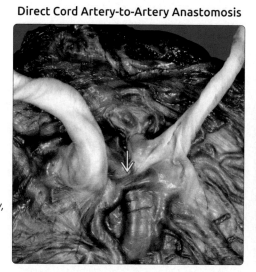

Macerated Acardiac Twin

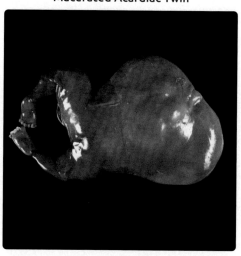

(Left) *Acardiac twinning is commonly associated with close approximation of the umbilical cords. There is a large artery-to-artery anastomosis ➡ noted between the 2 cords.* (Right) *This acardiac/acephalic twin was from a case of twin reversed arterial perfusion (TRAP). In TRAP, the acardiac twin shunts blood from the more normal pump twin. The pump twin dies in 50% of cases. (Courtesy S. Kostadinov, MD.)*

Nonmacerated Acardiac Twin

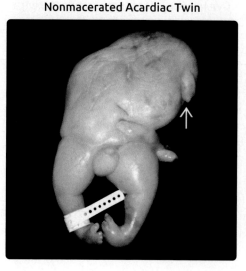

X-Ray of Acardiac Twin

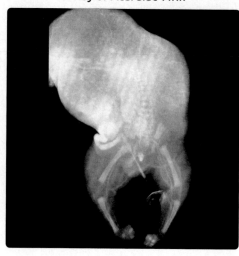

(Left) *This acardiac twin demonstrates well-formed lower extremities and relatively normal external male genitalia. There is only 1 rudimentary upper extremity ➡ and no cranial formation.* (Right) *Specimen radiographs help define anatomy of acardiac or conjoined twins to better guide dissection. Radiopaque dye was injected into the vasculature.*

Thoracoomphalopagus Conjoined Twins

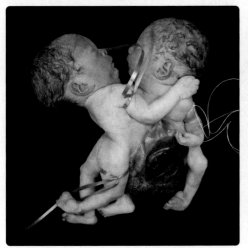

Dicephalus Conjoined Twins

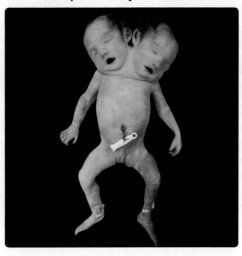

(Left) *These thoracoomphalopagus twins at 33 weeks were initially diagnosed on US at 15-weeks gestation. There were 2 hearts in an "upstairs-downstairs" configuration. The large abdominal wall defect contained a shared liver.* (Right) *Dicephalus conjoined twins have, on rare occasions, survived until adulthood.*

Parasitic Twin Attached to Abdomen

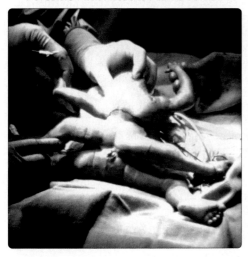

Surgically Removed Parasitic Twin

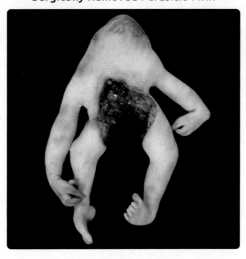

(Left) *This parasitic twin with 4 extremities was attached to the abdomen and pelvis. There were no shared organs and separation was possible.* (Right) *This image shows the parasitic twin after surgical separation. (Courtesy S. Rossmann, MD, PhD.)*

Fetus in Fetu

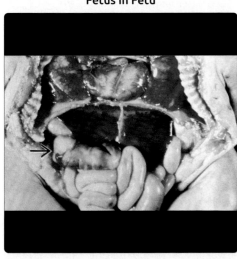

Fetus in Fetu With Umbilical Cord Structures

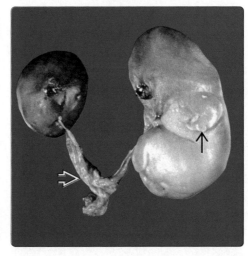

(Left) *The inked abdominal mass ➡ is an internal twin, a.k.a. fetus in fetu (FIF). FIFs have been reported at multiple sites in the body, though most are found in the retroperitoneum. An FIF is distinguished from a teratoma by the presence of an axial skeleton.* (Right) *This FIF consists of 2 amorphous masses connected by umbilical cord-like structures ⇨. One showed elements of an axial skeleton with a poorly developed upper extremity ➡. The other was more similar to an acardiac twin.*

TERMINOLOGY

Synonyms

- Selective fetal growth restriction
- Selective intrauterine growth restriction (sIUGR)
- Twin birth weight discordance
- Discordant severe IUGR

Definitions

- Selective or isolated fetal growth restriction
  o Occurring in absence of twin-twin transfusion syndrome (TTTS)
  o Various definitions for discordant growth in twins
    - > 20% or > 25% discordance in estimated fetal weight or birth weight
    - >10% discordance in abdominal circumference
    - Severe IUGR of 1 twin with estimated fetal weight or birth weight below 10th percentile
- Placental mass
  o Proportion of placental territory dedicated to 1 twin; in monochorionic twin placentas, defined by twin's chorionic plate vessel distribution

EPIDEMIOLOGY

Incidence

- More common in monochorionic than in dichorionic twins
- Incidence depends on definition used
  o Monochorionic twins
    - Estimated incidence of selective (non-TTTS) severe intertwin growth discrepancy: 15-46%
  o Dichorionic twins
    - Estimated incidence of severe intertwin growth discrepancy: 7-26%

ETIOLOGY/PATHOGENESIS

Monochorionic Twins

- Uneven distribution of placental mass between 2 twins
- Markedly eccentric or velamentous cord insertion of 1 or both twins

- Possible contribution of intertwin vascular anastomoses

Dichorionic Twins

- Placental factors
  o Uneven placental sizes
  o Abnormal (peripheral) cord insertion of 1 or both twins
  o Discordant placental implantation and uteroplacental perfusion
  o Discordant placental parenchymal pathology
- Other factors (discordant)
  o Genetic growth potential
  o Structural or chromosomal fetal anomalies
  o Congenital infection
  o Sex (usually not > 10% birth weight discordance)

CLINICAL IMPLICATIONS

Prognosis

- Significant risk of intrauterine death or neurologic adverse outcome for both smaller and larger twin
  o Outcome determined by onset and severity of discordance, degree of growth restriction, interval growth, and amniotic fluid volume of smaller twin
    - Risk highest when presenting in 2nd trimester
  o In monochorionic gestations
    - Death of small fetus may be followed by postmortem acute fetofetal transfusion from normally grown twin to dead fetus, resulting in death (15-20%) or severe neurological damage (20-30%) of larger twin
    - Normally grown twin may suffer neurologic impairment even if both twins are born alive due to acute fetofetal transfusion episodes in utero
- Highly variable clinical evolution
  o In monochorionic pregnancies: Classification in 3 types based on umbilical artery Doppler of IUGR twin
    - Correlation with clinical evolution and patterns of placental anastomoses
    - Type I sIUGR: Positive diastolic flow
      □ Generally good outcome
      □ Mild discordance in placental territories &/or large number of intertwin anastomoses

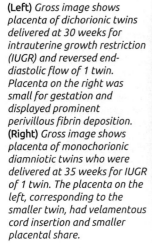

(Left) Gross image shows placenta of dichorionic twins delivered at 30 weeks for intrauterine growth restriction (IUGR) and reversed end-diastolic flow of 1 twin. Placenta on the right was small for gestation and displayed prominent perivillous fibrin deposition. (Right) Gross image shows placenta of monochorionic diamniotic twins who were delivered at 35 weeks for IUGR of 1 twin. The placenta on the left, corresponding to the smaller twin, had velamentous cord insertion and smaller placental share.

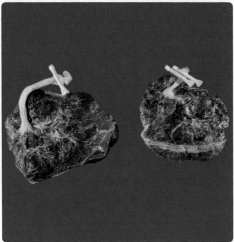

Growth Discordance: Dichorionic Twins

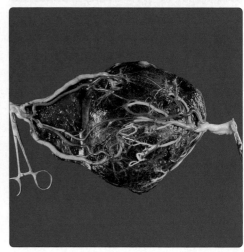

Growth Discordance: Monochorionic Twins

- – Type II sIUGR: Persistently absent or reversed end-diastolic flow
  - □ High risk for fetal deterioration before 30-weeks gestation, neurological damage, perinatal mortality
  - □ Placental territory of IUGR twin very small; few and small intertwin anastomoses
- – Type III sIUGR: Intermittently absent/reversed end-diastolic flow
  - □ Apparently benign evolution but potential for unexpected fetal demise of IUGR fetus and neurological damage of 1 or both twins
  - □ Large intertwin artery-to-artery anastomoses; short distance between cord insertion sites

Management

- Individualized, chorionicity- and gestational age-dependent options
  - o Expectant management
  - o Fetoscopic laser coagulation
  - o Selective feticide or termination of pregnancy
  - o Delivery

MACROSCOPIC

General Features

- In monochorionic and dichorionic placentas
  - o Uneven placental sharing
    - – Smaller share usually associated with smaller twin
  - o Peripheral (velamentous or marginal) cord insertion of at least 1 twin
    - – Peripheral cord usually associated with smaller twin
  - o Single umbilical artery of 1 (usually smaller) twin
- In monochorionic placentas
  - o Intertwin choriovascular anastomoses
    - – Proposed correlation with outcome of selective (non-TTTS) twin growth discrepancy
      - □ Type I sIUGR: Many anastomoses
      - □ Type II sIUGR: Few and small anastomoses
      - □ Type III sIUGR: Large artery-to-artery anastomoses
    - – Higher frequency of intertwin vein-to-vein anastomoses
- In dichorionic placentas
  - o Placental parenchymal lesions (discordant)
    - – Infarcts, fibrin deposition, retroplacental hematoma
    - – Predominantly (not exclusively) in smaller twin territory

MICROSCOPIC

Histologic Features

- In monochorionic and dichorionic placentas
  - o Discordant villous maturation
    - – Usually accelerated villous maturation in association with smaller share &/or peripheral cord
- In dichorionic placentas
  - o Placental parenchymal lesions, mainly in territory of smaller twin
    - – Infarcts
    - – Subchorionic fibrin deposition
    - – Retroplacental hematoma
    - – Fetal thrombotic vasculopathy

DIFFERENTIAL DIAGNOSIS

Twin-to-Twin Transfusion Syndrome

- In monochorionic twins
- Definition based on clinical (ultrasound) criteria: Oligohydramnios/polyhydramnios
- Increased frequency of uneven placental sharing and abnormal cord insertion
- Typical patterns of intertwin choriovascular anastomoses
  - o Decreased frequency of artery-to-artery anastomoses
  - o Increased frequency of vein-to-vein anastomoses

Anomalies or Infection

- Appropriate ancillary studies may be indicated
  - o Discordant chromosomal anomalies
  - o Structural fetal anomalies
  - o Congenital infection

DIAGNOSTIC CHECKLIST

Clinically Relevant Pathologic Features

- Relative distribution of placental territory if single disc
- Individual placental weights if separate discs
- Cord insertion types
  - o Paracentral
  - o Eccentric
  - o Marginal
  - o Velamentous
- Parenchymal lesions
  - o Gross and microscopic, estimation of proportion of parenchymal involvement
- Intertwin choriovascular anastomoses
  - o To be described as in all monochorionic placentas
  - o Potential correlation with outcome of selective, non-TTTS growth discordance

SELECTED REFERENCES

1. Khalil A et al: Consensus definition and essential reporting parameters of selective fetal growth restriction in twin pregnancy: a Delphi procedure. Ultrasound Obstet Gynecol. ePub, 2018
2. Konno H et al: Roles of venovenous anastomosis and umbilical cord insertion abnormalities in birthweight discordance in monochorionic-diamniotic twin pregnancies without twin-twin transfusion syndrome. J Obstet Gynaecol Res. 44(4):623-629, 2018
3. Bennasar M et al: Selective intrauterine growth restriction in monochorionic diamniotic twin pregnancies. Semin Fetal Neonatal Med. 22(6):376-382, 2017
4. Buca D et al: Outcome of monochorionic twin pregnancy with selective intrauterine growth restriction according to umbilical artery Doppler flow pattern of smaller twin: systematic review and meta-analysis. Ultrasound Obstet Gynecol. 50(5):559-568, 2017
5. Breathnach FM et al: Fetal growth disorders in twin gestations. Semin Perinatol. 36(3):175-81, 2012
6. Kent EM et al: Placental pathology, birthweight discordance, and growth restriction in twin pregnancy: results of the ESPRiT Study. Am J Obstet Gynecol. 207(3):220, 2012
7. De Paepe ME et al: Placental characteristics of selective birth weight discordance in diamniotic-monochorionic twin gestations. Placenta. 31(5):380-6, 2010
8. Valsky DV et al: Selective intrauterine growth restriction in monochorionic twins: pathophysiology, diagnostic approach and management dilemmas. Semin Fetal Neonatal Med. 15(6):342-8, 2010
9. Eberle AM et al: Placental pathology in discordant twins. Am J Obstet Gynecol. 169(4):931-5, 1993

TERMINOLOGY

Abbreviations

- Twin-twin transfusion syndrome (TTTS)

Definitions

- Complication of monochorionic twinning
  - Sometimes termed twin oligohydramnios-polyhydramnios sequence (TOPS)
- Characterized by chronic fetofetal blood transfusion from donor twin to recipient twin through placental vascular communications
  - Hemodynamic imbalance leads to oligohydramnios (donor)/polyhydramnios (recipient)
- Diagnosis of severe chronic TTTS based on strict antenatal ultrasound criteria
  - Monochorionicity
  - Asymmetric distribution of amniotic fluid across intertwin membrane

EPIDEMIOLOGY

Incidence

- 20% of all twin pregnancies are monochorionic
- 9-15% of monochorionic twin pregnancies are complicated by severe TTTS

Natural History

- Mortality > 70% for untreated midtrimester TTTS
  - Donor twin dies first in > 60% of cases
  - Risks for surviving twins: Death due to exsanguination in low-pressure circulation of dead or dying co-twin, neurologic or cardiac anomalies, and hypoxic-ischemic lesions in limbs, intestines, liver, and lungs

ETIOLOGY/PATHOGENESIS

Complex and Multifactorial Condition

- Placental and fetal contributory factors
- Secondary hemodynamic, hematologic, and hormonal imbalances

Placental Contributions

- Intertwin vascular anastomoses
  - Present in virtually all monochorionic placentas
  - Artery-to-artery (AA) anastomoses: Protective
    - Superficial and bidirectional
    - May compensate for hemodynamic balances created by uneven artery-to-vein (AV) anastomoses
  - Vein-to-vein (VV) anastomoses: Possibly detrimental
    - Superficial and bidirectional
  - AV anastomoses: Possibly detrimental
    - Deep penetration of chorionic plate by unpaired artery of one twin and unpaired vein of other twin
    - Obligatorily unidirectional
    - May create hemodynamic imbalance, especially in absence of AA anastomoses
- Cord insertion
  - Increased risk of TTTS associated with velamentous or marginal cord insertion
- Placental sharing
  - Increased risk of TTTS associated with uneven placental sharing

Fetal Contributions

- Donor twin
  - Hypovolemic and oliguric
  - Activation of renin-angiotensin system
    - Paradoxic decrease of renal and placental perfusion
    - Renal tubular dysgenesis: Absence or poor development of proximal convoluted tubules
  - Anemic, pale (often)
- Recipient twin
  - Hypervolemic and polyuric
  - Upregulation of endothelin-1 and atrial natriuretic peptide
    - Cardiovascular anomalies (recipient-twin cardiomyopathy)
  - Polycythemic, plethoric (often)
- Presentation of donor and recipient twins may be altered (reversed) by acute peripartum events or following demise of one twin

Twin-Twin Transfusion Syndrome

Ultrasound

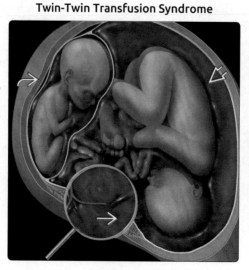

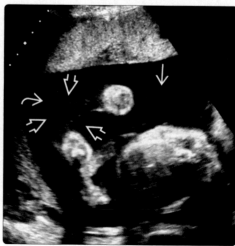

(Left) Growth-discordant monochorionic twins are shown with a unidirectional arteriovenous shunt ➡ from a growth-restricted, oligohydramniotic donor ➡ to a larger, hypervolemic, and polyhydramniotic recipient ➡. (Right) Ultrasound shows oligohydramnios ➡ and polyhydramnios ➡. The thin intertwin membrane ➡ is "shrink wrapping" the donor ("stuck twin"). The donor fluid is more echogenic. (Courtesy A. Kennedy, MD.)

CLINICAL IMPLICATIONS

Clinical Presentation

- Most clinically relevant during 2nd trimester of pregnancy
- Usually incidental finding during routine ultrasound
  - Oligohydramnios/polyhydramnios

Imaging Findings

- Monochorionic pregnancy
- Oligohydramnios-polyhydramnios

Staging of Twin-Twin Transfusion Syndrome

- Used to determine optimal management strategy
  - Based on ultrasound studies, including Doppler
  - Quintero staging system most widely used
    - Stage I: Polyhydramnios [maximum vertical pocket (MVP) ≥ 8 cm] in recipient twin and oligohydramnios (MVP ≤ 2 cm) in donor twin
    - Stage II: Same as stage I + nonvisualization of filling of donor bladder
    - Stage III: Same as stage I or stage II + critically abnormal Doppler studies
    - Stage IV: Ascites or frank hydrops in either fetus
    - Stage V: (Impending) demise of either fetus
  - Adaptations (e.g., Cincinnati system) include echocardiographic and hemodynamic indices

MACROSCOPIC

General Features

- Monochorionic twin placenta: Single disc, thin, 2-layered intertwin membrane (amnion only), intertwin vascular communications
- No pathognomonic TTTS features
- Overall: Increased frequency of uneven sharing, peripheral cord insertion, absence of AA anastomoses, and presence of VV anastomoses

Specimen Handling

- Routine examination of twin placenta
- Examination of choriovascular intertwin anastomoses
  - ± dye injection
  - Anatomic hallmarks of choriovasculature
    - Arteries superficial to accompanying veins
    - AA and VV anastomoses superficial and direct
    - AV anastomoses deep and indirect
  - Large AA and VV anastomoses identifiable without injection
- Injection of chorionic vasculature
  - Not routinely indicated for all monochorionic placentas
  - Potential indications
    - Examination of placenta following fetoscopic laser coagulation of TTTS
    - Monochorionic twin pregnancies with atypical course

MICROSCOPIC

General Features

- Poorly described; variable
  - Dependent on timing and degree of syndrome
    - Confounded by perinatal or postmortem acute twin-twin transfusion and associated placental anatomic features (implantation anomalies, cord insertion)
- Donor twin
  - Large and edematous (immature) villi, small and atrophic (hypermature) villi, amnion nodosum, increased erythroid precursors
- Recipient twin
  - Appropriately mature villi
  - Fewer erythroid precursors
  - ± edema

DIFFERENTIAL DIAGNOSIS

Discordant Severe Intrauterine Growth Restriction

- Uneven placental sharing
- Peripheral cord insertion

Twin Reversed Arterial Perfusion Sequence

- Acardiac fetus
- Single large AA and VV shunts

Twin Anemia-Polycythemia Sequence

- Large intertwin difference in hemoglobin levels without TOPS
- Spontaneous or after laser coagulation
- Small and few anastomoses, AA anastomoses usually absent

Acute Perinatal Twin-Twin Transfusion Syndrome

- Clinical presentation highly variable
- Occurs during birth
- Usually large AA &/or VV anastomoses present

DIAGNOSTIC CHECKLIST

Clinically Relevant Pathologic Features

- Relative distribution of placental territory
- Cord insertion types
- Presence/absence of AA and VV anastomoses
  - Description of AV imbalance potentially relevant in absence of AA anastomoses
- Confirmation of chorionicity
- Parenchymal lesions (type and extent)

SELECTED REFERENCES

1. Couck I et al: The placenta in twin-to-twin transfusion syndrome and twin anemia polycythemia sequence. Twin Res Hum Genet. 19(3):184-90, 2016
2. Kontopoulos E et al: Twin-to-twin transfusion syndrome: definition, staging, and ultrasound assessment. Twin Res Hum Genet. 19(3):175-83, 2016
3. Zhao DP et al: Veno-venous anastomoses in twin-twin transfusion syndrome: a multicenter study. Placenta. 36(8):911-4, 2015
4. De Paepe ME et al: What-and why-the pathologist should know about twin-to-twin transfusion syndrome. Pediatr Dev Pathol. 16(4):237-51, 2013
5. De Paepe ME et al: Placental markers of twin-to-twin transfusion syndrome in diamniotic-monochorionic twins: a morphometric analysis of deep artery-to-vein anastomoses. Placenta. 31(4):269-76, 2010
6. De Paepe ME et al: Demonstration of placental vascular anatomy in monochorionic twin gestations. Pediatr Dev Pathol. 5(1):37-44, 2002
7. Denbow ML et al: Placental angioarchitecture in monochorionic twin pregnancies: relationship to fetal growth, fetofetal transfusion syndrome, and pregnancy outcome. Am J Obstet Gynecol. 182(2):417-26, 2000

Discordant Growth

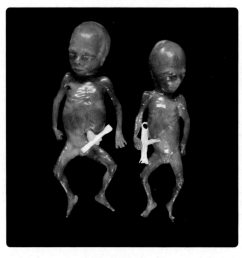

Discordant Organ Growth

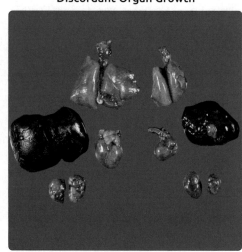

(Left) *In this case of diamniotic monochorionic twin-twin transfusion syndrome (TTTS) twins at 20-weeks gestation, the recipient twin is shown on the left and the smaller donor twin on the right.* **(Right)** *Organ overview highlights the striking difference in organ sizes between the twins, particularly affecting the heart and lungs. The organs of the recipient twin are shown on the left.*

Placenta of TTTS

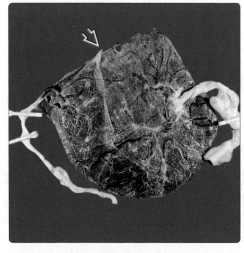

Placenta Following Vascular Injection

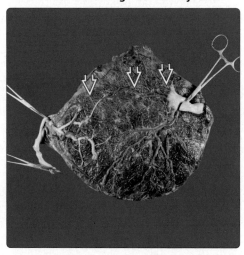

(Left) *Diamniotic monochorionic twin placenta from a TTTS pregnancy shows a thin and velamentously inserted cord of donor twin (left), larger and paracentrally inserted cord of recipient twin (right), and uneven sharing of the placental mass. The dividing membrane ➡ is shown.* **(Right)** *Same placenta is shown after vascular injection using the following color code: Left twin (donor): Artery is red, and vein is yellow; right twin (recipient): Artery is red, and vein is green. An artery-to-artery (AA) anastomosis is present ➡.*

Intertwin Anastomoses

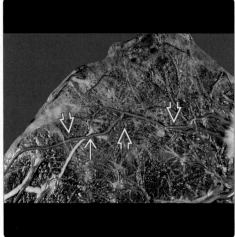

Deep Intertwin Anastomoses

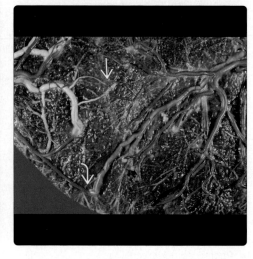

(Left) *Closer view of the upper portion of the placenta shows the superficial AA anastomosis ➡ as well as a deep artery-to-vein (AV) anastomosis from the recipient twin (right) to the donor twin (left) ➡.* **(Right)** *The lower portion of the placenta displays deep AV anastomoses from the recipient to the donor twin ➡ and a deep AV anastomosis from the donor to the recipient twin ➡.*

Placenta Following Vascular Injection

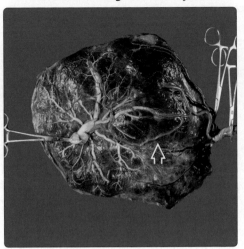

Large Intertwin Anastomoses

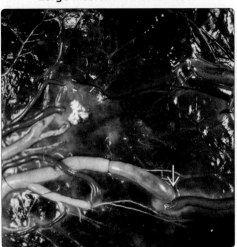

(Left) *Diamniotic monochorionic twin placenta from a TTTS pregnancy has been injected as follows: Recipient twin (left): Artery red and vein yellow; donor twin (right): Artery red and vein black. Donor twin has the smaller placental share, a velamentous cord insertion, and a magistral (nonbranching) vascular pattern. An AA anastomosis is present ➡.* **(Right)** *Closer view of the midportion of the placenta shows a large AV anastomosis from the donor twin (right) to the recipient twin (left) ➡.*

Recipient Twin Histology

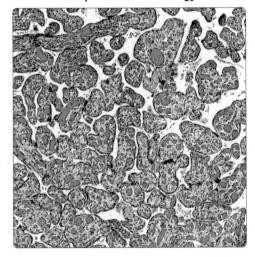

Donor Twin Histology

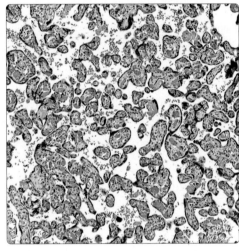

(Left) *Representative micrograph of placental parenchyma of the recipient twin shows relatively immature chorionic villi, chorangiosis, and the presence of nucleated erythroid precursors.* **(Right)** *Parenchyma of the donor twin shows accelerated villous maturation and prominent syncytial knots.*

Placenta Following Vascular Injection

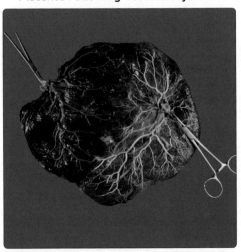

Deep Intertwin Anastomoses

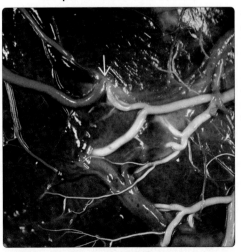

(Left) *In this TTTS twin placenta, superficial AA and vein-to-vein anastomoses are absent, which necessitated the use of 4 dyes for vascular injection [left twin (donor): Artery is red, and vein is black; right twin (recipient): Artery is yellow, and vein is green]. Donor twin has a marginal cord insertion.* **(Right)** *Closer view demonstrates a large, deep AV anastomosis from the donor twin to the recipient twin ➡.*

TERMINOLOGY

Abbreviations

- Twin anemia-polycythemia sequence (TAPS)

Definitions

- Complication of monochorionic twinning
- Characterized by large intertwin difference in hemoglobin and reticulocyte levels in absence of significant amniotic fluid discordance
  - Presence of oligohydramnios/polyhydramnios is diagnostic of twin-twin transfusion syndrome (TTTS)
- 2 forms of TAPS
  - Spontaneous TAPS
  - Postlaser TAPS
    - Iatrogenic, following laser treatment for TTTS

EPIDEMIOLOGY

Incidence

- Spontaneous TAPS
  - 3-6% of monochorionic twin pregnancies
- Postlaser TAPS
  - In up to 16% of TTTS pregnancies after incomplete laser treatment

Natural History

- Few concrete data on perinatal and long-term morbidity
- Reported neonatal outcomes range from isolated intertwin hemoglobin differences to cerebral injury and neonatal death
  - Donors: Hypoalbuminemia and hypoproteinemia, renal dysfunction, cerebral injury
  - Recipients: Polycythemia-hyperviscosity syndrome with secondary skin and limb necrosis, thrombocytopenia, cerebral injury
- Long-term neurodevelopmental outcome remains unknown

ETIOLOGY/PATHOGENESIS

Unique Placental Angioarchitecture

- Few, small intertwin anastomoses
  - Chronic and gradual blood transfusion results in highly discordant hemoglobin levels (donor anemic, recipient polycythemic)
  - Gradual character of transfusion prevents hemodynamic/hormonal imbalance and secondary development of oligohydramnios-polyhydramnios

CLINICAL IMPLICATIONS

Clinical Presentation

- Spontaneous TAPS
  - Typically after 26-weeks gestation
- Postlaser TAPS
  - Typically within 1 to 5 weeks after laser surgery
  - Usually former recipient becomes anemic and former donor becomes polycythemic

Diagnosis

- Antenatal
  - Based on Doppler ultrasound criteria
    - Interwin difference in middle cerebral artery peak systolic velocity (MCA-PSV)
      - MCA-PSV > 1.5 multiples of median (MoM) in donor
      - MCA-PSV < 1.0 MoM in recipient
  - Proposed antenatal TAPS staging
    - Stages 1-5, based on intertwin MCA-PSV difference and presence/absence of fetal compromise (abnormal Doppler flow, hydrops, intrauterine demise)
- Postnatal
  - Suspected in presence of large intertwin hemoglobin difference (> 8 g/dL)
  - Additional criteria proposed to differentiate between TAPS and acute peripartum TTTS
    - Increased reticulocyte count in donor (evidence of chronic anemia)

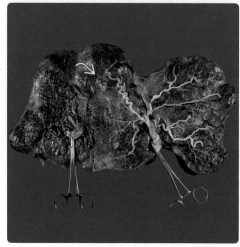

Twin Anemia-Polycythemia Sequence
Placenta: Fetal Surface

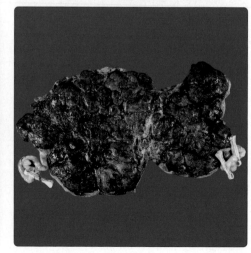

Twin Anemia-Polycythemia Sequence
Placenta: Maternal Surface

(Left) *Vascular injection of this diamniotic-monochorionic twin placenta from a pregnancy complicated by twin anemia-polycythemia sequence (TAPS) demonstrates the near-complete separation of the 2 vascular beds. A single, small artery-to-vein anastomoses is indicated* ➤. *Left twin (recipient) artery is red, and vein is green; right twin (donor) artery is yellow, and vein is black.* (Right) *The maternal surface of the placenta demonstrates marked color discordance with sharp demarcation of the placental territories.*

Twin Anemia-Polycythemia Sequence

□ Expressed as ratio of donor reticulocyte count over recipient reticulocyte count (proposed cut-off value for TAPS: > 1.7)
- Presence of (residual) intertwin anastomoses (diameter < 1 mm)
  □ Usually detected by vascular injection
o Proposed postnatal TAPS staging: Based on degree of intertwin Hb difference

Management

- No consensus on optimal management

MACROSCOPIC

General Features

- Monochorionic twin placenta: Single disc, thin 2-layered intertwin membrane, intertwin vascular communications
- Typical TAPS angioarchitecture
  o Few and small artery-to-vein (AV) anastomoses (3-4 per placenta, on average)
    - Frequently located along periphery of placenta
  o Artery-to-artery (AA) anastomoses: In 10-20% of TAPS placentas, small (< 1 mm)
  o Vein-to-vein (VV) anastomoses: In < 10% of TAPS placentas
- Some have intertwin color difference on maternal side of placenta
  o Anemic twin: Pale parenchyma
  o Polycythemic twin: Dark red parenchyma

Specimen Handling

- Routine examination of twin placenta
- Examination of choriovascular intertwin anastomoses
  o ± dye injection
  o Anatomic hallmarks of choriovasculature
    - Arteries superficial to accompanying veins
    - AA and VV anastomoses superficial and direct
    - AV anastomoses deep and indirect
  o Large AA and VV anastomoses identifiable without injection
- Injection of chorionic vasculature
  o Facilitates identification of small AV anastomoses

MICROSCOPIC

General Features

- No specific histopathologic features
  o In some, congestion (polycythemic twin) vs. increased numbers of circulating erythroid precursors (anemic twin)
  o Confounded by peripartum events
  o Influenced by associated placental anatomic features

DIFFERENTIAL DIAGNOSIS

Twin-Twin Transfusion Syndrome

- Also chronic fetofetal blood transfusion from 1 twin (donor) to other (recipient)
  o More severe condition resulting in hemodynamic/hormonal imbalance and secondary development of oligohydramnios in donor twin and polyhydramnios in recipient twin [twin oligohydramnios-polyhydramnios sequence (TOPS)]

o May be associated with intertwin hemoglobin differences: Hemoglobin level donor < recipient
- Primarily clinical diagnosis based on well-established antenatal ultrasound criteria
- Placental findings associated with increased risk for TTTS
  o Absence of AA anastomoses
  o Presence of VV anastomoses
  o Uneven placental sharing
  o Peripheral insertion of 1 or both cords
  o Unbalanced AV anastomoses (especially in absence of AA anastomoses)

Acute Peripartum (or Perinatal) TTTS

- Acute shift of blood volume between monochorionic twins during delivery
  o Resulting from blood pressure differences associated with uterine contractions, delayed cord clamping, or changes in fetal position around delivery
- Clinical presentation ranges from subtle intertwin hemoglobin differences to hypovolemic shock (donor) and polycythemia (recipient)
- Placental findings
  o Large superficial AA &/or VV anastomoses

Acute Perimortem TTTS

- Acute shift of blood volume between monochorionic twins after intrauterine death of 1 twin
  o Resulting from exsanguination from surviving twin into low-pressure circulation of dead or dying cotwin
- Placental findings
  o Large superficial AA &/or VV anastomoses

DIAGNOSTIC CHECKLIST

Clinically Relevant Pathologic Features

- Presence/number/direction/size of intertwin AV anastomoses
- Presence/absence of AA and VV anastomoses
- Relative distribution of placental territory
- Cord insertion types
- Presence/absence of color difference basal plate
- Confirmation of chorionicity
- Parenchymal lesions (type and extent)

SELECTED REFERENCES

1. De Paepe ME et al: Redness discordance in monochorionic twin placentas: correlation with clinical and placental findings. Placenta. 60:54-60, 2017
2. Couck I et al: The placenta in twin-to-twin transfusion syndrome and twin anemia polycythemia sequence. Twin Res Hum Genet. 19(3):184-90, 2016
3. Tollenaar LS et al: Twin anemia polycythemia sequence: current views on pathogenesis, diagnostic criteria, perinatal management, and outcome. Twin Res Hum Genet. 19(3):222-33, 2016
4. Paepe ME: Examination of the twin placenta. Semin Perinatol. 39(1):27-35, 2015
5. de Villiers SF et al: Placental characteristics in monochorionic twins with spontaneous versus post-laser twin anemia-polycythemia sequence. Placenta. 34(5):456-9, 2013
6. de Villiers S et al: Arterio-arterial vascular anastomoses in monochorionic twin placentas with and without twin anemia-polycythemia sequence. Placenta. 33(3):227-9, 2012
7. Lopriore E et al: Placental characteristics in monochorionic twins with and without twin anemia-polycythemia sequence. Obstet Gynecol. 112(4):753-8, 2008
8. Robyr R et al: Prevalence and management of late fetal complications following successful selective laser coagulation of chorionic plate anastomoses in twin-to-twin transfusion syndrome. Am J Obstet Gynecol. 194(3):796-803, 2006

TERMINOLOGY

Abbreviations

- Twin-twin transfusion syndrome (TTTS)

Definitions

- Fetoscopic laser coagulation of communicating vessels (FLOC)
  o Laser beam used to photocoagulate intertwin vascular communications
  o Interruption of hemodynamic imbalance by "dichorionizing" initially monochorionic placenta
    - Prevents shifting of blood volume between twins
    - Provides functional separation of both circulations in case of subsequent fetal demise of 1 twin

EPIDEMIOLOGY

Incidence of TTTS

- 9-15% of all monochorionic twin pregnancies are complicated by severe TTTS

Natural History

- Mortality > 70% for untreated midtrimester TTTS
- In case of single fetal demise, risks for surviving twin
  o Death due to exsanguination in low-pressure circulation of dead or dying co-twin
  o Neurologic or cardiac anomalies
  o Hypoxic-ischemic lesions in limbs, intestines, liver, and lungs

CLINICAL IMPLICATIONS

Fetoscopic Laser Coagulation of Communicating Vessels

- Treatment of choice for severe TTTS diagnosed before 26-weeks gestation
- Superior in terms of survival (76% survival of at least 1 twin), neurologic outcome, and gestational age at delivery
- Different technical approaches exist
  o Nonselective approach

  - Coagulation of all vessels crossing the intertwin membrane
  o Selective approach (Quintero)
    - Most common
    - Coagulation of intertwin vascular anastomoses only
    - Preservation of paired vessels (belonging to a single fetus) traversing intertwin membrane
  o Sequential selective approach
    - Coagulation of artery-to-vein (AV) anastomoses from donor to recipient, followed by those from recipient to donor
  o Superselective approach
    - Coagulation of suspected causative AV anastomosis only
  o Solomon technique
    - Increasingly more common
    - Coagulation of entire vascular equator (anastomoses and intervening parenchyma)
- Postcoagulation complications linked to presence of residual anastomoses
  o Persistent TTTS
  o Recurrent TTTS (5-14%)
  o Reversal of TTTS
    - Donor becomes recipient and vice versa
  o Twin anemia-polycythemia sequence (TAPS)
    - Incidence of iatrogenic form of TAPS: In up to 16% of TTTS pregnancies after incomplete laser treatment
      □ Incidence reduced by Solomon procedure
    - Attributed to residual anastomoses, mostly small and peripheral
    - Paradoxically, former recipient anemic; former donor polycythemic
  o Demise of 1 or both twins

Serial Amnioreduction

- Repetitive amniodrainage of the polyhydramniotic sac of the recipient twin
- 65% survival of at least 1 twin

Alternative Options

- Expectant management

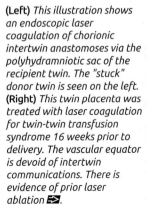

(Left) This illustration shows an endoscopic laser coagulation of chorionic intertwin anastomoses via the polyhydramniotic sac of the recipient twin. The "stuck" donor twin is seen on the left.
(Right) This twin placenta was treated with laser coagulation for twin-twin transfusion syndrome 16 weeks prior to delivery. The vascular equator is devoid of intertwin communications. There is evidence of prior laser ablation ➡.

Laser Coagulation of Intertwin Anastomoses

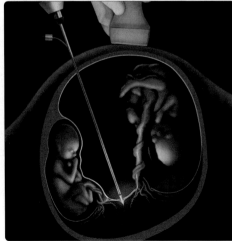

Twin-Twin Transfusion Syndrome Placenta After Laser Coagulation

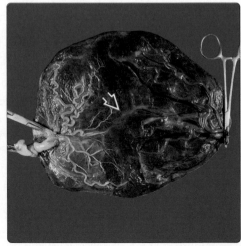

- Amniotic septostomy
  - Puncture of intertwin membranes to, temporarily, equilibrate amniotic fluid volume
- Elective preterm delivery
- Selective reduction of 1 fetus
- Pregnancy termination

MACROSCOPIC

General Features

- Monochorionic twin placenta: Single disc, thin 2-layered intertwin membrane (amnion only), (remnants of) intertwin vascular communications
- Pathologic findings following laser coagulation vary
- Dependent on time interval between intervention and delivery
  - Within 1 month after laser coagulation
    - Foci of laser impact usually identifiable
    - Located along recipient side of membrane
    - Hemorrhagic vessels with abrupt interruption of dye filling
  - > 1 month after laser coagulation
    - Regional or complete absence of intertwin anastomoses
    - Associated subchorionic fibrin deposition
- Dependent on treatment approach
  - Selective laser coagulation
    - Subtle lesions limited to chorionic vessels
  - Solomon technique
    - Extensive, full thickness placental necrosis along vascular equator

Specimen Handling

- Routine examination of twin placenta
- Examination of choriovascular intertwin anastomoses
  - No standardized guidelines for examination of postcoagulation placenta
  - If indicated, color-coded dye injection of chorionic vasculature
    - Anatomic hallmarks of choriovasculature
      □ Arteries superficial to accompanying veins
      □ Artery-to-artery (AA) and vein-to-vein (VV) anastomoses superficial and direct
      □ Artery-to-vein (AV) anastomoses deep and indirect
  - Description of residual anastomoses
    - More frequent along placental periphery
  - Description of evidence of laser coagulation
    - Abrupt interruption of chorionic vessels filling with dye
    - Coagulated vessels typically located along recipient side of intertwin membrane

MICROSCOPIC

General Features

- Selective laser coagulation
  - Evidence in/around intertwin anastomoses
    - Varying degrees of vascular necrosis
    - Focal intervillous hemorrhage and fibrin deposition
    - Associated avascular villi &/or infarction
- Solomon technique

  - Extensive full thickness infarction and necrosis

DIAGNOSTIC CHECKLIST

Clinically Relevant Pathologic Features

- General placental anatomic features associated with TTTS risk
  - Relative distribution of placental territory
  - Cord insertion types
    - Paracentral
    - Eccentric
    - Marginal
    - Velamentous
- Evidence of laser coagulation
- Presence of residual intertwin vascular communications
  - Presence/absence of (residual) AA and VV anastomoses
  - Presence, number, direction of (residual) AV anastomoses
- Confirmation of chorionicity
- Parenchymal lesions
  - Gross and microscopic, estimation of proportion of parenchymal involvement

SELECTED REFERENCES

1. Knijnenburg PJC et al: Incidence of and risk factors for residual anastomoses in twin-twin transfusion syndrome treated with laser surgery: a 15-year single-center experience. Fetal Diagn Ther. ePub, 2018
2. Quintero RA et al: Laser treatment of twin-to-twin transfusion syndrome. Twin Res Hum Genet. 19(3):197-206, 2016
3. Slaghekke F et al: Solomon technique versus selective coagulation for twin-twin transfusion syndrome. Twin Res Hum Genet. 19(3):217-21, 2016
4. Paepe ME: Examination of the twin placenta. Semin Perinatol. 39(1):27-35, 2015
5. De Paepe ME et al: What-and why-the pathologist should know about twin-to-twin transfusion syndrome. Pediatr Dev Pathol. 16(4):237-51, 2013
6. Chalouhi GE et al: Specific complications of monochorionic twin pregnancies: twin-twin transfusion syndrome and twin reversed arterial perfusion sequence. Semin Fetal Neonatal Med. 15(6):349-56, 2010
7. Lopriore E et al: Residual anastomoses in twin-to-twin transfusion syndrome treated with selective fetoscopic laser surgery: localization, size, and consequences. Am J Obstet Gynecol. 201(1):66, 2009
8. De Paepe ME et al: Placental findings after laser ablation of communicating vessels in twin-to-twin transfusion syndrome. Pediatr Dev Pathol. 7(2):159-65, 2004
9. Senat MV et al: Endoscopic laser surgery versus serial amnioreduction for severe twin-to-twin transfusion syndrome. N Engl J Med. 351(2):136-44, 2004
10. Quintero RA et al: Selective versus non-selective laser photocoagulation of placental vessels in twin-to-twin transfusion syndrome. Ultrasound Obstet Gynecol. 16(3):230-6, 2000
11. De Lia JE et al: Fetoscopic neodymium: YAG laser occlusion of placental vessels in severe twin-twin transfusion syndrome. Obstet Gynecol. 75(6):1046-53, 1990

TERMINOLOGY

Definitions

- ≥ 3 fetuses
  - Separate or shared discs
  - Separate or shared chorionic sacs
  - Separate or shared amniotic sacs

EPIDEMIOLOGY

Incidence

- Increased incidence of multiple births in developed nations over past 3 decades
  - Older maternal age distribution
  - Increased use and availability of fertility therapies
    - Assisted reproductive technologies (ART) [e.g., in vitro fertilization (IVF)]
    - Non-ART treatments (e.g., ovulation stimulation)
- Recent relative decline in rate of triplet and higher order multiple birth rates since 1998 peak
  - Improved ART procedures with transfer of fewer embryos per IVF cycle
  - Multifetal pregnancy reduction
- Birth rates in United States in 2016: 101 triplets or higher order multiple births per 100,000 live births

Natural History

- Increased risk for premature birth and intrauterine growth restriction
- Increased risk for poor neurodevelopmental outcome and neonatal death
- Spontaneous reduction of multifetal pregnancy
  - Usually in first 11-12 weeks of pregnancy
  - "Vanishing twins"
- Selective reduction of multifetal pregnancy
  - Usually in 1st trimester of pregnancy (after 12 weeks)

ETIOLOGY/PATHOGENESIS

Natural Higher Multiple Births

- Increased maternal age

Patterns of Placentation in Triplets

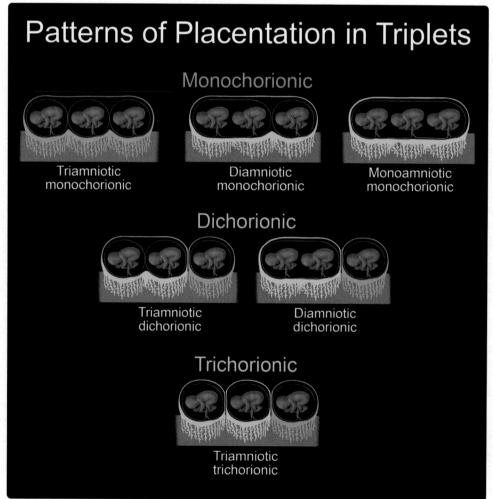

Triplets may be monochorionic, dichorionic, or trichorionic with all possible combinations of amniotic sacs. Monozygous triplets may be monoamniotic, diamniotic, or triamniotic. Dizygous triplets may be dichorionic or trichorionic. Trizygous triplets must be trichorionic. Combinations of monozygous and polyzygous multiples are common. Multichorionic placentas may be separate or fused. (Modified from Pathology of Placenta, 2e.)

Iatrogenic Higher Multiple Births

- ART
- Ovulation induction

CLINICAL IMPLICATIONS

Prognosis

- Increased risk for maternal complications
  - Preterm labor and delivery
  - Gestational hypertension and preeclampsia
  - Gestational diabetes
  - Placental abruption
  - Excessive postpartum bleeding
- Increased risk for fetal or neonatal complications
  - Fetal demise
  - Intrauterine growth restriction
  - Prematurity
  - Neurodevelopmental delay
- Predictors of outcome in higher order multiples
  - Maternal height
  - Parity (previous full-term, non-low-birth-weight outcome)
  - Type of placentation
    - Risks higher for triplets with mixed chorionicity than trichorionic triplets
    - Monochorionic multiples: At risk for twin-twin transfusion syndrome, twin anemia polycythemia syndrome, and selective intrauterine growth restriction
  - Number of fetuses

MACROSCOPIC

General Features

- Triplets may be any combination of zygosity and chorionicity
  - Triamniotic-trichorionic
  - Triamniotic-dichorionic
  - Triamniotic-monochorionic
  - Diamniotic-dichorionic
  - Diamniotic-monochorionic
  - Monoamniotic-monochorionic
- Higher order multiple placentas are usually fused, at least in part, due to space limitations
- Unfavorable placental implantation
  - Marginal or velamentous cord insertion common
  - Intertwin placental growth discordance common
- Examination of higher order multiple placentas is extension of examination of twin placentas
  - Chorionicity
  - Amnionicity
  - Cord insertion
  - Relative placental weights or sizes
  - Chorionic vascularity
  - Vascular intertwin anastomoses (between monochorionic twins)
- Examination after spontaneous or selective multifetal pregnancy reduction
  - Identification and description of reduced fetuses

MICROSCOPIC

General Features

- Variable
  - Influenced by associated placental anatomic features
    - Cord insertion
    - Placental size
  - Potentially confounded by chronic or acute twin-to-twin transfusion (between monochorionic twins)

DIAGNOSTIC CHECKLIST

Clinically Relevant Pathologic Features

- Intertwin relationships
  - Terminology includes number of amnions and number of chorions, followed by description of twins in monochorionic relationship (if applicable)
  - e.g., quadramniotic-trichorionic quadruplet placenta, diamniotic-monochorionic for quadruplets A and B
  - Confirmation of chorionicity
    - Sampling and microscopic analysis of intertwin membranes
- Description of individual placentas
  - Similar to twin placentas
  - Size of placenta
    - Weight (if separate disc)
    - Dimensions of individual placentas (if fused discs)
    - Relative distribution of placental vascular territory (between monochorionic twins)
  - Cord insertion type
  - Intertwin choriovascular anastomoses
    - Presence/absence of artery-to-artery (AA) &/or vein-to-vein anastomoses (between monochorionic twins)
    - Optional: Presence/number/direction of AV anastomoses (especially in absence of AA anastomoses)
  - Parenchymal lesions (type and extent)
- In case of spontaneous or selective multifetal pregnancy reduction, description of higher order placenta should include both original status and status at delivery
  - Description of remnants of reduced fetuses, if identified

SELECTED REFERENCES

1. Anthoulakis C et al: Risks of miscarriage or preterm delivery in trichorionic and dichorionic triplet pregnancies with embryo reduction versus expectant management: a systematic review and meta-analysis. Hum Reprod. 32(6):1351-1359, 2017
2. Committee on Ethics: Committee opinion no. 719: multifetal pregnancy reduction. Obstet Gynecol. 130(3):e158-e163, 2017
3. Downing M et al: Perinatal and neonatal outcomes of triplet gestations based on chorionicity. AJP Rep. 7(1):e59-e63, 2017
4. Martin JA et al: Births in the United States, 2016. NCHS Data Brief. 1-8, 2017
5. Razaz N et al: Perinatal outcomes in multifetal pregnancy following fetal reduction. CMAJ. 189(18):E652-E658, 2017
6. Sato Y et al: Incidences of feto-fetal transfusion syndrome and perinatal outcomes in triplet gestations with monochorionic placentation. Fetal Diagn Ther. 40(3):181-186, 2016
7. Practice Committee of Society for Assisted Reproductive Technology; Practice Committee of American Society for Reproductive Medicine: Elective single-embryo transfer. Fertil Steril. 97(4):835-42, 2012
8. Wen SW et al: Maternal morbidity and obstetric complications in triplet pregnancies and quadruplet and higher-order multiple pregnancies. Am J Obstet Gynecol. 191(1):254-8, 2004
9. Fox H and Sebire NH: Pathology of the placenta. Philadelphia: Saunders Elsevier. 355, 2007

Triamniotic-Trichorionic Triplet Placenta

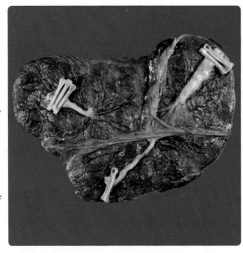

Diamniotic-Dichorionic Triplet Placenta

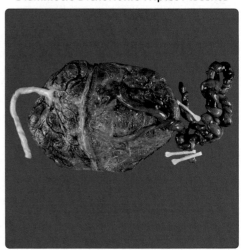

(Left) This triamniotic-trichorionic single disc triplet placenta from an in vitro fertilization (IVF) gestation was delivered at 32 weeks following preterm premature rupture of membranes. Cord A (single clamp) has a membranous insertion into the dividing membrane between triplets A and B (double clamps). (Right) This diamniotic-dichorionic triplet pregnancy (twins B and C: Monoamniotic) was complicated by fetal demise of triplets B and C, attributable to severe cord entanglement.

Triamniotic-Dichorionic Triplet Placenta

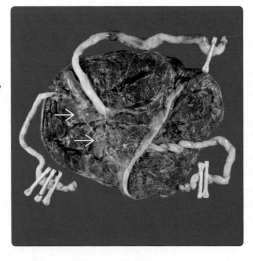

Triamniotic-Dichorionic Triplet Placenta

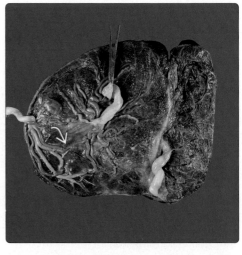

(Left) This triamniotic-dichorionic, single-disc, 30-week triplet placenta shows a thick intertwin membrane between triplets A (1 clamp) and C (3 clamps) on one side, and triplet B (2 clamps) on the other side. A thin intertwin membrane ➡ is present between monochorionic triplets A and C. (Right) The placenta underwent vascular injection using the following color code: Triplet A: Artery red and vein green; triplet C: Artery red and vein yellow. A superficial artery-to-artery anastomosis is present ➡.

Triamniotic-Trichorionic Triplet Placenta

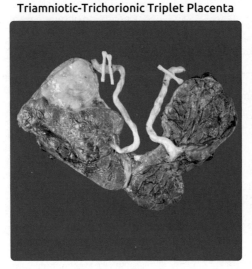

Triamniotic-Trichorionic Triplet Placenta With Fetus Papyraceus

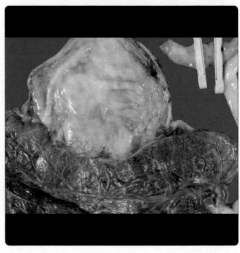

(Left) This triamniotic-trichorionic triplet placenta was delivered at 35-weeks gestation following elective reduction of the gestation to twin pregnancy. (Right) In the same case, a closer view shows a largely mummified fetus papyraceus.

Ultrasound of Quadruplet Pregnancy

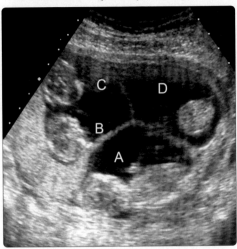

Quadramniotic-Quadrichorionic Quadruplet Placenta

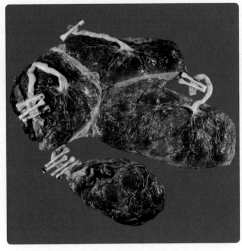

(Left) *US shows a triamniotic-trichorionic quadruplet pregnancy. There is no membrane between B and C, the monoamniotic pair. Fetuses B and C died at 28 weeks, and the cause of death was undetermined. Quads A and D were delivered by C-section at 36 weeks. (Courtesy A. Kennedy, MD.)* (Right) *These IVF-associated quadruplets were delivered at 33 weeks due to growth restriction of quads B and C. Shown is the quadramniotic-quadrichorionic double-disc quadruplet placenta.*

Quadruplet Placenta With Dual Fetal Demise

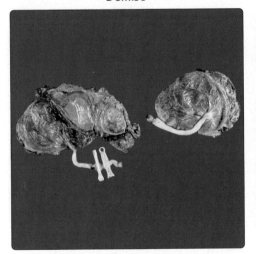

Quadruplet Placenta With Dual Fetal Demise

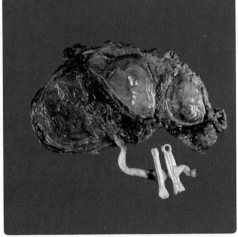

(Left) *This IVF-associated quadruplet pregnancy underwent early demise of 2 quads, resulting in spontaneous reduction to a twin pregnancy. The exact nature of the original quadruplet pregnancy cannot be determined (likely quadramniotic-quadrichorionic). The surviving quads are diamniotic-dichorionic. Preterm labor resulted in delivery at 24 weeks.* (Right) *A closer view shows the 2 fetus papyracei ("vanishing twins").*

Quadruplet Placenta After Selective Reduction

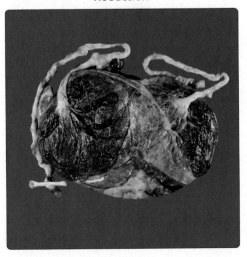

Quadruplet Placenta After Selective Reduction

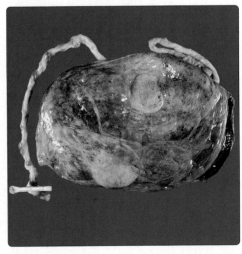

(Left) *This IVF-associated originally quadruplet pregnancy underwent selective reduction to twin pregnancy. The remaining twins are separated by a thick dividing membrane and display separate choriovascular networks, consistent with a diamniotic-dichorionic relationship.* (Right) *Closer examination reveals the presence of 2 mummified fetus papyracei deeply embedded in the placental membranes.*

TERMINOLOGY

- Direct causes of maternal death: Obstetric complications or treatment
- Indirect causes of maternal death: Preexisting disease or disease developing during gestation exacerbated by pregnancy

CLINICAL ISSUES

- USA maternal mortality rising in 21st century, global maternal death rate falling
  - USA ranks 60th worldwide
- Most frequent direct causes of maternal death include
  - Obstetric hemorrhage, 11-27% of deaths
  - Hypertensive disorders (preeclampsia), 14-22% of deaths
  - Embolization, 8-20% of deaths (thromboembolic and amniotic)
    - Thromboembolic disease and amniotic fluid embolism (AFE)
  - Infection, 4-13% of deaths

- Abortive outcome, including ectopic pregnancy, 8% of deaths

MICROSCOPIC

- Postpartum hemorrhage (PPH)
  - Uterine atony may be associated with retained placenta, acute or chronic endomyometritis, or abruption often with Couvelaire uterus
  - Delayed PPH, subinvolution of maternal spiral arteries or retained placenta
- AFE: Often diagnosis of exclusion
  - Fetal squames in small pulmonary arteries and capillaries, nonuniform distribution
    - Often coated with granular debris, associated with mucin ± fatty material from vernix caseosa
    - Cytokeratin staining, mucin stains, and oil red O may be useful
  - Accumulation of leukocytes and platelets in small pulmonary arteries and capillaries

---

Maternal Sepsis

(Left) *Sudden decompensation occurred immediately after delivery. Focal fibrin and neutrophils noted in the maternal intervillous space without chorioamnionitis were associated with maternal sepsis.* (Right) *Gram staining revealed large numbers of gram-positive cocci within the intervillous space. Culture was positive for Streptococcus pyogenes.*

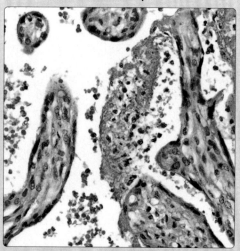

Maternal Sepsis Due to *Streptococcus*

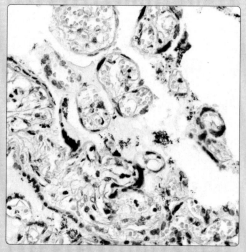

Necrotizing Fascitis Due to Group A *Streptococcus*

(Left) *Section of the uterine wall demonstrates necrotizing fascitis and maternal sepsis. Colonies ➡ of group A Streptococcus organisms are present in the devitalized myometrium.* (Right) *Septic abortion demonstrated massive ➡ bacterial overgrowth and neutrophils in the maternal intervillous space. The organism cultured was group B Streptococcus.*

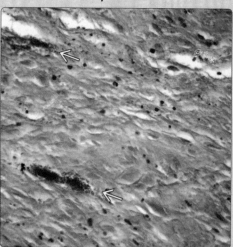

Septic Abortion Due to Group B *Streptococcus*

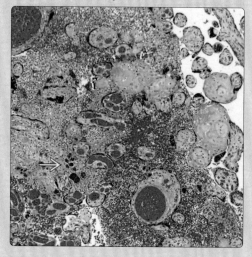

TERMINOLOGY

Definitions

- World Health Organization (WHO) and International Classification of Diseases definition of **maternal death**
  - Death of woman while pregnant (at any gestational age)
  - Within 42 days of end of pregnancy (any duration or site of pregnancy)
  - From any cause related to or aggravated by pregnancy or its management
    - Excluding accidental or incidental causes
- **Late maternal death** (WHO): Occurring > 42 days but < 1 year after end of pregnancy
- Surveillance methods and definitions vary, making accurate identification and classification of maternal deaths difficult
  - 25% of deaths occur antepartum, 28% intrapartum, and 36% postpartum
- **Direct causes**: Result of interventions, omissions, and improper handling or as result of causal chain that starts from series of conditions directly associated with pregnancy
- **Indirect causes**: Death due to preexisting disease or disease developing during gestation and not due to direct gestational causes but due to physiologic effects of gestation
- **Nongestational**: Death during gestation as result of external violence, suicide, or other random event; may account for 1/2 of deaths during pregnancy

CLASSIFICATION

Direct Causes of Maternal Death

- Hypertensive disorders, 14-22% of deaths
  - Hypertension affects 10% of pregnancies
  - Gestational hypertension: ≥ 140/90 mm Hg after 20 weeks
  - Preeclampsia (PE): 5% of pregnancies; ≥ 140 mm Hg systolic or 90 mm Hg diastolic on 2 occasions (4-6 hours apart) or one reading ≥ 160/90 mm Hg after 20 weeks
    - Proteinuria, ≥ 1+ on dipstick, ≥ 300 mg/24 hours, spot protein:creatinine ratio ≥ 0.30; can have PE without proteinuria
    - PE with severe features ≥ 160/110 mm Hg, severe headache, visual changes, seizures, thrombocytopenia (< 100,000/μL), nausea, vomiting or epigastric pain (liver capsular hemorrhage or rupture), transaminitis (2x upper limits, low 100s), worsening renal function tests, decreased urine output, pulmonary edema, multiorgan system dysfunction
    - Hemolysis, elevated liver enzymes, low platelets (HELLP) now considered subtype of PE with severe features; however, 15% of HELLP do not have hypertension
  - Chronic hypertension, ≥ 140/90 prior to 20 weeks
    - Chronic hypertension with superimposed PE; preexisting hypertension with new onset proteinuria, worsening of preexisting proteinuria, or development of abnormal lab tests
  - Eclampsia (seizures) occurs in 1.4% of pregnancies
- Embolization, 8-20% of deaths
  - Thromboembolic disorders; pregnancy is hypercoagulable state, especially postoperative
    - Risk for pulmonary embolism increased 6-10x during pregnancy, 10-20x during 6-week postpartum period
    - Incidence, 0.5-2.0/1,000 pregnancies; 24% of women with deep vein thrombosis will develop PE, and 15% with PE will die
  - Amniotic fluid embolism (AFE) 5-15% of maternal deaths
    - Incidence 1/8,000 deliveries
    - Maternal mortality, 11-61%; 85% of survivors have permanent neurologic damage
    - Neonatal mortality, 7-44%; 50% of survivors have permanent damage
  - Air, bone marrow, fat, trophoblasts, decidua, or fetal tissue emboli
- Obstetric hemorrhage, 11-27% of deaths
  - Postpartum hemorrhage (PPH) is defined as blood loss > 1,000 mL, vaginal or cesarean delivery, incidence 2.8-3.3% of deliveries
- Infection, 4-13% of deaths
  - Group A *Streptococcus* is most common organism
- Abortive outcome, 8% of deaths
  - Ectopic pregnancy
    - Incidence of death 0.5/100,000 live births; decline in mortality over past 4 decades
    - Cause of death: Hemorrhage, shock, and renal failure
    - Increased incidence in African Americans
    - Increased risk < 25 and > 35 years of age
  - Unsafe abortion circumstances, complications of curettage
    - Misoprostol can be purchased from internet and is being used to abort 2nd-trimester pregnancy with increased risk for bleeding, sepsis, and retained products of conception
  - Intrauterine fetal demise, increased risk for endometritis, rarely death due to hypofibrinolysis, "dead baby syndrome"
- Peripartum cardiomyopathy (PPCM), 1 in 3,000-4,000 live births, incidence 0.05%
  - Left ventricular dysfunction between last month of pregnancy and first 5 months postpartum
  - Diagnostic criteria, ejection fraction < 45%, &/or fractional shortening < 30%, end-diastolic dimension > 2.7 cm/m² body surface area
  - Etiology unknown with consideration for: Viral myocarditis, abnormal immune response to pregnancy, autoimmune, abnormal response to hemodynamic stress of pregnancy, accelerated myocyte apoptosis, cytokine-induced inflammation, malnutrition, genetic factors, excessive prolactin production, abnormal hormonal function, increased adrenergic tone, myocardial ischemia
    - Genetic studies have linked genes of idiopathic dilated cardiomyopathy with some cases of PPCM
- Fatty liver of pregnancy
  - Incidence 1/10,000-100,000 pregnancies
  - Association with fetal fatty acid oxidation defect [long-chain 3 hydroxyacyl-coenzyme A dehydrogenase deficiency (LCHAD)], less often short- or medium-chain deficiency
- Complications of anesthesia

- o Increasing use of general anesthesia with increasing rate of cesarean delivery, increased risk for aspiration of gastric contents
  - o High regional block
  - o Toxicity of local anesthetics
- Delivery outside hospital, prolonged or obstructed labor

Indirect Causes of Maternal Death

- Cardiovascular disease, 16-25% of deaths
  - o In pregnancy, heart rate increases 10-30 bpm, cardiac output increases by 30-50%, cardiac size increases 30%
  - o Cardiomyopathy
  - o Arrhythmias
  - o Coronary artery disease, acute myocardial infarction, artery dissection
  - o Prolonged QT syndrome
  - o Myocarditis, endocarditis
  - o Hypertension
- Indirect maternal infections, 10%
- Stroke
- Pulmonary hypertension rare but associated with 23% maternal mortality when severe
- Asthma
- Anemia (severe < 7 g/dL)
- Diabetes
- High prepregnancy BMI, especially class 3 obesity, BMI ≥ 40
- Mental disorders and diseases of nervous system
  - o Postpartum depression occurs in ~ 20% of pregnancies
  - o Epilepsy; due to risk of congenital malformations, women may discontinue antiseizure medications

Nongestational Death

- Homicide 7%
  - o Most often in younger, disadvantaged women, usually early in pregnancy
  - o Method in decreasing order: Gunshot, stabbing, strangulation, blunt force head injuries, burns, falls, toxic exposure, drowning
- Suicide 5%
  - o Most often in older, more advantaged women; most often opioid overdose; possibly accidental
- Accident, most commonly motor vehicle

ETIOLOGY/PATHOGENESIS

Risk Factors for Maternal Mortality

- Extreme ends of reproductive age range, especially > 40 years
- 1st pregnancy or > 3-5 pregnancies
- Unplanned pregnancy
- Single
- Undereducated
- Ethnicity, non-Hispanic African American, 3-4x greater
- Poverty, transportation, quality of care, ≤ 4 prenatal visits
- Obesity, especially class 3, BMI > 40
- Severe anemia, sickle cell disease
- Previous stillbirth or emergency cesarean delivery
- Smoking
- Diabetes

CLINICAL ISSUES

Epidemiology

- USA maternal mortality 1982: 7.5/100,000 live births
- USA maternal mortality 2011-2013: 17/100,000 live births
  - o USA ranks 60th worldwide
  - o Leading cause is cardiovascular disease and other maternal conditions
  - o Decline in infection, hemorrhage, anesthetic complications, and hypertensive disorders
- USA Department of Health and Human Services healthy people 2010 goal, ≤ 3.3/100,000 live births
- Global maternal mortality in 2015, 216/100,000 live births (300,000 deaths)

Presentation

- Acute PPH occurs in 11% of deliveries, delayed PPH in 1-3% of deliveries
  - o 77% due to uterine atony, rarely due to cervical or uterine lacerations or uterine rupture
  - o Risk: Older age, obesity, previous cesarean delivery
- PE, most are asymptomatic, may have hypertension, headache, visual disturbances, right upper quadrant pain, excessive weight gain, edema
  - o Increased risk with previous PE, chronic renal disease, hypertension, diabetes, autoimmune disorders, age > 40 years, long interpregnancy interval, obesity, multifetal pregnancy, infertility
  - o Currently we cannot predict or prevent PE, delivery is only cure
    - – Number of maternal serum markers are being investigated but currently are not sensitive or specific enough to be used as routine screening test
  - o Leading causes of death in PE: Intracranial hemorrhage, abruption with disseminated intravascular coagulopathy (DIC), acute renal failure, hypertensive crisis, pulmonary edema, ischemic brain injury
  - o Ruptured subcapsular hepatic hematoma, secondary to fibrin in liver arterioles with hepatic necrosis, mortality 18-86%
  - o Women with history of pregnancy-associated hypertension have increased risk for late mortality from all causes, especially Alzheimer, diabetes, ischemic heart disease, and stroke
- Embolization
  - o AFE; dyspnea, cyanosis, acute hypoxia, acute hypotension, hemorrhage or coagulopathy, altered consciousness, restlessness, seizures, sudden profound and unexpected shock due to cardiovascular collapse
    - – Pathogenesis unknown, amniotic fluid gains entry into circulation, mainly through venous channels of endocervical region
    - – Physical obstruction to pulmonary arterioles and alveolar capillaries
    - – Release of primary or secondary endogenous mediators
      - □ Meconium in amniotic fluid may be more toxic
    - – Risk: ≥ 35 years old, multifetal pregnancy, eclampsia, polyhydramnios, placenta previa, abruption, induction of labor, nonvertex presentation, cesarean delivery, cervical laceration or uterine rupture, manual removal of placenta, tumultuous labor

- 13% occur prior to onset of labor, 70% during labor or < 2 hours after delivery, rarely up to 48 hours
- Phase 1: Anaphylactoid reaction
  - Tryptase releases in large quantities during mast cell degranulation, can be measured in postmortem serum (> 110 μg/L) and in lung by IHC
  - Sudden pulmonary hypertension and right-sided heart failure
  - Decreased serum levels of C3 and C4
- Phase 2: Severe hemorrhage
  - Amniotic fluid produces thromboplastin-like effect, activates extrinsic pathway, induces platelet aggregation, and activates complement cascade, resulting in DIC
  - Left-sided heart failure
  - Endothelial activation and leakage
  - Thromboembolism, sudden onset of dyspnea and tachypnea, pleuritic chest pain, nonproductive cough, apprehension or sensation of impending doom
    - Pregnancy is state of hypercoagulability; risk for thrombosis is 5-10x higher during pregnancy and 10-20x higher for 6 weeks postpartum
    - May be increased in hereditary thrombophilia (protein C or factor V Leiden deficiency) or acquired defects (antiphospholipid antibody)
    - Risk: > 35 years old, higher parity, multifetal pregnancy, obesity, prolonged immobilization, pelvic trauma, surgery during pregnancy, including cesarean, history of previous thromboemboli, PE
    - 24% of women with deep venous thrombosis will develop pulmonary emboli, 15% mortality
  - Embolization of trophoblasts
    - Normal physiologic deportation of trophoblasts during gestation is part of immune tolerance
      - Increased deportation in PE, abruption, or trauma
    - Rare cases of excessive trophoblasts in pulmonary vasculature associated with maternal death during labor or within first 24 hours after delivery
    - Complete hydatidiform molar villi have been found in lung vessels
  - Embolization of fetal tissues or decidua
    - Rare complication of evacuation of products of conception
  - Bone marrow or fat emboli are usually complication of resuscitation and rib fractures
- Infection
  - Septic shock results in cardiovascular collapse and multiple organ dysfunction with death within 24-48 hours of onset; severe sepsis may cause same findings with more protracted course 7-14 days of onset
    - Necrotizing fasciitis, myometritis, or toxic shock, due to group A *Streptococcus pyogenes*
  - Increased incidence of maternal death during H1N1 influenza epidemic of 2009
- PPCM
  - Dilated cardiomyopathy with reduced left ventricular systolic function
  - Risk: ≥ 25 years old, non-Hispanic African American, multifetal gestation, severe anemia, chronic hypertension, pregnancy-related hypertension, obesity

- Mortality 10-14%, most improve and 1/2 completely recover 3-6 months after disease onset; those who do not may have thromboembolic events
- ~ 50% have recurrence of left ventricular dysfunction and heart failure in subsequent pregnancies
- Cardiac murmur, severe tricuspid insufficiency, mild to moderate pulmonary insufficiency, shift of interventricular septum leftward, and impaired left ventricular filling
- Cough, brown sputum (hemosiderin), pulmonary venous congestion, pulmonary edema, or pleural effusion
- Fatty liver of pregnancy
  - Occurs during 3rd trimester, often associated with PE or fetal fatty acid oxidation abnormality
  - Present with nausea and vomiting, which are key features that may help differentiate it from PE
    - Features similar to HELLP, elevated ammonia, transaminases < 1,000, decreased glucose, increased bilirubin and LDH from hemolysis, decreased fibrinogen, schistocytes due to DIC
  - 10-85% maternal mortality, often secondary to hepatic rupture
  - 40% fetal mortality, related to maternal complications or underlying fatty acid oxidation abnormality (LCHAD)
- Stroke, incidence 1.6/100,000, usually hemorrhagic due to high systolic pressure, PE
- Increased risk for spontaneous coronary artery dissection
- Hematopoietic
  - Increased risk associated with sickle cell disease due to acute crisis, splenic sequestration, pulmonary embolism, or infection
  - Thrombotic thrombocytopenic purpura/hemolytic-uremic syndrome; presents with renal dysfunction and mental status changes

MICROSCOPIC

Histologic Features

- PPH
  - Uterine atony may be associated with retained placenta, acute or chronic endomyometritis, or abruption often with Couvelaire uterus
  - Delayed PPH, generally associated with subinvolution of maternal spiral arteries or retained placenta
- PE, endothelial injury
  - Renal, glomerular endotheliosis, seen in all glomeruli, but severity varies; changes may last up to 6 months postpartum
    - Glomerular endothelial swelling resulting in bloodless glomeruli, obliteration of endothelial fenestrae
    - Immunofluorescence positive for multiple complement components, immunoglobulins and C4d
    - May have features of thrombotic microangiopathy
  - Liver periportal/portal necrosis and sinusoidal fibrin with hepatic arterial medial necrosis, thrombosis, subcapsular hematoma, hepatic rupture
  - CNS, perivascular edema, highlighted by histiocyte and platelet markers, hemosiderin, small vessel thrombosis, parenchymal necrosis, hypoxic damage in posterior parietal-occipital brain
  - Cardiac, subendocardial "flame" hemorrhages
  - Lung, pulmonary edema

- o DIC, fibrin and platelet microthrombi in small vessels, microinfarcts
- o Placenta, atheroma of maternal spiral arteries
- Embolization
  - o AFE, often diagnosis of exclusion
    - − Veins of cervix and lower uterine segment may contain fetal squamous cells
    - − Lung, edema, atelectasis, congestion
      - □ It is presumed that small amount of amniotic fluid is normally present in pulmonary vasculature
      - □ Fetal squamous cells (cytokeratin positive), often coated with granular debris in small pulmonary arteries and capillaries, distribution is not uniform in lung, may persist for week after delivery
      - □ Small pulmonary arteries and capillaries with accumulation of leukocytes and platelets
      - □ Mucinous material (Alcian blue or mucicarmine positive)
      - □ Meconium from gastrointestinal tract (TKH-2 staining, can also be measured in serum)
      - □ Fatty material from vernix caseosa (oil red O positive)
      - □ Increased mast cells (tryptase can also be measured in serum)
    - − May have microthrombi in lung and other organs due to DIC
  - o Thromboemboli
    - − Embolized clots from pelvic or deep leg veins, usually massive saddle emboli within main pulmonary arteries
  - o Excessive embolization of trophoblasts when seen in 80% of capillaries
  - o Bone marrow or fat emboli, commonly seen after resuscitation due to rib fractures (oil red O positive)
  - o Embolization of decidual tissue (PAS diastase resistant, vimentin positive), may include invasive trophoblasts (human placental lactogen and cytokeratin positive)
  - o Embolization of complete hydatidiform molar villi (HCG positive)
- Infection, sepsis
  - o Maternal intervillous space of placenta may have increased neutrophils entrapped in fibrin
  - o Usually associated with severe chorioamnionitis, acute villitis, or endometritis
- Complications of abortion
  - o Septic abortion, perforation of uterus, injury to bowel, and embolization of fetal or placental tissues
- PPCM
  - o 30% show healing myocarditis, mild inflammation within myocardium with foci of necrosis and variable amounts of hypertrophy and fibrosis, while only 9% of idiopathic dilated cardiomyopathy has inflammation
  - o High helper:supressor T-cell ratio in peripheral blood
- Fatty liver of pregnancy
  - o Microvesicular, central zonal steatosis, ballooning degeneration may mask lipid; no necrosis, no inflammation
  - o Extramedullary hematopoiesis, giant mitochondria may be present due to adaptive or degenerative response to altered metabolic environment

DIAGNOSTIC CHECKLIST

Clinically Relevant Pathologic Features

- Careful gross and extensive microscopic examination of uterus
- AFE are present in small pulmonary arterioles and capillaries; not in larger vessels like usual pulmonary emboli

Pathologic Interpretation Pearls

- May need special stains to confirm AFE
- May need special stains or cultures to confirm maternal sepsis

SELECTED REFERENCES

1. Howell EA: Reducing disparities in severe maternal morbidity and mortality. Clin Obstet Gynecol. 61(2):387-399, 2018
2. Creanga AA et al: Pregnancy-related mortality in the United States, 2011-2013. Obstet Gynecol. 130(2):366-373, 2017
3. Hecht JL et al: The pathology of eclampsia: an autopsy series. Hypertens Pregnancy. 36(3):259-268, 2017
4. Hirshberg A et al: Epidemiology of maternal morbidity and mortality. Semin Perinatol. 41(6):332-337, 2017
5. Lisonkova S et al: Association between prepregnancy body mass index and severe maternal morbidity. JAMA. 318(18):1777-1786, 2017
6. MacDorman MF et al: Trends in maternal mortality by sociodemographic characteristics and cause of death in 27 states and the district of columbia. Obstet Gynecol. 129(5):811-818, 2017
7. Nair M et al: Indirect maternal deaths: UK and global perspectives. Obstet Med. 10(1):10-15, 2017
8. Tamura N et al: Amniotic fluid embolism: pathophysiology from the perspective of pathology. J Obstet Gynaecol Res. 43(4):627-632, 2017
9. de Cosio FG et al: Late maternal deaths and deaths from sequelae of obstetric causes in the Americas from 1999 to 2013: a trend analysis. PLoS One. 11(9):e0160642, 2016
10. Moaddab A et al: Health care disparity and state-specific pregnancy-related mortality in the United States, 2005-2014. Obstet Gynecol. 128(4):869-75, 2016
11. Theilen LH et al: All-cause and cause-specific mortality after hypertensive disease of pregnancy. Obstet Gynecol. 128(2):238-44, 2016
12. Buschmann C et al: Maternal and pregnancy-related death: causes and frequencies in an autopsy study population. Forensic Sci Med Pathol. 9(3):296-307, 2013
13. Bhattacharyya A et al: Peripartum cardiomyopathy: a review. Tex Heart Inst J. 39(1):8-16, 2012
14. Herbst J et al: Cardiovascular conditions and the evaluation of the heart in pregnancy-associated autopsies. J Forensic Sci. 55(6):1528-33, 2010
15. Conde-Agudelo A et al: Amniotic fluid embolism: an evidence-based review. Am J Obstet Gynecol. 201(5):445.e1-13, 2009
16. Abboud J et al: Peripartum cardiomyopathy: a comprehensive review. Int J Cardiol. 118(3):295-303, 2007
17. Delmis J et al: Sudden death from trophoblastic embolism in pregnancy. Eur J Obstet Gynecol Reprod Biol. 92(2):225-7, 2000
18. Rolfes DB et al: Acute fatty liver of pregnancy: a clinicopathologic study of 35 cases. Hepatology. 5(6):1149-58, 1985
19. Filippi v., et al: Reproductive, Maternal, Newborn and Child Health: Disease Control Properties. 3rd edition. Washington, DC: The International Bank for Reconstruction and Development / The World Bank, 2016

Glomerular Endotheliosis in Preeclampsia

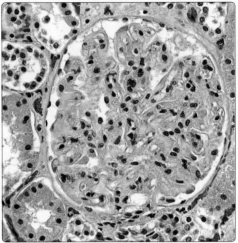

Hepatic Necrosis Due to Preeclampsia

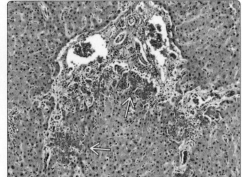

(Left) *Glomerulus from a woman with preeclampsia shows swollen capillaries of endotheliosis.* (Right) *Hepatocyte necrosis ➡ in the portal region (zone 1) of the liver is characteristic of preeclampsia.*

Hepatic Rupture Associated With Preeclampsia

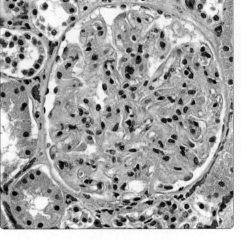

Atheroma of Maternal Spiral Artery

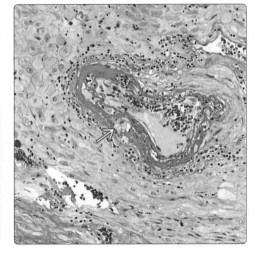

(Left) *Case of severe preeclampsia, complicating a multifetal pregnancy, shows hepatic capsule rupture. This section shows microvesicular steatosis ➡ and a large area of hepatocyte necrosis ➡. (Right) The implantation site in the uterus may show decidual arteriopathy, like this maternal spiral artery with acute atheromatosis. There is a thick layer of fibrinoid necrosis ➡, and there are foamy macrophages and perivascular lymphocytes.*

Massive Retroplacental Hematoma, Gross

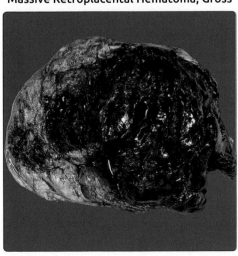

Multiple Infarcts of Different Ages

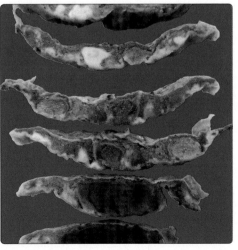

(Left) *A large retroplacental hematoma is characteristic of preeclampsia and may be associated with fibrinolysis and postpartum hemorrhage. (Right) A placenta with multiple, nonmarginal infarcts of different ages is characteristic of preterm preeclampsia.*

(Left) *Amniotic fluid embolus (AFE) characteristically involves the small arterioles. Note the lack of blood within the vessel, which is filled with neutrophils and rare fetal squamous epithelial cells* ➡.
(Right) *AFE with an abundant mucinous component and granular debris is consistent with meconium staining of the amniotic fluid.*

Amniotic Fluid Embolus

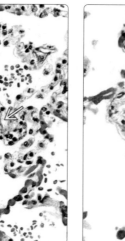

Amniotic Fluid Embolus

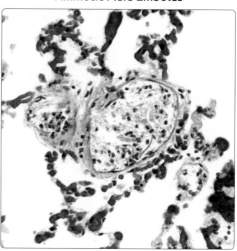

(Left) *Alcian blue stain of the lung shows the extent of amniotic fluid within arterioles and alveolar capillaries.*
(Right) *Pancytokeratin staining highlights the plate-like* ➡ *fetal squamous cells from the amniotic fluid. The stain is also positive within the alveolar lining cells.*

Amniotic Fluid Embolus, Alcian Blue

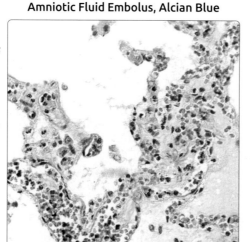

Aminotic Fluid Embolus, CK-PAN

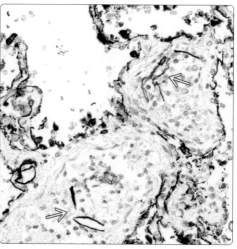

(Left) *Section from a uterine vein contains fetal squamous cells and inflammatory debris in a case with postpartum hemorrhage. This finding may or may not be associated with AFE.* **(Right)** *Higher magnification of the same vein shows platelet aggregates, neutrophils, and fetal squamous cells* ➡.

Uterine Vein With Amniotic Fluid Debris

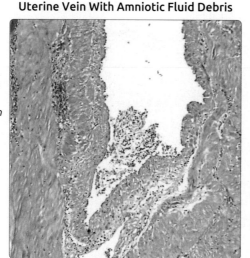

Uterine Vein With Amniotic Fluid Debris

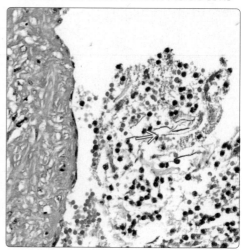

Syncytiotrophoblast in Maternal Pulmonary Artery, HCG

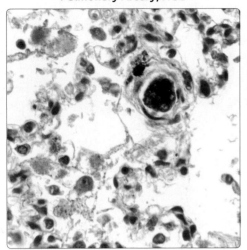

Bone Marrow Emboli

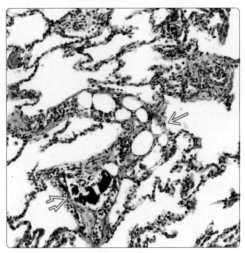

(Left) *Syncytiotrophoblasts are always found in the lung during pregnancy, stained here with human chorionic gonadotropin. When present in large numbers, they may be responsible for maternal death.* (Right) *Fat ➡ and bone marrow ➡ embolism are most likely secondary to resuscitation. Other etiologies for maternal death should be sought.*

Massive Pulmonary Embolus

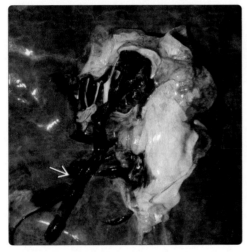

Pulmonary Embolus

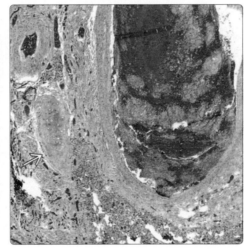

(Left) *Pregnancy is a state of hypercoagulability with marked increased risk for pulmonary emboli. This is a gross photograph of a massive pulmonary embolus from deep venous thrombi. A portion of the clot ➡ has been pulled out of the distal vasculature. (Courtesy D. Wolf, MD and M. Anzalone, MD.)* (Right) *Pulmonary embolus with lines of Zahn filling and distending a large pulmonary artery is shown. Note the cartilage ➡ of the adjacent proximal airway.*

Small Thrombosed Pulmonary Artery

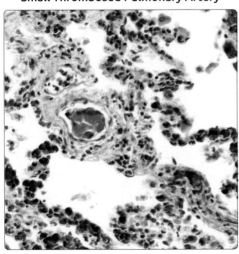

Fetal Tissue Embolized Into Uterine Vein

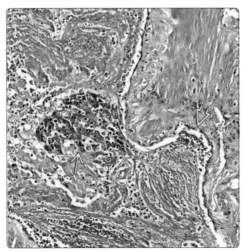

(Left) *Small vessel thrombus may be a component of preeclampsia or associated with disseminated intravascular coagulopathy (DIC).* (Right) *Stain shows an elective abortion with massive hemorrhage after the procedure. Thrombi and embolized fetal tissues ➡ (liver) were present in the veins ➡ of the uterus.*

Uterine Rupture Gross

Disrupted Uterine Vessels

(Left) *Spontaneous uterine rupture occurs most commonly at the lateral, lower uterine segment in the region of the uterine artery.* (Right) *Section taken from the area of uterine rupture shows acute hemorrhage and devitalization of the myometrium.*

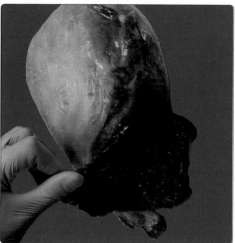

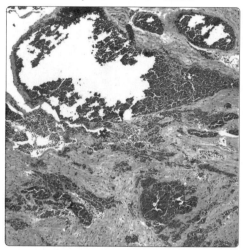

Rupture Ectopic Pregnancy

Ruptured Ectopic Pregnancy

(Left) *This image shows the result of a ruptured ectopic pregnancy. Villous tissue is extending out of the rupture site. There were 2,000 mL of blood within the abdominal cavity. (Courtesy D. Wolf, MD and M. Anzalone, MD.)* (Right) *A clot is present in the dilated fallopian tube lumen ➡, flattening the tubal epithelium. Larger cells within the tube's muscular wall are invasive trophoblasts ➡ of the implantation site. The embryo usually expelled into the abdominal cavity is not identified.*

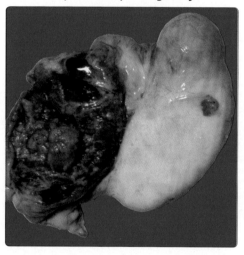

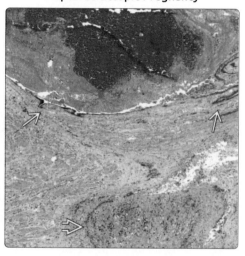

Complete Hydatidiform Mole

Fatty Liver of Pregnancy

(Left) *A complete hydatidiform mole was the cause of a massive maternal hemorrhage and death, in this case.* (Right) *Fatty liver of pregnancy may be a complication of preeclampsia or fetal fatty acid oxidation defect. There is diffuse microvesicular steatosis, no necrosis, and no inflammation.*

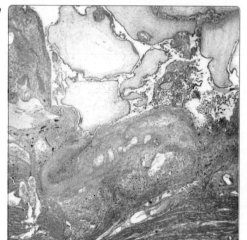

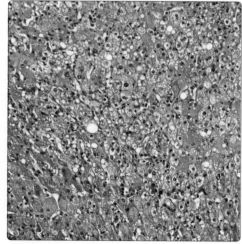

Acute Dissection of Coronary Artery

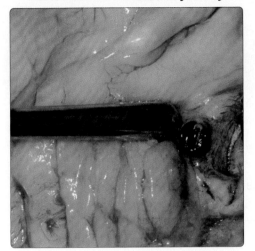

Acute Dissection of Coronary Artery

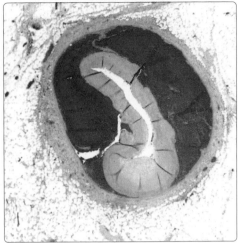

(Left) *Acute dissection of the coronary artery is an indirect cause of death during pregnancy. (Courtesy D. Wolf, MD and M. Anzalone, MD.)* (Right) *Microscopic photograph of the perivascular hemorrhage secondary to dissection of the coronary artery is shown.*

Myocardial Scarring

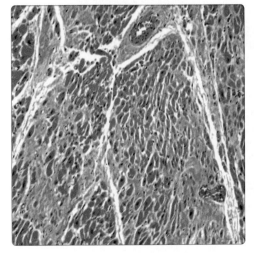

Maternal Malignancy Metastatic to Placenta

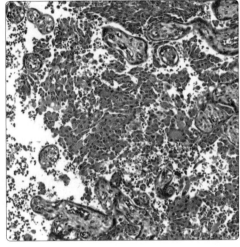

(Left) *Maternal death was indirectly due to cardiomegaly and myocardial scarring due to chronic hypertension, obesity, and coronary artery disease.* (Right) *Patient presented near term with an intrauterine fetal demise and DIC, which was thought to be due to "dead baby syndrome." She continued to have abnormal bleeding after delivery, which was found to be secondary to a widely metastatic tumor believed to be gastric in origin.*

Intrauterine Pregnancy at 5 Weeks, Gross

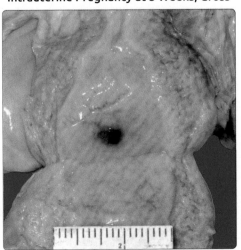

Implantation of Placenta at 5 Weeks

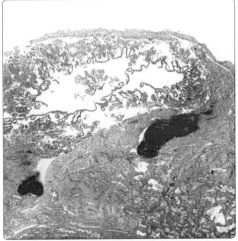

(Left) *A young woman who died from a drug overdose was found to have an intrauterine pregnancy of ~ 5 weeks. (Courtesy D. Wolf, MD and M. Anzalone, MD.)* (Right) *Section shows the implantation at ~ 5 weeks.*

TERMINOLOGY

Definitions

- Early postpartum hemorrhage (PPH): Hemorrhage within 24 hours of delivery
  - > 1,000 mL estimated blood loss after either vaginal or cesarean delivery
  - Alternative definitions include > 10% decrease in hematocrit, decrease in hemoglobin ≥ 2 g/dL, or need for red blood cell transfusion
- Late PPH: Hemorrhage 24 hours to 6 weeks after delivery
- Cesarean hysterectomy: Hysterectomy performed at same time as delivery of baby
- Postpartum hysterectomy: Hysterectomy performed some time after delivery of baby

EPIDEMIOLOGY

Incidence

- Incidence of PPH after vaginal delivery: 4-11%
- Incidence of PPH after cesarean section: 2-4%

ETIOLOGY/PATHOGENESIS

Early Postpartum Hemorrhage

- Clinical risk factors for PPH
  - Primiparity, previous cesarean delivery, previous PPH, fever during labor, smoking during pregnancy (increased incidence for previa), induction of labor, Pitocin, long duration of pushing, instrumented delivery
- Uterine atony 40-56%
- Placenta accreta 20-64%
  - Placenta previa is frequently associated with accreta
- Retained placenta occurs in 0.4-3.5% of deliveries (manual removal > 30 minutes after delivery)
  - Retained placenta does not always mean accreta
    - Portion of placenta or accessory lobe left behind
    - Possible increase for PPH when membranes are left behind
- Infection: 11%
- Lacerations of cervix, vagina, or myometrium

- Abruption, often associated with DIC
- Uterine rupture: 1/1,000 deliveries
- Uterine inversion: 1/2,250 deliveries
  - May be associated with placenta accreta or excessive traction on cord with placental delivery
- Hemorrhagic disorders
  - Thrombocytopenia
  - Hemophilia A, von Willebrand disease
  - Preeclampsia with severe features (hemolysis, elevated liver enzymes, low platelets)
  - Hypofibrinogenemia associated with abruption or intrauterine fetal demise
  - Amniotic fluid embolus

Late Postpartum Hemorrhage

- Retained placenta, placenta accreta
- Subinvolution of maternal vessels
- Infection
- Gestational trophoblastic disease

CLINICAL IMPLICATIONS

Prognosis

- PPH accounts for 11-27% of maternal deaths
- Uterine rupture and abruption is associated with high perinatal morbidity and mortality

Reporting

- Postpartum hysterectomy may be considered unintended procedure, "sentinel event"
- Communication with obstetrics team is essential to ensure sentinel event policy is in compliance with Joint Commission standards

MACROSCOPIC

General Features

- Nearly 1/2 of specimens will be supracervical hysterectomies
  - Supracervical hysterectomy is faster procedure with decreased length of stay

(Left) *This bisected uterus shows complete placenta previa* ➡️ *and placenta accreta* ➡️. *Placenta accreta is identified during pregnancy with increasing frequency. Management may include cesarean hysterectomy.* (Right) *This supracervical hysterectomy was performed for postpartum hemorrhage after a vaginal delivery. The endometrial cavity is large and the myometrium is thin and flabby, consistent with atony.*

Placenta Previa and Accreta

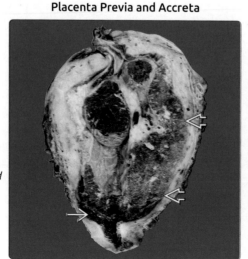

Uterine Atony

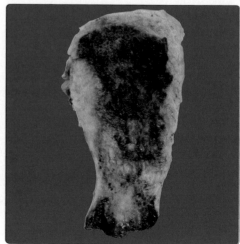

- o Cervix may be submitted separately
- Placental implantation site is usually area of pathology and is often difficult to identify grossly
  - o At term, implantation site in pregnant uterus is 20 cm in diameter; after uterus contracts post partum, it is only ~ 5 cm
  - o Areas of lush, spongy tissue are usually not implantation decidua
  - o Once implantation site is identified microscopically, gross specimen can be revisited for additional sections as needed
- Specimen radiographs may be useful when there has been use of embolization with Gelfoam, beads, or coils

Specimen Handling

- Proper orientation is critical and may be difficult due to distortion
  - o Differentiate anterior and posterior orientation
    - − Round ligament inserts anterior to fallopian tubes
    - − Anterior peritoneal reflection is higher than posterior; can be obscured in supracervical hysterectomy
    - − Hysterotomy incision is usually on anterior surface
    - − Planned cesarean hysterectomy often has fundal or even posterior hysterotomy
  - o Differential inking of abnormalities or for right-left orientation should be considered
- Obtain gross photographs prior to and during dissection
- Document current hysterotomy incision, if present, and whether open, sutured, and if intact
- Note presence or absence of cervix and whether it is closed or gaping
  - o Examine cervix for lacerations, particularly at lateral margins
  - o Note presence of clots or whether placental tissues are present in or over internal os
  - o History of prior cervical dysplasia warrants submission of entire cervix
- Identify prior surgical scars and adhesions
  - o Uterus heals remarkably well without significant gross scarring
  - o Submit areas that may represent placental extension into adjacent structures in placenta percreta for microscopic examination
- Note hematomas on serosa, into myometrium (Couvelaire uterus) adnexal structures, or within vascular pedicles
- Bivalve uterus along coronal plane; fixation is useful prior to taking microscopic sections
  - o Note size of endometrial cavity
  - o Note thickness of uterine wall at fundus and lower uterine segment
  - o Note appearance of endometrium; document clots, retained membranes, or villi
    - − Retained placenta may be obscured by blood clot
  - o Map endometrial cavity to identify implantation site and associated pathology
    - − Submit from cervix to fundus at 2-3 cm intervals to assure full coverage
  - o Submit sections from areas normally deficient in decidua; these are likely sites of placenta accreta
    - − Lower uterine segment, cornua of fallopian tubes, areas of prior incisions, and overlying leiomyomas

Placenta Accreta

- Uterus with in situ placenta with typical features of placenta accreta, increta, or percreta found on gross and microscopic exam

Separately Delivered Placenta

- Maternal surface may show incomplete cotyledons, suggesting retained placenta
- Fetal surface may have disrupted vessels at margin, suggesting missing accessory lobe

MICROSCOPIC

Implantation Site

- Identified by presence of invasive trophoblasts in decidua and myometrium with maternal spiral arteries adapted for pregnancy
- Look for evidence of residual placental villi
  - o Placenta accreta evidenced by adherence of villi and basal fibrin to myometrium with no intervening decidua

Endometrium

- Acute endometritis is associated with uterine atony ± clinical chorioamnionitis
- Submucosal leiomyomas may be associated with peripartum hemorrhage with causes other than atony

Myometrium

- Current hysterotomy site has localized myometrial necrosis with minimal neutrophilic infiltrate and hemorrhage
- Previous hysterotomy site usually shows minimal fibrosis, rarely residual suture material and serosal adhesions
- Adenomyosis is slightly more common in peripartum hysterectomy with possible increase in uterine atony
- Lymphoplasmacytic inflammation in myometrium and maternal spiral arteries may be seen with uterine atony

Cervix

- Vaginal delivery is associated with mild acute hemorrhage and moderate edema of cervix
- Uterine atony is associated with acute inflammation of cervix

SELECTED REFERENCES

1. Keating J et al: The association between ragged or incomplete membranes and postpartum haemorrhage: a retrospective cohort study. Aust N Z J Obstet Gynaecol. ePub, 2018
2. Greenbaum S et al: Underlying mechanisms of retained placenta: evidence from a population based cohort study. Eur J Obstet Gynecol Reprod Biol. 216:12-17, 2017
3. Endler M et al: Macroscopic and histological characteristics of retained placenta: a prospectively collected case-control study. Placenta. 41:39-44, 2016
4. Hernandez JS et al: Placental and uterine pathology in women undergoing peripartum hysterectomy. Obstet Gynecol. 119(6):1137-42, 2012
5. Forna F et al: Emergency peripartum hysterectomy: a comparison of cesarean and postpartum hysterectomy. Am J Obstet Gynecol. 190(5):1440-4, 2004

Placental Evaluation in Special Circumstances

Serosal Appearance of Placenta Increta

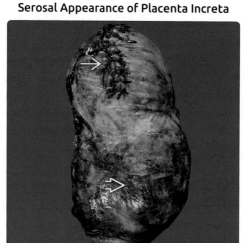

Placenta Increta

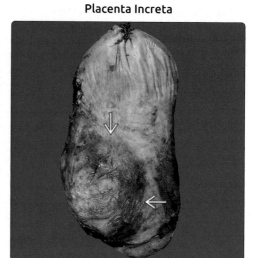

(Left) *This cesarean hysterectomy was planned for known placenta previa and accreta. The hysterotomy incision ➡ is fundal. Bluish discoloration and bulging ➡ in the left lower uterine segment is due to placenta increta or percreta. Tortuous vessels on serosa are common.* **(Right)** *The posterior aspect of the same uterus shows that the abnormal placental implantation ➡ extends to the posterior surface as well.*

Placenta Previa

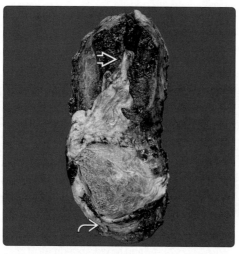

Complete Placenta Previa

(Left) *The anterior half of the uterus has free membranes ➡ entrapped in the hysterotomy incision. The placenta overlies the internal cervical os ➡.* **(Right)** *The posterior aspect of the same uterus has a nearly equal share of placenta as the anterior, consistent with complete placenta previa.*

Placenta Increta

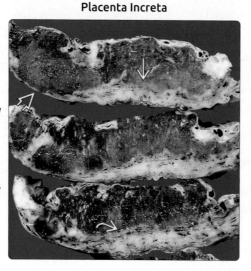

Placenta Accreta

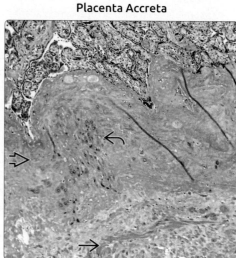

(Left) *Serial sections of the uterus and in situ placenta show focal severe thinning ➡ of the myometrium (increta). Focally there is no distinct separation ➡ between the placenta and myometrium (accreta). Basal plate fibrin ➡ is seen elsewhere.* **(Right)** *Placenta accreta shows the villous tissue separated from the myometrium ➡ only by basal plate fibrin (Nitabuch fibrinoid) ➡ with rare invasive trophoblasts ➡. There is a total absence of decidualized endometrium.*

Sampling Postpartum Hysterectomy

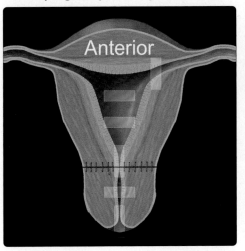

Postpartum Hysterectomy After Sectioning

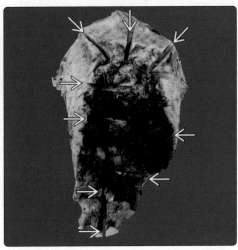

(Left) This diagram shows suggested sections in blue to assure identification of the implantation site. Sections also include areas with known deficiency of decidualization: Lower uterine segment, current and prior cesarean section incision, and cornua of the fallopian tubes. (Right) This bivalved uterus shows a thick myometrium and adherent blood clot. Sections submitted for microscopic examination ➡ were taken at regular intervals to assure identification of the implantation site.

Sampling Postpartum Hysterectomy

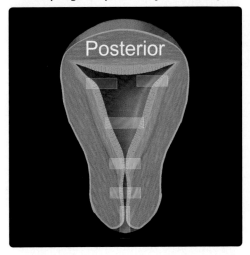

Cornual Placenta Accreta

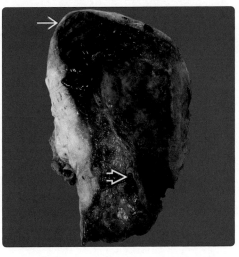

(Left) The posterior uterus should also be systematically sectioned to identify the placental implantation site. The normal site of placental implantation is fundal and posterior. (Right) This specimen shows cornual placenta accreta ➡ with overlying blood clot. Villi are not readily visible. Placental membranes ➡ are noted in the midbody. Retained membranes are rarely associated with postpartum bleeding but may be a source of infection.

Bladder Mucosa

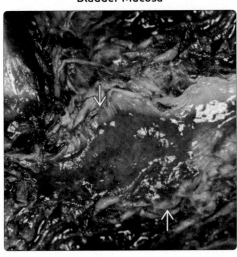

Adhesions in Lower Anterior Uterine Segment

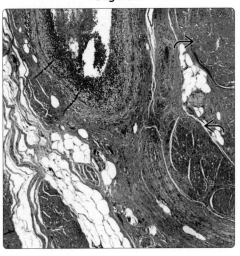

(Left) The anterior surface of this uterus shows dense adhesions and red urinary bladder mucosa ➡. A small portion of the bladder was removed at the time of hysterectomy due to inability to create a plane between the uterus and bladder. (Right) Dense adhesions on the anterior uterus are a common finding associated with a history of previous cesarean. This adhesion has a portion of urinary bladder smooth muscle ➡. Bladder mucosa is usually not present.

Round Cervical Os

Slit-Like Cervical Os

(Left) *This separately submitted cervix shows a round os, consistent with no prior vaginal delivery.* (Right) *This slit-like os is consistent with a parous cervix, but this pregnancy was delivered via cesarean with a nonlabored cervix.*

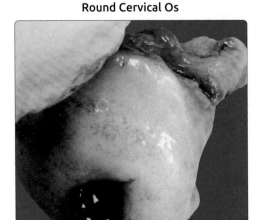
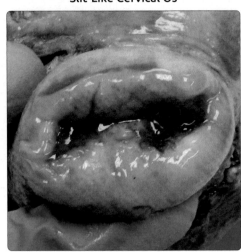

Hemorrhagic Cervical Os

Cervical Pregnancy

(Left) *This hemorrhagic, edematous cervix is from a recent vaginal delivery. A small cervical laceration would be very difficult to identify in this type of specimen.* (Right) *Extensive disruption of the endocervix was associated with excessive hemorrhage due to a cervical pregnancy in this case.*

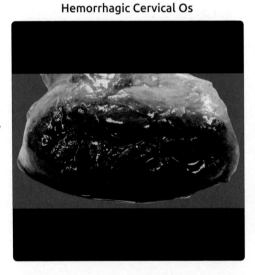
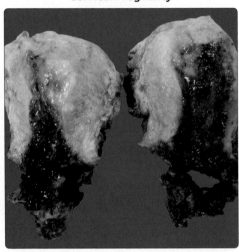

Vascular Anatomy

Uterine Rupture

(Left) *This illustration of the cervical and uterine vasculature shows the vulnerability of the lateral lower uterine segment and cervical regions.* (Right) *This gross photograph shows massive uterine rupture involving the lateral aspect of the lower uterine segment and endocervix. The ectocervix* ➡ *is partially detached.*

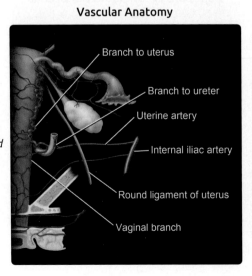

Branch to uterus

Branch to ureter

Uterine artery

Internal iliac artery

Round ligament of uterus

Vaginal branch

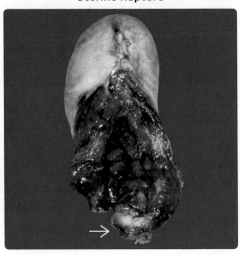

Abruption

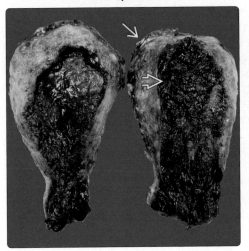

Dissecting Hemorrhage

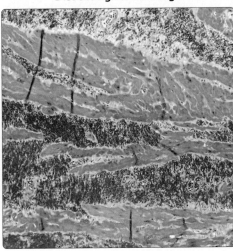

(Left) This uterine cavity is enlarged with a thin, flabby myometrium, consistent with atony. Early postpartum hemorrhage occurred after acute abruption with fetal demise at 35 weeks and vaginal delivery. The dusky myometrium ➡ suggests a Couvelaire uterus (extension of the retroplacental hematoma into myometrium to serosa). The implantation site was located beneath the adherent clot ➡. (Right) Extensive acute hemorrhage dissects between myometrial fibers on microscopic exam.

Acute Endometritis

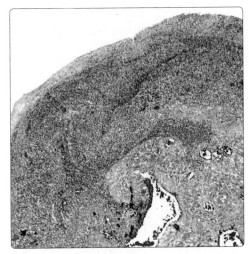

Acute Myometritis

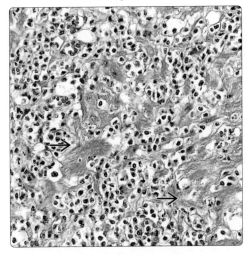

(Left) This case of uterine atony was associated with severe acute endometritis. The placenta showed severe necrotizing chorioamnionitis. (Right) The same case also had severe acute myometritis. The neutrophils extend deeply into and between the myometrial smooth muscle fibers ➡. Acute chorioamnionitis is associated with dysfunctional uterine contractions and uterine atony even without such severe inflammation as seen here.

Perivascular Infiltrates

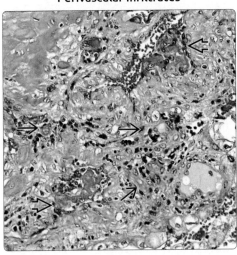

Chronic Inflammation

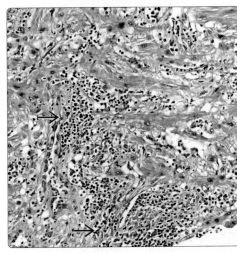

(Left) Uterine atony may be associated with abnormal chronic inflammation. Plasma cells ➡ are found within the deep endometrium. This is not from the implantation site, as the maternal vessels are not adapted for pregnancy. They contain fibrin thrombi ➡, suggestive of maternal coagulopathy. (Right) This section is from an atonic peripartum hysterectomy and shows a moderate lymphocytic infiltrate ➡ extending into the myometrium.

Postpartum Hemorrhage

TERMINOLOGY

- Postpartum hemorrhage (PPH)
- Early PPH occurs in first 24 hours after delivery
  - > 1000 mL after either vaginal or cesarean delivery
- Late PPH occurs 24 hours to 6 weeks after delivery

ETIOLOGY/PATHOGENESIS

- Uterine atony
  - Overdistended uterus: Multifetal pregnancy, macrosomia, polyhydramnios
  - "Overworked" uterus: Prolonged labor, Pitocin, grand multiparity, precipitous delivery
  - Infection: Chorioamnionitis
  - Relaxed uterus: Tocolytics (magnesium sulfate), general anesthesia
  - Adenomyosis
- Retained placenta
  - Accessory lobe, bilobate placenta, or accreta
- Lacerations: Cervix, vagina, or inner myometrium

- Instrumented or uncontrolled vaginal delivery
- Uterine rupture
  - Can occur in scarred and unscarred uterus
  - Cervical lacerations at 3- and 9-o'clock positions
- Hemorrhagic disorders
  - Thrombocytopenia, disseminated intravascular coagulopathy for any reason
  - Inherited thrombophilia
  - Preeclampsia
- Late PPH
  - Subinvolution maternal spiral arteries
  - Placenta accreta
  - Infection
  - Gestational trophoblastic disease

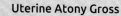

Uterine Atony Gross

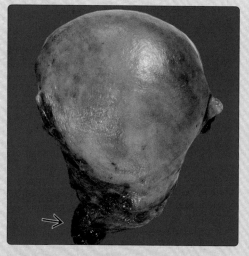

Uterine Atony With Enlarged Endometrial Cavity Gross

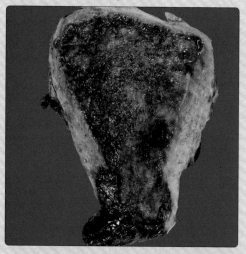

(Left) The atonic uterus is enlarged and flabby. There is a ➡ blood clot extending through the cervix. (Right) The atonic uterus has a very large endometrial cavity and thin myometrium, consistent with decreased contractility. Retained placenta is rarely visible on gross examination.

Postpartum Hysterectomy

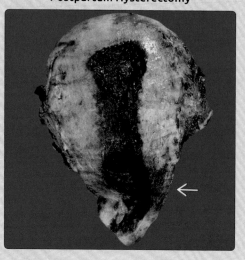

Postpartum Hysterectomy With Retained Placenta

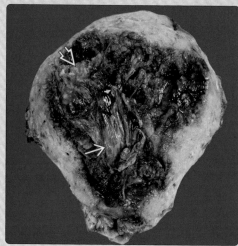

(Left) This uterus has a small endometrial cavity with thick myometrium, features of normal contractility. There is ➡ increased hemorrhage in the lower uterine segment. (Right) The uterus has features of atony with a large endometrial cavity and thin myometrium. There is a large amount of ➡ retained placenta, and ➡ shiny membranes are apparent as well. This was a case of undiagnosed placenta accreta where there was an unsuccessful attempt to remove the placenta manually after delivery.

TERMINOLOGY

Abbreviations

- Postpartum hemorrhage (PPH)

Definitions

- Early PPH occurs in first 24 hours after delivery
  - \> 1000 mL after either vaginal or cesarean delivery
    - Incidence after vaginal delivery: 4-8%
    - Incidence after cesarean delivery: 2%
    - Bleeding may occur prior to, with, or after delivery of placenta
  - Because amount of bleeding is difficult to estimate, following have been proposed to indicate PPH
    - Decrease in hematocrit of > 10%
    - Need for red blood cell transfusion
- Late PPH occurs 24 hours to 6 weeks after delivery; occurs in 0.23-1.00% of pregnancies
- Cesarean hysterectomy is performed at same time as cesarean delivery of baby
- Postpartum hysterectomy is performed some time after vaginal or cesarean delivery of baby

ETIOLOGY/PATHOGENESIS

Early Postpartum Hemorrhage

- Uterine atony accounts for 40-56% of early PPH
  - Overdistended uterus
    - Multifetal gestations, macrosomia, or polyhydramnios
  - "Overworked" uterus
    - Arrest of dilation or descent &/or prolonged 2nd stage of labor
    - Induction of labor or augmentation with oxytocin
    - Grand multiparity, parity > 7
    - Precipitous delivery
  - Infection
    - Chorioamnionitis results in dysfunctional uterine contractions
  - Relaxed uterus
    - Use of tocolytics, terbutaline, magnesium sulfate, or general anesthesia
  - Other risk factors
    - Prior PPH
    - Advanced maternal age ≥ 35 years
    - Preeclampsia
    - Abruption
    - Placenta previa
    - Instrumented vaginal delivery
- Genital lacerations account for 20% of early PPH
  - Cervical lacerations often at 3- and 9-o'clock positions, may extend into cervix from lower uterine segment
  - Risk factors include uncontrolled or traumatic vaginal delivery, shoulder dystocia, and operative vaginal delivery (vacuum or forceps)
- Uterine rupture, occurs in 1/1,000-3,000 deliveries
  - May occur prior to onset of labor or during labor and delivery
  - Occurs in scarred and unscarred uteri
    - Highest risk is with previous classic cesarean hysterotomy incision

- Most common location in scarred uterus is area of previous hysterotomy incision
    - Incidence with trial of labor after cesarean, 0.2-0.8%
  - Increased risk with high parity
  - Increased risk with overstimulation with oxytocin
- Uterine inversion, occurs in 1/2,000-2,500 deliveries
  - Accompanied by hemorrhage and shock
  - Predisposing factors include: Myometrial weakness, fundal placental implantation, short umbilical cord, excessive traction on umbilical cord with delivery of placenta, accreta, manual removal of placenta
- Bleeding diathesis
  - Thrombocytopenia: Pregnancy induced or idiopathic thrombocytopenia purpura
  - Inherited coagulopathy such as hemophilia A or von Willebrand disease
  - Coagulopathy associated with hypertensive disorders such as preeclampsia or HELLP syndrome
- Disseminated intravascular coagulopathy
  - Hypofibrinogenemia with retention of dead fetus (usually for > 4 weeks, does not occur with death of only 1 twin)
  - Amniotic fluid embolus syndrome, usually with rapid or tumultuous labor, sudden onset of shortness of breath
  - Abruption, especially with large retroplacental hematoma

Early or Late Postpartum Hemorrhage

- Retained placenta: Accounts for 10% of PPH
  - Accessory lobe or bilobate placenta with portion left behind
  - Placenta adherens (failed contraction of myometrium behind portion of placenta)
  - Trapped placenta (detached placenta trapped behind closed cervix)
  - May form polypoid endometrial mass (placental polyp)
- Placenta accreta: Accounts for 20-64% of hemorrhage
  - Increasing incidence in past few years as incidence of cesarean delivery has increased
    - 35% risk with prior cesarean and placenta previa
    - 18-60% risk with prior uterine curettage
  - Increased risk with history of manual placental removal or prior retained placenta
  - Marked risk with pregnancy after endometrial ablation
- Adenomyosis
  - Common pathology, rarely associated with uterine atony and PPH

Late Postpartum Hemorrhage

- Retained placenta
- Subinvolution of uterine arteries
  - Most commonly occurs 2nd week postpartum
  - Etiology is unknown
    - Immune factors, increased expression of bcl-2 oncoprotein, which inhibits apoptosis and prolongs cell survival
    - May be present with retained placenta
- Dehiscence of cesarean scar
- Leiomyoma or adenomyosis
- Gestational trophoblastic disease

- Placental site nodule, usually associated with dysfunctional uterine bleeding or infertility; rarely hemorrhage
- Chronic endomyometritis
- Increased risk with history of early PPH

CLINICAL ISSUES

Presentation

- Sudden massive vaginal bleeding and shock
- Constant seepage
  - Postpartum uterus may hold up to 1,000 mL of blood
- Hemoperitoneum associated with lacerations or uterine rupture

Treatment

- Surgical approaches
  - Direct uterine massage or bimanual compression
  - Uterine or vaginal packing or use of balloon tamponade
  - Curettage to remove any placental fragments and treat subinvolution
  - B-Lynch compression sutures
  - Ligation of internal iliac arteries (hypogastric) and uterine arteries
  - Endovascular therapy, such as embolization or balloon occlusion
  - Identify and repair lacerations
  - Hysterectomy
- Drugs
  - Uterotonics; oxytocics (Cytotec, Hemabate), Methergine
  - Treat coagulation abnormalities with appropriate blood components

Prognosis

- PPH is one leading cause of maternal mortality
  - Placenta accreta has 4-6% maternal mortality
  - Uterine rupture is associated with maternal morbidity
    - High fetal morbidity and 50-70% fetal mortality
  - Amniotic fluid embolus is associated with high maternal and fetal mortality
  - Uterine inversion is associated with 13-41% maternal morbidity and mortality
    - Symptoms of shock far exceed amount of blood loss

MACROSCOPIC

General Features

- Uterine atony
  - Boggy uterus, large endometrial cavity, may be isolated to lower uterine segment, generalized thin myometrium
- Placenta accreta
  - Uterus may be boggy or contracted
  - Accreta may be grossly visible but is usually microscopic
- Abruption
  - Couvelaire uterus with extension of blood into myometrium, visible through serosa
  - Retroplacental hematoma
- Infection
  - Generally appears atonic; placenta may have chorioamnionitis
  - Late PPH due to infection may be associated with myometrial abscess or necrosis
- Uterine inversion

- Endometrial surface extends out through cervix
- Subinvolution of maternal spiral arteries
  - Uterus is usually boggy with large thrombosed vessels visible on cut surface beneath endometrium

MICROSCOPIC

Histologic Features

- Uterine atony
  - Variable pathology
    - Acute endomyometritis, usually associated with chorioamnionitis
    - Microscopic placenta accreta
    - Chronic endomyometritis
    - Fibrinoid necrosis of maternal vessels in implantation site with perivascular lymphocytes
- Placenta accreta
  - Villi adjacent to myometrium without intervening decidua
  - Must identify placental implantation site, which may need to be extensively sampled
  - Very difficult diagnosis to make on curettage samples, due to lack of orientation
- Abruption
  - May have significant bleeding into myometrium, extending to serosal surface (Couvelaire uterus)
  - Retroplacental hematoma may result in hypofibrinogenemia
- Subinvolution of maternal spiral arteries
  - Normal involution occurs by proliferation of fibroblasts that initially obliterate vessel lumen
    - Reendothelialization occurs with development of patent lumen and smooth muscle reform within 8-10 weeks
    - Some of arterial smooth muscle is replaced by connective tissue, and there is fragmentation and duplication of elastica with late calcification of vessel wall
  - Subinvolution is associated with large, patent vessels, and thrombi of varying ages
    - Abnormal vessels may be adjacent to normally involuted vessels
  - Retained placenta will also result in some degree of subinvolution of maternal vessels in vicinity of retained tissue
  - Can be diagnosed on curettage specimen
- Amniotic fluid embolus
  - Amniotic fluid debris within small vessels and capillaries of lungs
  - Amniotic fluid debris in vessels in cervix and lower uterine segment

SELECTED REFERENCES

1. Mousa HA et al: Treatment for primary postpartum haemorrhage. Cochrane Database Syst Rev. 2:CD003249, 2014
2. Bateman BT et al: The epidemiology of postpartum hemorrhage in a large, nationwide sample of deliveries. Anesth Analg. 110(5):1368-73, 2010
3. Weydert JA et al: Subinvolution of the placental site as an anatomic cause of postpartum uterine bleeding: a review. Arch Pathol Lab Med. 130(10):1538-42, 2006

Placenta Previa With Acute Marginal Hematoma Gross

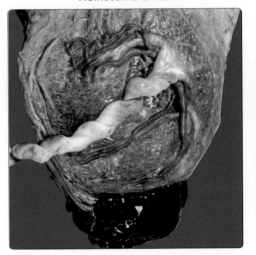

Placenta Previa

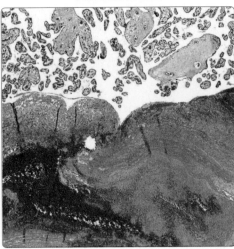

(Left) *Placenta previa may grossly be associated with an acute marginal hematoma. Usually there will be a combination of recent and remote hemorrhage noted on microscopic examination.* (Right) *Most often, the portion of placenta over the cervix in placenta previa is associated with microscopic evidence of remote and recent marginal hemorrhage.*

In Situ Placental Abruption Gross

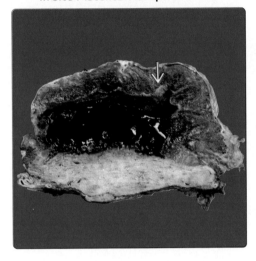

Acute Placental Abruption

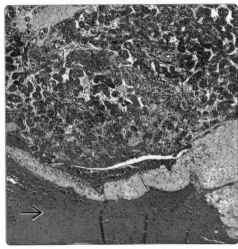

(Left) *In situ placental abruption is present in this cesarean hysterectomy. The patient had known placenta accreta and presented with preterm labor that was most likely secondary to abruption in the normally implanted portion of the placenta. The basal plate with ➡ Nitabuch layer of fibrin can be seen at the base of the placenta.* (Right) *Acute placental abruption may be associated with a retroplacental hematoma ➡ and villous stromal hemorrhage.*

Couvelaire Uterus Gross

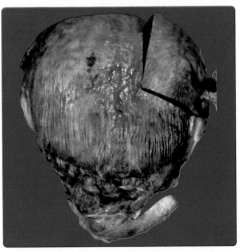

Couvelaire Uterus Cut Surface Gross

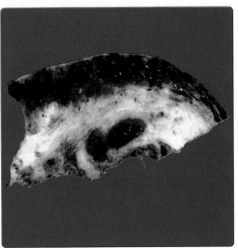

(Left) *This is a Couvelaire uterus with a large amount of blood evident beneath the serosal surface. There is extension of blood from the retroplacental area through the myometrium to the serosa, rather than accumulation of blood behind the placenta.* (Right) *The cut surface of the Couvelaire uterus has extensive hemorrhage, mostly noted beneath the serosal surface.*

(Left) *Image shows uterine atony after a term vaginal delivery. Note the large endometrial cavity and thin myometrium. There is no grossly evident residual placental tissue in the uterus.* **(Right)** *Sections from the uterus did reveal focal placenta accreta. Accreta may be microscopic, necessitating identification and extensive sectioning of the placental implantation site. The delay between delivery and hysterectomy has resulted in acute villous ischemia. Note the ➡ chronic inflammation at the implantation site.*

Atonic Uterus Gross

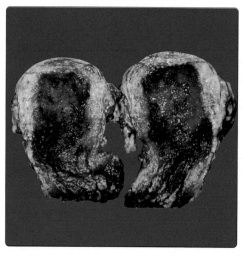

Microscopic Placenta Accreta

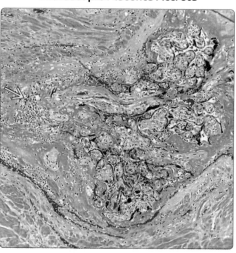

(Left) *This is a section of a uterine vein from the cervical region of a postpartum hysterectomy specimen. The lumen contains abundant acute inflammation and squamous epithelial cells ➔ that are presumed to be of fetal origin.* **(Right)** *This lung section shows fetal squamous cells ➔ within small vessels, diagnostic of amniotic fluid embolus. Just as in the uterine cervix, there may be a large number of inflammatory cells, particularly eosinophils, associated with the emboli.*

Amniotic Fluid in Uterine Vein

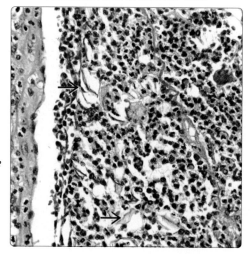

Amniotic Fluid Embolus Lung

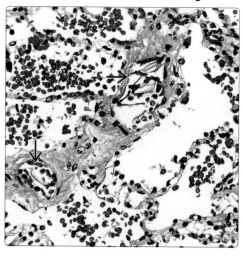

(Left) *This hysterectomy was performed for delayed postpartum hemorrhage. The specimen shows a large blood clot in the region of the uterine cornu. Underneath the clot there was a portion of retained placenta.* **(Right)** *The cornu of the uterus is an area with deficient decidua and is prone to abnormal implantation. This image shows placenta accreta with avascular villi ➡ adjacent to the myometrium.*

Cornual Placenta Accreta Gross

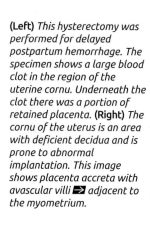
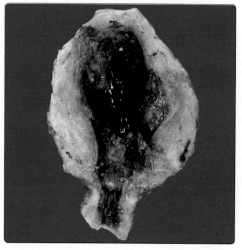

Delayed Postpartum Hemorrhage, Avascular Villi, Placenta Accreta

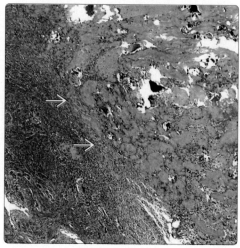

Hysterotomy Breakdown Due to Infection

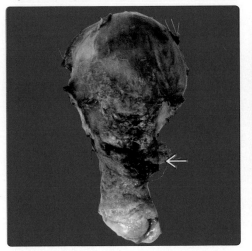

Group A *Streptococcus* Myometritis

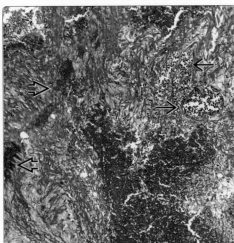

(Left) *A postpartum hysterectomy was performed several days after cesarean delivery. A large defect in anterior uterus is seen in the area of previous hysterotomy incision ➡️. There was severe acute chorioamnionitis in the previously delivered placenta.* (Right) *This section shows acute endomyometritis with large aggregates of neutrophils ➡️ and clouds of coccoid bacteria ➡️. The organism in this instance was group A Streptococcus, which may also be associated with necrotizing fascitis and toxic shock.*

Acute Myometritis

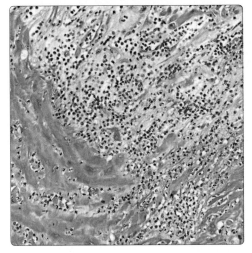

Chronic Endomyometritis

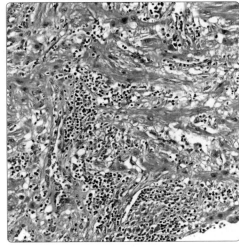

(Left) *Uterine atony in this postpartum hysterectomy was secondary to acute chorioamnionitis with acute endomyometritis.* (Right) *Chronic endomyometritis may also be associated with uterine atony. Abnormal maternal vessels are usually found as well. The placenta may also have chronic villitis and features of decreased uteroplacental blood flow.*

Group A *Streptococcus* Sepsis

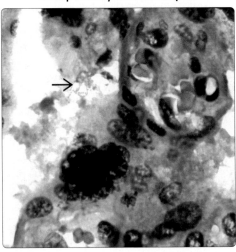

Group A *Streptococcus* Sepsis

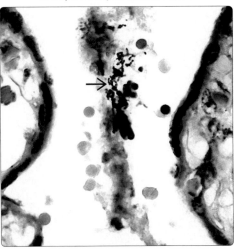

(Left) *Maternal shock and hemorrhage may rarely be associated with maternal sepsis. Rare cocci in chains ➡️ are present within the maternal intervillous space without a significant inflammatory reaction.* (Right) *Gram stain highlights the large number of gram-positive cocci ➡️ within the maternal intervillous space. The organism identified by maternal blood culture was group A Streptococcus.*

B-Lynch Compression Sutures Gross

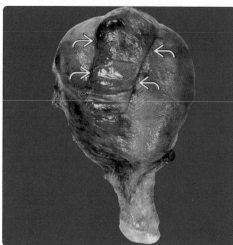

Compression Sutures in Uterus Gross

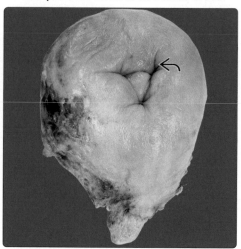

(Left) *Classic B-Lynch compression sutures* ➡ *are placed through the uterus in an attempt to reduce postpartum hemorrhage and prevent the need to perform a hysterectomy.* (Right) *Sutures* ➡ *were placed through the uterus in an alternative fashion in an attempt to stop postpartum hemorrhage.*

Placenta Percreta Gross

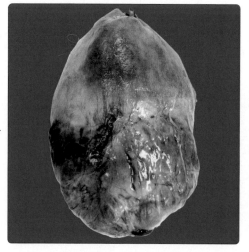

Gelfoam Within Uterine Vessels

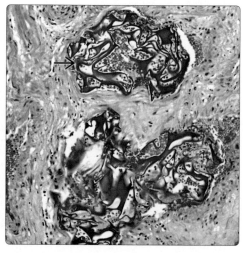

(Left) *The severity of placenta percreta in this case was evident at the time of delivery. In order to prevent excessive blood loss, Gelfoam embolization of maternal vessels was performed after the baby was delivered to reduce blood loss during the hysterectomy.* (Right) *This is the microscopic appearance of Gelfoam* ➡ *in uterine vessels.*

Uterine Inversion Gross

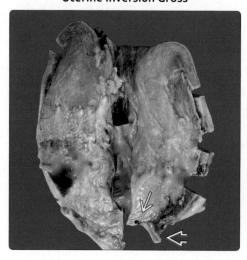

Uterine Inversion

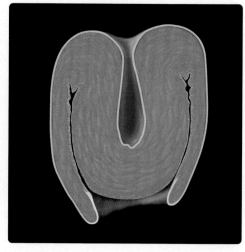

(Left) *Bivalved uterus which has already had tissue removed for histopathology is shown. The distorted uterus is difficult to orient, as the* ➡ *fundal endometrium is now protruding through the* ➡ *cervix.* (Right) *Graphic illustration of uterine inversion shows the fundus protruding through the cervix. The serosa is blue, endometrium pink, and cervix yellow.*

Complete Hydatidiform Mole Gross

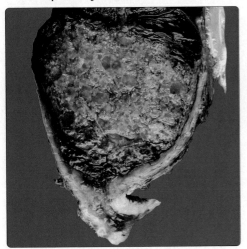

Complete Hydatidiform Mole

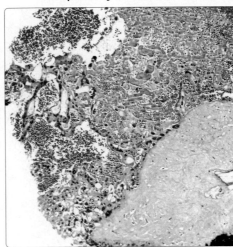

(Left) *Delayed postpartum hemorrhage may rarely be due to a complete hydatidiform mole, as seen here. The implantation site of the complete mole is prone to extensive hemorrhage.* (Right) *The rare residual villus with atypical trophoblast proliferation after evacuation of complete hydatidiform mole may also be associated with hemorrhage.*

Leiomyomatous Uterus

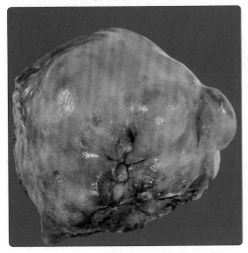

Leiomyomatous Uterus Gross

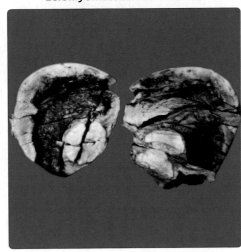

(Left) *Multiple leiomyomas may be associated with postpartum uterine atony. The leiomyomas may prevent the hysterotomy incision from proper closure.* (Right) *There is only one large leiomyoma, but the uterus shows features of atony. The leiomyoma is yellow and soft, which is consistent with infarction. Leiomyomas commonly infarct during pregnancy and may be associated with uterine pain.*

Postpartum Atony With Adenomyosis

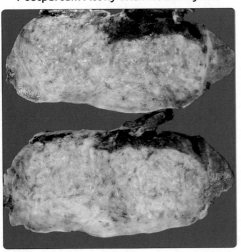

Adenomyosis

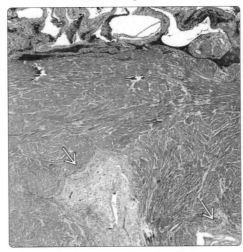

(Left) *Adenomyosis is a common finding in hysterectomy specimens and may also be associated with uterine atony and postpartum hemorrhage. The myometrium has a trabeculated appearance and may have small bloody cysts, not seen in these sections.* (Right) *This postpartum hysterectomy was preformed due to atony and hemorrhage. The only abnormality found was multifocal ➡ adenomyosis. This area is not from the placental implantation site.*

Laceration of Cervix and Lower Uterine Segment Gross

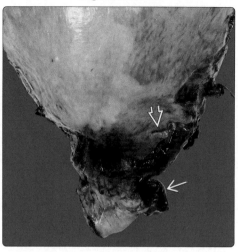

Cervix Post Vaginal Delivery

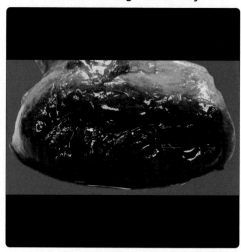

(Left) *Vaginal delivery occurred with brisk postpartum hemorrhage. A cervical laceration* ➡ *was found that extended into the* ➡ *lower uterine segment, necessitating a hysterectomy.* (Right) *The cervix after a vaginal delivery has moderate edema and acute submucosal and stromal hemorrhage. This may make identification of a laceration difficult.*

Vascular Anatomy of the Uterus

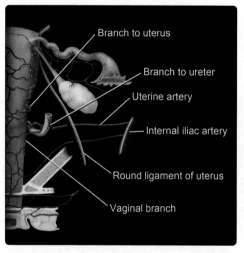

Branch to uterus

Branch to ureter

Uterine artery

Internal iliac artery

Round ligament of uterus

Vaginal branch

Uterine Rupture Gross

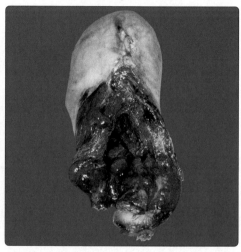

(Left) *Graphic that shows the location of the uterine artery branches. The origin at the lateral uterus is particularly problematic when the uterine rupture involves this area.* (Right) *Uterine rupture most often occurs at the 3- and 9-o'clock positions of the uterus in the area of the uterine arteries, which results in massive hemorrhage.*

Retained Products of Conception

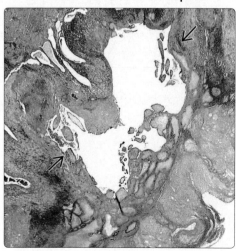

Retained Placenta D&C

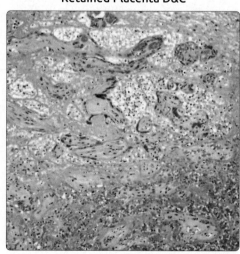

(Left) *The pathology of dysfunctional uterine bleeding can be similar to delayed postpartum hemorrhage with retention of products of conception, sometimes not clinically recognized. This case was found to be secondary to a retained empty gestational sac* ➡. (Right) *Delayed postpartum hemorrhage in this case was associated with retained villous tissue. There is extensive fibrin deposition and necrosis, which would suggest that the villi were not associated with accreta.*

Subinvolution of Maternal Spiral Arteries Gross

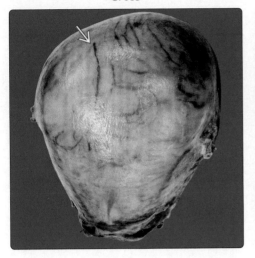

Subinvolution of Maternal Spiral Arteries

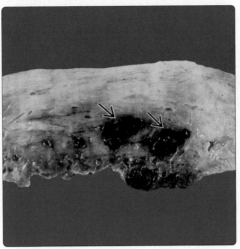

(Left) This hysterectomy was performed 2 weeks after delivery due to maternal hemorrhage and disseminated intravascular coagulation (DIC). Note the ➡ extensive thrombosis of maternal vessels, visible through the serosa. These thromboses are most likely secondary to the DIC. Classic features of subinvolution were present at implantation site. (Right) This section of the uterus shows large thrombosed myometrial vessels ➡ in a case of subinvolution of maternal spiral arteries and delayed postpartum hemorrhage.

Subinvolution of Maternal Spiral Arteries

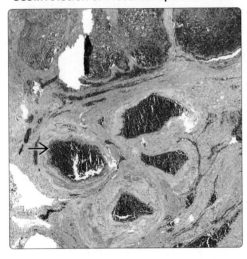

Subinvolution of Maternal Spiral Arteries

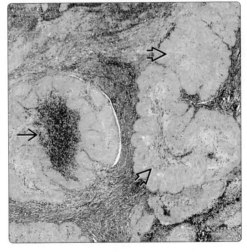

(Left) The maternal spiral arteries ➡ shown here have no involutional changes. They remain dilated with fibrin in the walls instead of normal involution with fibroblast proliferation and vascular smooth muscle. (Right) This image shows delayed involution of 1 vessel ➡, immediately adjacent to normally involuted vessels with fibroblast proliferation ➡. The vessels are surrounded by fibrinoid and a few residual invasive trophoblasts, consistent with the recent pregnancy.

Normal Involution of Maternal Spiral Artery

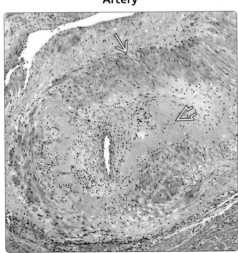

Subinvolution of Maternal Spiral Arteries, D&C

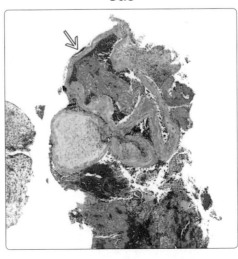

(Left) This spiral artery shows near complete involution 10 weeks postpartum with reformation of the ➡ vascular smooth muscle and a central endothelial-lined lumen. There is still evidence of the recent pregnancy with ➡ fibrinoid material. (Right) Image shows dysfunctional bleeding 12 weeks post D&C for spontaneous abortion. Repeat curettage shows ➡ maternal vessels that have not involuted. Hysterectomy often treats subinvolution of maternal spiral arteries, but curettage may also be diagnostic & therapeutic.

SECTION 4
Appendix

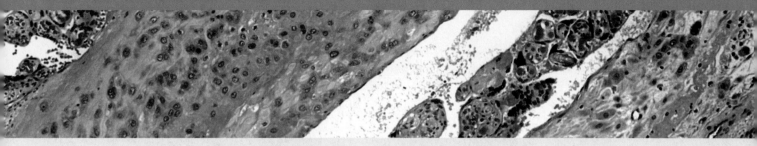

Reference Charts for Placental Evaluation

Sample Templates for Placental Evaluation

Reference Weights for Trimmed Singleton Placentas

Gestational Age (Weeks)	3rd Percentile	10th Percentile	25th Percentile	Mean	75th Percentile	90th Percentile	97th Percentile	Fetal:Placental Weight Ratio
21	102	**114**	128	143	158	**172**	184	2.5
22	107	**122**	138	157	175	**191**	206	2.8
23	88	**120**	152	187	220	**260**	285	3.2
24	90	**129**	153	198	228	**280**	304	3.3
25	112	**142**	169	206	242	**270**	298	3.7
26	122	**160**	184	223	260	**300**	325	3.9
27	108	**154**	186	235	280	**330**	362	4.2
28	184	**210**	238	270	302	**331**	357	4.8
29	201	**229**	259	293	327	**357**	385	5.2
30	220	**249**	281	316	352	**384**	413	5.2
31	239	**269**	303	340	377	**411**	441	5.5
32	258	**290**	325	364	403	**438**	470	5.9
33	278	**311**	347	387	428	**464**	497	6.0
34	296	**331**	369	411	453	**493**	526	6.2
35	317	**352**	391	434	477	**516**	551	6.4
36	336	**372**	412	457	501	**542**	578	6.6
37	353	**391**	432	478	524	**566**	603	6.8
38	370	**409**	452	499	547	**589**	628	6.9
39	386	**426**	470	519	567	**611**	651	7.1
40	401	**442**	487	537	587	**632**	673	7.2
41	414	**456**	502	553	605	**651**	693	7.2

Formalin fixation may increase weight by 5-8%, and prolonged refrigeration may decrease weight. Although a large series provides untrimmed weights from delivery room, significant variation in the amount of adherent blood, length of cord received, etc. make untrimmed weights a less reliable method for evaluation of placentas submitted to pathology. Weights are trimmed weights from fresh placentas. Placentas comprising the data for ages 23-27 weeks (Hecht et al) were selected from premature births with normal fetal growth (i.e., cases with fetal birth < 2 standard deviations below the mean were excluded). The placentas from the excluded cases in general showed features of uteroplacental malperfusion. Placentas comprising the data for gestational ages 21-22 weeks and 28-41 weeks were characterized as uncomplicated deliveries, excluding cases with intrauterine growth restriction, prolonged rupture of membranes, amniotic fluid infection sequence (chorioamnionitis), pregnancy-induced hypertension, infarcts, perivillous fibrin deposition, or thrombi.

SELECTED REFERENCES

1. Hecht JL et al: Reference weights for placentas delivered before the 28th week of gestation. Placenta. 28(10):987-90, 2007
2. Pinar H et al: Reference values for singleton and twin placental weights. Pediatr Pathol Lab Med. 16(6):901-7, 1996
3. Kalousek DK et al: Pathology of the human embryo and previable fetus: an atlas. New York: Springer, 1990
4. Kraus FT et al: Placental Pathology (Atlas of Nontumor Pathology). 3rd ed. American Registry of Pathology, 2005

Reference Weights for Trimmed Twin Placentas

Gestational Age (Weeks)	3rd Percentile	10th Percentile	25th Percentile	Mean	75th Percentile	90th Percentile	97th Percentile
19	131	**161**	185	210	239	**263**	289
20	143	**166**	190	218	245	**270**	292
21	152	**176**	202	231	260	**286**	310
22	166	**191**	219	251	282	**310**	336
23	181	**210**	241	276	311	**343**	371
24	200	**232**	267	307	346	**382**	414
25	221	**257**	297	341	386	**426**	462
26	243	**284**	330	380	430	**475**	516
27	268	**314**	365	421	478	**528**	574
28	293	**345**	401	464	527	**584**	635
29	320	**377**	439	509	579	**641**	698
30	346	**409**	478	554	631	**700**	762
31	373	**441**	516	600	683	**758**	826
32	399	**472**	554	644	734	**815**	889
33	424	**503**	590	687	783	**870**	949
34	447	**531**	624	727	830	**923**	1,007
35	469	**558**	656	764	873	**971**	1,059
36	489	**582**	684	798	912	**1,014**	1,107
37	505	**602**	708	827	945	**1,051**	1,148
38	519	**619**	728	850	972	**1,082**	1,181
39	529	**631**	743	868	993	**1,105**	1,207
40	537	**639**	753	879	1005	**1,118**	1,221
41	539	**642**	756	882	1009	**1,123**	1,226

All data is from unfixed, trimmed placental discs (after cord and membranes have been trimmed away). Majority of data is from "normal" twin placentas, free of common pathologic changes. For each gestational age, these data encompass combined weight of dichorionic placentas with separate discs, weight of dichorionic fused placental discs, and monochorionic twin placentas. The 3rd and 97th percentiles are calculated as -2 standard deviations and +2 standard deviations from the mean, respectively.

SELECTED REFERENCES

1. Hecht JL et al: Reference weights for placentas delivered before the 28th week of gestation. Placenta. 28(10):987-90, 2007
2. Pinar H et al: Reference values for singleton and twin placental weights. Pediatr Pathol Lab Med. 16(6):901-7, 1996

Reference Weights for Trimmed Triplet Placentas

Gestational Age (Weeks)	10th Percentile	Mean	90th Percentile
20	226	253	285
21	257	284	320
22	289	319	345
23	331	361	400
24	371	406	445
25	408	456	498
26	444	509	558
27	480	564	630
28	516	621	697
29	553	673	772
30	591	738	849
31	631	797	925
32	674	855	1,000
33	719	911	1,072
34	768	965	1,139
35	821	1,017	1,200
36	940	1,108	1,297
37	1,007	1,147	1,330

The weights for each gestational age include trichorionic separate discs weighed in aggregate and trichorionic fused, as well as all combinations of dichorionic fusion or monochorionicity for the respective triplet placentas.

SELECTED REFERENCES

1. Pinar H et al: Triplet placentas: reference values for weights. Pediatr Dev Pathol. 5(5):495-8, 2002

Reference Values for Fetal and Placental Growth From 8- to 20-Weeks Gestation

Postmenstrual Gestational Age	Mean Placental Weight (g) (95% CI)	Mean Umbilical Cord Length (mm)	Fetal Crown Rump Length (mm)	Fetal Foot Length (mm) ± SD	Fetal:Placental Weight Ratio
8	1.6 (0.0-3.7)	20	14	4	0.18
9	15.2 (13.3-17)	33	20	5	0.25
10	28.8 (27.2-30.4)	55	26	6	0.38
11	42.4 (41.1-43.8)	92	33	7	0.58
12	56.1 (54.8-57.3)	126	40	9	0.65
13	69.7 (68.4-71.0)	158	48	12 ± 2	0.72
14	83.3 (81.8-84.8)	188	56	17 ± 3	0.73
15	96.9 (95.2-98.6)	215	65	19 ± 1	0.80
16	110.5 (108.5-112.5)	240	75	22 ± 2	1.00
17	124.2 (121.8-126.5)	264	88	25 ± 3	1.29
18	137.8 (135.0-140.5)	287	99	28 ± 2	1.63
19	101.0	309	112	29 ± 4	1.78
20	112.0	330	125	33 ± 2	2.23

CI = confidence interval; SD = standard deviation. Placental weight data for 19- and 20-weeks gestation are from a separate reference; note that mean placental weight is smaller than one would expect from weeks 8-18. Foot length can be used to assess fetal growth in disrupted fetuses.

SELECTED REFERENCES

1. Weissman A et al: Sonographic measurements of the umbilical cord and vessels during normal pregnancies. J Ultrasound Med. 13(1):11-4, 1994
2. Kalousek DK et al: Pathology of the human embryo and previable fetus: an atlas. New York: Springer, 1990
3. Boyd J et al: The Human Placenta. Cambridge: Heffer & Sons, 1970
4. Streeter CL: Weight, sitting height, head size, foot length and menstrual age of the human embryo. Carnegie Inst. Contrib. Embryol. 11:144, 1920

Singleton Placenta Gross Evaluation and Dictation Template

Dictation	Applicable Notes
The specimen is received (fresh/fixed) labeled with (patient's name, medical record number). It consists of a single placental disc with attached umbilical cord and fetal membranes.	Note if any part of the specimen is detached or fragmented.
The (tan/gray/white/green) umbilical cord measures ____cm in length by ____cm in maximum diameter. It shows ___ coils and inserts (centrally/eccentrically/marginally/in membranes). It contains (2/3) vessels on cut section.	Recording the total number of coils allows calculation of the coil index (# of coils/10 cm), facilitating a diagnosis of hypercoiling or undercoiling. If the cord inserts in the membranes, measure the distance of intramembranous course of vessels to disc and note if intact/disrupted. Marginal insertion is insertion within 1 cm of nearest margin. Peripheral is > 1 but < 3 cm of the nearest margin. Describe cord abnormalities (e.g., true knots, thrombi, other lesions) if present. Cut off cord 1.0-1.5 cm above insertion and take section of fetal end for cassette A1 and placental end (~ 5 cm from insertion) for cassette A2.
The (translucent/tan/yellow/green-tinged) (glistening/dull) fetal membranes attach (normally at disc margin/circumvallate for ___% of circumference/circummarginate for ___% of the circumference). The area of membrane rupture is located ____cm from closest placental margin.	Completeness of the membranes should be noted. Note color and opacity. Describe membrane abnormalities if present. Delete sentence on area of membrane rupture if C-section with intact membranes or if membranes are excessively torn. Take 1 or 2 membrane rolls for cassette A1; cut off membranes.
The (round/oval/irregularly shaped) trimmed placental disc weighs ____g and measures ____ x ____ x ____cm. The fetal surface is (steel gray/blue/purple/yellow/green) with (normal/magistral) dispersion of chorionic plate vessels.	Describe vascular abnormalities (e.g., thrombi, disruptions) if present. Describe any other abnormalities of the chorionic plate appearance. Take section of chorionic plate with vessels 1-2 cm away from cord insertion for cassette A2.
The maternal surface appears (intact/disrupted).	Note if cotyledons appear complete. Identify and measure any adherent blood clot or indentation and note any shaggy extensions that could be myometrial fibers.
Serial sectioning through placental disc at 1-cm intervals reveals (spongy/firm) (dark red/pink/tan) parenchyma with (no grossly identifiable lesions or note lesions).	Common parenchymal lesions include tan areas, firm areas, regions of pallor, or hematomas. The greatest diameter of the lesion as well as its location (central, peripheral, at margin) should be noted. Give an estimated percentage of parenchyma affected by the gross lesion(s). Take 2 full-thickness representative sections of normal-appearing disc parenchyma (chorionic plate through maternal surface) for cassettes A3 and A4, taken within the central 2/3 of the disc. Sample any grossly identified lesions in additional cassettes (A5, etc.). In cases wherein maternal malperfusion is suspected (e.g., premature, intrauterine growth restriction infant, small placenta, preeclampsia, and related disorders), an additional cassette from maternal surface is useful for identifying maternal decidual arteriopathy. These may be either 4-5 perpendicular shallow wedge sections or en face sections.
Representative sections are submitted as follows: A1: Umbilical cord, fetal end, and 2 membrane rolls; A2: Umbilical cord, placental end, and chorionic plate section near cord insertion; A3-4: Placenta, full-thickness sections; A5, etc.: Cord lesions, membranous vessels, parenchymal lesions, &/or maternal surface wedge sections.	

This form provides a dictation template as well as basic instruction in gross evaluation of singleton placenta. These recommendations generally follow the Amsterdam placental workshop group consensus statement recommendations with slight modification: 3 full-thickness blocks, including 1 near the cord insertion is recommended by the Workshop. We find having 2 full-thickness blocks, 1 additional of chorionic plate vessels (with the cord in A2) and 1 with multiple wedge sections of the basal plate fulfills the recommended sampling and improves evaluation of chorionic plate vessels (as it is easier to embed) and basal plate.

SELECTED REFERENCES

1.   Khong TY et al: Sampling and Definitions of Placental Lesions: Amsterdam Placental Workshop Group Consensus Statement. Arch Pathol Lab Med. 140(7):698-713, 2016

Twin Placenta Gross Evaluation and Dictation Template

Dictation	Applicable Notes
Specimen is received (fresh/fixed) labeled with (patient's name, medical record number). It consists of (a single/2 separate) placental disc(s) with attached umbilical cords and fetal membranes.	If dichorionic with 2 separate discs, use singleton template 1x for each twin.
Twin A umbilical cord is identified by a single clamp. Twin B umbilical cord is identified by 2 clamps.	Correct if different. If cords are not assigned, state this in the dictation. If unassigned, describe as "twin 1" and "twin 2"; "twin A" and "twin B" are clinical designations, not a random assignment.
Twin A umbilical cord is (tan/gray/white/green) and measures ____ cm in length by ____ cm in maximum diameter. It contains ___ coils and inserts (centrally/eccentrically/at margin/in membranes) and contains (2/3) vessels on cut section.	Count coils to calculate coil index (# of coils/10 cm) and determine if cord is overcoiled or undercoiled. If insertion is near margin, state how close. If in membranes, measure intramembranous course of vessels to disc and note if intramembranous vessels are intact or disrupted. Describe cord abnormalities (e.g., true knots, thrombi, other lesions) if present. Cut off cord 1.0-1.5 cm above insertion and take sections for cassettes A1, A2.
Fetal membranes: (translucent/tan/yellow/green tinged), (glistening/dull) of twin A attach (normally at disc margin/circumvallate for ___ % of circumference/circummarginate for ___ % of circumference). Area of membrane rupture is located ____ cm from closest placental margin.	Delete sentence on area of membrane rupture if C-section with intact membranes or if membranes are excessively torn. Note if membranes appear complete. Describe membrane abnormalities if present. Take twin A membrane roll for cassette A1.
Twin B umbilical cord is (tan/gray/white/green) and measures ____ cm in length by ____ cm in maximum diameter. It contains ___ coils and inserts (centrally/eccentrically/at margin/in membranes) and contains (2/3) vessels on cut section.	Repeat evaluation described for umbilical cord of twin A. Cut off cord of twin B 1.0-1.5 cm above insertion and take sections for cassettes A5, A6. Note any cord entanglement in monoamnionic twins.
Twin B fetal membranes are (translucent/tan/yellow/green tinged), (glistening/dull), and attach (normally at disc margin/circumvallate for ___ % of circumference/circummarginate for ___ % of circumference).	Describe membrane abnormalities if present. Take twin B membrane roll for cassette A5. If monoamnionic, i.e., if no dividing membrane, dictate 1 description for membranes and placenta of the twins. Otherwise, continue dictating separately.
Interplacental membrane is (thick/thin), (translucent/tan/yellow/green tinged), and has a (thick/delicate) interface with chorionic plate. Chorionic plate vessels (do/do not) cross under interface on chorionic plate.	Take interplacental membrane roll and T section for cassette A9. Cut off fetal membranes.
Placental disc is (round/oval/irregularly shaped), weighs ____ g, and measures ___ x ___ x ____ cm. Fetal surface is (steel gray/blue/purple). Chorionic plate vasculature for twin A has a (normal/magistral) dispersion and occupies ___ % of shared placental disc. Chorionic plate vasculature for twin B has a (normal/magistral) dispersion and occupies ___ % of shared placental disc.	Describe vascular abnormalities (e.g., thrombi, disruptions) if present. If monochorionic, identify any twin-twin anastomoses (arterial-arterial, venous-venous or arterial-venous, venous-arterial from twin A to twin B) on surface of placenta, if indicated. Remember, arteries cross over veins. Injection studies may facilitate this evaluation, if clinically appropriate. Arteries and veins should dive down into parenchyma in pairs. Any single penetrating vessel is suspicious for a deep arterial-venous anastomosis. Note that virtually all monochorionic twins have anastomoses.
Maternal surface appears (intact/disrupted).	Identify and measure any adherent blood clot, indentation. Note if cotyledons appear complete, if any shaggy extensions could be myometrial fibers, and if any differences in appearance between the 2 twin territories, especially pallor.
Serial sectioning through placental disc at 1-cm intervals reveals (spongy/soft/firm), (dark red/pink/tan) parenchyma with (no grossly identifiable lesions/or describe).	For parenchymal lesions, note parenchyma of which twin is involved. Note any differences in parenchymal color or texture between respective twin territories. Give estimated percentage of each twin's parenchyma affected by any gross lesion. Common parenchymal lesions include tan lesions, areas of pallor, areas of firmness, and hematomas. They should be described in terms of number of lesions, size, and location relative to margin or cord insertion. Two full-thickness representative sections of normal-appearing parenchyma are taken from central 2/3 of the twin territory. Lesions are sampled separately.
Representative sections are submitted as follows: A1: Twin A umbilical cord, fetal end, and membrane roll; A2: Twin A umbilical cord, placental end, and chorionic plate section near cord insertion; A3-4: Twin A placenta, full-thickness sections; A5: Twin B umbilical cord, fetal end, and membrane roll; A6: Twin B umbilical cord, placental end, and chorionic plate section near cord insertion; A7-8: Twin B placenta, full-thickness sections; A9: Interplacental membrane roll and T section; A10, etc.: Additional sections for grossly identifiable cord lesions, membranous vessels, parenchymal lesions, or decidua basalis wedge sections as needed. Note associated twin.	

This form provides a dictation template as well as basic instruction in gross evaluation of twin placenta.

Microscopic Description

Umbilical Cord

____	3 vessels, no abnormalities
____	Edema
____	Decreased Wharton jelly
____	Single umbilical artery
____	Umbilical vein vasculitis
____	Umbilical artery vasculitis
	Fetal inflammatory response grade: 1 (mild-moderate) ____, 2 (severe) ____
	Fetal inflammatory response stage: 1 (umbilical phlebitis) ____, 2 (umbilical vasculitis)____, 3 (subacute necrotizing funisitis or concentric umbilical perivasculitis) ____
____	Peripheral funisitis, GMS stain positive ____, negative ____
____	Umbilical vein thrombus (acute ____, organizing____, with vessel wall necrosis ____)
____	Umbilical artery thrombus (acute ____, organizing ____, with vessel wall necrosis____)
____	Meconium-associated vascular necrosis
____	Remnants present
	Other: _____

Fetal Membranes (Amnion and Chorion)

____	No abnormalities
____	Reactive amnion
____	Necrotic amnion
____	Amnion edema
____	Pigmented macrophages: Rare ____, or increased ____, in amnion____, in chorion ____
____	Membranous chorionic trophoblast hyperplasia with ____ or without ____ chorionic microcysts, pleomorphism ____
____	Acute chorionitis ____, acute chorioamnionitis ____
	Amniotic fluid injection sequence (AFIS) maternal inflammatory response grade: 1 (mild-moderate) ____, 2 (severe) ____
	AFIS maternal inflammatory response stage: 1 (acute chorionitis) ____, 2 (acute chorioamnionitis) ____, 3 (necrotizing acute chorioamnionitis) ____
____	Chronic chorioamnionitis
____	Amnion nodosum
	Other: _____

Membranous Decidua

____	No abnormalities
____	Acute inflammation: Mild ____, moderate ____, severe ____
____	Chronic inflammation: Plasma cell deciduitis ____, granulomatous deciduitis____, perivascular lymphoid infiltrate ____
____	Laminar decidual necrosis ____, decidual leukocytoclastic necrosis ____
____	Decidual arteriopathy: Mural hypertrophy ____, acute atherosis ____, fibrinoid necrosis ____
	Other: _____

Chorionic Plate

____	No abnormalities
____	Pigmented macrophages: Consistent with meconium ____, consistent with hemosiderin ____ (iron stain ____)
____	Acute subchorionitis ____ or chorioamnionitis ____; AFIS maternal inflammatory response grade: 1 (mild-moderate) ____, 2 (severe)____; stage 1 (if limited to subchorionitis) ____
____	Chronic chorionitis
	Other: _____

Chorionic Plate Vasculature

____	No abnormalities
____	Fetal vasculitis: Acute ____, eosinophilic/T cell ____; single vessel ____, multifocal ____
	AFIS fetal inflammatory response grade: 1 (mild-moderate) ____, 2 (severe) ____; stage 1 (chorionic plate vasculitis, **if umbilical artery is not involved**) ____

Microscopic Description (Continued)

____	Thrombus: Single ____, multiple ____, acute ____, organizing ____, occlusive ____, nonocclusive ____, intimal fibrin deposition ____ (recent ____, remote with calcification ____)
____	Marked dilation (> 4x diameter of adjacent vessels)
____	Meconium-associated vascular necrosis
____	Other

Fetal Stem Villi

____	No abnormalities
____	Acute villitis
____	Chronic villitis ____ with stem vessel obliteration ____
____	Thrombus: Single ____, multiple ____ (# ____), acute ____, organizing ____, occlusive ____, nonocclusive ____, intimal fibrin deposition ____ (recent ____, remote with calcification ____), stem vessel obliteration ____
	Ectasia
____	Chorangiomatosis: Focal ____, multifocal ____
	Other: _____

Terminal Villi

____	Appropriately developed for gestational age
____	Delayed villous maturation
	Accelerated villous maturation
	Increased fibrinoid necrosis of individual villi
____	Distal villous hypoplasia (focal ____, diffuse ____)
____	Increased syncytial knotting for age
____	Infarct: Single ____, multiple ____ (# ____), recent ____, or remote ____, with central hemorrhage ____
____	Villous edema: Focal ____, multifocal ____, diffuse ____
____	Chorangiosis
____	Intravillous hemorrhage
____	Chronic villitis
	Low-grade focal ____, multifocal ____, high-grade patchy ____ diffuse ____; basal ____, midparenchyma ____, subchorionic ____ with associated avascular villi ____ with increased perivillous fibrin ____ with plasma cells ____ (if present, CMV immunostain or PCR study positive ____, negative ____)
____	Villous stromal-vascular karyorrhexis: Single focus ____ or multiple foci ____, < 5/focus ____, 5-15/focus ____, or > 15/focus ____
____	Avascular villi: Single focus ____ or multiple foci ____, < 5/focus ____, 5-15/focus ____, or > 15/focus ____
____	Increased nucleated red blood cells (> 10/40x field at term)
____	Dysplastic villous changes: Irregular villous contours ____, hyperchromatic, enlarged stromal cells ____, abnormal vasculature ____
	Other: _____

Intervillous Space

____	Acute intervillositis: Focal ____, multifocal ____
____	Chronic histiocytic intervillositis: Focal ____, multifocal ____ with associated increased perivillous fibrin ____ with associated chronic villitis ____
____	Excessive perivillous fibrin: Focal ____, encasing basal villi (maternal floor infarction) ____, full-thickness involvement of at least 50% of parenchyma on slide (massive perivillous fibrin deposition) ____ with associated extravillous cytotrophoblast proliferation in fibrin ____
____	Intervillous thrombus: With ____ or without ____ nucleated red blood cells
____	Microabruption ____ or dissecting intervillous hemorrhage ____
	Other: _____

Basal Plate/Decidua Basalis

____	No abnormalities
	Maternal spiral arteries appropriately adapted for pregnancy ____ **or** no maternal spiral arteries sampled in decidua basalis ____
____	Decidual arteriopathy
	Persistence of smooth muscle ____, intraluminal trophoblast ____, mural hypertrophy ____, fibrinoid necrosis ____, acute atherosis ____, thrombus ____
____	Retroplacental hemorrhage ± hemosiderin-laden macrophages

Microscopic Description (Continued)

____	Myometrial cells adherent to basal plate without intervening decidua (occult placenta accreta)
____	Diffuse decidual leukocytoclastic necrosis
____	Acute deciduitis
____	Plasma cell deciduitis
____	Increased multinucleated trophoblast in decidua basalis
	Other: _____

Final diagnosis: In wording a final diagnosis, it is useful to report the trimmed placenta weight and whether it is small, large, or appropriate for gestational age. Placental diagnoses may require significant clinical correlation. A header diagnosis, such as "changes of intrauterine infection/inflammation" or "severe maternal vascular malperfusion," is useful, followed by the individual features warranting that diagnosis. Do not forget significant gross features, such as cord abnormalities, circumvallation, or marginal abruption, which should be included in the final diagnosis. This template includes common significant changes in placental pathology and is provided for use in routine surgical pathology practice. It does not detail all possible pathologic changes in the placenta. Uncommon but significant lesions (e.g., chorangioma, placental mesenchymal dysplasia) should also be recognized and noted appropriately.

SELECTED REFERENCES

1. Khong TY et al: Sampling and Definitions of Placental Lesions: Amsterdam Placental Workshop Group Consensus Statement. Arch Pathol Lab Med. 140(7):698-713, 2016

Guidelines for Submission of Placentas to Surgical Pathology for Use in Labor and Delivery Room

Maternal Indications for Placental Examination (Check All That Apply)

____	Systemic disorder with clinical concern for mother or infant (e.g., preeclampsia, diabetes; please specify)	____	Severe oligohydramnios
____	Premature delivery (< 37 weeks)	____	Severe, unexplained polyhydramnios
____	Gestational age ≥ 42 weeks	____	Unexplained or recurrent pregnancy complications
____	Peripartum fever or infection	____	Invasive procedures with potential placental injury
____	Clinical concern for infection during pregnancy	____	History of substance abuse
____	Prolonged (> 24 hours) rupture of membranes	____	Nonelective pregnancy termination
____	Unexplained 3rd trimester or excessive bleeding	____	Severe maternal trauma
____	Abruption	____	Thick or viscid meconium

Fetal/Neonatal Indications for Placental Examination (Check All That Apply)

____	Admission or transfer to other than level 1 nursery	____	Infection or sepsis
____	Stillbirth or perinatal death	____	Major congenital anomalies, dysmorphic phenotype, or abnormal karyotype
____	Hydrops fetalis	____	Discordant twin growth (> 20% weight difference); **please indicate cords A and B**
____	Compromised clinical condition (cord pH < 7, Apgar < 7 at 5 minutes, ventilatory assistance > 10 minutes, hematocrit < 35%)	____	Multiple gestation with same-sex infants, fused placentas
____	Birth weight < 10th percentile or > 95th percentile	____	Vanishing twin beyond 1st trimester
____	Seizures	____	

Placental Indications for Placental Examination (Check All That Apply)

____	Physical abnormality (e.g., mass, vascular thrombosis, abnormal color, retroplacental hematoma, malodor, amnion nodosum, extensive infarction)	____	Umbilical cord lesions (e.g., marginal or velamentous insertion, thrombosis, torsion, true knot, single artery)
____	Small or large placenta for gestational age	____	Excessively long or short umbilical cord (e.g., length < 32 cm or > 100 cm at term)

Placental Examination Requested by Staff Physician

	Please specify concern		

There are no absolute indications for placental pathology examination from the American College of Obstetrics and Gynecology with the exception of cases of stillbirth. The indications above are modified from the College of American Pathologists practice guidelines for examination of the placenta. Placenta storage in a refrigerator for ≥ 3 days before disposal is recommended in case a neonatal condition warrants placental examination.

The Royal College of Pathologists of the United Kingdom published guidelines in 2017 that present a more conservative, evidence-based approach to placenta triage. Full gross and microscopic examination is recommended at a minimum for stillbirth, fetal growth restriction < 3rd percentile, gestational age < 30 weeks, maternal fever > 38°C, or severe fetal distress requiring admission to a neonatal intensive care unit. For all other conditions, the extent of examination (e.g., storage only, gross only, gross with sections taken for histology but no microscopic examination, full gross and microscopic examinations) is to be determined by local resources and the value placed on placental examination in these situations by the local obstetricians. Storage is for a short period of time (e.g., 2 weeks). Full examination can be requested at any time while placenta is stored.

SELECTED REFERENCES

1. Langston C et al: Practice guideline for examination of the placenta: developed by the Placental Pathology Practice Guideline Development Task Force of the College of American Pathologists. Arch Pathol Lab Med. 121(5):449-76, 1997
2. Cox P et al: The Royal College of Pathologists. Tissue pathway for histopathological examination of the placenta.

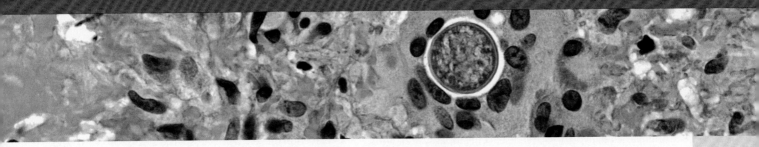

INDEX

A

INDEX

G

H

I

INDEX

INDEX

N

O

P

INDEX

X

Y

Z